MEDICAL
LABORATORY MANUAL
FOR
TROPICAL COUNTRIES

Volume I
Second Edition

Monica Cheesbrough FIMLS Tech RMS

Tropical Health Technology

Butterworths

London   Boston   Durban   Singapore   Sydney   Toronto   Wellington

First published in 1981
Second edition 1987 (copublished by Tropical Health Technology and Butterworths)

ELBS edition 1987

© Monica Cheesbrough 1987

British Library Cataloguing in Publication Data

Cheesbrough, Monica
    Medical laboratory manual for tropical
    countries.—2nd ed.
    Vol. 1
    1. Tropical medicine—Laboratory manuals
    I. Title
    610′.28   RC961

    ISBN 0-407-00402-5

Library of Congress Cataloging in Publication Data

Cheesbrough, Monica.
    Medical laboratory manual for tropical countries.

    Includes bibliographies and index.
    1. Tropical medicine--Handbooks, manuals, etc.
2. Diagnosis, Laboratory--Handbooks, manuals, etc.
I. Title.   [DNLM: 1. Tropical Medicine--laboratory
manuals.   WC 25 C515m]
RC961.5.C53   1987   616.9′88′3   87-6399
ISBN 0-407-00402-5 (v. 1)

Photoset by Image Plus of Lewes and Fakenham Photosetting Ltd, Norfolk
Printed in Great Britain at the University Press, Cambridge

Volume I
Contents

Preface

This new edition of Volume I reflects the needs of district laboratories in developing countries and the ideas and requests made by those involved in training and working in intermediate level laboratories.

The most frequently received request was for the inclusion of more artwork, particularly for colour plates to assist in the identification of parasites. We have therefore increased the number of colour plates from 7 to 58 and also strengthened the artwork of other parasites, particularly of the intestinal protozoa.

Other features of the new edition are the inclusion of Summary Method Sheets of the important clinical chemistry tests, and a greater coverage of quality assurance, safety, and laboratory equipment. The parasitology and clinical chemistry sections have been updated. A greater emphasis has been placed on the major parasitic diseases such as malaria, filariasis, African trypanosomiasis, Chagas' disease, leishmaniasis, and schistosomiasis. This is in keeping with new laboratory training curricula that have been introduced in several developing countries.

Details of the non-profit *Tropical Health Technology Laboratory Equipment Service to Developing Countries* are included in the back of the book. Regrettably it has not been possible to continue the inclusion of loose sheets in the back cover. To do so would have involved a considerable increase in the price of the book. As with the first edition, every possible effort has been made to keep the price of the new edition as low as possible.

At the request of many overseas technologists and tutors, a suggested *Code of Professional Conduct* for laboratory personnel has been included. The purpose of such a Code is to identify those personal qualities and skills which a medical laboratory technologist needs to work competently, compassionately and in harmony with other health professionals in serving the sick and building an effective National Health Service.

The author hopes that this new edition of Volume I will assist in the growth of reliable indigenous laboratory services and that those using the Manual will continue to share their ideas for future editions. Sharing and applying more effectively our resources and knowledge, will enable us to improve and extend our service to the sick and build healthy communities.

January 1987   Monica Cheesbrough

Acknowledgements

In preparing the second edition of Volume I, I have received the help and encouragement from many working in, or associated with, medical laboratory work and training in developing countries. I express my thanks to all who have sent ideas and comments for the new edition.

I also acknowledge with gratitude the assistance received from:

Dr John M. Jewsbury, Senior Lecturer at the Liverpool School of Tropical Medicine and Hygiene for helping to revise the parasitology section, supplying text and artwork for several of the Chapters, and for proof-reading. My thanks are also due to Dr Carol Homewood, formerly of the Liverpool School of Tropical Medicine and Hygiene, who also helped to revise the text and artwork of the parasitology section.

Mr Anthony Moody, Chief Laboratory Scientific Officer, and staff of the laboratory of the Hospital for Tropical Diseases in London, for carrying out practical work, supplying artwork and details of techniques, and for commenting on the text of the parasitology chapters.

Dr David Godfrey of the Tsetse Research Laboratory, University of Bristol, and Dr Roy L. Rickman of the WHO Tropical Disease Research Centre in Ndola Zambia, for helping to revise the chapter on African trypanosomiasis.

Dr. A. Michael Miles, of the Departamento de Parasitologia, Instituto Evandro Chagas, Fundação Serviços de Saúde Pública, Belém, Brazil, and Dr. Rodney Hoff of the Dept of Tropical Public Health, Harvard University, USA, for commenting on and contributing material for the chapter on Chagas' disease.

Professor Ralph Lainson of the Wellcome Parasitology Unit, Section of Parasitology, Instituto Evandro Chagas, Fundação Serviços de Saúde Pública, Belém, Brazil, for helping to revise the chapter on leishmaniasis.

Professor Leonard J. Bruce-Chwatt, of the Wellcome Museum of Medical Science in London, for comments on the malaria chapter.

Dr David Warhurst of the Pathology Dept of the Hospital for Tropical Diseases, London, for assisting in the revision of the protozoa chapter.

Dr Charles Mackenzie of the Wolfson Tropical Pathology Unit, London School of Hygiene and Tropical Medicine, for checking the filariasis chapter.

Dr Christopher C. Draper of the London School of Hygiene and Tropical Medicine for assisting in the revision of the immunodiagnosis of parasitic infections.

Dr N. R. H. Burgess, Senior Lecturer in Entomology, Royal Army Medical College, London, and Mr Kenneth G. V. Smith, Head of Medical Insects, of the Department of Entomology, British Museum, for commenting on the entomology chapter and kindly supplying artwork.

Mrs Barbara Cooper-Poole, formerly Senior Medical Laboratory Scientific Officer, British Technical Co-operation Southern Regions Health Project, Mbeya, Tanzania, for reading and commenting on the laboratory diagnosis of helminth infections.

Mrs A. C. Rijpstra of the Institute of Tropical Hygiene of the Royal Tropical Institute of the Netherlands, for kindly supplying artwork for the parasitology section.

Dr Callum G. Fraser, Biochemist and Senior Lecturer of the Department of Biochemical Medicine, Ninewells Hospital and Medical School, Dundee, for assisting in the revision of the clinical chemistry section, kindly contributing new text, and for proof reading.

Dr Brian Seaton, Principal Consultant, Clin-Lab Services, for contributing text and artwork and assisting in the preparation of the chapter on Quality Assurance in clinical chemistry.

Mr David Browning, Laboratory Manager, United Kingdom WHO Collaborating Centre for Research and Reference Services in Clinical Chemistry, for commenting on the chapter Quality Assurance in clinical chemistry.

Dr Peter Hill, Biochemist of Derbyshire Royal Infirmary, and Dr Howard Worth and Mr Robert P Hill of Clinical Chemistry, King's Mill Hospital, Sutton-in-Ashfield, for suggestions and practical work regarding clinical chemistry colorimetric methods.

Dr Geoff Gill, Clinical Biochemist, Freeman Hospital, Newcastle upon Tyne, for assisting in the revision of the interpretation of clinical chemistry tests.

Sister Cecile Benoot of Lilongwe Laboratory Training School, Malawi, for valuable comments and suggestions regarding the clinical chemistry section and other chapters.

Acknowledgement is also due to the US Army Academy of Health Sciences in Texas, US Department of Health, Education and Welfare, and Center for Disease Control, for permission to use artwork from their Study Guides and other publications to illustrate the parasitology and anatomy and physiology sections of the manual.

I would like to express my special gratitude to Mr Martin Cannon and Director of the Huntingdon Research Centre, Cambridgeshire, for generously photographing and processing artwork for much of the equipment section of the book and for providing some of the plates in the parasitology section.

Mr Warren L. Johns, Laboratory Advisor to the Aguaruna and Huambisa Indian Council, Peru, for suggestions regarding the content of the new edition and kindly assisting in the production of artwork.

I thank Mr Simon Janes of Image Plus, Lewes, for his interest in the project and skill in phototypesetting.

I should also like to acknowledge the assistance of Fakenham Photosetting for their careful origination of artwork and page makeup and Buralls of Wisbech and Saxon Photo Litho for their skilled processing and reproduction of the colour section.

To my father I express my special thanks for his encouragement, new ideas, and even greater committment to the project, and to my sister Mary for her skills and suggestions regarding text and artwork formats.

I should also like to acknowledge the continued involvement of the Overseas Development Administration in the production of the Manual and generous support, making possible the availability of the Manual at low cost and its greater circulation in developing countries.

Gratitude is also due to our co-publisher Butterworths for organizing and co-ordinating the printing and binding of the manual and assisting in its distribution.

Author

Acknowledgements for Colour Section:
Please see page 288.

TROPICAL HEALTH TECHNOLOGY

Registration Form

If you would like to receive information about new techniques and equipment as this becomes available, complete the form below and return it to us.

NAME ....

OCCUPATION ....

ADDRESS ....

....

....

....

Do you have any comments about this edition of Volume I and have you any suggestions for future editions?

....

....

....

Mail completed form to: *Tropical Health Technology*
14 Bevills Close
Doddington, March
Cambridgeshire UK PE15 0TT

SECTION I

INTRODUCTION TO THE LABORATORY

Laboratory Services
in Tropical and Developing Countries

1:1 ROLE OF THE LABORATORY IN HEALTH CARE AND TRAINING OF LABORATORY PERSONNEL

If the entire network of a laboratory service is to be dependable and contribute effectively to health care and disease prevention, every member of its workforce needs to:

■ Understand the role of the laboratory and its integration into the nation's health service.

■ Receive a good training and be well motivated.

■ Follow a *Professional Code of Conduct*.

■ Experience job satisfaction and have opportunities for continuing education and career development.

Role of the laboratory and its integration into the health service

The laboratory forms an integral part of a nation's health service. It gives the service a scientific foundation by providing accurate information to those with the responsibility for:

— treating patients and monitoring their response to treatment.
— deciding health priorities and allocating resources.
— monitoring the development and spread of infectious and dangerous pathogens.
— investigating preventable premature loss of life.
— deciding effective control measures against major prevalent diseases.

Without reliable laboratory support:

— patients are less likely to receive the best possible care.
— resistance to essential drugs will continue to spread.
— the sources of disease may not be identified correctly.
— epidemics and the spread of major communicable diseases will not be checked reliably.
— valuable financial and human resources may be diverted to ineffective control measures.

The degree to which a laboratory service performs its important functions and contributes to a higher standard of health care and the prevention of disease, depends on how well its service is recognized and how well it functions with the other components of the health service.

Recognition of the role of the laboratory by health authorities is essential and the correct proportion of available funds must be allocated to:

— training laboratory workers and the development of a professional career structure.
— running the diagnostic, investigative and disease control components of the laboratory service.
— extending laboratory services to where they are needed.

Equally important is the responsibility of the laboratory service to:

— develop and enforce a *Professional Code of Conduct*.
— train appropriately its workers and provide opportunities for continuing education.
— provide and maintain reliable diagnostic and epidemiological services.
— ensure the community becomes involved and has access to its services.

All members of a national health service *must work as a team* and learn to apply their combined skills and the nation's available resources to achieve the highest level of health care for their people.

Training of laboratory workers

Basic training should be undertaken nationally in accordance with a country's health needs, available resources, and laboratory working environments. A trainee should be taught the technical skills, knowledge, and attitudes required to perform reliably and confidently the functions of the type of laboratory in which he or she will serve. Performance needs to be assessed during training and supervised adequately after training.

Selection and content of a curriculum
In selecting a curriculum for training medical laboratory personnel in developing countries, the following are important considerations:

☐ About 80% of the health problems in developing countries are due to malnutrition and infectious diseases such as malaria, trypanosomiasis, leishmaniasis, hookworm disease, schistosomiasis, filariasis, leprosy, tuberculosis, pneumonia, diarrhoeal and dysenteric diseases, measles, hepatitis, and sexually transmitted diseases.

It is therefore essential that all laboratory curricula reflect the importance of techniques to investigate infectious diseases and provide information about the transmission, control and prevention of these diseases. Community based laboratory workers should receive special training in how to teach disease prevention and health protection. All laboratory workers should be encouraged to become promotors of health.

☐ Resources are often extremely limited in developing countries and supplies may be difficult to obtain.

Laboratory workers need therefore to be trained to work economically, to make the best use of resources, and to order supplies in good time. Curricula should include basic laboratory economics, how to estimate running costs, and how to plan for future needs. Also included should be how to order laboratory supplies correctly, keep stock records, and store reagents and chemicals correctly.

☐ In peripheral laboratories, the workload is usually high and results are often required urgently. Working hours are frequently long and irregular. There is little opportunity to test specimens in planned batches. Responsibilities are great with no opportunity to consult a specialist technician or pathologist.

Laboratory personnel working in district laboratories must therefore be trained to work responsibly with a high degree of organization and coordination, calmly and efficiently through emergencies and interruptions. Training in communication skills is essential.

☐ In many developing countries, laboratories are often in remote places without mains electricity or with only intermittent and fluctuating electrical supplies. Climatic factors may interfere with the performance of equipment and service and engineers are not usually available to maintain equipment.

Curricula for all laboratory personnel in developing countries must therefore include the principles of operation, care, preventive maintenance and servicing of essential laboratory equipment.

☐ In a developing country, reliable referral back-up systems are required to provide as full a laboratory service as possible to patients and to operate a cost-effective service.

Curricula should therefore include training in the collection, packing and dispatching of specimens safely, and how to keep reliable records of specimens sent and results received.

Training programmes

All laboratory personnel should receive an organized and carefully planned training, consistent with the work to be undertaken, working situation and responsibilities to be assumed. A training programme must be task-orientated (competency-based).

Having decided the curriculum for each type of course and written the educational objectives, the following are important guidelines regarding the structuring of medical laboratory training programmes:

☐ Allow adequate time and opportunity for both learning and assessment. Both trainees and tutors need to be assured of progress during training. For a trainee or tutor to discover whether he or she has been successful only at the end of a course has little advantage.

The knowledge, skills, and work attitudes of trainees need to be assessed throughout training and tutors should vary their methods of evaluation to produce maximum responses from trainees.

☐ Integrate carefully the theory and practical parts of the programme and follow a logical sequence. The theory should be relevant and applied, enabling trainees to perform their tasks intelligently, reliably and confidently. The teaching of unnecessary knowledge should be avoided.

☐ Choose carefully where the various parts of the training programme are to be conducted. Part of the training must take place in the field. Only in the real situation can a trainee learn:

— how to apply the skills that have been learnt.
— how to use the equipment that is provided in the field.
— how to organise and co-ordinate his or her work in a busy laboratory and cope with emergency conditions of work.
— how to approach and communicate with patients and their relatives, medical and nursing staff, and fellow laboratory workers.
— how to apply the *Professional Code of Conduct* for laboratory personnel (see later text).

On-the-job experience is usually best carried out towards the end of training when trainees can benefit most from their experience and still have the opportunity to return to their training centre to discuss their experiences and difficulties, and obtain further tuition if required. Tutors must ensure that the time a trainee spends in the field is supervised and assessed.

☐ Use appropriate and effective teaching methods and teaching aids. Consideration will need to be given to the educational background of trainees and available resources.

Whenever possible, teaching aids should be prepared locally. If outside aids are available in the form of manuals, charts, posters, slide sets, tapes, models, films or videos, these must be evaluated carefully by tutors and adapted to meet local situations. With the introduction of simple to operate and less expensive video cameras, 'play-back' equipment, and long playing reusable tapes, training centres should consider making their own sound videos to teach trainees important techniques, the use of equipment, and communication skills.

Note: The structuring of a competency-based training programme and other important aspects of training laboratory workers in developing countries can be found in the paper presented by Alex McMinn at the 1986 IAMLT Congress in Stockholm, and published in *Laboratory in Health Care, Developing Country Proceedings*. The Proceedings also includes other papers presented by laboratory tutors from various countries, related to training, quality assurance, safety and other aspects of medical laboratory work in developing countries. A limited number of free copies (courtesy of Sponsors of the Programme) are available to tutors in developing countries from Tropical Health Technology, 14 Bevills Close, Doddington, March, Cambridgeshire PE15 0TT, UK.

Professional code of conduct

A suggested *Code of Professional Conduct* for medical laboratory personnel is shown on the opposite page. The *Code* includes those attitudes and practices which characterize a responsible laboratory worker and which are necessary to ensure that a person works to a recognized standard which those using the laboratory service can expect to receive.

Above all a *Code of Professional Conduct* can keep alive motivation and remind us that the Medical Laboratory Profession is primarily dedicated to the service of the sick and promotion of good health care.

Upgrading and continuing education

For all laboratory personnel there should be opportunities for upgrading and career develop-

ment according to an individual's abilities and the recognized career structure of the indigenous laboratory service. The career structure and organization of a laboratory service must be based on national health needs and priorities and be sufficiently flexible to allow for future change.

In a developing country, continuing education is particularly important if high standards of work are to be maintained. Laboratory personnel often need to work in remote places with little opportunity to discuss their work with more experienced staff and to learn about new techniques.

Some of the ways of providing continuing education in developing countries are as follows:

☐ Conducting short refresher courses at regular intervals to evaluate existing techniques and to introduce new improved techniques.

☐ Developing a national *Medical Laboratory Association* with regional and district meetings to exchange views, discuss laboratory investigations of prevalent diseases, and bring about greater communication between laboratories.

☐ Circulating a simple national *Laboratory Newsletter* to which both trained laboratory workers and trainees can contribute their ideas. Such a newsletter could also be used to circulate information about new techniques and important advances relevant to national health problems.

1:2 STRUCTURING OF A LABORATORY SERVICE IN A DEVELOPING COUNTRY

A laboratory service network consists of:

■ Community-based primary health care laboratories
■ District hospital laboratories
■ Regional (provincial, base) hospital laboratories
■ Central and public health laboratory

The various activities of these laboratories need to be clearly defined and carefully coordinated. Good communication channels and effective back-up referral systems between laboratories are essential. The network needs to be operated reliably and cost-effectively with resoures being distributed according to the needs of the *entire* network.

Activities of community-based primary health laboratories

Community-based primary health care laboratories are becoming increasingly important

CODE OF PROFESSIONAL CONDUCT FOR MEDICAL LABORATORY PERSONNEL

1   Place the well-being and service of the sick above your own interests.

2   Be loyal to your medical laboratory profession by maintaining high standards of work and striving to improve your professional skills and knowledge.

3   Work scientifically and with complete honesty.

4   Do not misuse your professional skills or knowledge for personal gain.

5   Never take anything from your place of work that does not belong to you.

6   Do not disclose to a patient or any unauthorized person the results of your investigations.

7   Treat with strict confidentiality any personal information that you may learn about a patient.

8   Respect and work in harmony with the other members of your hospital staff or health centre team.

9   Be at all times courteous, patient, and considerate to the sick and their relatives.

10   Promote health care and the prevention and control of disease.

11   Follow safety procedures and know how to apply First Aid.

12   Do not drink alcohol during laboratory working hours or when on emergency stand-by.

13   Use equipment and laboratory ware correctly and with care.

14   Do not waste reagents or other laboratory supplies.

15   Fulfill reliably and completely the terms and conditions of your employment.

with the reorganization of health services which is taking place in many developing countries. Essential health care facilities which at one time were only available to a minority of the population are now becoming *community-based* and accessible *to all*.

The work of the community-based primary health laboratory is to support primary health care in investigating, controlling, and preventing major diseases in the community, and in promoting health care by integrated health education.

Without laboratory support for primary health care, diseases are often misdiagnosed or remain undiagnosed until they are advanced and accompanied by serious complications which require hospitalization of patients.

Staff
A laboratory in a primary health care centre will usually be staffed by a laboratory worker or a local community health worker trained to examine specimens microscopically, perform appropriate diagnostic and screening tests, collect and refer specimens for specialist tests, and participate in community health education.

Depending on the workload of the health centre, one or two laboratory aids may also be required.

Functions
The main functions of a comunity-based primary health laboratory are as follows:

☐ To investigate by referral or testing on site, important diseases and health problems affecting the local community. Depending on geographical area such investigations will usually include:
   Bacterial diseases: Tuberculosis, leprosy, meningitis, cholera, gonorrhoea, syphilis, vaginitis, urinary tract infections, respiratory tract infections, bacillary dysentery and relapsing fever.
   Parasitic diseases: Malaria, schistosomiasis, lymphatic filariasis, loiasis, onchocerciasis, African trypanosomiasis, Chagas' disease, leishmaniasis, amoebic dysentery, giardiasis, strongyloidiasis, trichuriasis, hookworm disease, and any other locally important parasitic diseases.
   Other causes of illhealth: Anaemia, sickle cell disease, diabetes, and skin mycoses (fungal infections).

☐ To collect and refer specimens for testing to the district laboratory, including:
   — water samples from sources used by the community.

— faecal specimens for the investigation of major enteric pathogens.

— serum for antibody tests, particularly to investigate syphilis and other important communicable diseases.

— specimens for biochemical testing to investigate major liver, kidney, metabolic, and deficiency diseases.

— specimens for culture and sensitivity to diagnose and assist in the treatment and control of important bacterial infections.

☐ To notify the district hospital at an early stage of any laboratory result of public health importance and send specimens for confirmatory tests.

☐ To screen pregnant women for anaemia, proteinuria and malaria, and refer serum for antibody testing to exclude, e.g. active syphilis.

☐ To promote health care and assist in community health education by, e.g. demonstrating microscopically the parasites of important local diseases and explaining the transmission and spread of such pathogens and how infection can be prevented.

☐ To keep careful records which can be used by health authorities in health planning, particularly of the incidence and intensity of major parasitic infections.

☐ To assist district and regional epidemiologists and sanitary officers in checking water supplies and performing surveys aimed at controlling local diseases.

☐ To request from the district laboratory on a regular basis, further supplies of reagents, standards, controls, stains, specimen containers, and laboratory request forms.

☐ To send a simple informative monthly report to the district laboratory of the work carried out and results obtained in the primary health laboratory.

Activities of district hospital laboratories
These laboratories have an important role in supervising the work of the peripheral community-based laboratories, testing referred specimens, and performing a range of tests compatible with the work of the district hospital.

Staff
A district laboratory is usually staffed by at least one laboratory technician and depending on work-

load, by two to four assistants and several aids. The staff of the district laboratory should also include a laboratory tutor to train and supervise the work of primary health laboratory workers.

Functions
The main functions of a district hospital laboratory are as follows:

☐ To perform a range of tests relevant to the medical, surgical, and public health activities of the district hospital.

☐ To support the work of the community-based laboratories by:
— testing referred specimens.
— providing reagents, controls, standards, stains, specimen containers, stationery, and other essential laboratory supplies.
— visiting each primary health centre once a month to inspect and discuss the investigations being performed, quality control, records, safety procedures, and maintenance of equipment.
— training community health laboratory workers and organizing refresher courses.

☐ To refer specimens to the regional laboratory that cannot be tested in the district laboratory or are more economically tested in batches in the regional laboratory.

☐ To notify the regional laboratory of any result of public health importance and to send specimens for confirmatory tests.

☐ To participate in the external quality assurance programme organized by the regional laboratory.

☐ To prepare a report every 3 months to send to the regional laboratory of the work and needs of all the laboratories in the district.

Regional hospital laboratories
The main role of the regional laboratory is to assist and supervize the district laboratories, to test referred specimens and to perform a range of specialist and other tests as required by the work of the regional hospital.

Staff
A regional laboratory is usually staffed by one co-ordinating (chief) laboratory officer, an experienced specialist trained technician and two or three technicians in each department, laboratory tutors, a safety officer, a stores officer, clerical staff, and several aids according to the workload.

Functions
The main functions of the regional laboratory are as follows:

☐ To perform a range of tests as required by the medical and health needs of the region.

☐ To operate a regional blood transfusion centre.

☐ To prepare reagents, controls, clinical chemistry standards, and specimen containers.

☐ To investigate epidemics and perform tests of public health importance in the region.

☐ To support the work of the district hospital laboratories in the region by:
— testing referred specimens.
— providing reagents, standards, controls, chemicals, blood grouping antisera, antihuman globulin, blood collecting packs, stationery, specimen containers, and other essential supplies.
— delivering tested donor blood for use in the district hospitals and collecting blood donated in the district for testing in the regional transfusion centre.
— visiting each district hospital laboratory every 3 months to discuss with the technical and medical staff the work of the laboratory, to inspect records and quality control charts, install and demonstrate any new equipment, and to ensure that safety measures are being followed.
— training laboratory tehnicians and organizing refresher courses.

☐ To send specimens that require specialist investigation to the central and public health laboratory.

☐ To participate in the external quality assessment programme organized by the central laboratory.

☐ To prepare a report every 6 months to send to the central and public health laboratory of the work and needs of all the laboratories in the region.

Central and public health laboratory
This laboratory is responsible for the planning, expenditure, and co-ordination of the national laboratory service. It has equally important roles in ensuring the reliability of the service, the appropriateness of its technology, training and motivation of its workforce, and ensuring that the

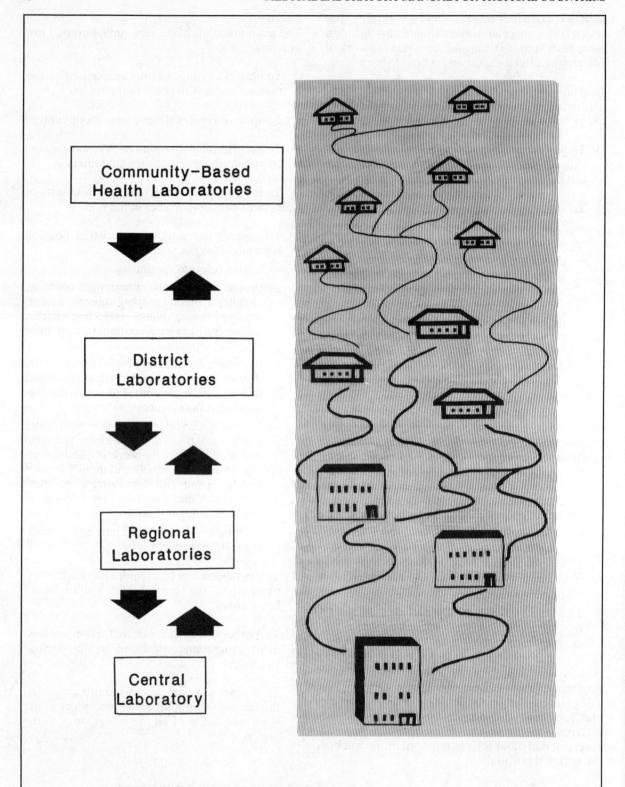

Fig. 1.1   Laboratory Service network in a Developing Country based on health needs and population distribution.

service extends into areas of health needs and its facilities are made available to as many people as possible.

The central and public health laboratory is also responsible for the prompt laboratory investigation of epidemics and outbreaks of serious illness among communities.

Staff

A central laboratory is staffed by a director (pathologist), a senior co-ordinating officer, several senior technologists and technicians, a senior safety officer, laboratory tutors, a finance officer, a stores officer, clerical staff, and several aids according to the size and workload of the laboratory.

Functions

The main functions of a central and public health laboratory are as follows:

☐ To formulate a *Professional Code of Conduct* for medical laboratory personnel.

☐ To perform a range of specialist tests not normally undertaken in the regional laboratories, such as viral, histopathological, cytological, immunological, nutritional, metabolic, forensic and genetic investigations.

☐ To carry out appropriate research into important national health problems.

☐ To organize a national blood transfusion service.

☐ To evaluate new technologies, standardize techniques, and test the appropriateness of new equipment.

☐ To purchase supplies and equipment for the national laboratory service and to organize an efficient system of requisition, distribution, and maintenance of equipment.

☐ To prepare control sera, blood grouping antisera, antihuman globulin, complex biochemical reagents and culture media that require standardization and are more economically prepared in the central laboratory.

☐ To communicate and collaborate with International Organizations in promoting laboratory standards and a *Code of Safety* for indigenous medical laboratories.

☐ To train specialist technicians and to organize laboratory teaching seminars.

☐ To prepare, and where required, translate appropriate training manuals for the different laboratory training programmes.

☐ To prepare laboratory request forms, record sheets, order forms, and other essential stationery which require standardization.

☐ To prepare and distribute an annual report on the activities of the country's laboratory service, to co-ordinate the work of the laboratory service within the national health programme, and to prepare a budget for presentation to health authorities.

☐ To support the work of the regional hospital laboratories by:

— providing control sera, certain standardized reagents, chemicals, bacteriological media constituents and ready-prepared complex media, blood grouping antisera, antihuman globulin, blood collecting packs, standardized stationery, specimen containers, and other essential laboratory supplies.

— visiting each regional laboratory every six months to discuss with the medical and technical staff the work and needs of all the laboratories in the region, to check records and quality control measures, service major equipment, install and demonstrate any new complex equipment, and ensure that safety measures in each department are being followed.

— co-ordinating an external quality assessment programme in parasitology, bacteriology, haematology, blood transfusion, and clinical chemistry.

Note: The structure of a developing country laboratory service based on health needs is illustrated in Fig. 1.1.

1:3 EFFECTIVE COMMUNICATION IN THE LABORATORY

If a laboratory service is to function smoothly, reliably, and effectively, laboratory workers must be able to communicate well.

Communication
By definition, communication is the accurate passing on or sharing of information.

In communicating, it is important to consider the:
— nature of the information being communicated.

— person or persons to whom the information is being communicated.

— most effective way of communicating the information.

In laboratory work there are three main ways of communicating information, by:

■ Writing
■ Speaking
■ Actions

Written communication

To be effective, written communication needs to be:

☐ presented legibly and neatly.
☐ expressed clearly and simply.

Writing legibly and neatly

In laboratory work, serious consequences may result when hand-written figures or words are read incorrectly because of poor handwriting or untidy corrections. An illegibly written report may result in a patient receiving incorrect treatment.

The presentation of well-written and neat reports not only avoids errors, misunderstandings, and frustrations, but also inspires confidence in those using the laboratory. Before issue, all reports should be checked by the most senior member of staff.

To promote standardization and neatness of reporting, the use of rubber stamps is recommended but care must be taken to ensure the stamp is positioned well and sufficient ink is used.

Writing clearly and simply

Opportunities for laboratory personnel to develop written skills should be provided during training.

A trained laboratory technologist needs to know how to write clear reports and instructions with regard to test methods, use of equipment, preparation of reagents, safety measures, collection of specimens, laboratory policies, notices, agendas for meetings, budgets, work reports, and requisitions for laboratory supplies.

Laboratory personnel should be encouraged to contribute to newsletters and journals.

Spoken communication

Important aspects of spoken (verbal) communication include:

— clarity of speech,
— tone of voice,
— ability to speak informatively.

Clarity of speech

The main requirement of spoken communication is that the words spoken can be heard distinctly by the person to whom they are addressed. A barrier to effective spoken communication is background noise. Noise should therefore be kept to a minimum when speaking, e.g. reduce the speed of a centrifuge.

It is particularly important to speak clearly when addressing patients. Hesitant and mumbled instructions lead to misunderstandings and a lack of confidence by patients.

Tone of voice

A kind and understanding tone of voice may greatly help a patient, especially a child, to feel less frightened, whereas a loud and impatient tone of voice may cause fear and add to the suffering of a patient. A laboratory worker should always try to reassure patients by explaining simply the procedure of a test and, without disclosing professional information, seek to answer patients' queries.

It is particularly important to communicate well in difficult situations, for example when called to crossmatch blood during a night emergency. Under these circumstances it is essential for the laboratory worker not only to function rapidly and reliably but also to reply calmly and patiently to anxious relatives and blood donors.

Spoken communication is influenced by temperament and fatigue, but a courteous response based on a respect for all persons should always be possible.

Ability to speak informatively

This is particularly important when giving the results of tests by telephone or directly to a medical officer or nurse. An understanding of the clinical significance of investigations is required.

If a laboratory worker does not have sufficient information to answer a question about a report, the questioner should be referred to a more experienced member of staff. If unable to reply and no other person is available, the laboratory person must advise that he or she is unable to assist. Inaccurate information must *never* be communicated.

The ability to speak informatively is also required when attending hospital interdepartmental meetings to discuss laboratory policies.

Action communication

Communication through bodily manner and actions (body language) is particularly important when relating to patients.

A pleasant friendly manner and a neat clean appearance inspire confidence whereas an impatient aggressive manner or an untidy appearance can make patients nervous and afraid. When unable to speak the language of a patient, facial expressions and actions become extremely important in reassuring a patient. A smile and a caring look and action can inspire trust.

Action communication is also important among staff members if a pleasant working environment is to be maintained.

Guidelines for effective communication

The following are among the guidelines for effective communication which Shirley Pohl presented at a Congress of the International Association of Medical Laboratory Technologists:

☐ Seek to clarify your ideas before communicating.

☐ Consider the total physical and human setting whenever you communicate. Meaning and intent are conveyed by more than words alone.

☐ When you communicate, be mindful of the overtones as well as the basic content of your message.

☐ Take the opportunity when it arises, to convey something of help or value to the receiver.

☐ Follow up your communication.

☐ Be sure your actions support your communications.

☐ Seek not only to be understood but to understand and be a good listener.

☐ Communicate for tomorrow as well as today.

1:4   LABORATORY POLICIES

By laboratory policies are meant those decisions which are taken in consultation with medical and nursing staff to enable a laboratory to operate reliably, effectively, and in harmony with other departments of the hospital or health centre.

Such policies usually cover:

■ Laboratory hours and emergency work.
■ Range of tests to be performed and the referral of specimens.
■ Collection of specimens.
■ Workload capacity of the laboratory.
■ Delivery of reports.
■ Reporting of results and record keeping (see 1:6).
■ Safety measures (see Chapter 2).

Laboratory hours and emergency work

As far as possible there should be definite laboratory working hours. In peripheral laboratories it is often more difficult to maintain working hours because of large out-patient clinics and the emergency nature of much of the work.

Outside of normal working hours, each laboratory should organize a system for testing urgent specimens. Only those investigations that are essential for the immediate care and assessment of a patient should be requested urgently.

Written details of the emergency laboratory service ('on call' service) should be circulated to all those concerned. Laboratory staff that participate in the emergency service must be able to work efficiently and reliably without supervision.

Range of tests to be performed and referral of specimens

In deciding which tests should be undertaken in a district hospital or primary health centre laboratory the following are important considerations:

☐ What is the clinical value of each investigation and which tests should have priority because they are needed to:
  — establish a diagnosis,
  — assess a patient's condition and prognosis,
  — judge whether to refer a patient to a centre with more facilities,
  — select a suitable treatment and follow a patient's response to it,
  — prevent and control serious disease in a community,
  — assist health authorities to plan cost-effectively.

☐ What is the level of experience and training of the laboratory staff? If required, can further training be obtained?

☐ How well is the laboratory equipped and can equipment be operated reliably and safely?

☐ Can the tests be controlled adequately, i.e. can tests be performed with adequate precision and accuracy?

☐ What are the costs involved, especially the cost of reagents, standards, controls and of running and maintaining essential equipment?

☐ Is it possible to refer specimens for testing, especially those that are non-urgent and can be more economically and reliably tested in batches in a larger laboratory? If able to refer, can specimens be preserved and transported safely? How quickly can the results of referred tests be known?

Collection of specimens

The correct collection of specimens is essential for reliable test results. Written instructions regarding the collection of routine and urgent specimens must be issued by the laboratory to all those responsible for the collection of specimens from inpatients and outpatients.

There should be an organized system for the collection of routine specimens from wards. Specimens for urgent analysis should be delivered to the laboratory as soon as possible.

A request form must accompany every specimen. This should provide essential patient information, and a clinical note regarding diagnosis and treatment. Those responsible for collecting samples must check that every specimen is clearly labelled with the patient's name and hospital number, date and time of collection, and that the name and number agree with what is written on the request form. Clerical mistakes can have serious consequences.

Any specimen found to be unsuitable must not be accepted by the laboratory for testing. When an error of collection has been made, a note indicating how to correct the fault should accompany the returned form. If the investigation is required urgently, every effort must be made by both the laboratory and ward staff to obtain a repeat specimen as soon as possible. Laboratory staff should encourage medical and nursing staff to seek advice if they are uncertain about the collection of specimens for particular investigations.

Note: Instructions regarding the collection of specimens for biochemical analyses can be found in 26:7. Information regarding the collection of microbiological specimens can be found in Volume II of the Manual.

Workload capacity of a laboratory

The workload capacity of a laboratory must be matched to the number of staff and to their level of training, and to the size of the laboratory and its facilities.

If the amount of work requested is beyond the capabilities of a laboratory, this must be brought to the attention of the medical officer with overall responsibility for the laboratory. When workload is excessive, the testing of specimens becomes unreliable and safety measures tend to be ignored. Too little work can also lead to unreliable test results due to a lack of concentration.

Delivery of reports

All results before they leave the laboratory must be checked by the most experienced member of the laboratory's technical staff. Any unexpected result should be investigated and repeated if necessary. It is important for laboratory workers to understand the clinical significance and accepted reference values ('normal' range) of the tests they perform.

A clinically serious abnormal result should be brought to the attention of the medical officer concerned as soon as possible. When a result is phoned, it is advisable to request the person receiving the report to repeat back the name of the patient and test result, to make sure that the report has been heard correctly. A written report should follow as soon as possible.

There should be an organized system for the delivery of reports to wards and clinics and from referral laboratories to the peripheral hospitals and community health centres. To avoid any loss of reports and to keep the results of tests confidential, all forms should be placed in marked envelopes or in closed folders which can be returned to the laboratory for re-use.

1:5　SI UNITS

In this manual, SI units (Système International d'Unités) are used in test methods, preparation of reagents, and reporting of test results. This is in accordance with a World Health Organization resolution which recommends the adoption of the International System of units by the medical community throughout the world.[1]

The International System of Units has been developed and agreed internationally in the interests of world health. It overcomes language barriers, enabling an exchange of health information within a country and between nations to be made without the misunderstandings which arise when each country, or even a separate hospital within a country, uses its own units of measurement for reporting tests. It is therefore important for health authorities and laboratories to adopt the new system of units. They are not difficult and are already being used in most medical publications and journals, by the manufacturers of chemicals and reagents, and by most scientific and medical organizations.

SI base units

The International System of Units was presented in 1960 by a General Conference of Weights and Measures. It is based on the *metre-kilogram-second* system and replaces both the foot-pound-second (Imperial) system and the centimetre-gram-second (cgs) system.

There are seven SI base units, i.e. metre, kilogram, second, mole, ampere, kelvin, and candela.

The symbols for these units and what they measure are listed in Table 1.1. All other units are derived from these seven base units. Some SI derived units have been given special names.

Table 1.1

SI base units	Symbol	Quantity measured
metre	m	length
kilogram	kg	mass
second	s	time
mole	mol	amount of substance
ampere	A	electric current
kelvin	K	temperature
candela	cd	luminous intensity

SI derived units

SI derived units consist of combinations of base units. Table 1.2 gives examples of SI derived units.

Table 1.2

SI derived unit	Symbol	Quantity measured
square metre	m^2	area
cubic metre	m^3	volume
metre per second	m/s	speed

Named SI derived units

Special names have been given to those derived units with complex base combinations. Examples of these are listed in Table 1.3.

Table 1.3

Named derived unit	Symbol	Quantity measured
Hertz	Hz	frequency
joule	J	energy, quantity of heat
newton	N	force
pascal	Pa	pressure
watt	W	power
volt	V	electric potential difference
degree Celcius	°C	Celcius temperature

SI Unit prefixes

To enable the measurement of quantities larger or smaller than the base units or derived units, the SI Unit system also includes a set of prefixes. The use of a prefix makes a unit larger or smaller.

Example

If the prefix milli (m) is put in front of the metre this would indicate that the unit should be divided by a thousand, i.e. 10^{-3}. The way of expressing this would be 10^{-3}m, or mm.

If however the prefix kilo (k) were used this would

indicate that the unit should be multiplied by a thousand, i.e. 10^3. This would be expressed 10^3m, or km.

The range of SI unit prefixes are listed in Table 1.4.

Table 1.4

Prefix	Symbol	Function	DIVIDE BY:
deci	d	10^{-1}	10
centi	c	10^{-2}	100
milli	m	10^{-3}	1 000
micro	μ	10^{-6}	1 000 000
nano	n	10^{-9}	1 000 000 000
pico	p	10^{-12}	1 000 000 000 000
femto	f	10^{-15}	1 000 000 000 000 000

Prefix	Symbol	Function	MULTIPLY BY:
deca	da	10^1	10
hecto	h	10^2	100
kilo	k	10^3	1 000
mega	M	10^6	1 000 000
giga	G	10^9	1 000 000 000
tera	T	10^{12}	1 000 000 000 000
peta	P	10^{15}	1 000 000 000 000 000

Note: With the exception of 10^{-2} and 10^2, the prefix values increase or decrease by multiplying or dividing by 1000.

Litre (l)

The SI derived unit of volume is the cubic metre (m^3). Because this is such a large unit, the litre (l) although not an SI unit, has been recommended for use in the laboratory.

The litre is equal to a cubic decimeter (1 dm^3)

Volume measurements are made in litres or multiples and submultiples of the litre, e.g. dl (10^{-1}l), ml (10^{-3}l), μl (10^{-6}l).

One litre is therefore equivalent to 10 dl, 1 000 ml, or 1 000 000 μl. One dl is equivalent to 100 ml, and 1 ml to 1 000 μl (see also Appendix III tables).

Table 1.5

SI unit	Old unit
dl	100 ml
ml or cm^3	cc
μl	lambda
nl	—
pl	$\mu\mu$l

Gram (g)

The kilogram (kg) is the SI unit for mass and the gram (g) is the working unit.

Formerly the gram (g) was written gramme, or gm.

Mass measurements are made in grams or in multiples and submultiples of the gram, e.g. mg $(10^{-3}g)$, μg $(10^{-6}g)$, ng $(10^{-9}g)$, pg $(10^{-12}g)$.

One g is therefore equivalent to 1 000 mg, 1 000 000 μg, or 1 000 000 000 ng. One mg is equivalent to 1 000 μg (see also Appendix III tables).

Table 1.6

SI unit	Old unit
kg	k, kilogramme
g	gm, gramme
mg	mgm
μg	gamma
ng	mug
pg	$\mu\mu g$

Metre (m)
The SI unit for length is the metre (m) and measurements of length are made in metres or in mm $(10^{-3}m)$, μm $(10^{-6}m)$, nm $(10^{-9}m)$.

One m is therefore equivalent to 1 000 mm or 1 000 000 μm and 1 mm is equivalent to 1 000 μm or 1 000 000 nm (see also Appendix III tables).

Table 1.7

SI unit	Old unit
nm	$m\mu$
μm	μ (micron)

Mole (mol)
The mole (mol) is the SI unit for amount of substance and measurements of the amounts of substances are made in moles, or in mmol $(10^{-3}mol)$, μmol $(10^{-6}mol)$, or nmol $(10^{-9}mol)$.

One mol is therefore equivalent to 1 000 mmol, 1 000 000 μmol, or 1 000 000 000 nmol. One mmol/l is equivalent to 1 000 $\mu mol/l$ (see also Appendix III tables).

Formerly, the results of tests expressed in mmol/l or $\mu mol/l$ were expressed in mg/100 ml or $\mu g/100$ ml. The formula used to convert mg/100 ml to mmol/l is as follows:

$$mmol/l = \frac{mg/100\ ml \times 10}{molecular\ weight\ of\ substance}$$

Where the molecular weight of a substance cannot be accurately determined (e.g. albumin), results are expressed in g/l.

Table 1.8

SI unit	Old unit
mol	M
mmol	mEq
μmol	μM
nmol	nM

International unit (U)
This unit is used to express enzyme activity. It is explained in 27:6.

Applications of SI units in clinical chemistry
The application of SI units in clinical chemistry is described in 27:7. The reference ranges of biochemical tests in SI units, with the factors used to convert the former units to the new units, are listed in 27:9.

The use of SI units in the preparation of solutions with formulae and examples to convert percentage and normal solutions into mole per litre (mol/l) solutions, are given in 24:5. The method of diluting mole per litre solutions is described in 24:6.

Note: Further information about the meaning and application of SI units can be found in the publication *The SI for the Health Professions*[2]

1:6   REPORTING LABORATORY TESTS AND KEEPING RECORDS

Standardization in the reporting of laboratory tests contributes to the efficiency of a laboratory service and is of great value when patients are referred from one hospital to another.

Whenever possible, request forms and other laboratory printed stationery should be prepared and issued by a central stationery office.

Use of rubber stamps
When stationery is not supplied from a central source, standardization in presenting and reporting results can be achieved by the use of rubber stamps. Adequate ink must be used and the stamp must be positioned carefully.

Keeping records in the laboratory
A record of all test results must be kept by the laboratory as carbon copies, work sheets, or in simple exercise books. Whichever system is used, it must enable patients' results to be found quickly. Records of tests are also required when preparing work reports and estimating the workload of the laboratory.

If carbon copies or work sheets are used these must be dated and filed systematically each day.

If exercise books are used, backing cards which are headed and ruled can be placed under pages to avoid having to rule and head each page separately. The cards must be heavily ruled so that the lines can be seen through the pages of the book. Separate books each with its own cards can be pre-

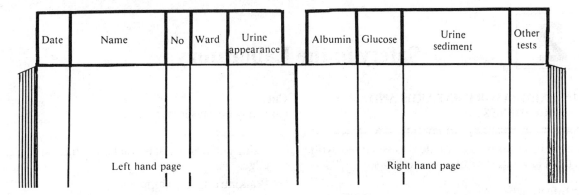

Date	Name	No	Ward	Urine appearance		Albumin	Glucose	Urine sediment	Other tests
	Left hand page							Right hand page	

Fig. 1.2 Example of an exercise book with card inserts to record test results. The lines from the ruled cards show through the pages of the book.

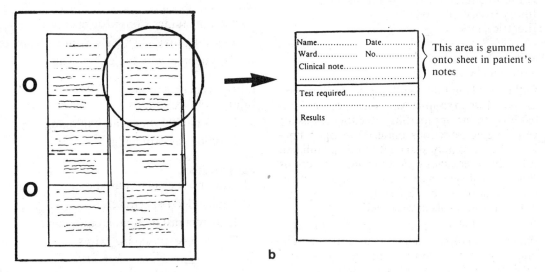

Name................ Date............
Ward............... No..............
Clinical note..........................
....
Test required......................
....
Results

This area is gummed onto sheet in patient's notes

a   b

Fig. 1.3 Transferring laboratory results into the hospital notes of a patient.
a Sheet in patient's notes on to which laboratory report forms are gummed or stapled.
b Close-up of a simple laboratory form. A rubber stamp can be used to print the upper part of the form.

pared to record the results of haematological, bacteriological, clinical chemistry, urine and faecal tests. An example of the cards which could be used in a Urine Analysis Record Book is shown in Fig. 1.2.

Recording laboratory results in patients' notes
When resources are limited, an inexpensive reliable way of recording laboratory results in patients' notes is to report results on small stamped forms and attach these to a sheet of paper reserved for laboratory results in each patient's notes. The forms can be prepared from yellow X-ray film wrapping paper if no other paper is available. If the pieces of paper are arranged as shown in Fig. 1.3, several reports can be attached to one sheet.

The system sometimes used in district hospitals of 'charting' laboratory results from laboratory record books into patients' notes is not recommended. It is not only time-consuming but can give rise to serious errors when results are not copied correctly or fully.

References
1 Resolution WHA 30.39 adopted by the thirteenth World Health Assembly, May 1977.
2 World Health Organization. *The SI for the Health Professions*, WHO, Geneva, 1977.

Recommended Readings
Guilbert, J. J. *Educational Handbook for Health Personnel* (English and French), World Health Organization, Geneva.

Abbatt, F. A. and McMahon, R. *Teaching Healthcare Workers*, McMillan publishers, 1985. Available at low cost (£2.50) from TALC, PO Box 49, St Albans, Herts, AL1 4AX, United Kingdom.

McMinn, A. and Russell, G. J. *Training of Medical Laboratory Technicians: A Handbook for Tutors* (English and French), World Health Organization, Geneva.

2   Safety in the Laboratory

2:1   LABORATORY HAZARDS AND ACCIDENTS

The main hazards and accidents associated with medical laboratory work are as follows:

- Infection
- Burns
- Cuts
- Harmful effects of toxic chemicals
- Injury from explosions
- Electric shock

Infection

Infection can be caused by:

- ☐ Pathogens being inhaled in aerosols (airborne droplets) when snap-closing specimen containers, dispensing or pipetting infectious fluids, or centrifuging infectious material in open buckets. Aerosols may also be formed and inhaled following breakages or after spilling infectious fluids. Breakages in centrifuges can be particularly hazardous if the centrifuge is opened before the aerosols have settled.

- ☐ Pathogens being ingested from contaminated fingers, or in food that has been contaminated, e.g. by being stored in a laboratory refrigerator. Care should be taken to avoid the fingers or other parts of the body touching infected material.

  Mouth-pipetting specimens and cultures is one of the commonest ways of ingesting pathogens.

- ☐ Pathogens entering the skin through needle punctures, cuts, scratches, insect bites, sores or other open skin lesions. Laboratory workers must always handle infected needles with great care.

Note: Laboratory-acquired infections are more fully discussed in Chapter 33 in Volume II of the Manual.

Burns

Burns may be caused by:

- ☐ Flammable chemicals and stains, or by reagents catching alight.

- ☐ Fires from spirit lamps, Bunsen burners, lighted tapers (e.g. when heating Ziehl-Neelsen stain), or from faulty electrical equipment or overloaded circuits. Spirit burners should not be used in direct sunlight because in bright light the flame can be difficult to see.

- ☐ Corrosive chemicals being spilt on the skin or ingested when mouth-pipetting.

Cuts

Cuts may be caused by:

- ☐ Breakages.
- ☐ Using glassware that is cracked or has damaged edges.
- ☐ Walking on glass chippings.

Harmful effects of toxic chemicals

Harmful effects of toxic chemicals can be caused by:

- ☐ Inhaling fumes from toxic chemicals.
- ☐ Ingesting toxic chemicals by mouth-pipetting.
- ☐ Skin contact with toxic chemicals.

Injury from explosions

Injury from explosions can be caused by:

- ☐ Incompatible chemicals exploding.
- ☐ Leaking gas exploding.

Electric shock

Electric shock can be caused by:

- ☐ Faulty electrical circuits.
- ☐ Incorrect installation of equipment.
- ☐ Touching exposed live wires.

Factors contributing to laboratory accidents

While a poorly designed laboratory and overcrowding can increase the risk of accidents occurring, most laboratory accidents are the result of bad laboratory practices due to:

— poor training,
— lack of concentration,
— noisy environment,
— untidy working and not using racks to hold containers,
— allowing the working bench to become cluttered,
— carelessness and neglect,
— overwork and fatigue,
— hot and humid climatic conditions,
— hurrying to finish work 'on time'.

Accidents are also more likely to occur when working under emergency conditions, especially during night hours.

Every laboratory no matter how small should establish an appropriate *Code of Safe Laboratory Practice*. The head of the laboratory or a person designated as Safety Officer should ensure that this

Code is followed and adequate protection exists for all those working in and visiting the laboratory, i.e. technical staff, laboratory aids, cleaners, outpatients and other visitors.

The following aspects of laboratory safety are covered in this Chapter.

Note: Classification of microorganisms into Risk Groups I, II, III, and IV and a more detailed coverage of safety in microbiological laboratories can be found in Chapter 33 in Volume II of the Manual.

2:2 SAFE LABORATORY DESIGN AND ORGANIZATION

The following are among the features of a safely designed and organized laboratory:

☐ Adequate floor, bench, and storage space for staff to work safely.

☐ A floor that is well constructed with a surface that is non-slip, impermeable to liquids, and resistant to those chemicals used in the laboratory. It should be bevelled to the wall and the entire floor should be accessible for washing. It should not be heavily waxed or covered with matting. Floor drains are recommended.

☐ Walls that are smooth, free from cracks, impermeable to liquids, and easily washable.

☐ A door at each end of the laboratory so that laboratory staff will not be trapped should a fire break out. The doors should open outwards and exit routes must never be obstructed.

Internal doors should be self closing and contain upper viewing panes.

☐ Adequate ventilation with windows that can be opened. Windows should be fitted with blinds and mosquito-proof screens.

☐ Sectioning of the laboratory into separate rooms or working areas with definite places for

patients, visitors, and the reception of specimens. There should also be an easily accessible, and suitable equipped First Aid area in the laboratory.

If a separate room for outpatients is not available, at least a small area should be partitioned off from the main testing area of the laboratory. Patients and visitors should not be allowed into the testing area of the laboratory.

The place selected for the reception of specimens must not be within the outpatient area. The specimen reception area must be equipped with a table or hatchway which has a surface that is impervious, washable, and resistant to disinfectants.

☐ Bench surfaces that are without cracks, impervious, washable, and resistant to the disinfectants and chemicals used in the laboratory.

Benches, shelving and cupboards need to be well constructed and kept free of pests.

Bench tops need to be kept as clear as possible to give maximum working area and to facilitate and encourage cleaning.

☐ Suitable storage facilities that include a well-ventilated, fireproof, locked store for the storage of flammable chemicals.

☐ A gas supply that is piped into the laboratory with the gas cylinder stored in an outside locked store.

☐ A room that is separate from the working area where refreshments can be taken and personal food and other belongings stored safely.

Wall pegs should be provided *in* the laboratory on which to hang laboratory coats.

Near to the staff room there should be a separate room with toilet and hand-washing facilities.

☐ An adequate number of handbasins in the laboratory with running water. Whenever possible, taps should be operated by wrist levers or foot pedals. Bars of soap should be provided, not soap dispensers.

Ideally paper towels should be used. If this is not possible small frequently laundered pieces of cloth should be provided. The use of a single large towel laundered once or twice a week should be avoided.

☐ Provision of protective safety cabinets and fume cupboards as required.

Note: The different types of microbiological safety cabinet are described in 33:5 in Volume II of the Manual.

□ A sufficient supply of wall electric points to avoid the use of adaptors.

□ Fire extinguishers sited at accessible points. These need to be of the dry chemical type. If extinguishers are not available, several buckets of sand must be provided.

□ As good illumination as possible, especially in the testing areas of the laboratory.

□ An adequate waste disposal area and a safe disposal system.

There should be a system for marking *HIGH RISK* specimens, discard containers, and hazardous chemicals and reagents.

Suitably labelled separate containers should be provided for the disposal of infected material, needles, syringes, and broken glassware. A simple warning symbol such as a red triangle can be used to mark containers in which infected material is placed.

Use of signs
Displaying suitable safety signs is a way of encouraging the practice of safety in the laboratory. Examples of prohibitive (do not) and command (do) signs are shown in Fig. 2.1. Prohibitive signs can be easily recognized because they are always crossed by a red line (see Fig. 2.1, upper).

Signs to label chemicals and reagents, e.g. *Flammable, Toxic, Corrosive, Harmful, Irritant, Oxidizing,* or *Explosive* are shown in 2:5.

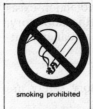 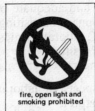 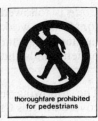
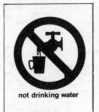 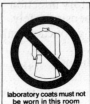 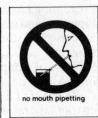
 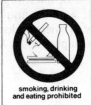 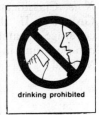

Fig. 2.1 Prohibition signs for wall display.
Courtesy of Jencons Scientific Ltd.

■ Disposing safely of specimens and contaminated material.

■ Being immunized against highly infectious pathogens.

Practice of personal hygiene
Laboratory staff must practice a high standard of personal hygiene. This includes:

□ Washing of hands and arms with soap and water before attending outpatients, visiting wards, after handling specimens and infected material, and when leaving the laboratory for a break, to take refreshment, or at the end of the day's work.

If there is a shortage of piped water, provision must be made for the storage of water, e.g. collection of rain water in tanks during the rainy season. It is not safe for a laboratory to function without an adequate water supply.

□ Wearing protective clothing over normal clothing or instead of it. The protective overall should be made of a fabric such as polycotton that can be bleached and frequently laundered and suitable for wearing in tropical climates. If available, an antistatic and flammable-resistant fabric should be used.

2:3 PREVENTING LABORATORY INFECTION

All specimens received in the laboratory should be regarded as potentially pathogenic not just specimens sent specifically for bacteriological culture. For example, a cerebrospinal fluid sent for measuring glucose or a blood sample sent for measuring haemoglobin may contain highly infectious microorganisms.

The following are the main ways that laboratory workers can prevent laboratory-acquired infections:

■ Practising personal hygiene and reducing contact with infected material.

■ Handling all specimens and infected materials with care.

■ *Never* mouth-pipetting.

The overall should give maximum protection to the major part of the body and be worn with fasteners, buttons or tape closed. A side closing design with *Velcro* type tape is preferable to a front opening because it gives better protection when working at the bench and enables the overall to be removed quickly should harmful or infectious material be spilt on it. *Velcro* tape is long-lasting and gives good closure providing it is kept free from fluff by being brushed with a dry stiff brush.

Soiled clothing should be placed in a special bag and not left in a cupboard or under a bench in the laboratory. Prior to laundering, the clothing and bag should be soaked overnight in 1% v/v domestic bleach.

Protective clothing should always be left in the laboratory and *never* taken home or worn in a room where refreshments are taken.

When attending outpatients or inpatients, a clean overall should be worn.

☐ Wearing closed shoes and not walking barefoot.

☐ Not eating, drinking, chewing gum, smoking, or applying cosmetics in any part of the laboratory.

Food or drink should never be stored in a laboratory refrigerator.

☐ Not licking gummed labels or placing pens, pencils or other articles near the mouth, eyes, or in hair.

☐ When handling specimens or cultures which may contain highly infectious pathogens, protective gloves should be worn and if indicated the work should be undertaken in a safety cabinet (see 33:5 in Volume II of the Manual).

☐ Covering any cuts, insect bites, open sores, or wounds with a water-proof adhesive dressing. Insect bites if particularly irritating should be treated.

Safe handling of specimens and infectious material
Special precautions need to be taken when collecting specimens, especially blood specimens, and when testing specimens and handling infected material.

Safe collection of blood specimens
Safety measures involved in the collection of blood include the careful handling and disposal of syringes, needles and prickers and not collecting capillary blood by mouth-suction (see 2:4).

Specimen containers must be leak-proof. A special carrying tray should be used for collecting blood. It should have separate compartments for holding clean equipment, specimens, and contaminated articles.

When collecting blood from patients suspected of having a highly infectious disease such as hepatitis, AIDS, or viral haemorrhagic fever, protective gloves and a plastic apron (over laboratory overall) should be worn.

Needle pricks are a common source of laboratory-acquired hepatitis. Immediately after use, a used needle should be carefully inserted back into its guard and not left exposed in a carrying tray.

Used syringes (if not of the disposable type) must be soaked overnight in 1% v/v hypochlorite solution (domestic bleach diluted 1 in 5) before being cleaned. Non-disposable prickers and needles should be soaked in a glutaraldehyde disinfectant or if unavailable, in 70% v/v alcohol or 10% formalin solution before being cleaned (metal is attacked by bleach). Disposable needles and syringes should be incinerated. Prior to incineration they should be discarded into jars or metal cans, not into cardboard boxes because the sharp ends may penetrate the card.

Note: Other hazards associated with the use of syringes and needles are covered in 33:4 in Volume II of the Manual.

Safe testing of specimens and handling of infected material
The careless handling of specimens, cultures and other infected material may result in the contamination of fingers and working surfaces, and particularly in the formation of aerosols (airborne droplets). The inhaling of infected aerosols is a common cause of infection.

How aerosols are formed
The following are the main ways in which aerosols can be formed:

— Pouring off supernatant fluids, especially from a considerable height into a discard container. A safe way of discarding supernatant fluids is by pouring the fluid down the side of a funnel the end of which is immersed in disinfectant solution in the discard container.

— Vigorous tapping of a tube to resuspend a sediment. This should be avoided and a Pasteur or plastic bulb pipette used to mix the sediment.

— Rapid snap-closing of specimen or culture tubes instead of using screw-cap or other safe cap containers.

— Heating a contaminated wire loop in the hottest part of a Bunsen burner flame. Protection can be given by using a hooded Bunsen burner (see Plate 33.3 in 33:4 in Volume II of the Manual).

Using a long springy loop which is not properly closed can also lead to aerosols being formed.

— Rapid rinsing out of Pasteur or plastic bulb pipettes, especially when the discard container is almost full.

— Vigorous shaking of unstoppered tubes in a rack. The tubes should always be closed first with tightly fitting caps. Inserting the rack of tubes in a plastic bag while shaking is recommended.

— Centrifuging specimens or infected fluids in open buckets, particularly when using an angled centrifuge and the tubes are more than three quarters full.

— Accidental dropping or spilling of specimens or infected fluids.

When an infected fluid is spilt, the affected area should be covered with a cloth soaked in a disinfectant such as 1% w/v (10 000 ppm) hypochlorite solution for 30 minutes. The room should be left to ventilate for 10 minutes before resuming work. Spillages are less likely to occur if racks are used to hold tubes and containers.

Following the breakage of a container in a centrifuge, at least 30 minutes should be left for the droplets to settle before opening the centrifuge. A glutaraldehyde disinfectant, 70% v/v alcohol, or 10% v/v formalin solution should be used to clean the centrifuge. Protective rubber gloves should be worn and forceps should be used to remove the broken glass.

Important: Specimens from patients who may have hepatitis, viral haemorrhagic fever, or acquired immune deficiency syndrome (AIDS), must be clearly marked HIGH RISK and preferably also have attached a warning symbol such as a red star or disc.

When working with material which may contain highly infectious pathogens, protective gloves should be worn and the work carried out in a suitable microbiological safety cabinet as described in 33:5 in Volume II of the Manual. Where indicated, specimens should be referred for testing to a containment or maximum containment laboratory (see 33:3 in Volume II of the Manual).

Note: The safe transport of specimens is described in 33:6 and 46:5 in Volume II of the Manual.

Strict prohibition of mouth-pipetting
Pathogens may be ingested during mouth-pipetting, either by direct aspiration or from the mouth ends of pipettes which have been contaminated from fingers or benches. Infection may also occur from aerosols produced when fluid is being sucked up or expelled from a pipette.

The use of a pipette with a piece of attached rubber tubing and mouth-piece is no safer than direct mouth-pipetting and should also be prohibited. A cotton wool plug in the top of a pipette is not an effective microbial filter.

There are many inexpensive ways to measure and dispense safely without mouth-pipetting. These are described in 2:4.

Safe disposal of specimens and contaminated material
Specimens, cultures and other material which may contain infectious pathogens and equipment used to test such material must be made non-infectious before being discarded or cleaned for reuse. Ideally all material should be sterilized to ensure the destruction or removal of all living forms (including spores). This, however, is not always possible and decontamination methods aimed at the destruction of the vegetative forms of pathogens may be all that can be achieved.

Laboratory waste which includes reusable articles may be decontaminated using disinfectants or by physical means.

Decontamination using hypochlorite disinfectants
Disinfectants must be used at the correct dilutions, not overloaded, and renewed when they are no longer active. For laboratory work, hypochlorite disinfectants are recommended because they are active against viruses as well as bacteria.

A hypochlorite disinfectant is an alkaline solution that contains chlorine. Sodium hypochlorite solution is readily available in most countries as domestic or laundry bleach (usually requiring dilution 1 in 5 in water) or as *Chloros* (requiring dilution 1 in 10 in water). At the correct strength, a hypochlorite solution kills bacteria and viruses, including hepatitis viruses.

Contaminated glassware requires soaking overnight. Discard containers must not be overcrowded. Infected articles must be completely immersed and pipettes filled. A hypochlorite disinfectant works by giving off free chlorine. It must therefore be prepared daily. A freshly made 1% w/v hypochlorite solution contains 10 000 parts per million (ppm) available chlorine and should be used for disinfecting blood spills and material containing much protein. For general use in discard containers and for the routine disinfecting of bench surfaces, a 0.25% w/v hypochlorite solution containing 2 500 ppm chlorine is adequate.

A hypochlorite solution should not be used for disinfecting metal equipment such as centrifuge buckets because the chemical corrodes metal. Metal articles can be disinfected using 10% v/v formalin solution (prepared from strong formalin solution) or a glutaraldehyde disinfectant prepared as instructed by the manufacturer. If these solutions are not available, 70% v/v alcohol can be used.

Caution: A concentrated hypochlorite solution must be stored in a cool place. If stored under warm conditions it will rapidly lose its available chlorine. It is a toxic chemical which must be prepared with care. It can damage the eyes, skin and lungs. Rubber gloves and goggles should be worn when diluting hypochlorite disinfectants.

Note: Further information about chemical disinfectants can be found in 33:6 in Volume II of the Manual.

Decontamination by autoclaving
Moist steam under pressure is the most effective means of achieving sterilization. A steam-operated gravity displacement autoclave is recommended. When unavailable, a pressure cooker type of sterilizer should be used. Details of electric, gas and kerosone operated autoclaves can be found in 48:1 in Volume II of the Manual.

Materials for autoclaving should be placed in wide shallow containers to assist in the removal of air and the penetration of heat. The chamber must not be overloaded with tightly packed articles. Sterilization of infected material is usually achieved at 121 °C for 20 minutes.

The operation of an autoclave must be carefully controlled using a thermocouple or commercially available autoclave indicators as explained in 33:6 in Volume II of the Manual.

Decontamination by incineration
If open burning is used to incinerate infected material, the waste should be placed in metal cans, e.g. kerosene tins or oil drums and these should be placed in the centre of a fierce wood or waste fire. The temperature will usually be high enough to kill all organisms and none can escape in smoke or air draughts.

If an incinerator is used, the combustion chamber must not be overfilled because this will prevent the destruction of *all* microorganisms in the waste. Living pathogens may then remain in the ash pit of the incinerator after burning has taken place.

Immunization
It is not possible or desirable to vaccinate laboratory workers against all the pathogens with which they may come in contact. The medical officer in charge of the laboratory should decide which vaccinations are required.

Protective inoculations are usually given against tuberculosis (when not Mantoux positive), typhoid, diphtheria, tetanus, poliomyelitis, and cholera.

An annual chest X-ray should also be available to laboratory staff.

District laboratories not equipped to handle highly infectious material, should refer any particular high risk specimen to a laboratory with adequate containment facilities (see 33:3 in Volume II of the Manual).

Laboratory biosafety manual for safety officers
Further information about the practice and management of safety with regard to infectious material, can be found in the 1983 WHO *Laboratory Biosafety Manual* available from World Health Organization, 1211 Geneva-27, Switzerland.

2:4 PIPETTING AND DISPENSING SAFELY

The safe pipetting and dispensing of specimens and reagents should receive a high priority in every laboratory. Worldwide, mouth-pipetting is now banned in most laboratories. Highly infectious pathogens can be found in specimens sent to the laboratory for testing and poisonous and corrosive chemicals are frequently required to analyze samples.

Changing to safer methods of pipetting and dispensing specimens and reagents can be achieved simply and economically as is described in this subunit. Besides the safety aspect, such changes often result in a higher standard of work because many pipetting and dispensing devices operate with great precision.

Accidents caused by mouth-pipetting
Mouth-pipetting can result in:

- Infection
- Poisoning, chemical burns, and other injuries from chemicals
- Cuts

Acquiring infection by mouth-pipetting
Commonly this occurs by:

— Accidentally sucking up specimens and cultures into the mouth.

— Putting a pipette in the mouth after its end has become contaminated from the fingers or a contaminated bench surface.

— Ingesting infected droplets which are produced as a specimen or culture is being sucked up.

Chemical injury caused by mouth-pipetting
Poisoning, chemical burns, and other injuries are

associated with mouth-pipetting toxic, corrosive, and irritant chemicals. The following are the main ways this can happen:

— Accidentally sucking up reagents into the mouth, e.g. when rapidly sucking up in a narrow bore pipette or when a reagent is contained in a dark brown bottle or opaque plastic container and the level of fluid cannot be seen clearly, resulting in air being drawn in and forcing the reagent up the pipette into the mouth.

— Putting a pipette in the mouth after its end has been in contact with a harmful reagent, disinfectant, or dry chemical, often carried on the fingers.

— Inhaling poisonous or irritating fumes, e.g. from acetic acid, concentrated hydrochloric acid, or formalin solution.

Cuts caused by mouth-pipetting
Cuts to the lips and mouth can occur when mouth-pipetting using a glass pipette with a chipped end.

Devices for pipetting and dispensing specimens
Most district laboratories will probably find that they need to use several different devices to cover the collection of capillary blood from patients and the measuring of venous blood, serum, urine and other specimens.

The devices described in this subunit for pipetting and dispensing specimens have been selected from a wide range that the author has tried. In evaluating each device, the author has considered its appropriateness for use in a district/regional hospital laboratory and a community-based laboratory. Considerations have included the effectiveness, ease of use, maintenance, and cost (inclusive of consumables and replacement parts) of a device.

Availability: The devices described in this subunit and shown in Plates 2.1 to 2.3 are available to developing countries from Tropical Health Technology (see Appendix IV, Capillary aspirators, Pipetters, Pipette fillers, Dispensers, Dilutor)

Simple bulb aspirator, see Plate 2.1b
This simple inexpensive device is suitable for use with graduated capillaries. The bulb has a hole which is left uncovered when the blood is being drawn into the capillary. The hole is covered with the finger when expelling and rinsing the blood from the capillary.

Thumb wheel aspirator, see Plate 2.1a
This device is particularly useful because it can be used with capillaries, shell-back pipettes (e.g. Sahli or WBC pipettes), and most small bore graduated pipettes, e.g. measuring up to 0.5 ml. It is extremely easy to use and control and is highly recommended to replace the dangerous practice of

mouth-pipetting using a mouth-piece and rubber tubing.

Pipetters (automatic pipettes), see Plate 2.1c
A wide range of pipetters to replace pipettes is available. Pipetters use plastic or glass tips and models are available for measuring single volumes or several different volumes. What are called positive displacement (solid interface) pipetters have a greater precision and accuracy than air displacement pipetters. The latter pipetters are considerably less accurate and precise when attempts are made to reuse the plastic tips which are meant to be disposable or to use plastic tips which are not specifically designed for the instrument but appear to fit it.

The pipetter shown in Plate 2.1c is a positive displacement pipetter. It is called a PDP 5 and can be set by the user to measure and dispense 5 different volumes. The model shown measures 20 μl (0.02 ml), 30 μl, 40 μl, 50 μl, and 60 μl. Another model measures 100 μl (0.1 ml), 120 μl, 150 μl, 175 μl, and 200 μl.

PDP 5 pipetters use glass capillaries which do not require changing or even washing between samples because a piston 'cleans' the side of the capillary as the specimen is dispensed. The piston protrudes from the end of the capillary to ensure that the entire measured volume is dispensed. When using any pipetter, the outside of the tip requires wiping before dispensing the volume. When dispensing, the tip should touch the side of the tube or other receiving container. Each PDP 5 model has its own capillaries but the same capillary can be used for measuring all five volumes.

When using a PDP 5, only a single downward stroke is needed to dispense the sample (some pipetters require an additional press to ensure complete emptying).

The capillary of a PDP 5 pipetter requires replacement only when it becomes damaged. A plastic guard is supplied to protect the capillary when the pipetter is not in use. At the end of a day's work, or more often if indicated, the capillary can be filled with a suitable disinfectant (e.g. domestic bleach diluted 1 in 10) and left to soak overnight. After soaking the capillary must be well rinsed with clean water. A further advantage of using a capillary, is that it can be examined to ensure that it is completely clean.

Capillaries, piston and wire are easily replaced. Calibration with the PDP 5 pipetter can be rapidly checked by simply unscrewing the calibrator device from the end of the pipetter, inserting it into the end of the capillary and adjusting a knob until it just touches the piston.

For details of availability of PDP 5 pipetters, see Appendix IV, Pipetters.

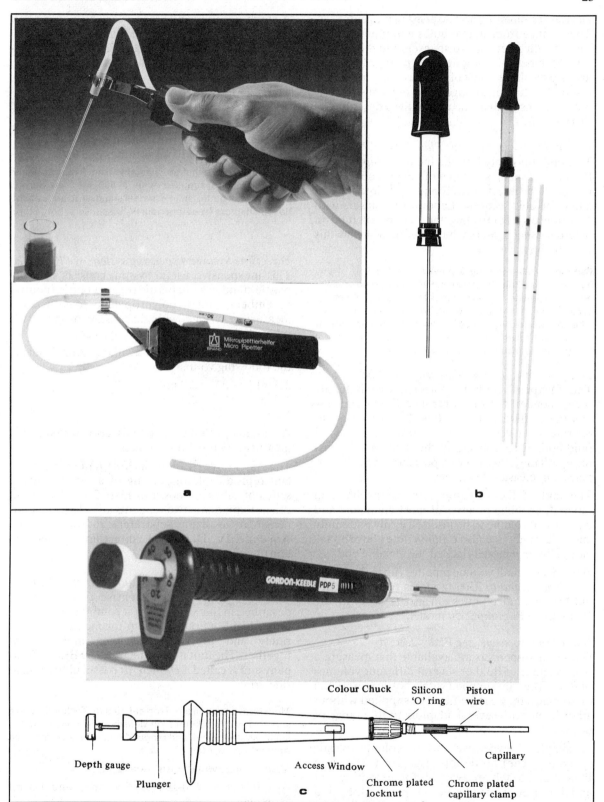

Plate 2.1   Equipment for measuring and dispensing specimens, e.g. blood, serum, plasma.
a   Thumb wheel aspirator for use with graduated capillaries or micro pipettes.
b   Rubber bulb for use with graduated capillaries.
c   Positive displacement pipettor with reusable glass capillary (see text).

Devices for pipetting and dispensing reagents

These range from simple bulbs and pipette fillers for use with pipettes, to dispensers and dilutors, to replace pipettes. Although macro type pipetters are also available, most of these use very wide bore disposable tips or syringes and are considerably more expensive than the alternatives described in this subunit.

PVC bulb pipette filler, see Plate 2.2a

This bulb fits easily into the hand. Its *tapered and flexible* end enables all types of pipettes up to 10 ml volume to be inserted easily and *safely* into the end and to be held securely. Laboratory workers with experience of controlling the volume of fluid in pipettes using a rubber bulb (teat), will find this PVC bulb easy to use.

Caution: When inserting a pipette into the end of any device, always hold the *upper* end, not the middle or lower end of the pipette. Serious injuries to the hand or wrist can occur when a long pipette is held *lower down* and breaks when it is pushed with force into the end of a bulb or other device, particularly when the end of the device is not tapered and is made of hard rubber or plastic.

Pi-pump 2500, pipette filler, see Plate 2.2b

This inexpensive plastic wheel device is highly recommended for the controlled filling and dispensing of fluid from pipettes. It is very easy to operate and gives excellent control of the level of fluid both when drawing up the fluid and dispensing it. All the fluid can be dispensed or it can be dispensed in measured volumes.

The end of the *Pi-pump 2500* is flexible and tapered, enabling pipettes of most diameters and up to 10 ml volume to be inserted easily and safely and held firmly (see also *Caution* note above). Previous *Pi-pump* models lacked this flexible end.

When using small volume pipettes (up to 2 ml), the 2 ml blue *Pi-pump 2500* model is recommended, but 1 ml and 2 ml pipettes can also be used with the 10 ml green *Pi-pump 2500* model.

Bottle top dispensers, see Plates 2.2c, d

Bottle top dispensers are available that measure a fixed volume of fluid or several different volumes of fluid. They are supplied with a bottle (reservoir) on to which they can be fitted or supplied without a bottle but with several adaptors to fit a range of bottles.

A simple, inexpensive, fixed volume plastic (polypropylene) bottle top dispenser is shown in Plate 2.2c. Models are available for measuring 3 ml and 4 ml (see Appendix IV, Dispensers). Such a dispenser has good reproducibility providing the top is pressed in a controlled way (as with any dispenser). A plastic bottle is provided which is made from high density polyethylene. This simple dispenser is suitable for dispensing many reagents in the laboratory.

A highly accurate and precise variable volume bottle top dispenser is shown in Plate 2.2d. It is manufactured by Brand Company. It is a rugged dispenser with an unbreakable plastic sidearm which has an attached closing cap. The plunger is made from PTFE. Models available are as follows:

— Measuring 0.1-0.5 ml volumes in 0.02 ml steps
— Measuring 0.4-2.0 ml volumes in 0.05 ml steps
— Measuring 1.0-5.0 ml volumes in 0.1 ml steps
— Measuring 2.0-10 ml volumes in 0.25 ml steps

Brand dispensers that are available from Tropical Health Technology are supplied with a 500 ml high density polyethylene bottle, stainless steel stand, and range of bottle top adaptors (see Appendix IV, Dispensers, bottle top).

Direct line Syringe dispensing system, see Plate 2.2e

This inexpensive useful system consists of a red plastic stand, 500 ml plastic reagent bottle (neutral or amber), and a polypropylene fixed volume measuring syringe with dispensing probe. PVC tubing links the reagent to the syringe.

Fixed volume syringes are available for measuring the following volumes:

0.5 ml	2.0 ml
1.0 ml	2.5 ml
1.5 ml	

A variable volume syringe is also available for measuring 0.1 to 1 ml volumes.

The system is particularly useful for the rapid, safe, and reproducible dispensing of a reagent into a series of tubes as shown in Plate 2.2e. The stand can accommodate two reagents and all the components are available separately at low cost (see Appendix IV, Dispensers, direct line syringe system).

Bottle top hand operated dilutor, see Plate 2.2f

This unit is the most expensive of the devices described in this subunit but it combines in a single unit a hand-operated system for measuring accurately and precisely, specimen and reagent together. The unit is manufactured by Brand Company and is called a *Diluette*. It has an unbreakable side arm.

Models available from Tropical Health Technology are supplied with a 500 ml high density polyethylene bottle, stainless steel stand, and range of bottle top adaptors (see Appendix IV, Dilutor).

Models are availabe for measuring:

— 0.02-0.1 ml (20-100 μl) specimen and 1-5 ml reagent
— 0.1-0.5 ml (100-500 μl) specimen and 1-5 ml reagent

If required, the unit can be used for measuring reagent only, e.g. to dispense haemoglobin diluting fluid when using capillary blood.

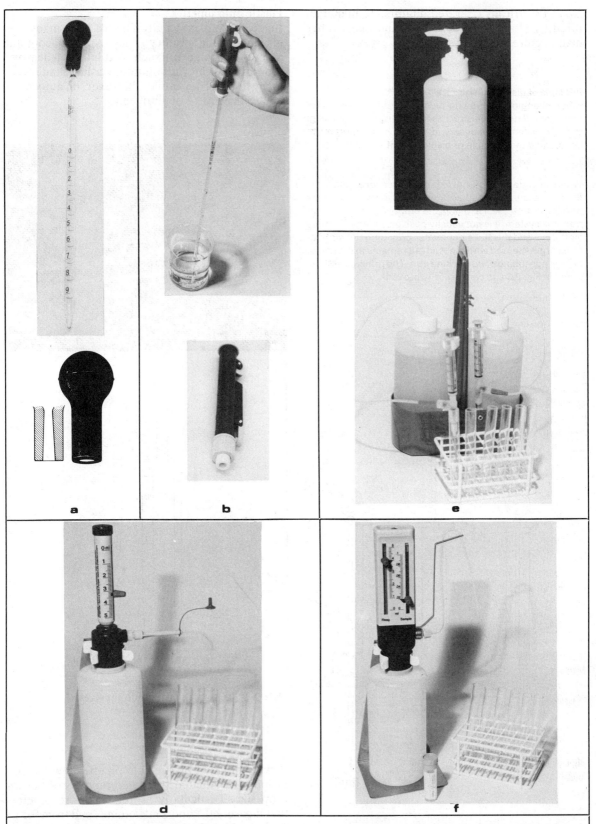

Plate 2.2 Equipment to measure and dispense reagents. a Bulb pipette filler, b Pi-pump pipette filler, c Polypropylene fixed volume dispenser, d Variable volume dispenser, e Direct fixed volume syringe system, f Hand operated dilutor.

Note: Electrically operated dilutors are manufactured by Hook and Tucker Ltd and many other manufacturers.

Principle of displacement

When changing from using pipettes to other devices for liquid handling which are based on displacement (e.g. syringe systems, dispensers, dilutors), it is important to understand the principle of displacement.

When using a syringe device, dispenser, or dilutor, the fluid is measured by displacement. Such a system requires priming before use, i.e. filling and emptying to remove air from the system. It is not usually possible to remove *every* air bubble and this does not matter providing the air bubble is *not* dispensed with the fluid but remains in the end of the syringe tubing or dispensing arm. The principle is illustrated in Fig. 2.3 and can be easily proved.

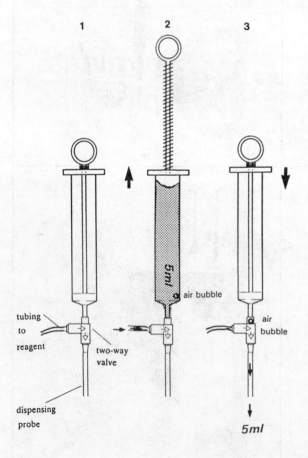

Fig. 2.3   Principle of displacement. Note the air bubble in the reagent (diagram 2). Providing this bubble is not dispensed with the reagent (diagram 3), the correct volume will be dispensed.

Plastic bulb pipettes

Inexpensive plastic bulb pipettes have many uses in a medical laboratory. They can be decontaminated in disinfectant such as diluted bleach or a sodium hypochlorite solution, washed, and reused many times. They cannot, however, be autoclaved or sterilized in a hot air oven.

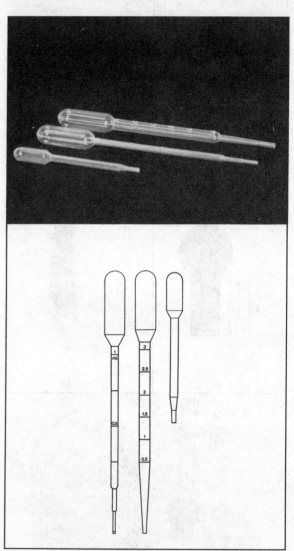

Plate 2.3   Reusable plastic bulb pipettes.

A wide range of plastic bulb pipettes is available, including graduated types and pipettes of known drop size. Particularly useful are those pipettes that measure 0.5 and 1 ml volumes and from 0.5 to 3 ml (see Plate 2.3). Small types are suitable for filling and transferring fluids from small bore tubes. For availability to developing countries, see Appendix IV, Plastic bulb pipettes.

2:5 SAFE USE AND STORAGE OF CHEMICALS AND REAGENTS

Even in the smallest laboratory, dangerous chemicals are used directly or incorporated into stains and reagents. These include highly flammable (easy to catch alight) chemicals such as ether or methanol, highly corrosive (able to attack the skin and destroy solid matter) chemicals such as phenol or sulphuric acid, or toxic (poisonous) and harmful chemicals such as formaldehyde solution. The correct handling and storage of hazardous chemicals is essential to prevent injury and damage.

Note: In tropical countries, it is particularly important to keep chemicals out of direct sunlight and avoid overheating in chemical stores and the laboratory. Overheating can decompose many chemicals, cause explosions, or the formation of toxic fumes.

Labelling of dangerous chemicals and reagents

To reduce accidents caused by chemicals, many countries have introduced legislation, requiring manufacturers to label dangerous chemicals with hazard symbols and to provide simple safety instructions. The six accepted danger symbols currently being used to label hazardous chemicals are shown in Fig. 2.2.

In addition to labelling stock bottles of chemicals with hazard warning signs, it is equally important to label those reagents prepared from dangerous chemicals. A guide to which reagents require hazard symbols are given in the following text and in the pages which describe the preparation of individual reagents in Appendix I.

Availability of hazard safety symbols

Self-adhesive labels with black official symbols on a yellow background (as shown in Fig. 2.2), measuring 38 × 38 mm are available at low cost to developing countries from Tropical Health Technology, (see Appendix IV, Hazard Safety labels).

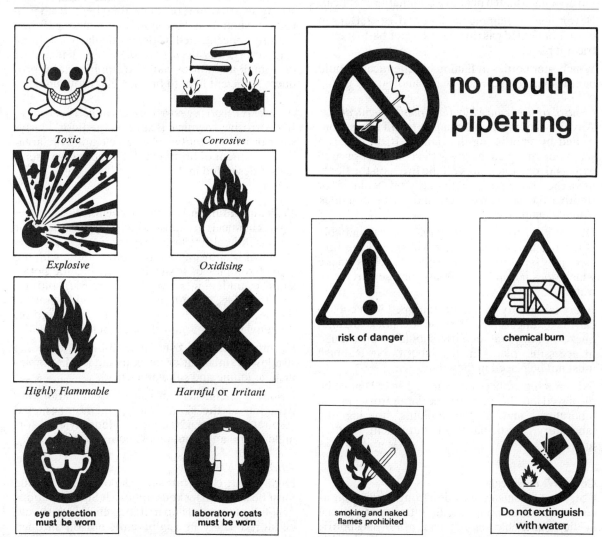

Fig. 2.2 Hazard warning symbols. *Courtesy of Jencons Scientific Ltd.*

Flammable chemicals
Flammable chemicals include ether, xylene, toluene, methanol, ethanol, other alcohols, glacial acetic acid, acetone, and acetic anhydride. Alcoholic Romanowsky stains and acid alcohol solutions are also highly flammable.

Storage
Flammable chemicals should be stored in a fire-proof metal box at ground level, preferably in an outside, cool, locked store. If a metal box is not available, at least a container well lined with tin foil should be used. Only small quantities of flammable solvents should be kept on laboratory benches and shelves.

Safe use
Before opening a bottle containing a flammable solvent, check that there is no open flame such as that from a Bunsen burner or burner unit of a gas operated fridge (including the pilot flame) within 6 feet. When using ether, allow a distance of 10 feet. Do not light a match near to a flammable chemical.

Never heat a flammable liquid over a Bunsen burner or lighted gas ring. Use a water bath or electric hot plate.

Winchester bottles of flammable chemicals should be transported in carriers with handles.

Control of fires caused by flammable chemicals
Any fire caused by a flammable liquid is best controlled by smothering the flames. If the fire is a small one on a bench, cover the container or area with a lid, or a thick cloth. If the fire is on the floor, use a chemical type fire extinguisher if available, or smother the flames with dry sand, earth, or a thick *woollen* blanket.

Do not pour water on the flames of a flammable liquid fire because the water will spread the fire, especially if it is caused by a solvent such as xylene which does not mix, but floats, on the surface of water.

Every laboratory should be equipped with chemical fire extinguishers. If these are not available, buckets of dry sand or earth should be positioned in accessible places in the laboratory. Rubbish must not be placed in these buckets.

'No smoking' notices (see Fig. 2.1 in 2:2) must be displayed on the door of the laboratory, in the laboratory, and in the building housing the laboratory, particularly in outpatient waiting areas.

Corrosive chemicals
Corrosive chemicals include strong acids such as concentrated sulphuric acid, nitric acid, glacial acetic acid, trichloroacetic acid, *ortho*-phosphoric acid, and caustic alkalis such as sodium hydroxide

(caustic soda), and potassium hydroxide (caustic potash).

Storage
Corrosive chemicals should be stored at low level to avoid any serious injury which could be caused if they were accidentally knocked off a shelf.

Safe use
Never mouth-pipette a corrosive chemical. Use a pipette filler, automatic pipetter, or dispenser (see 2:4). The accidental swallowing of a corrosive chemical can cause severe injury because such chemicals destroy living tissue.

Always pour a corrosive chemical at below eye level, slowly, and with great care to avoid splashing. When opening a container of a concentrated corrosive chemical, and when pouring it, wear a protective face visor or if unavailable, wear at least protective eyeshields.

The dissolving of a solid corrosive chemical such as sodium hydroxide in water or the diluting of a strong acid in water, produce great heat. Both procedures should be done slowly with mixing. When diluting concentrated acids, particularly sulphuric acid, always *add the acid to the water*. The adding of a small amount of water to sulphuric acid produces sufficient heat to break a glass container.

Accidents involving corrosive chemicals
If a corrosive chemical is spilt on the floor, always wear protective footwear when cleaning the area. The treatment of burns caused by corrosive chemicals is described in 2:7.

Toxic, harmful, and irritating chemicals
Toxic chemicals are those which can cause death or serious ill-health if swallowed or inhaled, or if the chemical is allowed to come into contact with the skin. Examples of toxic chemicals include potassium cyanide, mercury II (mercuric) nitrate, sodium azide, sodium nitroprusside, thiosemicarbazide, formaldehyde solution, chloroform, diphenylamine, barium chloride, and methanol.

Harmful chemicals can cause ill-health by being swallowed, inhaled, or by skin contact. Examples include iodine and sulphanilic acid.

Irritating chemicals can cause inflammation and irritation of the skin, mucous membranes, and respiratory tract. Examples include xylene, formaldehyde, and ammonia vapours.

Storage
Highly toxic chemicals such as potassium cyanide must be kept in a locked cupboard. Stock solutions or solids of harmful and irritating chemicals should be stored safely in a cupboard, not on an open shelf.

Safe use
Handle toxic, harmful, and irritating chemicals with great care. Wear protective gloves. Always lock away highly toxic chemicals immediately after use. Never leave a toxic chemical unattended. Always wash your hands after using a toxic or harmful chemical.

Chemicals with an irritating or harmful vapour should be used in a fume cupboard, or if this is not available, keep the laboratory well-ventilated while the chemical is being used. Never mouth-pipette any chemical. Always use a pipette filler, automatic pipetter or dispenser (see 2:4).

Accidents involving toxic or harmful chemicals
The first aid treatment for poisoning and injuries caused by harmful and irritating chemicals is described in 2:7.

Oxidizing chemicals
Oxidizing chemicals include chlorates, perchlorates, strong peroxides, potassium dichromate, and chromic acid.

Storage
Oxidizing chemicals must be stored away from organic materials and reducing agents. They can produce much heat when in contact with other chemicals, especially flammable chemicals.

Safe use
Handle oxidizing chemicals with great care. Most are dangerous to skin and eyes and when in contact with reducing agents.

Explosive chemicals
Heat, flame, or friction can cause explosive chemicals to explode. An example of an explosive chemical is picric acid, which must be stored under water. If picric acid is allowed to dry, it can become explosive. This can occur if the chemical is left to dry in pipes without being flushed away with an adequate amount of water.

Carcinogens
A chemical that can cause cancer by ingestion, inhalation, or by skin contact, is called a carcinogen.

Chemicals with proven carcinogenic properties include benzidine, *o*-tolidine, (*o*-toluidine is suspected),*o*-dianisidine, alpha- and beta- naphthylamine, nitrosamines, nitrosophenols, nitronaphthalenes, and selenite. The risk in handling these chemicals is proportional to the length and frequency of the exposure and the concentration of the chemical.

Storage
Carcinogens should be kept in closed containers* and labelled 'Carcinogenic, handle with special precautions'.

*Naphthylamines may vaporise to a dangerous extent at temperatures near to room temperature.

Safe use
Always wear protective plastic or rubber gloves, a face mask and eyeshields when handling carcinogenic chemicals. Carcinogens must not be allowed to come into contact with the skin because some carcinogens can be absorbed through the skin such as beta-naphthylamine.

After handling a carcinogen, wash well in cold water all the apparatus, bench, bottles and protective gloves (*before* removing them) and change your overall. Rinse your hands in cold running water before using soap.

Should a carcinogen come accidentally into contact with skin or the eye, immediately wash the affected part in cold running water for 5 minutes. If a spillage occurs on an overall or shoes, immediately remove the contaminated overall or shoes and wash in cold water.

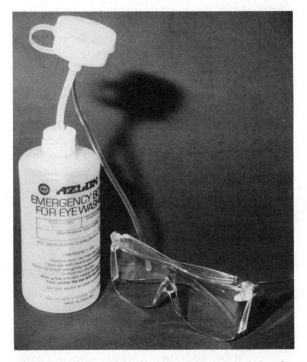

Plate 2.4 *Left:* **500 ml emergency eye wash bottle. Squeezing the bottle gently sprays the eye. The waste liquid flows through a tube to the sink or collecting vessel. Instructions for use are printed in green on the bottle.** *Right:* **Protective eyeshields with closed in sides. The goggles are made from polycarbonate.**

Properties and Storage of Some Dangerous Chemicals

KEY

a^1 **Flammable**: Store in a metal box at ground level, preferably in an outside store.

a^2 **Highly flammable**: Store in a metal box at ground level in a well-ventilated fire-proof outside store.

b **Corrosive**: Store at low level. Open the container with a cloth over the neck and cap. May cause severe burns.

c **Toxic** (poisonous): Store in a safe place. If highly toxic, store in a locked cupboard.

d **Injurious or irritating vapour**: Store in a well-stoppered bottle in a safe place.

e **Harmful**: Store in a safe place, not on an open shelf.

f **Oxidizing**: Store away from organic material, reducing agents, and flammable chemicals.

g **Explosive**: Handle with care, and read the instructions on the label regarding storage.

h **Deliquescent** (dissolves in water from the air): Store in a well-stoppered bottle.

i **Volatile** (vapourizing rapidly): Store in a well-stoppered bottle.

Chemical	Properties and storage
Acetic acid, glacial	a^1, **b, d** Store separate from oxidizing chemicals.
Acetone	a^2, **d, i** Must not be allowed to come into contact with chromic acid as this can cause a violent chemical reaction. Store in a cool place.
Ammonia solution	**b, d, i**
Barium chloride	**c**
Benzoic acid	**c, d** Do not expose to an open flame.
Chloroform	**c, d, i** Forms toxic carbonyl chloride on exposure to light. Always store in a dark bottle. Chloroform vapour is anaesthetic.
2,4-Dinitrophenyl-hydrazine	**c**

Diphenylamine	**c, d**
Ethanol, absolute	a^2, **e, i** Hygroscopic
Ethanolamine	**b, d**
Ether, diethyl	a^2, **i** May form explosive peroxidases when exposed to light. Always store in a dark bottle. Do not refrigerate. Use in a well-ventilated laboratory. Ether vapour is anaesthetic.
Formaldehyde solution	**c, d** Store separate from oxidizing chemicals.
Hydrochloric acid, concentrated	**b, d** In contact with air, it forms corrosive fumes. Violent chemical reaction can occur if in contact with chromic acid. Store separate from alkalis.
Hydrogen peroxide solution	**b, f** Store in a dark polythene bottle in a cool place. Decomposes in light and warmth.
Iodine	**e, i** Iodine attacks rubber (do not use rubber bungs).
Mercury	**c, d, i** Attacks lead piping and soldered joints.
Mercury II chloride	**b, c**
Mercury II nitrate	**c**
Methanol, absolute	a^2, **c, d, i** Hygroscopic
Nitric acid, concentrated	**b, d, f** Store in a well-stoppered dark bottle. Fire hazard when coming into contact with combustible materials. Store separate from alkalis.
P-Nitrophenyl	**e, f** Store separate from strong bases.

Phenol **b, c**
(carbolic acid) Hygroscopic. Oxidizes and
turns pink on exposure to
light. Store in a dark bottle
in a dry place.

o-Phosphoric acid **b, e**

Picric acid (solid) **a^1, c, g**
Explosive when dry, therefore make sure the chemical
is always covered with
water. Do not leave chemical to dry in pipes.

Potassium cyanide **c**
Highly toxic when inhaled,
swallowed, or in contact
with skin. Wear mask and
protective gloves when
handling. Always store in a
locked cupboard. Develops
highly toxic gas on contact
with acid.

Potassium **e**
dichromate Irritates eyes, respiratory
organs, and skin.

Potassium hydroxide **b, h**
Store separate from acids.

Potassium oxalate **c**

Silver nitrate **b, f**
Store always in a dark bottle.

Saponin powder **d, e**

Sodium azide **c**
Highly toxic when swal-
lowed. Develops highly
toxic gas upon contact with
acid. Sweep up spilled
chemical and wash away
remainder with a large volume of water.

Sodium hydroxide **b, h**
Store separate from acids.

Sodium nitro- **c**
prusside

Sulphanilic acid **e**

Sulphuric acid **b**
Hygroscopic, *never* add
water to the acid. Store
separate from alkalis.

Thiosemicarbazide **c**

o-Tolidine **c**
Carcinogen

Toluene **a^2, d**

o-Toluidine solution **a^1, c**
Reacts violently with acids.
Possibly carcinogenic.

Trichloroacetic acid **b, d, h**

Xylene **a^2, d, i**

Note: Always read the information supplied by a
manufacturer on the label of a bottle of chemical.

2:6 SAFE USE OF EQUIPMENT

Avoidance of accidents involving laboratory
equipment depends on the correct positioning,
installation, use, preventive maintenance, and regular servicing of equipment.

Positioning of equipment
Both convenience and safety must be considered
when positioning equipment in the laboratory. For
example, a Bunsen burner or gas ring must not be
placed near to where flammable reagents or stains
are stored, nor in direct sunlight which will make
the flame difficult to see. A piece of equipment
which is frequently used should not be placed at
the back of the bench where access is difficult.

The following points are also important:

- Avoid overcrowding a bench with equipment.
  Overcrowding will not only reduce the working
  area but also make daily disinfecting of the
  bench surface difficult and less likely to be done
  properly.
- Make sure that equipment which requires ventilation is positioned correctly. For example,
  refrigerators must not be placed close to a wall.
  The chimney aperture of a gas or kerosene
  operated refrigerator must not be obstructed in
  any way or positioned under a shelf. The same
  applies to the burner aperture of a flame emission spectrometer (flame photometer).
- If acid rechargeable batteries are used to operate equipment, position these with great care to
  prevent accidents from acid corrosion and fires
  from the crossing of leads over terminals. Hydrogen is evolved from acid batteries, therefore
  the laboratory must be well-ventilated especially when a battery is being recharged.

Installation of electrical equipment

The installation of electrical equipment must be carried out either by the supplier of an apparatus, or if this is not possible, by the hospital electrician or a trained laboratory equipment technician.

Important points of safety regarding the installation of electrical equipment include:

- Ensuring that the voltage of the new equipment is the same as that of the electricity supply in the laboratory. For those instruments that can be operated from both 100-120 volts and 220-240 volts, it is important to check that the voltage selector switch is in the correct position.

- Checking that the power required by the instrument does not exceed the power supply circuit of the laboratory, and that socket outlets are not overloaded. Multiple adaptors should not be used because these can lead to overloading and bad connections.

- Making sure that the equipment is wired correctly and that the plug carries a fuse of the correct rating. The wiring system should have a grounded conductor.

  The wire flex should not be longer than is necessary and it should not be frayed. It should contain no joins, and be kept clear of water, hot pipes, and surfaces which may become very hot. The flex should be checked regularly for signs of wear.

Safe use of electrical equipment

Whenever possible the use of an apparatus should be demonstrated by the supplier. If this is not possible, the operations and service manual (which must accompany the instrument) should be carefully studied before the equipment is operated. When put into routine use, written instructions and safety precautions should be displayed near to the instrument.

The following are important points with regard to the safe use of electrical equipment:

- When using an electrical piece of equipment, the hands must be completely dry and also the floor on which the operator is standing (water is a very good conductor of electricity). The treatment of electric shock is described in 2:7.

- The electricity supply to an instrument must be disconnected (by removing the plug from the wall socket) at the end of the day's work (excluding fridges and incubators). An instrument must *always* be disconnected when performing any maintenance such as fitting a new bulb.

- If a fuse should 'blow', do not automatically put in a new fuse until the circuit is checked to investigate why the fuse wire has melted.

  Should a fire break out due to an electrical fault, it should be controlled by a dry chemical type extinguisher or with dry sand. Water must never be used.

Mainenance and servicing of equipment

It is essential to maintain and service equipment regularly to ensure:

- Continued efficient functioning of the equipment and the avoidance of breakdowns which could interupt the laboratory service to patients.

- Safe operation of the equipment and the prevention of accidents due to worn flex, loose connections, worn components, or corroded parts (especially in humid climates).

A stock should be kept of the relevant replacement parts of all the equipment used in the laboratory, to avoid essential apparatus being put out of action while delivery of a compoment is awaited e.g. a new lamp or connector.

Whenever possible, larger laboratories should arrange for a member of staff to be trained as a laboratory instrument technician. Such a person can help to reduce the cost of servicing equipment and the frequency with which instruments fail.

Careful selection of equipment and standardization in the use of equipment (especially that used in rural laboratories) are important in helping to achieve regular servicing and avoiding equipment being out of action for long periods.

Note: The maintenance of individual items of laboratory equipment is described in Chapter 3.

2:7   FIRST AID

Knowing what to do immediately an accident occurs can help to reduce suffering and the consequences of serious accidents. In some situations, First Aid can be life saving.

Training in First Aid

All laboratory workers should receive a basic practical training in First Aid, with particular attention being paid to the types of accidents which may occur in the laboratory. They should also know what emergency action needs to be taken if an outpatient or blood donor collapses in the laboratory.

The training must include demonstrations and be given by a person qualified to teach First Aid.

First aid equipment

An adequately equipped *First Aid* box should be kept in the laboratory, in a place that is known and accessible to all members of staff. The box should be clearly marked e.g. with a red cross and preferably be made of metal or plastic to prevent it being destroyed by pests. The contents should be checked regularly by the Safety Officer.

A medical officer or First Aid worker should be consulted regarding the contents of the box. Although commercially prepared *First Aid* boxes are available, they are expensive and not necessary. It is advisable for the laboratory to prepare its own *First Aid* box to ensure that the contents are appropriate and can be replenished from hospital stocks.

A First Aid chart giving the immediate treatment of cuts, burns, poisoning, shock, and collapse, should be prepared by the Safety Officer and displayed in the laboratory.

Emergency treatment of cuts and bleeding

If the cut is small
— wash with soap and water,
— apply pressure with a piece of cotton wool,
— disinfect the area with a skin antiseptic such as tincture of iodine,
— cover with a water-proof dressing.

If the cut has been caused by contaminated glassware
— encourage bleeding,
— seek medical advice.

If there is serious bleeding from a limb
— raise the injured limb to reduce the bleeding,
— apply pressure with a clean dressing backed with cotton wool,
— bandage the dressing in position,
— immediately seek medical assistance.

Bleeding from the nose
— seat the person upright with the head slightly forward,
— tell the person to pinch firmly the soft part of their nose for about 10 minutes and breathe through their mouth,
— if the bleeding does not stop, seek medical advice.

Emergency treatment of burns

Heat burns
— immediately plunge the burnt area into cold water or apply a pad soaked in cold water to the affected part for 10 minutes.
— cover with a dry dressing.

Note: If more than a minor burn, seek medical treatment.

Chemical burns of the skin
— wash immediately in running water,
— neutralize with a suitable chemical as follows:
   If an *acid* burn, neutralize with sodium bicarbonate powder.
   If an *alkali* burn, neutralize with boric acid powder.
— seek medical attention.

Chemical injury to the eye
— wash the affected eye as quickly as possible under running tap water or with water from an eye wash-bottle,
— neutralize with a suitable chemical as follows:
   If an *acid* injury, neutralize with 5% sodium bicarbonate solution.
   If an *alkali* injury, neutralize with 5% acetic acid or vinegar diluted 1 in 5.
— immediately seek medical attention.

Emergency treatment for poisoning

Swallowing of an acid or alkali
— immediately rinse the mouth well with water,
— neutralize with a suitable chemical as follows:
   If *acid* has been swallowed, neutralize by drinking 8% w/v magnesium hydroxide suspension (milk of magnesia).
   If an *alkali* has been swallowed, neutralize by drinking lemon juice or 5% acetic acid.
— drink three or four cups of water,
— seek medical attention.

Note: When an acid or alkali has been swallowed, do not encourage vomiting.

Swallowing of other poisonous chemicals
— rinse out the mouth well with water,
— depending on the chemical swallowed, take a suitable chemical antidote under medical supervision.

Note: Always seek medical advice and treatment after swallowing toxic or harmful chemicals.

Swallowing of infected material
— immediately seek medical treatment.

Mouth-pipetting: This is the main cause of the accidental swallowing of chemicals or infected material in laboratories. Mouth-pipetting should be banned from all laboratories (see also 2:4).

Fainting

Emergency treatment of a faint is as follows:

— lay the person down and raise the legs above the level of the head (see Fig. 2.4),
— loosen clothing at the neck, chest, and waist,
— make sure the room is well-ventilated,
— reassure the person as consciousness is regained,
— gradually raise the person to the sitting position. Sips of drinking water may be given

Note: If breathing becomes difficult, place the person in the position shown in Fig. 2.5. This is called the *recovery position*.

Electric shock

— immediately turn off the electricity from the *mains*,
— if the person has collapsed, send immediately for medical help and if the person is not breathing, give artificial respiration until assistance arrives.

Important: On no account try to free an electrocuted person from the electrical contact without using some form of insulation material, such as *thick* cloth, folded laboratory coat, folded newspaper, or strip of rubber. If insulation is not used, the person rescuing will also be electrocuted.

Emergency resuscitation when a person stops breathing

If a person stops breathing following an electric shock or for any other reason, artificial respiration must be applied *as soon as possible* (if the the brain is deprived of oxygen for more than about 4 minutes, permanent brain damage will occur). The person may also require heart compression if there is circulatory arrest.

Mouth-to-mouth respiration

There are several ways to perform artificial respiration. The most effective is mouth-to-mouth:

1. Lie the unconscious person on the floor. Supporting the neck, tilt the head backwards with the chin pushed upwards as shown in Fig. 2.6.

   This position will keep the person's airway open (see Fig. 2.6).

2. If the person does not start to breathe, begin immediately mouth-to-mouth respiration:

   — open your mouth wide and take a deep breath,
   — pinch the person's nostrils together with your fingers,

— press your lips around the person's mouth,
— blow into the person's mouth (air will pass to the lungs) until the chest is seen to rise.
— remove your mouth and watch the chest fall,
— repeat the inflation at the normal rate of breathing, i.e. 10-15 times per minute.

Note: Give the first few breaths *rapidly* to saturate the person's blood with oxygen.

Heart not beating

3. If after the first two inflations, natural breathing is not restored, check whether the heart has stopped beating.

   Indications that the heart has stopped beating are:

   • Person remaining or becoming grey-blue.
   • No carotid pulse being felt (see Fig. 2.7).
   • Pupils of the eye appearing widely dilated.

   Take immediate action to restart the heart while *at the same time* continuing mouth-to-mouth respiration:

   — Begin external heart compression by placing the heel of your hand on the lower half of the person's breastbone and cover this hand with the heel of your other hand as shown in Fig. 2.8 (the palms and fingers of your hand should be raised away from the person's chest).
   — With your arms straight, press down rapidly (once every second), looking to see whether there is an improvement in the person's colour (indicating a return of circulation). If there is no improvement, continue compression and mouth-to-mouth respiration.

   If resuscitating by yourself, apply 15 heart compressions followed by 2 quick lung inflations and then repeat.

   If you have help, apply 5 heart compressions, followed by 1 deep inflation. The person carrying out the mouth-to-mouth respiration should feel for a carotid pulse.

4. Once natural breathing has been restored and the heart is beating, place the person in the recovery position (see Fig. 2.5). This is important because the person may vomit and in this position there will be no danger of choking.

5. Obtain further medical assistance at the earliest opportunity.

Note: Other forms of resuscitation will be required if it is not possible to apply mouth-to-mouth respiration. Alternative methods should therefore be learnt.

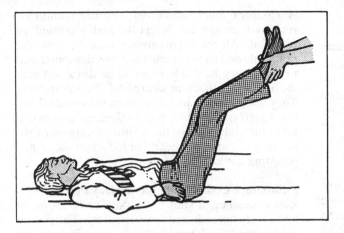

Fig. 2.4. Position in which to place a person who has fainted.

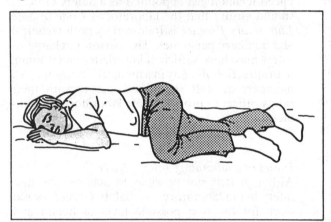

Fig. 2.5   The recovery position.

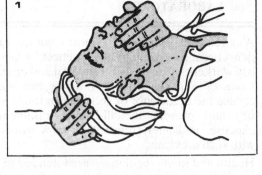

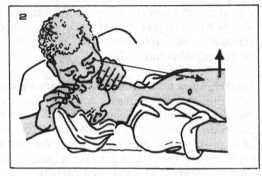

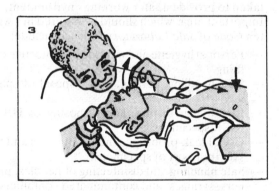

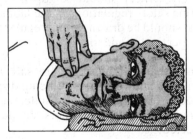

Fig. 2.7   Feeling for the carotid pulse.

Fig. 2.6   Mouth to mouth respiration during emergency resuscitation. If the heart has stopped beating, perform external heart compression (see text for details).

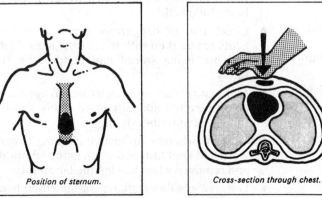

Position of sternum.

Cross-section through chest.

Fig. 2.8   Position of hands over lower breast bone when performing external heart compression.

Acknowledgement: Illustrations are reproduced by permission of St John   Ambulance Association.

2:8   CODE OF SAFETY FOR DISTRICT LABORATORIES

As already explained in 2:1, most laboratory accidents occur as a result of bad practices by laboratory workers. A carefully formulated and operated *Code of Safe Laboratory Practice* can greatly reduce the occurrence of accidents in the laboratory and prevent the ill-health, disablement, expense, and interference with work associated with such accidents.

Health and safety regulations are intended to protect patients, laboratory technical staff, and those who clean and visit the laboratory, from acquired infections and injury caused by chemicals, broken glassware, fire, explosions, faulty electrical equipment, and other hazards.

Formulating a Code of Safe Laboratory Practice

To formulate an *effective Code of Safe Laboratory Practice* it is necessary to understand the main causes of laboratory accidents (see 2:1). Every laboratory should then analyze whether its work practices are contributing to or helping to avoid such accidents, and what realistic actions can be taken to provide a safer working environment.

Important areas which should be covered in a written *Code of Safe Laboratory Practice* include:

— Personal hygiene and wearing of protective clothing.
— Safe handling, testing, and disposal of specimens.
— Identifying, testing, and disposing of HIGH RISK specimens.
— Use of leak-proof specimen containers and the safe transport of specimens.
— Safe handling and disinfecting of needles, prickers, syringes, and contaminated containers.
— Safe pipetting and dispensing of specimens and reagents.
— Methods of reducing aerosol production and spillages.
— Labelling of dangerous chemicals.
— Safe handling and storage of chemicals.
— Ways of reducing fire hazards.
— Selection and correct use of fire fighting apparatus.
— Operation and maintenance of laboratory equipment.
— Ways to reduce injury from broken glassware.
— Improvements in the layout of the laboratory to promote a safer working environment and to give better protection to outpatients.
— Use of protective gloves, eyeshields, face masks, and other safety equipment.
— First aid measures.
— Immunizations.
— Recording and analyzing of laboratory accidents.

A *Code of Safe Laboratory Practice* should be reviewed at regular intervals and modified as required. All the regulations should be sensible, practical, and clearly explained and demonstrated to laboratory staff. They should be discussed with the medical officer in charge of the laboratory. They should not make unreasonable demands on ward staff or patients. Safety devices introduced into the laboratory must not create hazards because of their complexity or incorrect use, e.g. a pipetting device.

Enforcing a Code of Safe Laboratory Practice

Every member of staff has a duty to be aware of laboratory hazards and to work safely. The person in charge of the laboratory, or a qualified experienced technologist appointed as a Safety Officer, should ensure that the laboratory's *Code of Safe Laboratory Practice* is followed by both technical and auxiliary personnel. The person in charge of safety must have sufficient knowledge and training in the practice of safety in a medical laboratory. All members of staff should co-operate with their safety officer to provide a safe laboratory environment.

Duties of a laboratory safety officer

Although it is not possible to achieve absolute safety in the laboratory, the Safety Officer should work for the best possible level of health and safety.

The Safety Officer should set up a system for monitoring safety regulations in the laboratory. A check list should be drawn up and regular (but random) inspections made to:

● Ensure that test methods are safe and that specimens and reagents are being disposed of correctly. The method of disinfecting and of cleaning specimen containers should also be inspected.

● Check whether the safety precautions for identifying and testing HIGH RISK specimens are being followed.

● Check that all dangerous chemicals and reagents are marked with the correct hazard label and are being stored and handled by staff safely.

● Make sure that specimens and reagents are being pipetted and dispensed safely and that there is no mouth-pipetting.

● Observe whether protective clothing is being worn and kept fastened when in the laboratory and removed when leaving the laboratory.

● Observe whether staff are washing their hands after handling specimens or dangerous chemicals and before leaving the laboratory, and whether running water and soap are always available.

- Note whether other safety regulations are being kept such as no smoking, eating, drinking or chewing gum in the laboratory. The laboratory fridges should be inspected for food and drink.

- Check whether safety equipment such as the First Aid box, eyewash bottles, sand buckets, and fire extinguishers are in good order and well located in the laboratory, and that staff know the locations and how to use the equipment especially fire extinguishers.

- Ensure that corridors and exits from the laboratory are not being obstructed and that fire doors are being kept closed.

- Check whether the laboratory is being kept clean and that benches are being kept free of unnecessary equipment and personal property.

- Examine equipment for defects and observe whether it is being used correctly. Check also for cracked or chipped glassware.

- Observe whether safety regulations regarding patients and visitors to the laboratory are being followed.

During such inspections, the Safety Officer should take the opportunity of reviewing and discussing safety regulations with the staff, revizing First Aid and fire regulations, and modifying any regulations which are not helping to promote safety. If a laboratory accident has occurred recently, the causes of it should be discussed and if required new safety measures introduced to help prevent its recurrence.

The Safety Officer should instruct trainees and any new members of staff in the *Code of Safe Laboratory Practice* before they are allowed to work in the laboratory. It should also be the duty of the Safety Officer to check that electrical equipment is disconnected at the end of the day, that windows are closed and that the laboratory is locked securely. Care should be taken not to leave the laboratory unattended during working hours. If this is unavoidable, the laboratory should be locked until the staff return from the wards or outpatient clinic.

Safety equipment available from Tropical Health Technology

In addition to the range of pipetting and dispensing devices described in 2:4, the following are also available to developing countries at low cost from Tropical Health Technology Equipment Service:

- Eyeshields (goggles) made from break-resistant clear polycarbonate and fitted with side shields. They help to protect the eyes when preparing dangerous chemicals.

- Eye wash bottle, 500 ml made from polyethylene and supplied with spray. Squeezing the bottle gently sprays the eye. The waste liquid flows through a tube to the sink or collecting vessel. Instructions for use are printed in green on the bottle.

- Disposable plastic (polyethylene) gloves, medium size.

- Self-adhesive hazard labels for labelling dangerous reagents, as described in 2:5.

For further details, see Appendix IV, Eyeshields, Eyewash bottle, Gloves, Hazard safety labels

---

Recommended Reading

Report of a working party, headed by Sir James Howie. *Code of Practice for the Prevention of Infection in Clinical Laboratories and Post-Mortem Room.* London, 1979. Available from H. M. Stationery Office, 49 High Holborn, London WC1 England, approx. £1.75.

World Health Organization *Laboratory Biosafety Manual*, WHO, Geneva, 1983.

Health and Safety Commission. *Safety in Health Service Laboratory, Hepatitis B*, 1985. Available from Health and Safety Executive, St Hugh's House, Trinity Road, Bootle, Merseyside L20 3QY, UK.

Advisory Committee on Dangerous Pathogens. *LAU/HTLVIII Causative agent of AIDS and related conditions, Revised guidelines*, code VIA3, June 1986. Available from DHSS Store, Health Publications Unit, No. 2 Site, Manchester Road, Haywood, Lancs OL1U 2PZ, UK.

First Aid Manual

A copy of the St John Ambulance First Aid Manual, 4th edition 1982, can be obtained from Supplies Dept, St John Ambulance, St John's Gate, Clerkenwell, London, EC1M 4DA, United kingdom.

3

Equipment for a District Hospital and Health Centre Laboratory

3:1 SELECTION, MAINTENANCE, AND ORDERING OF EQUIPMENT

When selecting equipment for use in district hospital laboratories and health centre laboratories in developing countries, the following should be considered:

■ Will the equipment improve significantly the laboratory service to patients? This is the most important question and one which requires an honest discussion to define the value of a piece of equipment and differentiate between what is wanted and what is needed.

■ Is the cost of purchasing, running, and maintaining the equipment within the resources available?

■ Is the equipment suited to the type of laboratory and conditions under which it will be used? For example, what are the power requirements or is there any information available to show that the equipment will operate in a hot climate or under conditions of high atmospheric humidity?

■ Has the laboratory staff sufficient knowledge and experience to operate and maintain the equipment efficiently and safely? If not, will it be possible for the necessary training to be given. Aspects regarding the safe use of laboratory equipment are described in 2:6.

■ What parts of the equipment require regular replacement, e.g. bulbs, fuses, carbon brushes, thermostat, heating element, electrodes, deionising resins, wicks, washers, tubing, connectors, etc? What will be the cost of these replacement parts and how easy will it be to obtain them? In the event of a breakdown, will it be easy to repair the equipment and is there a realistic manufacturer's guarantee given with the instrument? One of the best ways of answering these questions is to obtain in advance of purchasing, a copy of the *Operations and Service Manual* from the manufacturer.

■ Does the equipment form part of a system? For example, is the operation of the instrument dependant on a continued supply of imported ready-made reagents or can it be operated using locally prepared reagents?

In a paper given by Desmond Philip during the 1986 IAMLT Congress (as part of a seminar on Appropriate Technology),[1] the following steps were suggested to achieve the successful purchasing of laboratory equipment:
— establish the need
— define the requirements
— define the resources
— call tenders
— evaluate tenders
— select
— purchase

A purchase should always be reviewed at a later stage.

Approach to new technologies

The development of automated and semi-automated laboratory equipment has in many instances greatly increased working capacity, speeded up test results, and improved the precision of many routine laboratory investigations such as cell counting, staining, pipetting and dispensing, and clinical chemistry assays.

While some developments have resulted in more rugged, safer, reliable, and useful equipment (as shown in this Chapter and in 2:4), other technologies have resulted in highly sophisticated and specialized equipment which is expensive to buy and maintain and not appropriate or required to investigate the health problems of developing countries. Johannes Vang of the World Health Organization has commented that 'we have to realize that most health technology is invented in a specific culture and does not transplant itself readily into a different culture unless we transform it somewhat or at least deal with it in a critical way, asking questions like:
— does it have any value for us?
— what are the costs for us if we adopt this technology?
— what else might we use our resources and efforts for?
— what do we have to give up for this new technology?
— can we modify it to suit our purposes without losing its efficacy?

Dr Vang concludes, 'let us improve our technology and use it wisely to create better health for those we serve'.[3]

Repair and maintenance of laboratory equipment

To facilitate the repair and maintenance of laboratory equipment in developing countries, the

World Health Organization makes the following recommendations:[2]

- Service manuals must be provided.
- Spare parts should be clearly listed.
- Daily care of equipment should be emphasised.
- Equipment should be demonstrated by manufacturers or their representatives.
- Laboratory staff should receive training in the relevant aspects of equipment operation and maintenance.
- To avoid interrupting essential laboratory services, there should be available suitable equipment to substitute when routine equipment needs to be repaired.

The same WHO document describes the organization of *A National Repair and Maintenance Service* with the following functions:

- To repair and maintain medical instruments, especially electrical, electronic, and optical.
- To give on-the-job training to technicians in repair and maintenance.
- To advise on the choice of equipment to be purchased with regard to durability, reliability, and correctness of specifications.
- To design and develop needed equipment.
- To maintain a library of repair and maintenance service manuals, instrument operation manuals, and other related periodicals and books.

Note: Guidelines regarding the maintenance of major items of laboratory equipment are covered in the subsequent subunits of this Chapter.

Ordering of laboratory equipment and supplies
The planned and correct ordering and purchasing of laboratory supplies are essential if a laboratory is to function reliably and avoid any discontinuity in its service.

The person in charge of purchasing laboratory equipment and supplies should be an experienced medical laboratory technologist who is well informed about the conditions under which the equipment and supplies will be used. As far as possible there should be standardization within a laboratory service of equipment and important supplies such as chemicals and essential reagents. Decisions about standardization must be made and reviewed in consultation with peripheral laboratories to ensure that equipment, chemicals, reagents, and other supplies are closely matched to local needs and facilities.

Ordering from a Central Store
In most developing countries, a system exists for invidual laboratories to obtain essential laboratory equipment and supplies from a Central Supplies Store. The features of such a system should include:

— The distribution to all laboratories of a clearly presented *Laboratory Supplies Catalogue*, requisition forms, and clear instructions on how to order.

— The employment of adequate staff to check purchased goods, to pack supplies safely, and dispatch goods speedily.

— The availability of trained equipment technicians to assist intermediate and peripheral laboratories to assemble and install equipment correctly.

— The provision for a laboratory to return to the Central Store a piece of equipment that has been damaged in transit and to receive a replacement speedily.

— The provision for a laboratory to order supplies, especially reagents, in emergency situations such as during an epidemic. This should include the possibility of a laboratory to purchase direct from a manufacturer.

Because supplies are usually ordered at monthly, 3 monthly or even 6 monthly intervals, it is *essential* for individual laboratories to plan ahead and to order in sufficient quantity and in good time. Each laboratory should keep an *Order Notebook* in which members of staff can write what is required or is likely to be needed in the near future. Always consider the shelf-life of reagents and expected life of the replacement parts of equipment.

When ordering, the correct catalogue number and other relevant specifications must be entered accurately on the requisition form. A record must be kept of what is ordered (dated carbon copy) so that this can be referred to when the goods are received.

Ordering direct from a manufacturer or supplier
To avoid wasting money and incurring unnecessary delays, it is essential to receive sufficient information from a manufacturer or a supplier *before* placing an order. This should include an adequate description of the goods, ordering information, current prices, expected delivery time and where relevant, a list of recommended spares and details of installation, demonstration, guarantee, and servicing arrangements.

When ordering, always use the supplier's catalogue number and give a description of the product. Make sure all the essential parts are ordered, e.g. a rotor head and buckets with a centrifuge, or the required optics for a microscope. These are often listed by manufacturers as 'Accessories' or 'Spares'.

Purchasing chemicals, reagents and stains
When ordering chemicals it is particularly important to obtain a catalogue and price list from a manufacturer to ensure that:
— the correct name of the chemical is used. Whenever possible, give the formula of the chemical. Some chemicals can be obtained in both hydrated and anhydrous forms and therefore the form required must also be stated.
— the amount you wish to order is available from a supplier. Unless a chemical is very expensive, it is unlikely to be available in small amounts, e.g. under 100 g. Many chemicals can only be obtained in minimum quantities of 250 g or 500 g.
— the shelf-life of the chemical is acceptable and that the conditions of storage can be met to ensure stability and safety.
— if needing to be imported, that national regulations will allow importation of the chemical and that it is not listed by the manufacturer as an unstable chemical which is unsuitable for export.
— the price of the chemicals can be afforded. Some companies may also have a minimum order value, making it impossible to buy just one or a few chemicals at a time.

Test kits
Guidelines regarding the purchase of clinical chemistry test kits can be found in 26:1.

When purchasing stains it is also important to obtain a supplier's catalogue to make sure the correct name of the stain is used, to know the form in which the stain is available, e.g. as a powder, liquid concentrate, or liquid ready-made stain, and to know the quantities available and prices. A few ready-made stains have a restricted shelf-life and may require storage at 2-8 °C.

Purchasing plastic-ware
As described in 3:2, a wide range of good laboratory plastic-ware is now available to replace most glassware. Articles made from polyethylene and polypropylene are recommended because they are inexpensive, break-resistant, and resistant to most of the chemicals used routinely in medical laboratories. Polypropylene can also withstand repeated autoclaving.

Plastic-ware is ordered as follows:

— *Flasks, cylinders, beakers*: Order by capacity. Available sizes usually include 50 ml, 100 ml, 250 ml, 500 ml, 1 litre. When ordering a flask, it is important to state whether a volumetric or Erlenmeyer (conical) flask is required.

— *Funnels*: Order by the size of the diameter across the top of the funnel, e.g. 65 mm, 90 mm, 115 mm, or 140 mm across. It is best to buy a funnel that has ribs to prevent air locks and to speed filtration.

— *Tubes*: Order by the diameter and length, e.g. 12 × 75 mm or 13 × 100 mm (different sizes are available from different manufacturers). If conical (centrifuge) tubes are required, this should be stated.

— *Cover glasses*: Order by size and thickness. For routine use No. 1½ cover glasses of size 20 × 20 mm or 22 × 22 mm are recommended. When ordering cover glasses for counting chambers, state the purpose (there is no need to give a size or thickness because these specifications are standardized for counting chambers).

Purchasing syringes, needles, blood lancets
For collecting blood, a Luer type polypropylene or Nylon syringe of 2.5 ml, 5 ml, or 10 ml capacity is recommended.

The recommended size of needle for collecting venous blood is 19 gauge. A supply of size 23 gauge needles should also be purchased for collecting blood from children.

Note: Certain manufacturers refer to a 19 SWG needle as size 18 (bore 1.016 mm), and a 23 SWG needle as size 22 (bore 0.610 mm).

When purchasing needles, it is also necessary in addition to stating the size, to specify that they must be of Luer mount and of the long bevel type. Whenever possible, disposable needles should be used (these are always of Luer mount).

Blood lancets (prickers) are ordered by the box (number in each box depends on the supplier). Stainless steel lancets can be autoclaved and re-used whereas plastic mounted prickers cannot be autoclaved.

Purchasing racks
When ordering racks, it is necessary to specify the following:
— Purpose of the rack, e.g. whether for tubes, bottles, or for draining slides.
— The number of holes or spaces required and size of the tube (length and diameter) or bottle diameter to be used in the rack (in mm).
— The material of the rack, e.g. whether plastic, metal, or nylon coated wire.

A supplier's catalogue will be required to know the sizes and types of rack available.

Purchasing haemocytometers (counting chambers)
Order according to the ruling required, e.g. Improved Neubauer (used for counting white blood cells) or Modified Fuchs-Rosenthal (used for counting cells in c.s.f.). To facilitate counting, haemocytometers which have clear 'bright' rules should be ordered.

It is usually best to order a few extra cover glasses. Two cover glasses are usually supplied with a haemocytometer.

3:2 LABORATORY PLASTIC-WARE

In recent years, important advances have been made in the use of plastic resins to produce a wide range of reliable plastic-ware to replace glassware in medical laboratories.

Much of the routine laboratory plastic-ware is of high quality, break-resistant, and therefore less expensive and safer to use than glassware. Plastic goods can also be transported at lower cost than glassware which is heavier and more easily broken. Most plastic-ware can be disinfected in 0.5 g% sodium hypochlorite or domestic bleach (diluted 1 in 5) and some plastics can also be autoclaved (see later text).

Resins used to produce laboratory plastic-ware
- Polyolefin resins which include:
  — Polyethylene (PE) in low density (LDPE) or high density (HDPE). LDPE is more transparent, less rigid and slightly less resistant to some chemicals than HDPE. Articles made from LDPE cannot be autoclaved. HDPE can withstand 120 °C for up to 15 minutes.

    LDPE is used for making wash bottles, dropper bottles, and plastic bulb pipettes. HDPE is recommended for reagent bottles. Amber (brown opaque plastic) bottles are usually available only in LDPE.

  — Polypropylene (PP), which is translucent, and can be autoclaved repeatedly. It is used for making flasks, cylinders, funnels, beakers, specimen containers, syringes, and other items.

  — Polymethylpentene (PMT, also known as TPX), which is transparent and can be autoclaved and sterilized in a hot air oven at 160 °C. It is mostly used for cylinders, flasks, and reagent bottles. It is more expensive than polypropylene and polyethylene.

- Styrene resins which include:
  — Polystyrene (PS), which is rigid, transparent, and not as durable or chemically resistant as polypropylene or polyethylene. It is used for making disposable laboratory ware. It cannot be autoclaved. When needing to be reused, containers and tubes can be chemically disinfected e.g. in bleach solutions.

- Vinyl resins which include:
  — Polyvinyl chloride (PVC), which can be clear or opaque. It is often used for tubing or for making trays, etc. It cannot be autoclaved.

- Fluoroplastics which include:
  — Polytetrafluorethylene (PTFE, Fluon, Teflon), which is opaque and can be sterilized by autoclaving and dry heat. It is resistant to all chemicals and has a low coefficient of friction. It is commonly used for making bearings, 'O' rings, and stirring bars.

  — PFA fluoropolymer, which has similar properties to PTFE but is translucent. Articles made from PFA are very expensive and not required in routine medical laboratories.

Note: The expected chemical resistance of the range of plastics commonly used in the production of laboratory plastic-ware is shown in Table 3.1.

Cleaning of plastic-ware
Immediately after use, laboratory plastic-ware should be soaked in water or if contaminated, soaked overnight in a suitable disinfectant e.g. in 0.5% w/v sodium hypochlorite, domestic bleach (usually requiring dilution 1 in 5), or *Chloros* (1 in 10 dilution), see also 2:2.

Most plastic-ware is best cleaned in a warm detergent solution, followed by at least two rinses in clean water, and ideally a final rinse in distilled water. The articles should then be left to drain and dry naturally or dried in a hot air oven, set at a temperature the plastic can withstand (see Table 3.2).

Abrasive cleaning powders should not be used for cleaning plastic-ware. Stains or precipitates are best removed using dilute nitric acid or 3% v/v acid alcohol.

Note: A range of plastic-ware is shown in Fig. 3.1 and in Plate 3.1 in 3:3.

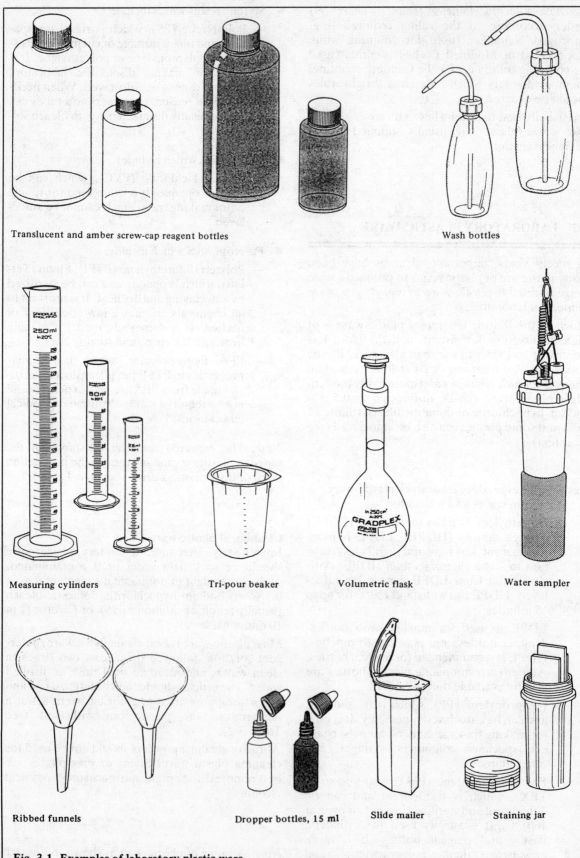

Translucent and amber screw-cap reagent bottles

Wash bottles

Measuring cylinders   Tri-pour beaker   Volumetric flask   Water sampler

Ribbed funnels   Dropper bottles, 15 ml   Slide mailer   Staining jar

Fig. 3.1 Examples of laboratory plastic-ware.

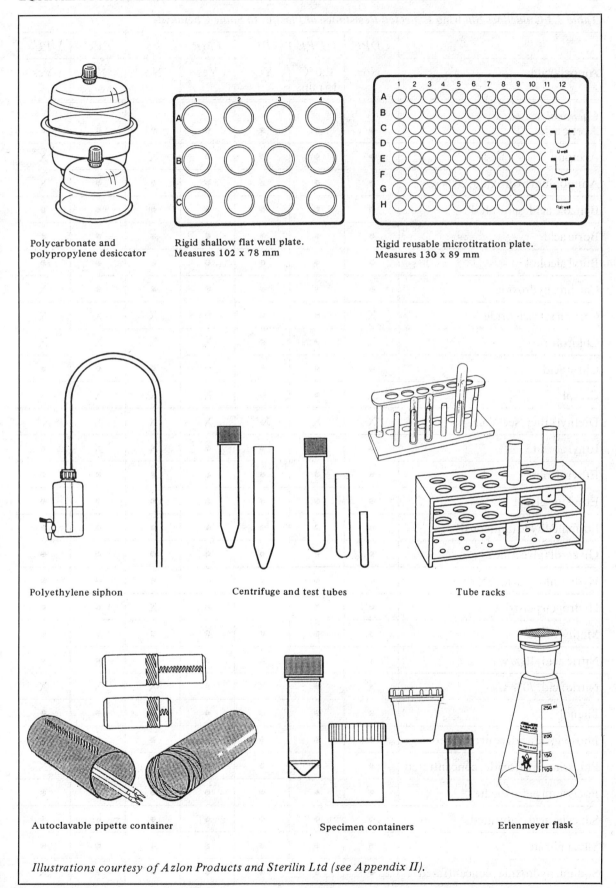

Polycarbonate and
polypropylene desiccator

Rigid shallow flat well plate.
Measures 102 x 78 mm

Rigid reusable microtitration plate.
Measures 130 x 89 mm

Polyethylene siphon

Centrifuge and test tubes

Tube racks

Autoclavable pipette container

Specimen containers

Erlenmeyer flask

Illustrations courtesy of Azlon Products and Sterilin Ltd (see Appendix II).

Table 3.1 Guidelines Showing Expected Resistance of Plastics to Some Chemicals

	LDPE	HDPE	PP	PMP	PS	PVC	PC
Autoclavable	No	120°C 15 mins	Yes	Yes	No	No	Yes
Chemical resistance Acetic acid	●	●	●	●	●	●	●
Acetone	●	●	●	●	X	X	X
Ammonium hydroxide, 28% w/v	●	●	●	●	●	●	X
Benzoic acid, saturated	●	●	●	●	●	●	●
Boric acid	●	●	●	●	●	●	●
Butyl alcohol	●	●	●	●	●	●	●
Calcium hydroxide	●	●	●	●	●	●	X
Carbon tetrachloride	X	●	●	●	X	X	X
Chloroform	X	●	●	X	X	X	X
Citric acid	●	●	●	●	●	●	●
Cresol	X	●	●	X	X	X	X
Diethyl ether, see *Note*	X	X	X*	X	X	X	X*
Ethyl acetate	●	●	●	●	X	X	X
Ethyl alcohol	●	●	●	●	●	●	●
Ethylene glycol	●	●	●	●	●	●	●
Formaldehyde (aqueous)	●	●	●	●	●	●	●
Glycerol (glycerine)	●	●	●	●	●	●	●
Hydrochloric acid, 35% v/v	●	●	●	●	●	●	●
Hydrogen peroxide	●	●	●	●	X	●	●
Methyl alchol	●	●	●	●	●	●	●
Nitric acid, 10% v/v	●	●	●	●	●	●	●
Nitric acid, 70% v/v	X	●	X	●	X	X	X
Phenol	●	●	●	●	●	●	●
Phosphoric acid, concentrated	●	●	●	●	●	●	●
Potassium hydroxide, concentrated	●	●	●	●	●	●	X
Potassium permangate	●	●	●	●	●	●	●
Salicylic acid, saturated	●	●	●	●	●	●	●
Silver nitrate	●	●	●	●	●	●	●
Sodium hydroxide, concentrated	●	●	●	●	●	●	X

Table 3.1 Guidelines Showing Expected Resistance of Plastics to Some Chemicals

	LDPE	HDPE	PP	PMP	PS	PVC	PC
Sodium hypochlorite, 0.5% w/v	●	●	●	●	●	●	X
Sulphuric acid, dilute	●	●	●	●	●	●	●
Sulphuric acid, concentrated	X	●	●	●	X	X	X
Toluene	X	●	●	X	X	X	X
Trichloroacetic acid	●	●	●	●	●	●	●
Trichlorethylene	X	X	X	X	X	X	X
Urea	●	●	●	●	●	●	X
Xylene	X	●	X	X	X	X	X

Key: ● = Resistant at 20 °C.   X = Appreciable reaction, not recommended.

LDPE = Low density polyethylene,   HDPE = High density polyethylene,   PP = Polypropylene,
PMP = Polymethylpentene (TPX),   PS = Polystyrene,   PVC = Polyvinyl chloride,
PC = Polycarbonate
Note: Tubes made from polypropylene (PP) or polycarbonate (PC) can be used with the formol ether concentration technique.

Acknowledgement: Above chart is mainly based on that which appears in the Azlon catalogue

Availability of plastic-ware: Manufacturers of laboratory plastic-ware include Azlon Products Ltd and Kartell Plastics Ltd. Nylon coated wire racks are manufactured by E. Lloyd and Company Ltd (for addresses, see Appendix II).

All the items shown in Fig. 3.1 are included in the Tropical Health Technology Equipment Service to Developing Countries (see Appendix IV under separate items).

Table 3.2 Temperature Resistance of Plastics

	Up to 15mins	Continuous
LDPE	95 °C	80 °C
HDPE[a]	120 °C	110 °C
PP[b]	140 °C	130 °C
PMP[b]	200 °C	180 °C
PS	70 °C	60 °C
PVC	80 °C	70 °C
PC[b]	140 °C	130 °C

a   Can therefore be autoclaved with care (up to 15 minutes).
b   Can therefore be autoclaved

3:3   EQUIPMENT FOR STAINING

Equipment required for staining includes:
- Stain and reagent dispensing containers
- Staining jars or racks and troughs
- Trough with rods
- Draining rack

Stain dispensing containers
A suitable container for holding and dispensing stains and reagents (acid alcohol, acetone, etc) is one that does not leak when dispensing, can be closed when not in use to prevent evaporation or moisture from entering, and can be easily opened without staining or contaminating the fingers with reagent.

Examples of containers which meet these specifications are shown in Plate 3.1. The spout top container is made from polyethylene. Capacities of the containers include 100 ml, 250 ml and 500 ml. The other container is a glass dropper bottle of the TK type. It has a ground glass stopper with a groove for dispensing. TK bottles are available in amber or plain glass, usually with a maximum capacity of 100 ml.

For dispensing water to wash smears, a plastic wash bottle as shown in Fig. 3.1 is recommended.

Availability: The spout top polyethylene container shown in Plate 3.1 is manufacturered by Kartell Plastics Ltd (see Appendix II). The 100 ml and 250 ml spout top containers, and 100 ml amber TK bottles are included in the Tropical Health Technology Equipment Service to Developing Countries (Appendix IV, see Stain dispensing containers).

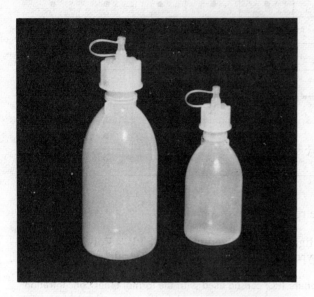

Plate 3.1   Leak-proof stain dispensing containers .

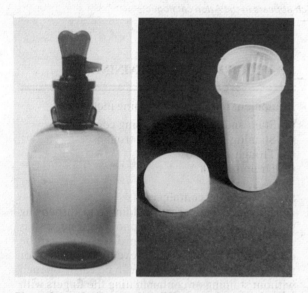

Plate 3.2   *Left:*   **Amber TK type dropper bottle.**
Right: **Polypropylene staining jar.**

Staining jars and troughs

When staining several slides together, a Coplin type staining jar can be used or alternatively a rack and staining trough.

A polypropylene Coplin staining type jar is shown in Plate 3.2. It can hold up to 10 slides when positioned back to back. The screw-cap lid is airtight.

A staining rack and trough with lid is shown in Plate 3.3. The unit is made in black polyacetal (resistant to stains and solvents, including xylene). The rack can hold up to 25 slides (extra racks can be obtained). The trough measures $100 \times 85 \times 55$ mm deep. The lid of the trough incorporates a simple draining rack.

Availability: Both the Coplin type jar and polyacetal rack and trough unit are manufactured by Azlon Products Ltd (see Appendix II). They are included in the Tropical Health Technology Equipment Service to Developing Countries (Appendix IV, see Slide staining jar, Slide staining tray and rack).

When needing to stain slides individually, two parallel rods across a sink or deep stainless steel staining trough is suitable as shown in Plate 3.4. The stainless steel rods have levelling screws.

Availability: The staining trough and rods are manufactured by Middlemass Fabricators Ltd (see Appendix II). The complete unit or the rods only are available to developing countries through the Tropical Health Technology Equipment Service (Appendix IV), see Staining trough with rods).

Slide draining rack

A simple stainless steel rack for draining slides is shown in Plate 3.5. It measures $200 \times 30 \times 40$ mm high.

Availability: The rack shown in Plate 3.5 is manufactured by Middlemass Fabricators Ltd (see Appendix II). It is included in the Tropical Health Technology Equipment Service to Developing Countries (Appendix IV, see Slide draining rack).

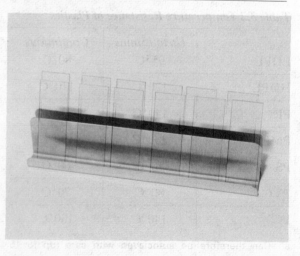

Plate 3.5   Stainless steel slide draining rack to hold two rows of slides.

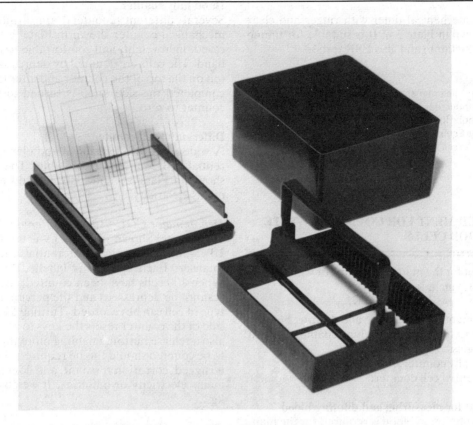

Plate 3.3 Polyacetal staining unit with draining rack.

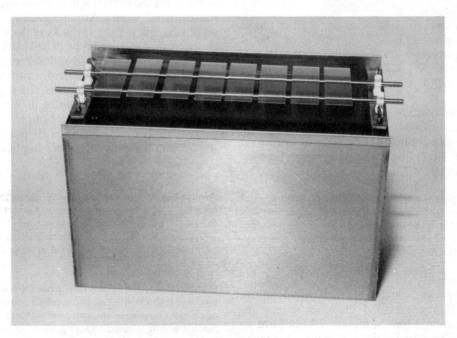

Plate 3.4 Stainless steel staining trough with rods.

Timers

A robust mechanical timer with ringer and clear dial is shown in Plate 3.6. It is suitable for timing staining reactions (and also ESR tests).

Availability: The timer shown in Plate 3.8 is manufactured by Smiths Industries and available from Arnold Horwell (see Appendix II). It is included in the Tropical Health Technology Equipment Service to Developing Countries (Appendix IV, see Timer).

3:4 EQUIPMENT FOR COUNTING WHITE BLOOD CELLS

Equipment for the manual counting of white blood cells (WBC) includes:

- Equipment for measuring and diluting blood.
- Haemocytometer (counting chamber) with cover glass.
- Hand tally counter.
- Differential cell counter.

Equipment for measuring and diluting blood

A 1 in 20 dilution of blood is required for the manual counting of white cells. This can be obtained by mixing 50 μl (0.05 ml) of blood with 0.95 ml of diluting fluid.

Measurement of blood

Systems for the safe measuring of 50 μl of blood include using a shell back 50 μl pipette or a 50 μl graduated glass capillary (reusable), with a thumb wheel aspirator or simple bulb aspirator as shown in Plate 2.1 in 2:4.

Measurement of diluting fluid

A 1 ml graduated pipette can be used with a pipette filler (see Plate 2.2 in 2:4) or a narrow bore 1 ml syringe with direct line to the reagent can be used as shown in Plate 3.7.

Use of bulb pipettes with bead: These pipettes are not recommended for diluting blood for white cell counts. It is difficult to obtain good mixing of the blood and therefore counts tend to be unreliable. The pipettes are also expensive and difficult to clean.

Haemocytometer

For counting white blood cells (and platelets), an Improved Neubauer ruled chamber is recommended. It should have a metallized platform so that the rulings are bright and clear. A special cover glass is used with the counting chamber (two are provided with a haemocytometer and extra ones can be purchased separately).

Hand tally counter

Several different counters are available. The mechanical counter shown in Plate 3.8 is plastic-cased, lightweight, and comfortable to hold in the hand. The cells are counted by depressing the button on the top of the counter and after the count is completed the side knob is turned to return the counter to zero.

Differential cell counter

A wide range of mechanical and electronic differential cell counters is available. The two types shown in Plate 3.9 and Plate 3.10 do not require mains electricity.

Denominator COU-0106 LT differential counter

The counter shown in Plate 3.9 is the COU-0106 LT 5-unit mechanical differential counter with totaliser. Each window is labelled by the user. When 100 cells have been counted, the keys lock (cannot be depressed) and the percentage of each type of cell can be recorded. Turning a knob on the side of the counter resets the keys to zero. There is also a release button, enabling more than 100 cells to be counted should this be required. The counter is rugged, corrosion resistant, and does not require mains electricity or batteries. It weighs only 0.85 kg.

Trumeter Universal differential counter

The counter shown in Plate 3.10 is the *Universal* electronic 6-unit counter with totaliser which operates from two 1.5v batteries. It takes very little power with the batteries being estimated to last for more than 2 years. After counting 100 cells, an audible signal is heard (the keys do not lock) and the percentage of each type of cell can be recorded. A reset button is then pressed to zero all the counters. The counter automatically switches itself off when not used for 20 minutes. The keys are labelled by the user. Three sets of blank removeable labels are supplied with each Counter. The *Universal* counter is compact and easily portable, weighing only 0.6 kg with batteries (supplied).

Availability: Graduated capillaries, aspirators, hand tally counter, and a range of differential counters (including COU-0106 LT) are available from Arnold Horwell Ltd. The *Universal* electronic counter is manufactured by Trumeter Company Ltd (for addresses see Appendix II).

Both the COU-0106 LT and *Universal* differential cell counters, and also a White Cell Counting Kit consisting of all the equipment for measuring and diluting blood, an Improved Neubauer bright-ruled counting chamber, and hand tally counter are included in the Tropical Health Technology Equipment Service to Developing Countries (Appendix IV, see White blood cell counting equipment, White cell counter).

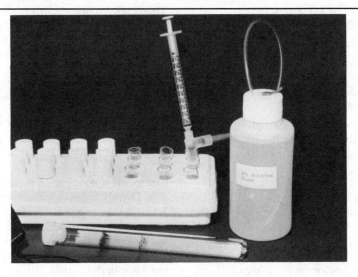

Plate 3.7 Direct line diluting fluid dispensing system

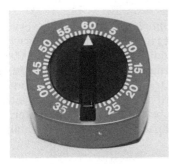

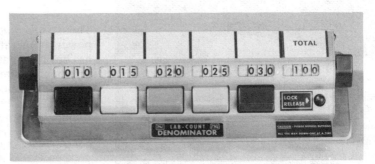

Plate 3.6 Interval timer

Plate 3.9 Mechanical WBC Differential counter.
Courtesy of Arnold R Horwell Ltd.

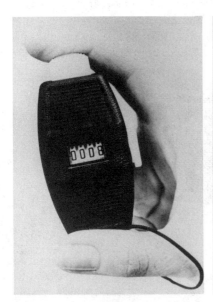

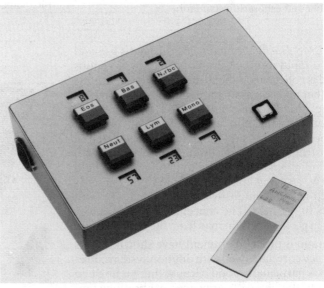

Plate 3.8 Hand tally counter
Courtesy of Arnold R Horwell Ltd

Plate 3.10 Electronic WBC differential counter
Courtesy of Trumeter Company Ltd

3:5 EQUIPMENT FOR MEASURING HAEMOGLOBIN

Systems for measuring haemoglobin include:

- Visual direct reading system which requires no dilution of the blood.
- Electronic, highly accurate haemoglobin meter which requires dilution of the blood and measures oxyhaemoglobin or cyanmethaemoglobin.

Visual direct reading system

An example of a visual direct reading system is the *BMS Haemoglobinometer* as shown in Plate 3.11. The system is particularly recommended for use in health centres and small hospital laboratories where only a few haemoglobins are measured.

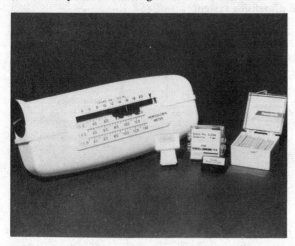

Plate 3.11 BMS haemoglobinometer, supplied with chamber and calibration standard.

The *BMS Haemoglobinometer* is easy to use and gives a rapid result. A drop of capillary or venous blood is collected on the surface of a reusable glass chamber and a saponin impregnated stick is mixed in the blood to haemolyze it. The chamber is pushed into the clip to give an even layer of haemolyzed blood and the unit is then inserted in the instrument. Looking through the eyepiece with the reading knob depressed to illuminate the field of view, a sliding knob on the side of the meter is moved until the intensity of light matches in both halves of the field. The concentration of haemoglobin in g/100 ml is then read from the upper scale.

Evaluations of the instrument have shown that its accuracy correlates well with dilution systems. Precision is particularly good because there is no need to dilute the blood. A grey glass calibration standard is provided to check the performance of the instrument. Extra chambers and supplies of saponin sticks are available.

The *BMS Haemoglobinometer* is available as a battery model which operates from two C size batteries or as a mains and battery operated model. The mains/battery model operates through a convertor adaptor.

Availability: The *BMS Haemoglobinometer* is manufactured by Buffalo Medical Specialties (see Appendix II). It is included in the Tropical Health Technology Equipment Service to Developing Countries (Appendix IV, see BMS Haemoglobinometer).

Electronic haemoglobin meter

The *Delphi haemoglobin meter* is shown in Plate 3.12. It is a rugged, electronic, battery or mains operated meter which gives a direct readout of haemoglobin measured by the cyanmethaemoglobin or oxyhaemoglobin technique. Two standards are supplied so that the user can calibrate the meter for either the cyanmethaemoglobin or oxyhaemoglobin technique. The instrument has been shown to operate reliably in tropical countries.

The *Delphi haemoglobin meter* uses very little power. It operates from a small 9v battery which it has been estimated gives in excess of 100 000 measurements. Alternatively, the meter can be used from a mains electricity supply through a converter adaptor. Standard size plastic or glass cuvettes of 10 mm lighpath are used with the meter. The instrument is compact and portable, weighing only 0.8 Kg.

Availability: The Delphi haemoglobin meter is manufactured by Delphi Industries Ltd (see Appendix II). It is included in the Tropical Health Technology Equipment Service to Developing Countries (Appendix IV, see Delphi Haemoglobin Meter).

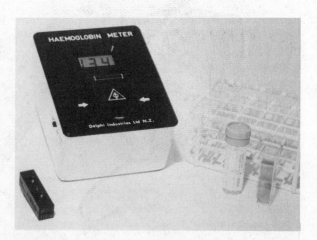

Plate 3.12 Delphi electronic meter for measuring oxyhaemoglobin or cyanmethaemoglobin. Supplied with standards (lower left).

3:6 EQUIPMENT FOR WEIGHING

Considerable savings can be made if a laboratory prepares most of its routine stains and basic reagents. To do this a scale or balance of adequate sensitivity that weighs accurately is required.

For the work carried out in most peripheral laboratories, a scale or balance having a sensitivity of 0.01 g (10 mg) will be adequate. For the preparation of some reference solutions, an analytical balance having a sensitivity of 0.001 g (1 mg) may be required.

A wide range of scales and balances is available including:

- Manually operated scales and balances.
- Direct read-out and top-loading electric balances.

Manually operated scales and balances
Among the range of manually operated balances and scales those manufactured by Ohaus are recommended.

Availability: Ohaus balances are manufactured by Ohaus Corporation (see Appendix II) and are available from many suppliers. The model 505 and model 311 are included in the Tropical Health Technology Equipment Service to Developing Countries (Appendix IV, see Balance, Ohaus).

— *Model 505* (see Plate 3.13) which is a small inexpensive scale having a sensitivity of 0.01g and capacity of 50.5 g. No separate weights are required. It is supplied with an anodized aluminium corrosion-resistant scoop of 76 mm diameter. It is rugged and easy to use. The foot screw is used to zero the scale. This model is recommended for use in small hospital laboratories and health centres.

— *Model 311* (see Plate 3.14) which has a sensitivity of 0.01 g and capacity of 311 g. No separate weights are required. A knob on the end of the beam on the pan side is used to zero the balance. This model is particularly recommended for district and regional laboratories.

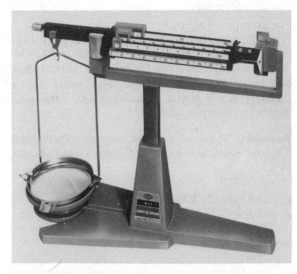

Plate 3.14 Ohaus 311 single pan balance with sensitivity of 0.01 g and capacity of 311 g.

— *Havard model* (see Plate 3.15) which is a trip type of balance with a sensitivity of 0.1 g and capacity of 2000 g. The weights are integral (below the pans). It is useful for weighing large quantities of chemicals and for balancing centrifuge tubes (when a centrifuge requires such fine balancing).

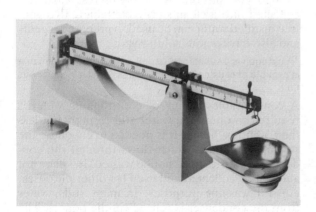

Plate 3.13 Ohaus small 505 scale with sensitivity of 0.01 g and capacity of 50.5 g.
Courtesy of Ohaus Corporation

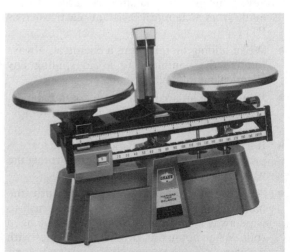

Plate 3.15 Ohaus Havard trip balance with sensitivity of 0.1 g and capacity of 2000 g.
Courtesy of European instruments

Direct read-out electric balances

Many of the direct read-out balances are of the electronic type, and are costly to purchase and maintain.

Electric direct read-out balances, however, are also available. These are less costly to purchase and maintain and are generally more robust than the electronic type.

An example of a direct read-out, mechanical electric balance with a capacity of 200 g and a sensitivity of 0.0001 g (0.1 mg) is the *Bosch model S2000/10*. An example of a top-loading mechanical electric balance with a direct read-out scale and a capacity of 170 g with a readability of 0.001 g (1 mg) is the *Bosch model P 115*.

Availability: The Bosch balances, models S2000/10 and P 115 are manufactured by Bosch Company (see Appendix II).

Use and care of a laboratory balance

A balance is a delicate instrument that requires practical instruction in its correct use. The following rules apply when using a balance:

- Read carefully the manufacturer's instructions and always handle a balance with care.
- Position the balance on a firm bench away from vibration, draughts, and direct sunlight.
- Make sure that the balance is level, adjusting if necessary the screws on which it stands. A spirit level or plumb line is often provided to assist in levelling the instrument.
- Before starting to weigh, zero the balance as directed by the manufacturer.
- Weigh chemicals at room temperature in a weighing scoop (if provided) or small beaker, never directly on a balance pan unless this is made from a chemical resistant plastic such as PTFE.
- When adding or removing a chemical, always remove the container to avoid spilling any chemical on the balance pan.
- When using an analytical double pan balance, bring the pans to rest before adding or removing a chemical.
- If using a box of weights, *always* use the forceps provided to add or remove weights. Protect the weights from dust and moisture.
- After completing the weighing, return the balance to zero weight. Use a small brush to wipe away any chemical which may have been spilt. When not in use, protect the balance with a cover.
- In humid climates, place a suitable desiccant such as silica gel inside the case of an analytical balance.

- Keep a small notebook by the balance in which to make the necessary weighing calculations and to record the date of preparation of reagents.

Maintenance of a balance

The accuracy of a balance should be checked regularly as recommended in the manufacturer's manual. If the balance is of the analytical double pan type, the knife edges should be checked periodically. When at rest the pans should not leave the stirrups. If separate weights are used, have the accuracy of these checked from time to time.

Note: A self-instructional sheet (LAB/85.7) giving the operating principles and use of an analytical balance is available from the Health Laboratory Unit, World Health Organization, Geneva.

3:7 STILLS, WATER FILTERS AND DEIONISERS

Laboratories in rural areas often have difficulty in obtaining good quality water to make reagents, especially for clinical chemistry tests. Chemically pure water can be obtained by:

- Distillation
- Deionisation

Distillation

This is a process by which impure water is boiled and the steam condensed on a cold surface (condenser) to give pure distilled water. The apparatus used to produce distilled water is called a still.

Distilled water is free from dissolved salts and should be clear, colourless, odourless, and tasteless. It will also be sterile and pyrogen-free* providing it contains only the condensed steam and is collected into a clean sterile container. Pyrogen-free distilled water can be used to prepare reagents and also intravenous solutions.

*A pyrogen is a substance, usually of bacterial origin, that is capable of causing fever if transfused in an intravenous fluid.

A considerable volume of cool running water is required to operate a water still (usually not less than 50 litres /hour). It is needed to condense the steam. The water which flows through the condenser to 'waste' need not be wasted. It will be hot and can be collected and used for other purposes, e.g. for washing purposes. In many stills, water from the condenser is reused (in the boiler). The manufacturer's instructions must be followed regarding the use and maintenance of a water still. Regular cleaning is essential.

Water stills

The *Watermatic SS 3.5 Still* is shown in Plate 3.16. It is a stainless steel still with a condenser made of borosilicate heat-resistant glass. It is capable of producing 3.5 litres of distilled water per hour. It uses a 2.75 kW heater and requires 50 litres of water/hour. The boiler is fed with preheated water from its own condenser. The boiler is fitted with an anti-splash baffle plate. The unit is easy to clean. The *Watermatic Still model SS 7.0* is capable of producing about 7 litres of distilled water per hour. It uses two 2.75 kW heaters.

Availability: The *Watermatic Still model SS 3.5* is available from Scientific Industries International Inc. (UK) Ltd (see Appendix II), priced approx. £199 (1986). The model SS 7.0 costs £295 (1986).

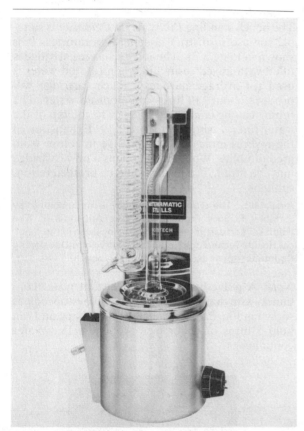

Plate 3.16 Watermatic bench standing still, measuring 630 x 200 x 280 mm. *Courtesy of Scientific Industries.*

The *Bibby W14S Still* is shown in Plate 3.17. It is made from Pyrex borosilicate glass and is capable of producing about 4 litres of distilled water per hour. The level of water in the boiler is automatically controlled and the water from the double coil condenser pre-heats the water before it enters the boiler. There is an automatic cut-out to prevent overheating. It is fitted with a 3 kW heater which is sheathed in Vycor for safety, longer life, and purity. It requires about 50 litres of water/hour to operate. It can be free-standing or wall mounted.

Availability: The *Bibby W14S Still* is available from J. Bibby Science Products Ltd (see Appendix II), priced £319 (1986).

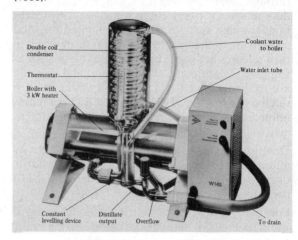

Plate 3.17 Bibby bench or wall mounted still measuring 435 x 215 x 400 mm. *Courtesy Bibby Science Products*

The *Manesty L4 Still* is shown in Plate 3.18. It is a wall mounted stainless steel still which is capable of producing 3.4-4.5 litres per hour. The consumption is 3 KW per hour. There is a water levelling device and the descending steam in the condenser tube pre-heats the ascending column of raw water. The still is fitted with an efficient system of baffles.

Availability: The *Manesty L4 Still* is available from Manesty Machines Ltd, (see Appendix II), priced £390 (1986).

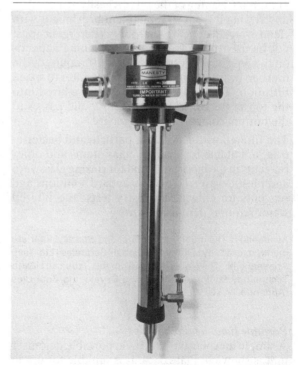

Plate 3.18 Manesty wall mounted still, measuring 760 mm long. *Courtesy of Manesty Ltd.*

Deionisation

This is a process in which impure water is passed through anion and cation exchange resins to produce ion-free water. Cations which may be present in the water such as calcium, magnesium, and sodium are exchanged by the cation resin which in turn releases hydrogen ions (H^+). Anions such as sulphate, bicarbonate, silica, nitrate, and chloride are exchanged by the anion resin which in turn releases hydroxyl (OH^-) ions. The hydrogen ions immediately combine with the hydroxyl ions to give ion-free water (H_2O).

Deionised water has a low electrical conductivity and is free from water-soluble salts but is not sterile or pyrogen-free. It must not therefore be used to prepare intravenous solutions.

For many district laboratories, the filtering of water combined with deionisation, is the most economical and often the only way to obtain chemically pure water. Mains electricity is not required and neither are the large volumes of running water needed to operate a water still. Before poor quality water is passed through a deioniser, it should be filtered first to remove organic particles otherwise the resins will become rapidly exhausted and require frequent changing.

Water filter

An easy to use and maintain gravity water filter made of nylon coated light-weight aluminium is shown in Plate 3.19. It is fitted with a self-steriliz-ing *Sterasyl* candle filter which has a long-life (6-12 months). Cleaning of the filter is easily achieved by unscrewing it from its mount and brushing it with clean water to unclog the pores (detergent must not be used). The frequency of cleaning depends on the type of water being filtered. If required, the unit can be fitted with more than one filter to speed filtration. The water to be filtered is poured into the top of the container, is filtered, and passes to the bottom compartment by gravity.

The filtered water, which is particle and bacteria-free, is suitable for making many stains and other reagents in the laboratory and for rinsing glassware and plastic-ware. To make standard solutions and reagents for clinical chemistry tests, the filtered water requires deionising.

Availability: The gravity water filter and *Sterasyl* filter are manufactured by Fairey Industrial Ceramics Ltd (see Appendix II). They are included in the Tropical Health Technology Equipment Service to Developing Countries (Appendix IV, see Water Filter).

Portable hand held deioniser

A simple inexpensive hand held portable deioniser unit is shown in Plate 3.20. It is suitable for use in small hospital laboratories and health centres. It consists of a polythene bottle containing a car-tridge filled with self-indicating mixed deionising resin (i.e. cations and anions). Squeezing the bottle dispenses the deionised water. The amount of resin in the bottle is sufficient to give about 15 litres of pure water when the bottle is filled with filtered water of average hardness. When needing replacement, the resin changes from blue to yellow. When this happens the exhausted resin must be discarded and the cartridge filled with new resin. The resin should be protected from sunlight.

Availability: The portable deioniser unit and resins are available from Arnold Horwell (see Appendix II) and other suppliers. The deioniser and resins (4 resins in a pack) are included in the Tropical Health Technology Equipment Service to Developing Countries (Appendix IV, see Deioniser, portable).

Bench deioniser

The bench standing *Bibby ADH Deioniser* is suitable for use in district hospital laboratories. It is shown in Plate 3.21. The ion exchange cartridge is filled with mixed resin and when filtered water is used (of average hardness), each cartridge will produce about 110 litres of deionised water. The tubing can be connected directly to the tap of the water filter shown in Plate 3.19. Exhaustion of the resin is indicated by a change in colour from green to blue. When this happens a new cartridge must be fitted. The resin should be protected from sunlight.

Availability: The *Bibby ADH Dioniser* is manufactured by J. Bibby Science Products Ltd (see Appendix II). The deioniser and cartridges of resin are included in the Tropical Health Technology Equipment Service to Developing Countries (Appendix IV, see Deioniser, bench).

Note: A polyethylene break-resistant water container with handle and removeable stopcock is shown in Fig. 3.2. It is hexagonal in shape and can hold 5 litres of water (see Appendix IV, Water container).

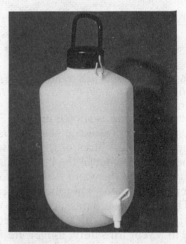

Fig. 3.2 Polyethylene 5 litre capacity water container with removable stopcock.

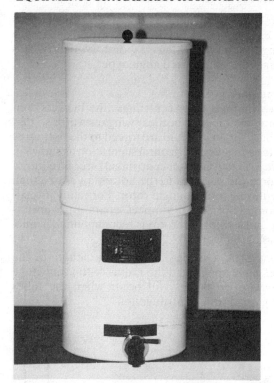
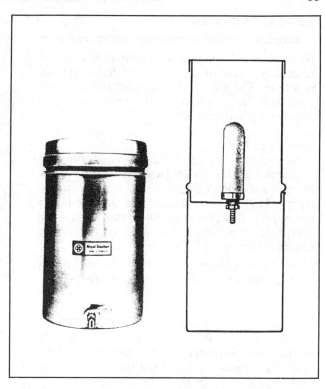

Plate 3.19 *Left:* **Assembled water filter.** *Right:* **Top of water filter fitted into base for easy transportation. Diagram shows the position of the candle filter during filtration.**
Photographs: Courtesy of Fairey Industrial Ceramics Ltd.

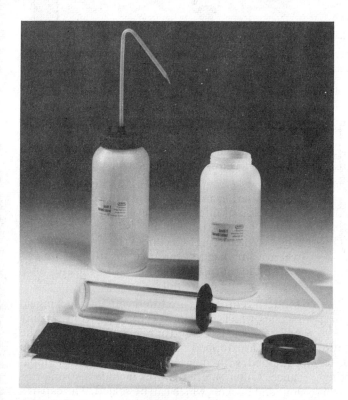

Plate 3.20 Hand held portable deioniser
Courtesy of Arnold R Horwell Ltd

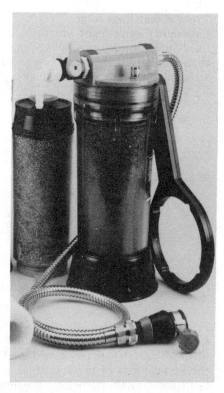

Plate 3.21 Bench deioniser unit
Courtesy of Bibby Science Products Ltd

3:8   CENTRIFUGES

By exerting a force greater than that of gravity, a centrifuge is able to sediment particles suspended in a fluid. The greater the centrifugal force (outward pull due to rotation), the more rapid and effective the sedimentation.

Centrifugal force

Until recently, the centrifugal force required to sediment particles in a fluid was indicated by giving the speed of centrifuging in revolutions per minute (rpm). The actual sedimentation achieved at a given speed, however, depends on the radius of the centrifuge. It is better, therefore, to specify the required relative centrifugal force (RCF).

Most manufacturers now specify the maximum RCF as well as the rpm of which a centrifuge is capable.

Calculation of maximum RCF
The maximum RCF, can be calculated from a knowledge of the rpm and the radius (in cm) of the centrifuge which is taken from the centre of the centrifuge shaft to the tip of the centrifuge tube:

$$RCF\ (g) = 1.118 \times radius \times rpm^2 \times 10^5$$

Note: A nomogram for calculating RCF is shown on p. 580.

Types of centrifuge rotor

Laboratory centrifuges are fitted with either a fixed-angle rotor or a swing-out rotor. Interchangeable fixed-angle and swing-out rotor heads are available with some centrifuges.

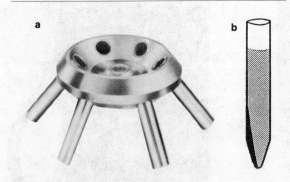

Plate 3.22   Centrifuging in a fixed angle rotor.

Fixed angle rotor
In a fixed-angle rotor centrifuge, the tube or bottle holders (buckets) are positioned at a fixed angle to the vertical axis of the centrifuge head. During centrifugation, the particles in the fluid are thrown to the side and bottom of the tube to give a slanted separation as shown in Plate 3.22 (b). Separation is

more rapid and generally greater centrifugal forces can be applied in a fixed-angle centrifuge than in a swing-out model. Many laboratory bench centrifuges are of the fixed angle type.

Swing-out rotor
In a swing-out rotor centrifuge, the buckets containing the tubes or bottles swing outwards so that the particles in the fluid are forced to the bottom of the tube to give a horizontal separation as shown in Plate 3.23 (b). Greater centrifugal force is required to force the particles to the bottom of a tube than when using a fixed-angle rotor. For many investigations, a horizontal compact separation is preferable and a swing-out rotor is recommended in microbiological work.

When using a swing-out rotor, the length of the tubes *must not* exceed the radius of the centrifuge otherwise breakages will occur when the tubes swing out during centrifugation.

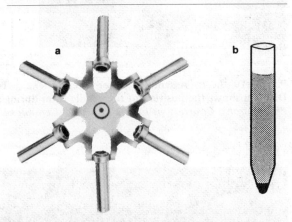

Plate 3.23   Centrifuging in a swing-out rotor.

Choosing a centrifuge

Safety, available facilities, capacity, cost, and maintenance are important considerations when choosing a centrifuge.

Safety
Among the hazards associated with centrifuges are the release of infected aerosols by opening a centrifuge before rotation has stopped, especially when centrifuging specimens in open tubes or when a breakage occurs and insufficient time is allowed for aerosols to settle. Other hazards arise when centrifuges are not balanced.

Modern centrifuges are fitted with interlocking lid catches which prevent a centrifuge from starting before the lid is secured or being opened before the rotor has stopped. Many centrifuges are also equipped with devices that warn against imbalance. Other safety features include a strong casing, and buckets which can be sealed. The cap of a sealed bucket should fit into, not onto, a bucket so that if a breakage occurs, any infected fluid will be centrifuged from the screw thread back into the bucket and not down the outside of the bucket.

Available facilities

When mains electricity is not available, it may be possible to operate a 110v or 220-240v centrifuge from a 12v battery using a transvertor but this takes considerable power from the battery. Alternatively, a centrifuge having a 12v motor or 9v motor (with adapter) can be used with a 12v battery (see later text).

Capacity

The size of centrifuge required will depend on the work-load of the laboratory. Most district laboratories will probably find that a swing-out rotor centrifuge which can hold 6 or 8 tubes will be adequate. It may also be helpful to have accessory buckets which can accept Universal type bottles. Smaller laboratories may also find it more economical to purchase a centrifuge for which a haematocrit (microhaematocrit) head attachment is available rather than buy a separate haematocrit centrifuge (see later text).

Cost

When evaluating the price of a centrifuge, it is important to note how a manufacturer details the costs to ensure that you arrive at the total cost involved. Most manufacturers give a price for the centrifuge without rotors or buckets. Rotors, buckets, and also cushions are usually priced separately. Models that have a brake or timer are often more expensive. Prices of centrifuges with similar specifications vary considerably from one manufacturer to another.

Maintenance

Always make sure an *Operations and Maintenance Manual* is supplied with a centrifuge. At the time of purchase, obtain a supply of important replacement parts such as carbon brushes and a few extra cushions for the buckets (these are easily lost). The irregular running of a centrifuge or 'sparking' is an indication that the carbon brushes require changing. If sparking occurs, a centrifuge must not be used until the brushes are changed because of the risk of fire and possible irreversible damage to the motor.

Types of centrifuge

Electric bench centrifuges

The *Clandon T51H centrifuge* is shown in Plate 3.24. This is a modern centrifuge which is supplied with an 8 place swing-out rotor and haematocrit head attachment. It is fitted with a brake, timer, safety catches, and rotor imbalance interlock. The casing is strengthened and lined to reduce noise

and increase safety. The button marked H III is used to operate the haematocrit rotor at 10 750 rpm) and the other two buttons marked I and II are used to control the speed of the swing-out rotor as follows:

Button I .... 1550 rpm (low speed)
I and II .... 4250 rpm (medium speed)
II .... 4800 rpm (high speed)

Availability: The *Clandon T51H centrifuge* is available from Clandon Scientific Ltd (see Appendix II). The price to developing countries is £399.50 (1986) which includes the swing-out rotor to take 8 tubes of 15 ml capacity, haematocrit rotor to take 24 capillaries, fitted brake, safety locks, and attached timer. Sealed buckets are available at extra cost.

Capillaries (plain or heparinised), sealant for capillaries and haematocrit (microhaematocrit) reader are included in the Tropical Health Technology Equipment Service to Developing Countries (Appendix IV, see Capillaries, Microhaematocrit reader).

Note: Other manufacturers of small bench centrifuges with swing-out rotors include Hettich Company (model *Universal*) and Gallenkamp (model *CFC-301*). Addresses are given in Appendix II.

Battery operated bench centrifuge

Even a small capacity 12v battery operated centrifuge requires considerable power and therefore the battery will require regular charging. The frequency of charging will depend on how often the centrifuge is used and the power requirements of other equipment being run from the same battery.

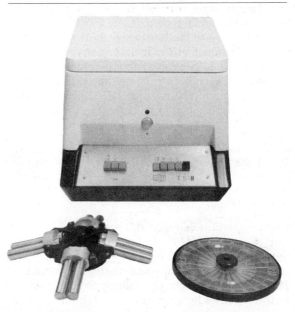

Plate 3.24 Electric bench centrifuge with swing-out and haematocrit rotors.
Courtesy of Clandon Scientific Ltd.

The *Hettich EBA 111 centrifuge* is shown in Plate 3.25. It can be operated from a 12v battery. It is a fixed-angle centrifuge (swing-out rotors for battery operation are not available). Model No. 2008 has a 4 place rotor, model No. 2009 has a 6 place rotor, and model No. 2030 has an 8 place rotor. Each rotor accepts tubes of 15 ml capacity. Greater care needs to be taken when using an EBA 111 centrifuge because it has none of the safety features found on electric centrifuges. At no time should the lid be removed before the rotor has come to rest.

Availability: *Hettich EBA 111* 12v battery operated centrifuges are available from Medin-Staal (see Appendix II). Model No. 2008 costs approx. £185, No. 2009 costs approx. £205 and No. 2030 costs approx. £230 (1986).

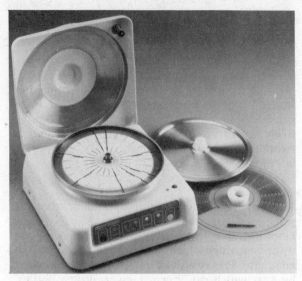

Plate 3.26 Electric haematocrit centrifuge. *Courtesy of LIC Medical.*

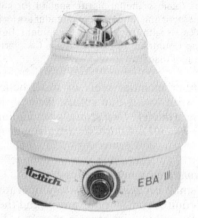

Plate 3.25 Hettich EBA 111 battery operated centrifuge.

Electric haematocrit centrifuges
The haematocrit (microhaematocrit) centrifuge shown in Plate 3.26 is the *LIC SH 2450 Hematocrit Centrifuge*. It is of modern design and incorporates a range of safety features including an interlocking tight-fitting lid. The rotor can accommodate up to 24 capillaries. The centrifuging time can be set for 3, 4, or 5 minutes and the RCF is 10 000. An haematocrit reader is provided.

Availability: The *LIC SH 2450 Hematocrit Centrifuge* is available from LIC Ltd (see Appendix II). It is priced approx. £525 (1986). Capillaries (plain and heparinised) and sealant are available from LIC or to developing countries from Tropical Health Technology Equipment Service (see Appendix IV).

Battery operated haematocrit centrifuge
The *Compur M1100 haematocrit centrifuge* is shown in Plate 3.27. This portable minicentrifuge can be operated from mains electricity or from a 12v battery through the appropriate converter adapter. It uses heparinised micro capillaries (9 μl volume) to measure the haematocrit (PCV). No sealant is required for the capillaries. After filling *completely* the capillary, it is placed in the rotor

and the central button is depressed which seals the capillary during centrifuging. The haematocrit rotor can accept up to 6 capillaries.

The *M 1100* is programmed to centrifuge for 3 minutes 20 seconds after which it turns itself off and the haematocrit (PCV) can be read using the scale on the rotor.

A *Plasma Rotor* is available as an accessory rotor for use with the M 1100 minicentrifuge. This can be used to obtain plasma for clinical chemistry tests. Larger capillaries (60 μl) are required for use with this rotor.

Availability: The *M 1100 Minicentrifuge* is manufactured by Compur-Electronic GmbH (see Appendix II). It is included in the Tropical Health Technology Equipment Service to Developing Countries (Appendix IV, see Haematocrit centrifuge M 1100). Special adaptors are required to operate the minicentrifuge from a 12v battery or from mains electricity. These adaptors, the plasma rotor, and the capillaries for use with the M 1100

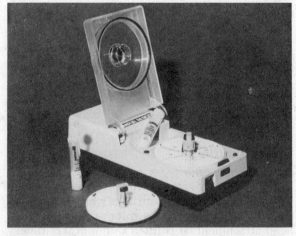

Plate 3.27 Battery and mains mini haematocrit centrifuge. Plasma rotor is also available. See also p. 594.

haematocrit and plasma rotors are also available to developing countries from Tropical Health Technology Equipment Service.

Use and care of a centrifuge

- Read carefully the manufacturer's instructions.
- Balance a centrifuge by positioning the buckets correctly, checking that each bucket contains its cushion, and ensuring that the contents of the buckets on each side of the centrifuge weigh the same.

  With balances of the self-balancing type, it is sufficient to check by eye that the level of fluid in the tubes matches providing the thickness of glass of the tubes is the same.
- When using a swing-out rotor, check that the tubes or bottles are of a suitable length and will not be broken when the buckets swing out.
- Before filling tubes or bottles, check that they are not cracked or chipped. Whenever possible use plastic-ware.
- When filling tubes or bottles, leave a space of at least 20 mm between the fluid and the rim of the container.
- Use capped tubes or bottles when centrifuging specimens or other material which may contain pathogens. If available, use buckets which can be sealed.
- Do not attempt to stop a centrifuge by hand because this can cause injury and will also damage the bearings.
- *Never* open a centrifuge until the motor has stopped and the buckets have come to rest otherwise infectious material may be sprayed into the laboratory. If possible, use a centrifuge with an interlocking safety catch which will allow opening only when rotation has stopped.
- Clean regularly the buckets and inside of a centrifuge using a cloth soaked in a non-corrosive disinfectant such as 2% w/v glutaraldehyde, 70% v/v alcohol, or 10% v/v formalin solution (do not use a hypochlorite solution because this corrodes metal). Wear protective rubber gloves.
- If a breakage occurs when centrifuging, do not open the centrifuge immediately. Allow at least 30 minutes for the droplets to settle. Wear protective gloves and use forceps and cotton wool swabs soaked in disinfectant to remove the broken glass. Clean the buckets and inside of the centrifuge before using it again.
- Every 3-6 months (depending on the age and condition of the centrifuge), inspect the centrifuge for corrosion and check the plug connections and flex for signs of wear. Follow the manufacturer's recommendation regarding other maintenance measures.

3:9 INCUBATORS, DRY BLOCK HEATERS, AND INCUBATORS

Incubation at controlled temperatures is required for bacteriological cultures and some blood transfusion, serological, haematological, and clinical chemistry tests. For bacteriological cultures, an incubator is required whereas for the other tests a dry heat block is recommended or if unavailable a water bath.

Incubators

Electric models
For the routine culturing of bacteriological specimens in most district laboratories, a small capacity gravity convection type incubator fitted with a hydraulic thermostat is adequate. An example of such an incubator is the *Gallenkamp Economy Incubator INA-300, size 1* as shown in Plate 3.28. It is supplied with shelves and has an inner glass door which closes on a gasket to reduce heat loss. The operating temperature range is 5 °C above ambient to 80 °C with a 0.5 °C fluctuation at 38 °C, and ±2 °C temperature variation at 38 °C. The walls and door of the incubator are glass fibre insulated. A hole is provided in the top of the incubator for the insertion of a thermometer. Air is circulated in the incubator by natural convection.

When a large capacity incubator is required, a model in which the air is circulated by a fan should be considered. A fan circulated type incubator is more expensive than a gravity convection type.

Availability: The *Gallenkamp Economy Incubator* shown in Plate 3.28 and other types of incubators are available from Gallenkamp (see Appendix II). Prices start at about £395 (1986). Wherever possible, a hospital should purchase through a local agent to ensure that the incubator is functioning correctly after being installed and that spares (e.g. thermostat) and servicing will be available.

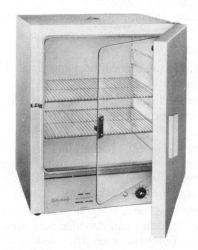

Plate 3.28 Gallenkamp Economy Incubator INA-300
575 x 590 x 490 mm. *Courtesy of Gallenkamp Ltd.*

Battery operated incubators

A simple inexpensive incubator which can be operated from a 12v battery is the *GQF laboratory incubator* as shown in Plate 3.29. The GQF incubator is made of thermal plastic which permits heating with a low wattage (30 watt) heater. The thermostat can be adjusted to operate over a temperature range of 28-42 °C, within ±0.5 °C. A thermometer can be fitted to the side of the incubator as shown in Plate 3.29. The inside chamber of the incubator measures 357 × 280 × 270 mm high.

Availability: The *GQF laboratory 12v incubator, No. L333/ 12* and centigrade scale thermometer No. 414 are available from GQF Manufacturing Company (see Appendix II). The incubator costs approx. US$ 100 (1986).

Note: Information about how to make a simple 12v incubator for incubating bacteriological cultures can be obtained from the HAMLO Group (see Appendix II).

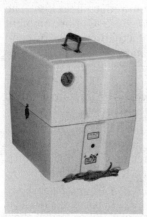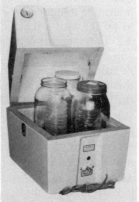

Plate 3.29 *Left:* **Battery operated incubator.**
Right: **Three candle jars containing culture plates inside the incubator.** *Courtesy of GQF Company.*

Use and care of an incubator
● Read carefully the manufacturer's instructions.
● Make sure the incubator is positioned on a level surface.
● Before incubating cultures and tests, check the temperature.
● Clean the incubator regularly, (making sure it is disconnected from the mains electricity supply).
● Every 3-6 months (depending on the age and condition of the incubator), check the incubator and flex for signs of wear and examine the connections inside the plug.

Follow the directions of the manufacturer regarding other maintenance measures. At the time of purchase, it is advisable to buy a spare thermostat and thermometer (if this is a special type).

Note: A Self-Instructional sheet (LAB/85.7) describing the operation and maintenance of a laboratory incubator is available from the Health Laboratory Unit of the World Health Organization, Geneva.

Dry heat blocks

Compared with a water-bath, a heat block is usually less expensive to buy and run, requires very little maintenance, and because water is not used there is no risk of moisture entering tubes and interfering with reactions.

A versatile heat block is the *Stuart Test Tube Heater SHT1* as shown in Plate 3.30. It operates over a temperature range of 8 °C above ambient to 100 °C. The power rating is 400 watts. The temperature is controlled by a solid state thermostat. Temperature fluctuation is ±0.1 °C. Four different aluminium blocks (each measuring 75 × 95 × 50 mm high) are available for use with the heater to accommodate a range of tubes from 10 mm to 19 mm in diameter (see Availability). There is also available a solid block without holes. The *Stuart Test Tube Heater* holds two blocks.

Availability: The *Stuart SHT1 Test Tube Heater* is available from Stuart Scientific Co Ltd (see Appendix II). Four different blocks are available to hold tubes of diameters 10 mm, 12 mm, 16 mm, and 19 mm. The 10 mm and 12 mm blocks have 20 places, the 16 mm block has 12 places, and the 19 mm block has 8 places. The range is included in the Tropical Health Technology Equipment Service to Developing Countries (Appendix IV, see Test tube heater).

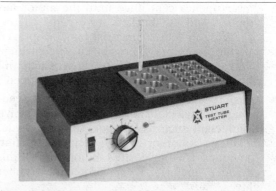

Plate 3.30 Stuart dry heat block containing two blocks with different hole sizes.
Courtesy of Stuart Scientific Ltd.

Use and care of a heat block
● Keep a thermometer in the heat block and check that the temperature is correct before use.
● Keep the correct number of blocks in the heater (models for holding 2 blocks or 3 blocks are available).
● Follow the manufacturer's instructions regarding the maintenance of the heater and blocks.

Water baths

A water bath is required to incubate bottles of culture media, liquids in flasks or other large containers, or when needing to incubate several racks of tubes.

A wide range of thermostatically controlled water baths of varying types and capacities is available. The heating unit may be enclosed in the casing of the bath or an immersion type of heater may be fitted. The more expensive water baths have a sensitive thermostat and a propeller to circulate the water and maintain it at the correct temperature throughout the bath.

A range of stainless steel economically priced water baths, which includes small capacity baths (4 litre, 5.5 litre), is available from M. Memmert Company (see Appendix II). Many other Companies with agents in developing countries such as Baird and Tatlock and Gallenkamp, supply medium to large capacity water baths.

Use and care of a water bath
- Fill the bath and *maintain its level* with clean rain water or chemically pure water. Do not use tap water because this will cause salts to be deposited and eventually damage the inner surface of the bath.
- Before incubating tests, always use a thermometer to check the temperature of the water.
- Ensure that the level of the water is above the level of whatever is being incubated.
- Do not use a lid when incubating uncapped tubes or bottles. Contamination and dilution of tests can occur due to condensation. To prevent loss of heat, the surface of the water around the incubating vessels can be covered with plastic spheres.
- Clean the water bath regularly, taking care not to damage the heating unit. Follow the manufacturer's instructions.
- Every 3-6 months check the bath for corrosion and the flex for wear. Check also the connections of the plug.

3:10 MIXERS AND ROTATORS

Mixers are not usually considered essential items of laboratory equipment because adequate mixing of most specimens and reagents can be achieved manually, especially in small laboratories. In busy district laboratories with a high work-load, however, the use of cell mixers and possibly magnetic stirrers should be considered. A rotator, however, is required for performing RPR card tests (see 45:2 in Volume II of the Manual).

Cell mixer

In haematology work, adequate mixing of anticoagulated blood specimens is essential if reliable results are to be obtained.

A rotary blood cell mixer is shown in Plate 3.31 (*Stuart SB1 Blood Tube Rotator*). This type of blood cell mixer is recommended in preference to the roller type because it gives better mixing of blood samples and is less expensive.

The disc of the mixer shown in Plate 3.31 is fitted with a single spring and can be adjusted for use with tubes from 9-19 mm in diameter. The disc can be stopped by hand for inserting or removing the specimens. The angle of the disc is fully adjustable from horizontal to vertical. As shown in Plate 3.31, it can hold up to 20 EDTA containers.

Availability: The mixer shown in Plate 3.31 is available from Stuart Scientific Ltd (see Appendix II). It is included in the Tropical Health Technology Equipment Service to Developing Countries (Appendix IV, see Mixer, blood cell.

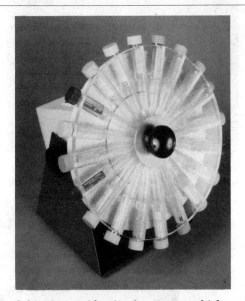

Plate 3.31 Stuart blood tube rotator which can be adjusted to take containers of different size.
Courtesy of Stuart Scientific Ltd.

Vortex mixer

Examples of vortex mixers are shown in Plate 33.4 on p. 20 in Volume II of the Manual. While such a mixer can achieve rapid and safe mixing of liquids in tubes, bottles, and flasks, the correct use of a vortex type mixer must be demonstrated to members of staff. The incorrect use of a vortex mixer can result in the loss of contents from a tube and possible injury depending on the fluid being vortexed.

Magnetic stirrers

A magnetic stirrer is particularly useful in the preparation of reagents and culture media, especially when combined with a hotplate. Plate 3.32 shows the *Stuart SM3 Magnetic Stirrer Hotplate*. The magnetic stirrer is of variable speed. The highest speed is 1300 rpm. The hotplate is of cast aluminium and measures 130 mm in diameter. It has a regulator and maximum temperature of 400 °C with a power rating of 400 watts. The magnetic stirrer is driven by a powerful magnet and the unit is supplied with two PTFE coated magnetic followers, one 20 mm long and the other of 40 mm (other sizes are available).

Availability: The *SM3 Magnetic Stirrer Hotplate*, complete with magnetic followers is available from Stuart Scientific Company Ltd priced approx. £113 (1987) (see Appendix II). The same Company also produces variable speed magnetic stirrers without a combined hotplate. The smallest unit (SM4) measures 90 × 160 × 90 mm high. It is supplied with one magnetic follower of 25 mm length and costs approx. £50.

Rotator

Most RPR (rapid plasma reagin) card tests require mixing of the specimen and reagent for 8 minutes at 100 rpm. The rotator *R50 Rotatest Minor* shown in Plate 3.33 has a fixed 100 rpm speed of rotation and is equipped with a timer. At the end of the preselected time a buzzer sounds. The rotator can also be used for mixing reagents on slides. The model shown operates from mains electricity.

Note: It is hoped that a 12v battery and mains operated rotator with lid, to accept two reusable RPR cards, will become available from Tropical Health Technology Equipment Service in 1987.

Availability: The *R50 Rotatest Minor* rotator is manufactured by Luckham Ltd (see Appendix II). It is included in the Tropical Health Technology Equipment Service to Developing Countries (Appendix IV, see Rotator).

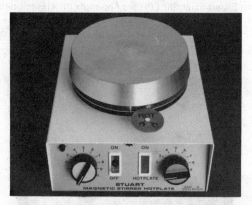

Plate 3.32 Stuart magnetic stirrer and hotplate. *Courtesy of Stuart Scientific Ltd.*

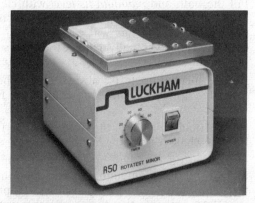

Plate 3.33 (*Upper*) Luckham rotator with speed of 100 rpm. *Courtesy of Luckham*

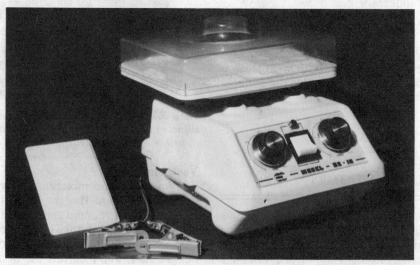

Plate 3.33 (*Lower*) Prototype of Chapman battery and mains rotator of variable speed up to 100 rpm with timer, lid, and reusable RPR plates.

3:11 pH METERS

The most reliable way to measure the pH of a solution is to use a pH meter. For an explanation of the meaning of pH, see 24:4. A pH meter measures the differences in potential (e.m.f.) between two solutions of different pH value.

Measuring pH using a hydrogen ion sensitive electrode

When two solutions containing hydrogen ions are separated by the bulb of a glass pH electrode that is hydrogen-ion sensitive, an electrical potential is developed across the thin glass separating the two solutions. If the solution inside the bulb is of fixed hydrogen ion concentration, the potential across the glass will change as the hydrogen ion concentration of the other solution varies. This difference in potential can be measured by making an electrical connection between the internal element of the glass electrode and a reference electrode (potential of which is known).

The reference electrode is usually a calomel electrode that has an electrical potential of 0.2415 volt at 25 °C (calibrated against the standard hydrogen electrode which has an electrode potential of zero). It consists of a mercury electrode covered with mercury I chloride (calomel) and a solution of mercury in saturated potassium chloride. The calomel electrode will maintain its specified potential providing its calomel and mercury content remain intact and its potassium chloride solution is kept saturated.

Many pH meters use what is called a combination pH electrode, i.e. an electrode in which the measuring glass electrode and the reference calomel electrode are combined into one unit.

The potential difference measurements of the meter are related to pH values by measuring the potential difference of a buffer solution, the pH of which is known exactly. This process is referred to as standardization.

Types of pH meter

A wide range of pH meters is available, including battery powered and mains electrically operated models. Modern pH meters are of the digital electronic type as shown in Plate 3.34.

The model shown is the portable digital *WPA pH meter CD60* which can be operated from mains electricity through an adaptor (as shown) or from a 9v PP3 dry battery. It reads pH values up to pH 14 in steps of 0.01. It is fitted with a temperature adjustment dial. There is no slope control. The electrode is of the combination type and has a plastic 'skirt' to protect it from damage. A low battery warning device is incorporated into the meter.

Should the power in the battery be insufficient, the display will show a '*LO BAT*' warning.

The *WPA pH CD60* meter is easy to use. The method is as follows:

1. Measure the temperature of the test solution. Adjust the temperature dial so that it reads the temperature of the test solution.

2. Using a wash bottle, wash the electrode using distilled or deionized water (when not in use the electrode must always be stored in an acid solution, e.g. pH 4 buffer).

3. Transfer the electrode to a beaker containing the standard buffer, i.e. buffer of known pH. The pH of the standard buffer should be close to the expected pH value of the test solution (buffers of pH 4, 7, or 9 are available for standardization). Adjust the buffer control knob to give the reading of the standard buffer.

4. Wash the electrode using distilled or deionized water and transfer it to the test solution. Record the pH reading.

5. Wash the electrode and replace it in a container of pH 4 buffer or 3% v/v hydrochloric acid solution.

Availability: The compact *WPA pH meter CD60* is manufactured by Walden Precision Apparatus Ltd (see Appendix II). It is included (complete with stand to hold the electrode, plastic beaker, and thermometer) in the Tropical Health Technology Equipment Service to Developing Countries (Appendix IV, see pH Meter).

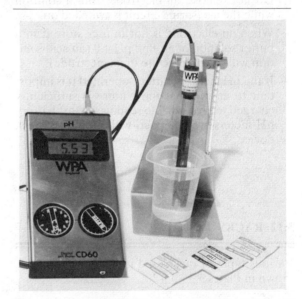

Plate 3.34 Mains and battery operated digital pH meter with combination electrode.

Care, and maintenance of pH meters

For the detailed use, care, and maintenance of a pH meter, it is important to consult the manufacturer's instruction manual.

The following are general guidelines regarding the care and maintenance of a pH meter:

— Handle the electrode (or electrodes) with great care. If the glass bulb is cracked or even scratched the electrode will need to be replaced.

Note: If the tip of an electrode is not provided with a protective 'skirt', a protective sheath can be easily made by boring or burning a hole of suitable diameter in a plastic bottle top through which the end of the electrode can be inserted.

— Use plastic containers to hold the buffer and test solutions. When measuring the pH, do not allow the electrode to touch the sides of the container.

— When an electrode is transferred from one solution to another rinse it with distilled or deionized water or with the test solution. Wiping the electrode with a tissue is not recommended because this may result in slight polarization and subsequent sluggishness of response.

— When measuring the pH of a solution, allow adequate time for the electrode to reach equilibrium before taking the reading.

— Always adjust the temperature calibration knob to the temperature of the test solution being measured (unless the meter automatically adjusts for temperature changes).

— Do not remove an electrode from a solution while the measuring circuit is switched on.

— When an electrode is not in use, store it in a buffer solution of around pH 4.0 (an acid solution will prolong the life of an electrode).

— If the pH meter is battery-operated it is important to ensure that the battery is sufficiently charged to give reliable readings. Most battery pH meters are equipped with a battery check device.

3:12 RACKS

Various types of racks used in the laboratory are shown in Plates 3.35-3.42.

Nylon coated wire racks

Nylon coated wire racks are rugged, easy to clean, lightweight, and generally less expensive than most other types of racks. They can also be used in the autoclave because nylon will withstand temperatures up to 125 °C.

Nylon coated wire racks are available for holding:

— Test tubes of 75-100 × 10-13 mm, see Plates 3.35 a and b.

— Conical (centrifuge) tubes of 100-125 mm in length, see Plate 3.36.

— EDTA and ESR containers, see Plate 3.37.

— Universal type containers, see Plate 3.38.

— Bijou bottles, see Plate 3.39.

Nylon coated wire racks are also available for draining glassware and plastic-ware (see Plate 3.40) and for carrying Winchester bottles (see Plate 3.41).

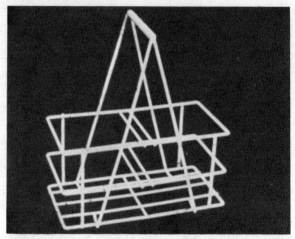

Plate 3.41 Polythene coated wire rack for carrying Winchester bottles. *Courtesy of Azlon Products Ltd.*

Plastic racks

A wide range of rigid plastic (polystyrene, polypropylene, ABS) racks is becoming available but some types are very expensive. Inexpensive rigid polystyrene racks are shown in Plates 3.42.

Availability: Nylon coated wire racks and other racks are available from Arnold Horwell Ltd (see Appendix II). The range shown in Plates 3.35-3.42 is included in the Tropical Health Technology Equipment Service to Developing Countries (Appendix IV, see Racks).

Other equipment and supplies for use in district laboratories and health centres

Equipment for pipetting and dispensing specimens and reagents is described in 2:4.

Details of smaller items of equipment and essential supplies for district hospital laboratories and health centres that are available from the non-profit Tropical Health Technology Equipment Service to Developing Countries can be found in Appendix IV.

Autoclaves

Autoclaves that can be operated from gas and kerosene as well as from mains electricity are described in Volume II of the Manual (p. 394).

Refrigerators and cold boxes

Details of refrigerators (and cold boxes will be described in Volume III of the Manual (Haematology and Blood Transfusion).

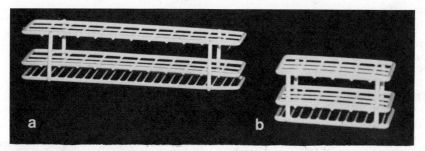

Plate 3.35 White nylon coated wire test tube racks to hold tubes 75-100 X 10-13 mm. *a* Holds 36 tubes *b* Holds 24 tubes.

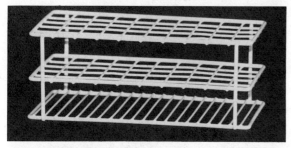

Plate 3.36 Nylon coated wire rack to hold 50 tubes 100-125 mm X 15-20 mm diameter.

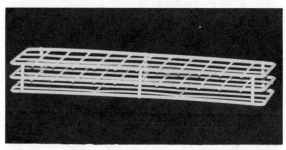

Plate 3.37 Nylon coated wire rack to hold 36 EDTA, ESR, or similar containers.

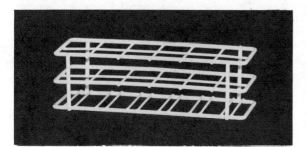

Plate 3.38 Nylon coated wire rack to hold 12 Universal type bottles.

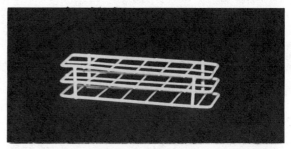

Plate 3.39 Nylon coated wire rack to hold 12 Bijou type bottles.

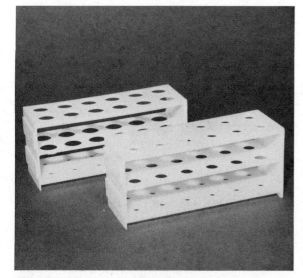

Plate 3.42 Rigid polystyrene racks.
Upper holds 12 tubes 100-125 X 15-20 mm.
Lower holds 12 tubes 100 X 11-13 mm.

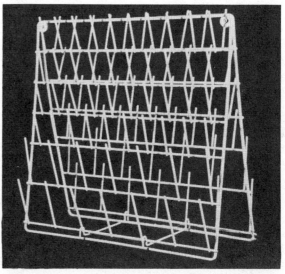

Plate 3.40 Free-standing polythene coated wire draining rack. Each side measures 510 X 480 mm.

References

1 Philip, D. Guidelines for equipment selection - Getting what you want and wanting what you get. Paper in *Laboratory in Health Care - Developing Country Proceedings of the 17th IAMLT Congress, 3-8 August 1986.* A limited number of copies are available from Tropical Health Technology, 14 Bevills Close, Doddington, March, Cambridgeshire, PE15 0TT, UK (free to developing countries, priced £5 to other countries).

2 World Health Organization. WHO Task Force on the Development of Appropriate Technology for Health in the Field of Laboratory Equipment, ATH/79.2, WHO, Geneva.

3 Vang, J. Introductory remarks to the seminar on Appropriate Technology and the use of technology in different cultures. Paper in *Laboratory in Health Care - Developing Country Proceedings of the 17th IAMLT Congress, 3-8 August, 1986.* For availability, see Reference 1.

4

Microscopy

4:1   THE PRINCIPLE OF THE MICROSCOPE

The microscopical examination of specimens is still the most reliable means of diagnosing many diseases especially those caused by parasites. It is essential for medical laboratory workers to know the working principle of a basic microscope and how to use and maintain one correctly. A microscope is one of the most expensive instruments used in a laboratory.

Working principle of a microscope
The microscope produces an enlarged image of the object which is examined through it. This enlargement is known as its magnification and is measured in diameters. For example, a magnifying lens which gives an image five times as large across as that of the object being seen through it, is said to have a magnification of five diameters, or simply 5×.

An ordinary magnifying glass is known as a simple microscope and this may have a magnification of 5×, 10×, perhaps 20× or even more. The laboratory microscope has magnifications much greater than this and is what is known as a compound microscope. A magnified image of the object is first produced by one lens and then this image is further enlarged by a second lens to give a still more highly magnified image. These two lenses are mounted one at each end of a tube. The first lens which is near the object is for this reason known as the objective lens, or simply the objective, while the second lens which is near the eye is known as the eyepiece lens, or simply the eyepiece (see Plate 4.1).

Total magnification of a microscope
The total magnification of a microscope is the magnification of its objective multiplied by that of its eyepiece. For example, using a 10× objective and a 10× eyepiece, the total magnification through the microscope is 100×. If a 100× objective is used with the same 10× eyepiece, it will give a total magnification of 1 000×.

Useful and empty magnification
If the eyepiece of a microscope is changed for another with a higher power, it gives an increased magnification from the objective. If this increased magnification brings further detail of the object into view, it is known as useful magnification. If

the magnification is still further increased there is a degree of magnification beyond which any further enlargement from the objective does not bring into view any more detail, but only a more highly magnified image which is increasingly blurred. This is known as empty or useless magnification.

The highest possible *useful* magnification of which an objective is capable depends on its resolving power.

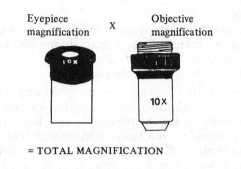

Eyepiece magnification   X   Objective magnification

= TOTAL MAGNIFICATION

Resolving power of a microscope
When two small dots in an object lie very close together, if their image is sharp it may be possible to see these with the microscope as two distinct dots. If, however, the image of each dot is blurred, they will run into each other and appear as one dot.

The ability of an objective to distinguish the dots separately and distinctly is known as its resolving power. The higher the resolving power of an objective, the closer can be the little dots in the object which it can separate in the image, i.e. the more detail can be seen in the structure of an object.

The resolving power of a microscope is therefore important. It is dependent on what is known as the numerical aperture (NA) of the objective. This is explained in 4:4.

Parts of a microscope
A microscope consists of:

- The microscope stand which is a support for all the other parts. It is described in 4:2.
- The mechanical adjustments of the microscope which are described in 4:3.
- The optics of the microscope which are described in 4:4.

4:2   THE MICROSCOPE STAND

The stand is the framework of a microscope. The main parts of the stand of a basic microscope are as follows:

☐ A tube which holds the objectives and the eyepiece.

☐ A body and its focusing mechanisms.

☐ An arm which supports the tube and body.

☐ A stage on which the specimen lies.

☐ A substage.

☐ A foot, or base, upon which the whole instrument rests.

Tube
The tube holds the eyepiece and objective in line and at the correct distance apart. It may also contain additional lenses, adjustment knobs, and slots for filters and other accessories.

The objective is screwed into the lower end of the tube by a standard objective thread which enables objectives to be interchanged. For laboratory work, three or even more objectives of different magnification are needed. These are screwed into what is known as a revolving nose-piece which allows any of the objectives to be swung quickly into place.

The eyepiece is inserted loosely into the upper end of the tube. This has a standard diameter so that all eyepieces are also interchangeable.

Tubelength
The tubelength of a microscope can often be adjusted by simply sliding the drawtube with its eyepiece up or down. Objectives are made to work best at a given tubelength. This is usually 160 mm.*

*A tubelength of 160 mm is the recommended DIN standard for tubelength measurement.

Body and arm
The tube is attached to the microscope by what is called the body. This contains the important focusing mechanisms (see 4:3).

The body of the microscope and the tube attached to it are supported at the correct height by a firm arm which may also provide a lifting handle for the microscope.

Stage and substage
The specimen to be examined (object) lies below the objective on a flat plate called the stage and is usually held in place by a pair of spring stage clips. In the centre of the stage there is a circular hole for light from below to pass through.

Mechanical stage
Most medical laboratory microscopes are equipped with what is called a mechanical stage. This enables specimens to be moved in a controlled way. The mechanical stage holds the slide in place and moves it systematically in straight lines either across or along the stage, slowly and smoothly, by the rotation of two knobs, one for each direction (X and Y movement). The knobs may project upwards from the stage or out to one side of it. There is often a measuring scale for each movement.

Substage
Immediately below the stage is the substage which holds a condenser lens with an iris diaphragm and a holder for light filters and stops (see 4:4).

Foot
This makes sure that the microscope rests firmly on the laboratory bench. The foot, or base, may take the form of a large block, or other form.

4:3   THE MECHANICAL ADJUSTMENTS OF A MICROSCOPE

The mechanical adjustments of a microscope include:

☐ Coarse and fine focusing adjustments.

☐ Condenser adjustments.

Coarse and fine focusing adjustments
The satisfactory operation of a microscope depends partly on the perfect movement of its coarse and fine focusing mechanisms (see Plate 4.1). For many microscopes, these focusing adjustments operate by a strip of metal sliding up and down in a matching slot. Careful lubrication is essential to give a smooth movement. This mechanism is often one which gives difficulty in hot humid climates.

Coarse adjustment
The coarse focusing adjustment is usually driven by a rack and pinion mechanism, controlled by a pair of large knobs positioned one on each side of the body. Rotation of these knobs moves the tube with its lenses, or in some microscopes the stage, up or down fairly rapidly.

Fine adjustment
While low power objectives can be focused by the coarse adjustment, high power objectives require a fine adjustment which moves the objectives or

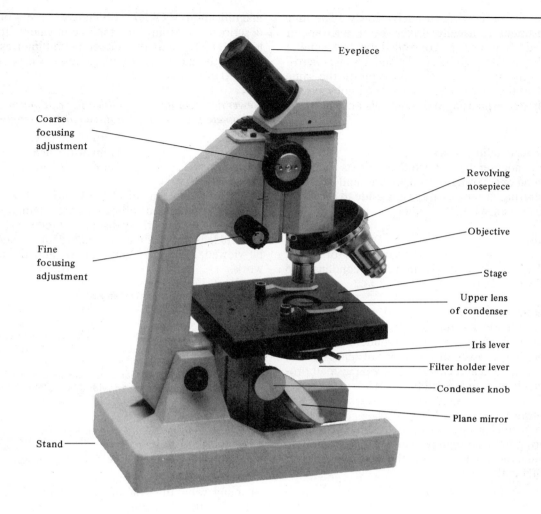

Plate 4.1 The main components of a monocular microscope.
Courtesy of Hampshire Micro.

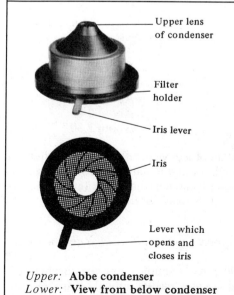

Upper: **Abbe condenser**
Lower: **View from below condenser**

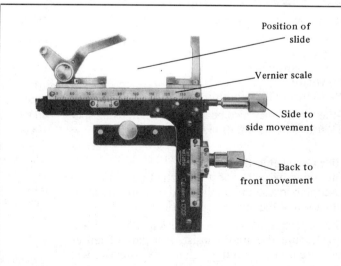

Mechanical stage which fits onto the stage of a microscope.

stage up or down extremely slowly. The fine adjustment is usually driven by a micrometer thread. It is usually controlled by two smaller knobs, one on each side of the body. Some microscopes incorporate the fine focusing on the same knob as the coarse adjustment. The knobs may be graduated in microns to show the distance moved.

Condenser adjustments

The condenser has adjustments for its focusing, opening and closing of its aperture, and often for its centring. It can also be swung aside to remove it or to exchange it with another.

Focusing

The condenser is focused usually by rotating a knob to one side of it. This moves the condenser up or down.

Adjustment of aperture

The condenser aperture is adjusted by the iris diaphragm which is just below the condenser. The iris diaphragm consists of a number of leaves which can be opened and closed by moving a small projecting lever (see 4:5 and Fig. 4.4).

Centring

In some microscopes the condenser can be centred to bring the illuminating beam of light accurately through the instrument. In others the condenser is permanently fixed.

4:4 THE MICROSCOPE OPTICS

The optics of a basic microscope include:

- Objectives
- Eyepiece
- Condenser and iris
- Mirror
- Source of illumination

Other optics may also be required when using special forms of illumination.

Microscope objectives

The objective is the most important part of a microscope because the quality and most of the magnification of the image depend on it.

The objective is never a single lens. A very low power objective may consist of a pair of lenses cemented together but a high power objective will consist of a number of carefully calculated lenses assembled together with great accuracy.

Modern objectives are described according to their magnification. Older objectives are often described according to their equivalent focal length (EFL), and this either in millimetres or inches (the meaning of EFL is described later in the text).

Newer descriptions in diameters	Older descriptions in equivalent focal lengths
10×	16 mm or 2/3 inch
40×	4 mm or 1/6 inch
100×	2 mm or 1/12 inch

For most routine medical work, 10×, 40× and 100× (oil immersion) objectives are adequate. A 20× or 25× long working distance objective is also a useful lens if specimens in capillary tubes need to be viewed, e.g. in trypanosomiasis and filariasis work.

Standardization of objective lengths

What are called DIN objectives are now available. DIN is the abbreviation used to describe the German published standards relating to the measurement of objectives and to other microscopical measurements. The DIN distance of an object to the shoulder of an objective is set at 45 mm. DIN objectives are longer than other objectives and should not therefore be interchanged with them. DIN objectives will only be parfocal with other DIN objectives.

Numerical aperture of an objective

Objectives are engraved not only with their magnification but also with their numerical aperture (NA).

In many ways the NA of an objective is more important than its magnification for upon the NA depends the highest resolving power and useful magnification (see 4:1) of an objective.

As a rule it can be taken that the total magnification of the microscope should not exceed the NA of the objective being used multiplied by 1 000. The following are the usual figures for the NA of the commonly used objectives:

Objective	NA
10×	About 0.25
20×	About 0.45
40×	About 0.65
100×	About 1.30

The NA of an objective is an exact figure that has been worked out mathematically from its equivalent focal length and lens diameter. It is not necessary to know the details of this calculation.

Equivalent focal length and working distance of an objective

The focal length of a simple lens is the distance between what is known as its optical centre and the point at which parallel rays of light passing through it come to a focus. An objective, however, is a complicated lens and it is not easy to know the exact position of its optical centre. The term equivalent focal length is therefore used instead. This is the focal length of a simple lens which has the same magnification as the objective.

The relationship between the NA of an objective and its equivalent focal length (EFL) and lens diameter, is shown in Fig. 4.1. The larger the lens diameter of the objective and the shorter its EFL, the wider is the cone of light entering the objective. The wider the angle of the cone of light, the higher is the NA of the objective which it illuminates and the greater is the objective's resolving power and useful magnification.

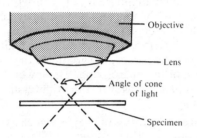

To show the angle of cone of light

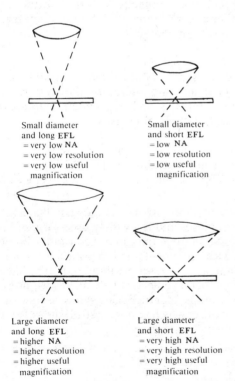

Small diameter
and long EFL
= very low NA
= very low resolution
= very low useful
  magnification

Small diameter
and short EFL
= low NA
= low resolution
= low useful
  magnification

Large diameter
and long EFL
= higher NA
= higher resolution
= higher useful
  magnification

Large diameter
and short EFL
= very high NA
= very high resolution
= very high useful
  magnification

Fig. 4.1 Relationship between the NA of an objective and its equivalent focal length (EFL) and lens diameter.

The equivalent focal length of an objective is not the same as its working distance, which is simply the distance between the front lens and the specimen it is examining (see Fig. 4.3). The importance of knowing the working distance of an objective when using a microscope is described in 4:5.

Aberrations of objectives
The edge of a lens gives a slightly higher magnification than its centre. This is called spherical aberration. Blue light is magnified slightly more than red and this is called chromatic aberration. When the image from a first lens is again magnified by a second lens, these aberrations are magnified also and the final image can be so blurred and edged with colour that it is useless.

While these aberrations cannot be avoided in a single lens objective they can be corrected by using a series of lenses mounted one behind the other, each made of a different special glass, carefully calculated and designed. The quality of an objective depends very much on how perfectly it has been corrected.

Achromats, fluorites (sometimes called semi-apochromats), and apochromats are the names given to objectives to describe their degree of correction.

Achromats
Achromatic objectives are the most widely used of objectives. In most achromats, chromatic aberrations are corrected for two wavelengths and spherical aberrations are corrected for one wavelength. Their working distances and NA's make these lenses suitable for the routine examination of most specimens.

Fluorites (semi-apochromats)
Fluorite objectives are engraved *Fl* and are more highly corrected and more costly than achromats. Chromatic and spherical aberrations are both corrected for two wavelengths. The use of fluorite gives these lens a higher NA (the higher the NA the greater the resolving power). A 50× fluorite immersion objective is a valuable lens for searching blood films because it has a wider field than the 100× oil immersion objective and a sharper image than high power dry objectives.

Apochromats
Apochromatic objectives are engraved *Apo*. They are very highly corrected and costly and only required for special work. Chromatic aberrations are corrected for three wavelengths and spherical aberrations for two. Their NA's are higher and therefore their images are sharper but only in focus in the central part of the field due to field curvature. Apochromatic objectives work very close to the top of the cover glass of the object. The thickness of the cover glass is therefore important.

Flatfield (plano) objectives

As their name implies, flatfield objectives correct for field curvature. Additional lenses are usually built into these objectives to flatten the image across the field, so that the entire field of view appears in focus at the same time. Plano, or flatfield, objectives are mainly used in photomicrography work. Achromats, fluorites or apochromats can be obtained as flatfield objectives but they are more expensive.

Spring-loaded objectives

The high power objectives (e.g. 40× and 100×) of most modern microscopes are spring-loaded, i.e. the front mount of the objective will be pushed in rather than pushed through a specimen if such an objective is accidentally pressed against a specimen when focusing. Spring-loaded objectives protect a specimen and the front lens of an objective from being damaged.

Working of oil immersion objectives

When a beam of light passes from air into glass it is bent and when it passes back from glass to air it is bent back again to its original direction. This has little effect on low power objectives but with high power lenses, this bending limits not only the amount of light which can enter the lens but also affects the NA of the objective and consequently its resolving power.

The bending effect and its limitations on the objective can be avoided by replacing the air between the specimen and the lens with an oil which has the same optical properties as glass, i.e. immersion oil. When the correct oil is used, the light passes in a straight line from glass through the oil and back to glass as though it were passing through glass all the way (see Fig. 4.2).

Some 50× objectives and all 100× objectives are used immersed in oil. Whenever possible the immersion oil recommended by the manufacturer of a microscope should be used.

Eyepiece (ocular)

The most common form of eyepiece is known as the Huygens eyepiece. This is the eyepiece normally used with achromatic objectives. It consists of two lenses mounted the correct distance apart with a circular diaphragm between which gives a sharp edge to the image. Huygenian eyepieces are available in a range of magnifications, usually 4×, 6×, 7×, 10×, 15× and sometimes as high as 20×. The higher the power, the greater is the total magnification of the microscope. The lower the power of the eyepiece, however, the brighter and sharper is the image.

There are other forms of eyepiece such as the more costly compensating eyepieces intended for use with fluorite and apochromatic objectives, but these are of no advantage when used with the ordinary achromatic objectives. It is important to use the eyepiece recommended by the manufacturer for use with the objectives supplied.

Wide-field eyepieces

These eyepieces enable a greater area of field to be examined and are therefore particularly useful when needing to search a specimen. They are often used with flatfield objectives.

Monocular and binocular microscopes

The instrument shown in Plate 4.1 is a monocular microscope because it has only one eyepiece (ocular).

A binocular microscope, as shown in Plate 4.2, has two eyepieces and is a widely used form of instrument. No more detail can be seen with a binocular than with a monocular microscope and a binocular instrument requires more illumination because the light in each eyepiece is halved. It has, however, the advantage that the image can be seen with both eyes at once, which is more restful when examining specimens for prolonged periods.

The adjustment of the head of a binocular microscope is described in 4:5.

Trinocular head

What is called a trinocular head attachment consists of an inclined binocular with a protruding tube and sliding prism. The additional tube is used for attaching a camera for photomicrography work.

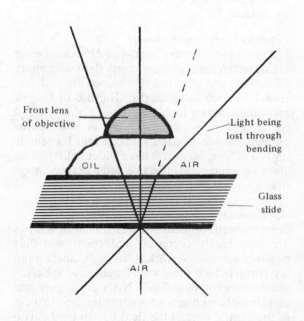

Fig. 4.2 The working of an oil immersion objective.
Courtesy of Churchill Livingstone publisher.

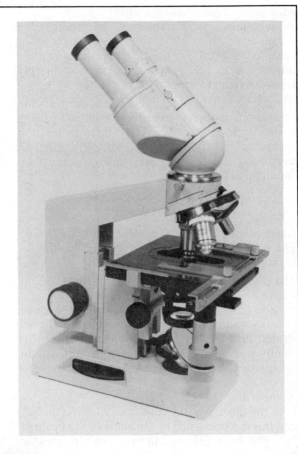

Plate 4.2 *Right:* **Binocular microscope with a fixed mechanical stage and a fine focusing wheel at the base of the instrument. A mirror is used to reflect the light.**
Courtesy of Technical and Optical Equipment.

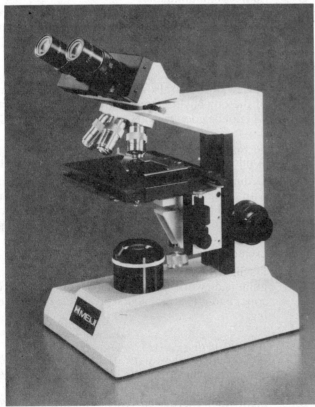

Plate 4.2 *Left:* **Binocular microscope with fixed mechanical stage and fine focusing combined with coarse focusing on the same knob. The illumination is built-in to the base of the instrument.**
Courtesy of Hampshire Micro.

Measuring eyepiece and graticule

A measuring, or micrometer, eyepiece is an eyepiece which is fitted with a disc which has a scale on it (graticule). The upper lens can be adjusted so that the graticule scale can be sharply focused on the specimen.

The measurement of each division of the graticule scale for each objective can be calculated by using a stage micrometer. The stage micrometer is a measured scale. Instructions for calibrating an eyepiece graticule from a stage micrometer can be found in 4:11.

Condenser and iris

The condenser is a large lens with an iris diaphragm. It is mounted below the stage.

The condenser lens receives a beam from the light source and passes it into the objective. It does not need to be highly corrected. It usually consists of two or sometimes three lenses and is highly curved so that light can pass to the objective at a sufficiently wide angle. For routine transmitted light microscopy, an Abbe type condenser is suitable.

Numerical aperture of the condenser

Like the objective, the condenser also has an NA and this is represented by the angle of the beam of light which passes from it to the specimen and so to the objective.

If the angle of this beam of light from the condenser matches that of the objective, the condenser will have the same NA as the objective, and will exactly fill it with light. In practice, however, the condenser must not fill completely the objective with light because glare will result. The angle to which the NA of the condenser must be reduced to avoid glare, depends on the type of specimen. Glare caused by using too large a condenser aperture destroys the quality of the image, and cells and microorganisms may be missed in unstained specimens (see also 4:6).

The angle of the beam of light entering the condenser is adjusted by the iris. The importance of reducing or increasing the condenser aperture when examining specimens is explained in 4:5.

Condenser with swing-out-top lens

Some microscopes are fitted with a condenser which has an upper lens which can be swung aside when using a very low power objective. This enables the light to fill the much larger field of view of the lower power objective. It is usually necessary also to lower the substage slightly.

Aplanatic condenser

This type of condenser has better correction for spherical aberration than the Abbe type and is therefore often used when an Abbe condenser is not adequate.

Achromatic condenser

This type of condenser is corrected for both chromatic and spherical aberration and is therefore expensive. It is only necessary for special forms of work.

Mirror

The mirror is situated below the condenser and iris (in microscopes without built-in illumination). It is circular and mounted so that it can be turned in any direction and will stay in place. The mirror reflects the beam of light from the light source upwards through the iris into the condenser. It generally consists of two mirrors, mounted back to back, one flat and the other curved inwards (concave).

The curved mirror is itself a form of low power condenser and it must never be used together with a condenser. Only the flat mirror should be used with the condenser and it is a good thing to cover over the curved mirror, perhaps with adhesive paper to prevent its being used accidentally.

The concave side of the mirror is used with very low NA objectives when a condenser is *not* used.

Sources of illumination

The form of illumination used with the microscope will depend on circumstances, whether the microscope is being used by day or after dark and whether electric current is available or not.

Whatever the source of light, it should fill the field of view. It should also fill the whole of the back lens of the objective regularly with light or the image will not be good (see also 4:6).

Daylight

A microscope must not be used in direct sunlight.

Ordinary daylight may be sufficient for some work with a monocular microscope, especially when reflected from a white painted sunlit board placed outside the laboratory, particularly if the light from this can enter through a small window to exclude glare.

Daylight, however, is scarcely enough for oil immersion work and rarely for a binocular microscope, and it is not of course available in the evenings.

Electric light

An ordinary 60 watt pearl electric bulb placed about 18 inches from the microscope is sufficient for most routine work and can be used by day or night when there is current, but a proper microscope lamp which shields the user from glare is recommended. Whenever possible, this should have a focusing condenser system, an adjustable field diaphragm, a mount to rotate the lamp with a locking clamp, lamp-centering screws, height and angle adjustments, and the lamp itself should have a tight, flat, coil filament.

Quartz halogen (quartz iodine) and other high intensity lamps are available and are very good light sources because they give excellent illumination and do not blacken like ordinary tungsten lamps. They do, however, give out considerable heat. Quartz halogen lamps can be used for some forms of transmitted fluorescence microscopy (see later text).

Many microscopes, especially binocular instruments, are now provided with correctly aligned built-in sources of illumination (see Plate 4.2) which use tungsten or quartz halogen lamps operating on 6, 8 or 12 volts through variable transformers.

Battery lamp
A 6 volt microscope lamp can also be connected to a 6 volt battery or to half of a 12 volt car battery. This enables a 6v built-in source of illumination (normally used through a transformer) to be used during the hours when mains electricity is not available.

Oil lamp
If neither daylight nor electricity is available, good work can be done with a kerosene oil lamp. The flame of an ordinary oil hurricane lamp gives an excellent illumination with the oil immersion lens, but it is rather small for the 40× and especially so for the 10× objective. If an oil lamp is used, great care must be used to make sure it is positioned well away from any flammable chemicals including alcohol-based stains, fixatives, and differentiating reagents (see 2:5). Whenever possible, the use of an oil lamp should be avoided.

Note: The light from an electric lamp and particularly from an oil lamp is rather yellow. It may be improved by the use of a blue daylight filter.

Filters
Light filters are used in microscopy as follows:

☐ To reduce the intensity of light when this is required. A neutral grey filter is used to decrease the brilliance of a light source.

☐ To increase contrast and resolution. A blue daylight filter is commonly used when using an electric 'yellow' lamp. This increases resolution by absorbing light rays of longer wavelengths and transmitting the shorter wavelengths. Green filters also increase resolution.

☐ To adjust the colour balance of the light to give the best visual effect.

☐ To provide monochromatic light, e.g. in some forms of phase contrast work.

☐ To absorb heat. A heat absorbing filter is used with medium and high intensity lamps.

☐ To transmit light of a selected wavelength, e.g. an exciter filter used in fluorescence microscopy (see 4:10).

☐ To protect the eye from injury caused by ultra violet light e.g. a barrier filter used in fluorescence microscopy (see 4:10).

4:5 ROUTINE USE OF A BASIC MICROSCOPE

A microscope must always be used with gentleness and care. The steps for its routine use are as follows:

1. Place the microscope on a firm bench so that it does not vibrate. Make sure it will not be exposed to direct sunlight because this would be unsuitable for illumination, bad for the instrument, and dangerously bright for the eyes.

   The user must be seated at the correct height for the convenient use of the microscope.

2. Select the source of light as described in 4:4.

   If this is a built-in source, all that is required is to switch this on. If it is not a built-in source, use the flat side of the mirror to reflect the light up through the condenser (to be adjusted later).

3. Place the specimen on the stage, making sure the underside of the slide is *completely dry*.

   Specimens are usually examined on standard 76 × 25 mm glass slides and if they are to be used with a dry lens, especially the high power, they must be mounted under a cover glass. For most routine work a No. 1½ cover glass is recommended. Alternatively, if the specimen is a smear to be examined with an oil immersion lens, spread a thin smear of oil on it which will enable it to be scanned first using a 10× or 40× objective.

   Specimens to be examined with an oil immersion objective may be either with or without a cover glass.

4. Select the objective to be used.

   It is usually better to begin examinations with the 10× objective. Once in focus all the other objectives should also be nearly in focus provided they are parfocal.

The 10× objective can be used for adjusting the illumination and for searching the specimen before using a higher power lens.

5. Focus the objective.

To do this, rack the objective carefully downwards using the coarse focusing knob and *looking at it from the side* until the lens is near the specimen but not touching it. Then while looking through the eyepiece, rack the objective slowly upwards, still with the coarse adjustment, until the image comes into view and is sharply focused.

6. If using daylight or a light source positioned in front of the microscope adjust the mirror until the illumination of the image is at its brightest.

7. Focus the condenser.

To do this, open fully the iris of the condenser and using the *condenser adjustment knob*, focus the condenser on the details of the light source, such as the lettering engraved on the bulb and then rack downwards until these details are *just out of focus*.

Alternatively, focus the condenser by partially closing the iris until its image (probably blurred and possibly off centre) appears in the field of view. Using the condenser knob, focus the condenser until the image of the diaphragm appears as sharp as possible (it may be fringed with colour which is unavoidable). The condenser will then be in focus. Centre it if it appears off centre, using the centring screws.

8. Adjust the aperture (opening) of the condenser iris according to the specimen being examined.

The wider the condenser aperture, the brighter will be the specimen and the smaller will be the details which can be resolved. The smaller the aperture, the greater will be the contrast.

Certain specimens, e.g. stained and mounted specimens give little glare and for these the condenser iris should be opened more widely giving a well illuminated image with fine detail. Other specimens, e.g. urine, unstained cerebrospinal fluid, and saline mounted faecal specimens, give much glare and require a reduced condenser iris to increase contrast (see Fig. 4.4).

9. Examine the specimen, moving it by the mechanical stage.

Note: The image of the specimen will be upside down and will move in the opposite direction to the slide.

10. For a higher magnification, swing the 40× objective into place. Focus the 40× objective, using the fine adjustment.

If for any reason the image is not visible, lower the objective *(while looking at it from the side)*, until it is nearly but not quite touching the specimen. Then looking through the eyepiece, focus upwards with the fine adjustment until the image comes into view.

Adjust the aperture of the condenser iris for this objective. The 40× objective requires the iris to be opened more widely than the 10×.

11. For the highest magnification, add a drop of immersion oil to the specimen and swing the 100× oil immersion objective into place. Open the iris fully to fill the objective with light.

Greater care must be taken when moving and adjusting this lens than with the 40×, because it is in focus when close to the specimen (see Fig. 4.3).

Note: If examining a stained smear directly with the oil immersion lens and it is not possible to focus it, remove the slide and check that the oil has been placed on the smear side of the slide and not by mistake on the underside of the slide.

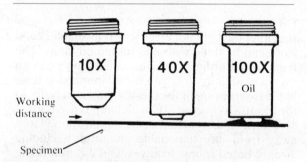

Fig. 4.3 To show the working distances of the commonly used objectives. Note the short working distances of the 40X and 100X oil immersion objectives.

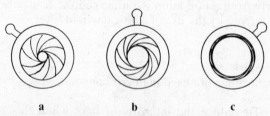

Fig. 4.4 Adjustment of the condenser aperture to give the best image when examining specimens.
a The iris diaphragm is almost closed, as when using the 10X objective.
b The iris diaphragm is about half opened, as when using the 40X objective.
c The iris diaphragm is opened widely, as when using the oil immersion objective.
Courtesy of Dr. J. McArthur.

Adjustment of a binocular head

When using a binocular microscope there are two adjustments to be made:

☐ Adjusting the distance between the eyepieces to match the separation of the user's eyes. This is done by sliding the two eyepieces nearer or further apart until the fields merge and can be seen comfortably by both eyes at the same time.

☐ Adjusting for any difference between the two eyes. To do this, first focus the specimen with one eye through the fixed eyepiece, then without altering the focusing of the microscope, adjust the other moveable eyepiece up and down until it also is in focus. This done, the two images should be identical and the microscope comfortable to use.

4:6 CRITICAL MICROSCOPY

It is possible with understanding and skill to adjust a microscope to give a perfect image so that, when required, this can be obtained to distinguish doubtful detail. Critical microscopy is the art of obtaining the highest possible resolving power and useful magnification of which an objective is capable.

To obtain critical microscopy it is necessary to understand:

■ Numerical aperture, upon which resolving power depends (see 4:4).

■ The principles of microscopical illumination.

■ What is meant by glare, how it can be avoided, and how to adjust the microscope to give the highest resolution with the minimum of glare.

■ The importance of using the correct tube length and cover glass thickness.

Illumination

Critical illumination provides a uniform illumination which just fills the field of view of the eyepiece, and no more, when the microscope condenser is focused.

At the same time it must almost fill the aperture of the objective uniformly and completely with light. This can be seen by removing the eyepiece and looking down the tube of the microscope. As described in 4:5, the iris diaphragm of the condenser also requires adjustment depending on the type of specimen being examined. Having checked that the objective is correctly illuminated, critical illumination can be carried out in one of two ways:

— By allowing the light from a regular source (sheet of illuminated opal glass or a white sunlit board) to pass through a small window or other aperture of the size just required to fill the field of view in the eyepiece.

— By using a small intense source of light and enlarging this to fill the field of view by using a lens at the correct situation between the source and the microscope, as used in most microscopes with built-in illumination.

By either method, some way should be used to adjust the size of the light source for each objective. When using the low power objective, the source of light must be quite large. It must be smaller for the high power dry objective, and smaller still for the oil immersion lens. This adjustment for size is best made by using a large iris diaphragm in front of the lamp and opening or closing it until it just fills the field of view in the eyepiece for each objective lens.

Glare

Glare in the microscope is caused by any light reaching the eye which does not go to make up the perfect image but interferes with the image.

Glare can be produced by:

☐ Stray light entering the eye from outside the microscope, e.g. from windows or other sources of light in the room. This can be called external glare.

☐ Using a larger source of illumination than is necessary i.e. one that illuminates more of the object than is seen in the field of view. This can be called illumination glare.

☐ Using a larger condenser aperture than is necessary, i.e. one which more than fills the objective with light. This can be called condenser glare.

☐ Reflection back and forth in the specimen, e.g. in water between a slide and cover glass or in air between a specimen and the front of the objective. This can be called mounting glare.

☐ Stray reflections from inside the objective, microscope tube, or eyepiece. This can be called mechanical glare.

All these added together can seriously spoil an image and therefore the more each one can be reduced the better.

Reducing glare

For critical microscopy it is important to try and reduce each source of glare. This can be attempted as follows:

— Reduce external glare by using the microscope

in a subdued light, preferably in a darkened part of the room. When this cannot be done, an eye-shade can help to exclude such glare.

— Avoid illumination glare by using a light source which can be adjusted to illuminate no more than the field of view. A different size of light source is needed for each objective, large for the lowest power, and small for the highest power objective.

— Diminishing condenser glare by reducing the condenser aperture. This will increase contrast in the microscope but at the expense of resolving power. If the other sources of glare are reduced, the condenser aperture does not have to be reduced so much.

— Reducing mounting glare when this is possible.

Some kinds of specimen give more glare than others. A stained blood film or bacterial stained smear with no cover glass and examined with an oil immersion objective, gives little glare and should be examined always with the iris as wide open as possible.

Unstained particles suspended in water beneath a cover glass give considerable glare. There are many reflections back and forth between cover glass and lens, and between cover glass and slide which are encouraged by the different refractive properties of the water and glass. Examination of c.s.f., urine, or a faecal specimen diluted with saline using a 10× objective, requires the condenser iris to be quite considerably reduced. This increases contrast with an unavoidable loss of resolution.

Note: Stray light from the instrument itself is more a problem for the manufacturer than for the user, but the source of such glare may sometimes be recognized by the user and corrected.

Tubelength and cover glass thickness
In routine work, tubelength and cover glass thickness are of little importance. Many microscopes, including binocular instruments, do not allow for any adjustment of tubelength.

In critical microscopy, however, the tubelength and cover glass thickness are important when using high power dry objectives such as the 20×, 40×, and those over 40× with a high NA. These high power dry objectives are generally calculated to work best with a cover glass thickness of 0.17 mm and a tube length of 160 mm.

For critical microscopy, the cover glass should not vary more than about 0.03 mm on either side of the correct 0.17 mm, and some workers use a micrometer gauge to check this. If the cover glass is too thick it can to a certain extent be compensated

for by decreasing the tubelength and if the cover glass is too thin the tubelength can be increased.

Summary of critical microscopy
To summarize, to achieve the highest resolution and useful magnification of an objective:

☐ The light source must be focused in the plane of the object and must just fill the field of view in the eyepiece.

☐ The cone of light must just fill the whole of the objective uniformly with the absence of glare.

This is critical illumination.

4:7 CARE, CLEANING, AND REPAIR OF A MICROSCOPE

A microscope is a delicate instrument both mechanically and optically and therefore it is necessary to treat it with care and to handle it gently. Always carry a microscope using both hands.

When not in use, a microscope should be protected from dust, moisture, and direct sunlight. Rather than keeping it stored in its wooden box it is generally better to keep it standing in place ready for use, but protected by a light cover. In humid climates it may be necessary to seal the microscope in a plastic bag with a drying agent overnight to avoid moulds growing on the lenses. During the day the drying agent (e.g. silica gel) will need to be redried in an oven. At the end of each day's work, the surface lenses of the objectives, eyepiece, and condenser, should be cleaned using lens tissue or a soft clean cloth.

Mechanical parts
No instrument of any kind should ever be forced. If any of the controls of a microscope begin to run hard, a touch of machine oil *may* be required. This must be machine oil not vegetable oils which become dry and hard. Always, read carefully the manufacturer's instructions regarding maintenance, especially the cleaning and lubrication of parts.

If a movement begins to run loose, e.g. a rack and pinion movement or dovetail, a smear of paraffin wax or candle grease may help. A movement which runs loose on a hot day may however be right on a cold day.

The use of a screwdriver on a microscope should only be attempted with caution because damage can be done by a person who is unskilled with delicate machinery.

Optics

The optics of the microscope also need care and attention. They should be examined occasionally with a magnifying glass for smears or dust, and kept cleaned. Always consult the manufacturer's manual.

Most objectives are now made with spring mounts for safety, but if not, it is particularly important to avoid striking the specimen with an objective (see 4:5).

After use, the immersion objective should be wiped with a piece of clean soft cloth or lens tissue.

The front surface of an objective can be examined through a magnifying glass or by using a Huygens eyepiece reversed. If the objective lens is dirty or smeared, it should be cleaned using a clean piece of soft linen or a piece of lens tissue. If a smear is difficult to remove it may be wiped with a very little xylene. Alcohol must *never* be used because this may dissolve the cement which is used to keep the lenses of an objective in place.

The inner surfaces of the objective lenses are less likely to be smeared and dirty and attempts to clean these should be avoided. Under no circumstances should an objective be unscrewed and dismantled.

Eyepiece

If on rotating an eyepiece in its tube, particles are seen to rotate with it, these are in the eyepiece. To discover which lens is dirty, the upper lens can be rotated without moving the rest of the eyepiece and it will at once be seen whether the dust is on the upper or the lower lens.

Generally the only lens to clean in an eyepiece is the upper one, but the lenses may be unscrewed to clean their inner surfaces if necessary using a soft clean piece of linen or lens tissue. The lenses should be removed, cleaned, and replaced separately to be sure that each returns to its right place.

Condenser and iris

The condenser should be kept clean and its focusing mechanism lubricated as instructed by the manufacturer. The iris diaphragm is very delicate, and generally if damaged or badly corroded, it is beyond repair.

Mechanical stage

The mechanical stage must be kept in good condition and its mechanism kept clean and well-lubricated.

The surface of the fixed stage *must* be kept dry and clean. If the under surface of a slide is wet or has oil on it, the slide will be difficult to move. This will increase the pressure on the movements of the mechanical stage with possible damage and breaking of the spring clip holding the slide in position.

Repair of the microscope

Except for obvious and simple measures, if a microscope becomes damaged optically or mechanically, it is better to return it or the damaged part to a reliable scientific instrument repairer or preferably to the manufacturer.

Note: If using a microscope with a built-in illumination and a lamp requires replacing, this can be done by the user. The manufacturer's manual should be consulted. Spare lamps should always be bought at the time a microscope is purchased.

4:8   PHASE CONTRAST MICROSCOPY

Transparent micro-organisms suspended in a fluid may be difficult and sometimes impossible to see. One method of making them more visible is to use what is called phase contrast.

Principle of phase contrast

A ray of light consists of waves travelling in a straight line. If two such rays of similar waves travel together, in step with each other, they are said to be in phase. They help each other and together they produce a brighter ilumination. If, however, the waves are out of step with each other they are said to be out of phase. They interfere with and hinder each other which results in a less bright illumination.

Phase contrast microscopy makes use of this ability of waves to help or hinder each other to produce variations in the intensity of illumination. Such variations increase the contrast in the microscopical image.

Phase contrast is obtained by placing in the condenser what is called an annulus and in the objective what is called a phase plate (see Fig. 4.5).

The annulus in the condenser is a plate which allows only a ring of light to pass into the microscope. The phase plate in the objective has a circle engraved in it or deposited on it, which matches the ring of light coming to it from the condenser. This circle on the phase plate has the effect of making the waves take a longer or a shorter 'step', so becoming out of phase with those waves which pass through the rest of the plate.

If the specimen is a clear fluid containing no micro-organisms or particles, the only light which reaches the eye is that which goes from the annulus through the circle on the phase plate. If, however, there are micro-organisms or particles in the fluid, these diffract and scatter the light coming from the annulus, so that it passes through the whole of the phase plate. The effect of this is that the light which comes from the fluid and only passes through the circle of the phase plate, is out of phase with, and interferes with the light which comes from the organisms, so making them and their structures stand out in contrast to their background.

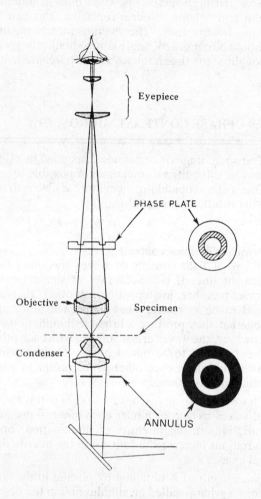

Fig. 4.5 To show the layout of a phase contrast microscope (the phase plate is not drawn to scale).
Courtesy of Vickers Instruments Ltd.

Equipment required

Phase contrast may be obtained from any power of objective on the microscope, but each objective requires a different size of phase plate and matching annulus. These are always made up as a unit and generally as part of a complete microscope. It is also necessary to have a telescope to examine the rings of both the annulus and phase plate during their adjustment (see later text).

Note: Phase contrast objectives can also be used for ordinary transmitted lighting. It is not therefore necessary to have two sets of objectives.

Setting up phase contrast

1. Illuminate the microscope in the usual way. Turn the required objective into place and focus it on the specimen.

2. Move the matching annulus into place.

3. Insert the telescope into the microscope in place of the eyepiece and adjust it until the two rings, one bright and one dark, are in focus.

4. Adjust the centering screws of the condenser until the bright ring of the annulus fits exactly into the darker ring of the phase plate.

5. Remove the telescope, replace the eyepiece, focus, and examine the specimen.

Value of phase contrast

Phase contrast is particularly useful for examining:

☐ Unstained bacteria, e.g. cholera vibrios in specimens and cultures.
☐ Amoebae in faecal preparations.
☐ Trypanosomes in blood, cerebrospinal fluid, and lymph gland fluid.
☐ Promastigotes of leishmanial parasites in culture fluid.
☐ *Trichomonas* species in direct smears and cultures.
☐ Urine sediments.

Phase contrast also facilitates the counting of platelets in a counting chamber.

Disadvantages

One disadvantage of phase contrast is that it produces what looks like a sheath or halo around each organism or particle and this can be mistaken for part of its structure and can be misleading. Guidance from an experienced microscopist is required in the beginning.

There is also a slight loss of resolution when using phase contrast but this disadvantage is not as great as the advantage of the increased contrast.

4:9   DARK-FIELD MICROSCOPY

Dark-field microscopy, which is also referred to as dark ground illumination, is another method of lighting micro-organisms suspended in fluid, enabling their structure and motility to be seen more clearly. It makes some living organisms visible which cannot be seen by ordinary transmitted lighting, e.g. the delicate spirochaetes of *Treponema pallidum*.

Principle of dark-field microscopy

In dark-field microscopy, the light enters a special condenser which has a central blacked-out area so that the light cannot pass directly through it to enter the objective. Instead, the light is reflected to pass through the outer edge of the condenser lens at a wide angle (see Fig. 4.6).

The only light entering the eye comes from the micro-organisms themselves, with no light entering the eye directly from the light source. In this way, small micro-organisms are seen brightly illuminated against a black background, like stars in a night sky or dust in a shaft of sunlight across a darkened room.

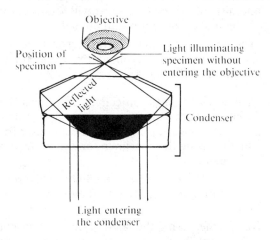

Fig. 4.6 Principle of dark-field microscopy.

Equipment required

The best form of dark-field microscopy is obtained by using a special dark-field condenser (dark ground condenser). Such a condenser is essential if wishing to examine specimens by dark-field microscopy using the 100× objective. When such high magnification is not required, adequate dark-field can be obtained for use with the 10× and 40× objectives by inserting a simple opaque disc, or stop, in the filter holder of the substage to prevent light passing through the condenser to the objective. This inexpensive method of obtaining dark-field microscopy is explained later in the text.

Equipment for the conventional method of obtaining dark-field
— An oil immersion dark-ground condenser with centring screws, to replace the ordinary microscope condenser.

— A funnel stop for insertion in the 100× objective to reduce its NA and exclude light coming directly from the source (see later text).

— A 6× or 10× eyepiece. The lower the power of the eyepiece, the brighter will be the image.

— A high intensity microscope lamp.
— Good quality slides that are not more than 1 mm thick, free from scratches, and *completely clean*.
— *Completely clean* cover glasses.

Setting up dark-field microscopy using a dark ground condenser

1. Remove the ordinary condenser from the microscope and insert the immersion dark ground condenser, clamp it in place and raise it to be about level with the stage surface.

2. Make a thin preparation using a clean slide and cover glass and a *small* drop of specimen.

   Note: It is important that the slide is not more than about 1 mm thick because of the short working distance of the condenser. Both the slide and cover glass must be perfectly clean and free of grease because the slightest smear will destroy the image and its dark background.

3. Place the specimen on the microscope stage, adding a drop of immersion oil between the slide and condenser.

4. Arrange the high intensity microscope lamp about 18 inches away and direct its beam to the middle of the mirror. Adjust the mirror so that the light passes upwards into the condenser.

5. Focus the *10× objective* on the specimen and adjust the mirror until the best light is obtained (which may not be much). Probably a small ring of light will be seen illuminating a part of the specimen.

6. Focus the condenser up or down, until the ring grows smaller and finally becomes a bright spot of light.

7. Centre the bright spot of light in the field by using the centring screws of the condenser.

8. Swing the 40× objective into place, focus it, and examine the specimen. If necessary, adjust the centring and focusing of the condenser.

9. If wishing to use the 100× oil immersion objective, swing this into place, oil immersed and with funnel stop inserted. Focus the specimen and if necessary again improve the condenser focusing and centring.

   Note: Because of the time and care that is required in setting up good dark-field microscopy, if a laboratory uses this form of illumination frequently, it is usually best to keep a microscope set up just for this purpose.

Making and use of dark-field stops for use with the 10× and 40× objectives

The stops must be made of a material such as metal or thick card through which light cannot pass. Two stops are required, one for use with the 10× objective and the other for use with the 40× objective. It is not possible to make a stop suitable for use with a 100× oil immersion objective.

The correct size of stop to use with each objective is that which just cuts out all the light entering the objective lens.

Note: All the materials to make dark-field stops for use with the 10× and 40× objectives are supplied in kit form, free of charge in the back of Volume II of the Manual.

Method of making stops using kit from Volume II

1. Locate the filter holder below the condenser of the microscope, and measure its *internal* diameter in mm. It will probably be 31, 32 or 33 mm.

2. Select from the sheet of clear filters provided the two which match the size of the filter holder (or nearest size). Carefully cut out both filters.

   Note: A ground glass filter or blue daylight filter is not suitable for making a dark-field stop.

3. Place each clear filter into the filter holder to make sure it fits well. Trim if required.

4. *Carefully* cut out the three sizes of stop provided for use with the 10× objective. Place these with one of the clear filters.

5. Carefully cut out the set of stops provided for use with the 40× objective and place these with the other filter.

6. Set up the microscope in the usual way to obtain the *best* illumination. Make sure the light source is centred.

7. Raise the condenser to its uppermost position.

8. Make a test specimen preparation on a slide by mixing a small amount of saliva taken from the side of the mouth (to include a few epithelial cells) and a small drop of a weak saline suspension of red cells. Cover with a cover glass.

   Important: The slide and cover glass must be completely clean and the preparation sufficiently thin.

9. Focus the preparation with the 10× objective in the usual way. Close sufficiently the condenser iris while focusing the specimen, and when focused open it *fully* again.

10. Select out of the three 10× stops provided, the one which gives the best dark-field, i.e. the brightest illuminated cells and particles against a black background.

    To find the best stop, place each in turn in the centre of the clear filter. The stop is centrally placed when its cross mark matches exactly that on the filter. Use a piece of plasticine, Blutak, or very *small* drop of immersion oil to hold the stop in position when trying it.

    Note: If the stop selected is too small, light will enter the objective and dark-field will not be achieved. If the stop size is too large, insufficient light will reach the specimen and the organisms or cells will be poorly illuminated and difficult to see (the same will also occur if the light source is not bright enough).

    When the stop which gives the best dark-field is selected, glue this permanently to the filter, and mark it 10×.

11. Change to the 40× objective, and focus the specimen (if the specimen shows signs of drying, make another). Adjust the condenser iris while focusing the specimen, and then open it *fully* again.

    If using a mirror to reflect the light, make sure the mirror is adjusted to give the best illumination.

    Note: When using the 40× objective, a bright and central illumination is *essential* to give good dark-field.

12. Select from the set of 40× stops provided, the one which gives the best dark-field. Position each stop carefully in the centre of the second clear filter using the same technique as described in step No. 10.

    To obtain good dark-field with the 40× objective, the stop *must* be of the correct size. This is why a range of 6 stops is provided from which to select the best. Slight adjustment of the filter holder may also be necessary to obtain good dark-field with the 40× objective. The source of light *must* be adequate.

    When the correct size of stop is selected for the 40× objective, glue it to the clear filter, and mark it 40x.

Problems associated with dark-field microscopy

Difficulties in using dark-field microscopy may arise from:

— Imperfect focusing or centring of a dark ground condenser.

— Using a lamp that is not sufficiently bright or correctly aligned.

— Using a slide or cover glass that is not completely clean.

— Too dense a specimen.

— A bubble in the immersion oil, or insufficient oil contact between the specimen and objective, or between the specimen and a dark ground condenser (when using a 100× oil immersion objective).

Value of dark-field microscopy
This form of microscopy is particularly useful for examining living micro-organisms such as:

☐ *Treponema pallidum* spirochaetes in chancre fluid, the movement of which cannot be seen by ordinary transmitted light.

☐ Borreliae in blood.

☐ Leptospires in urine.

☐ Microfilariae in blood because the sheath of the pathogenic species can be easily seen by dark-field.

☐ Vibrios and campylobacters in specimens and cultures.

4:10 FLUORESCENCE MICROSCOPY

Fluorescence microscopy is widely used in the immunodiagnosis of important bacteriological and parasitic diseases. Recent developments in the production of monoclonal reagents have made this form of microscopy more important and more widely used. Fluorescence is also of particular value in examining sputum and other specimens for tubercle bacilli using auramine. Acridine orange is also an excellent fluorochrome (fluorescent dye) for demonstrating some parasites and bacteria (see later text).

Principle of fluorescence
White light is composed of seven different colours, i.e. red, orange, yellow, green, blue, indigo, and violet. These form what is called the visible spectrum, each colour having its own wavelength, red the longest, and violet the shortest (see 25:1).

There are, however, other wavelengths which are not visible to the eye, including ultra-violet light which has a very short wavelength. Those that are very near to the ultra-violet are of a deep blue colour and only just visible.

In fluorescence microscopy, ultra-violet light or the just-visible deep blue light may be used to illuminate particles or micro-organisms which have been previously stained with fluorescing dyes (fluorochromes). These dyes transform the invisible ultra-violet light into visible light, or the just-visible deep blue light into much more visible yellow or orange light, by increasing their wavelength. This enables fluorescent stained organisms, cells, or their specific structures to be seen glowing (fluorescing) against a dark background.

The effect produced by a fluorochrome depends on its excitation and on the pH of the medium. A commonly used fluorochrome in immunofluorescence is fluorescin isothiocyanate (FITC) which produces a green fluorescence.

Light from a fluorescence lamp is first passed through an optical filter (a primary, or exciting filter) which removes all the unwanted colours (wavelengths) of light and passes only those which are required.

The light is then brought to the specimen by an immersion dark ground condenser (see 4:9) so that none of the unwanted and possibly dangerous ultra-violet light reaches the eye. Fluorescence, e.g. the golden yellow produced by auramine for demonstrating acid fast bacilli, is then given off by the specimen. This, coming to the eye to form the image must pass through a yellow filter (a secondary, or barrier filter) to filter off all light other than the actual fluorescence.

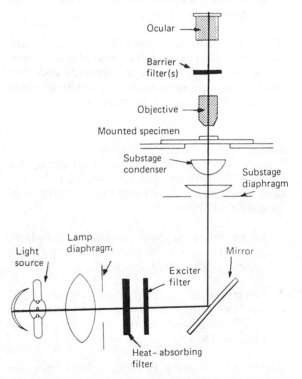

Fig. 4.7 Components of a fluorescence system.
Reproduced with modifications from Introduction to Medical Laboratory Technology. Courtesy Butterworth

Equipment required

It is usual for fluorescence equipment to be made as a unit, and generally as a complete fluorescence microscope. Otherwise the following are required:

— A fluorescence lamp, either mercury vapour or quartz iodine.

A mercury vapour lamp is expensive, heavy and bulky, requires mains supply, and can be a little dangerous. It requires about 20 minutes to warm up and if switched off it must cool before it is switched on again.

A quartz iodine (quartz halogen) lamp is much smaller and cheaper and can be run from a car battery or from a small mains transformer. It can be switched on and off without requiring a warming up or cooling down period. There are some fields of work for which a mercury lamp may be necessary, but for most fluorescence work a quartz iodine lamp is ideal.

— A primary, or exciting, filter. The transmission of this filter must match the emission peak of the fluorochrome being used (see *Note* below).

— A secondary, or barrier, filter.

— An immersion dark ground condenser, as described in 4:9.

— Liquid paraffin or other *non-fluorescing* immersion oil for the condenser and 100× oil immersion objective.

Note: The use of the correct filters is very important in fluorescence work. The correct filter combinations to use in fluorescent antibody tests and other fluorescent techniques are usually specified in test methods or by filter suppliers.

Setting up fluorescence microscopy

With a complete fluorescence microscope, the maker's instructions should be used for the particular instrument. Otherwise the following steps should be followed:

1. Set up the quartz iodine (quartz halogen) lamp in its housing in front of the microscope as for ordinary transmitted light work.

2. Insert the dark ground condenser, and using liquid paraffin or a non-fluorescing immersion fluid, focus and centre the condenser as explained in 4:9.

3. Insert the primary, or exciting, filter anywhere conveniently between the quartz iodine lamp and the condenser, possibly in the substage filter holder.

4. Insert the yellow barrier filter anywhere conveniently between the objective and the eye, possibly clipped on above the eyepiece.

5. Insert a specimen stained with the appropriate fluorochrome, focus, and examine. In the beginning, the help of an experienced person will be required to examine fluorescence preparations, particularly fluorescent antibody preparations.

Value of fluorescence microscopy

Important applications of fluorescence microscopy include:

☐ Examination of sputum and cerebrospinal fluid for acid fast bacilli (AFB) using an auramine staining technique (see 34:7 in Volume II of the Manual).

☐ Examination of acridine orange stained specimens for *Trichomonas vaginalis* flagellates, *Entamoeba histolytica* cysts (chromatoid bodies fluoresce), intracellular gonococci and meningococci, and other parasites and bacteria (see 34:13 in Volume II of the Manual).

☐ Immunodiagnosis using both indirect or direct fluorescent antibody tests, especially with monoclonal reagents which are highly specific.

Recent developments in fluorescence

Illumination for fluorescence has in recent years been improved by the use of reflected (incident) and the use of modern dichroic filters that transmit one wavelength and reflect another. These systems give excellent fluorescence but are very expensive.

4:11 MEASUREMENT USING A CALIBRATED EYEPIECE SCALE

The measurement of objects using a calibrated eyepiece scale (micrometer) is called micrometry. The eyepiece micrometer scale requires calibration from a measured scale engraved on a glass slide (stage graticule).

Required

— Eyepiece micrometer to fit into a Huygenian 10× eyepiece or if available a special measuring 10× eyepiece. A suitable line scale for the eyepiece micrometer is one that is divided into 50 divisions.

— Stage graticule to calibrate the eyepiece scale. A suitable scale for the stage graticule is one that measures 2 mm in length with each large division measuring 0.1 mm (100 μm) and each small division measuring 0.01 mm (10 μm).

Availability of eyepiece micrometer and stage graticule

An eyepiece micrometer with a line scale having 50 divisions can be obtained from Graticules Ltd, code No. E3, priced approx £12.50 (1986). When ordering, the diameter of the graticule required must be stated, e.g. to fit an eyepiece of internal measurement (when top lens screwed off) 16mm, 19 mm, or 21 mm.

A stage graticule measuring 2 mm in length with 0.1 mm and 0.01 mm divisions can be obtained from Graticules Ltd, code No. S22, price approx. £15.00 (1986).

Note: If a stage graticule is not available it is possible to calibrate an eyepiece micrometer scale using a haemocytometer (counting chamber).

Method of calibrating an eyepiece micrometer

The eyepiece micrometer will require calibration for each objective of the microscope at which measurements will be required. For parasitology, the scale should be calibrated for the 40× objective and for haematology it is useful to calibrate for the 100× objective. A table can be prepared for each objective giving the measurements for 1 to 50 divisions of the eyepiece scale.

The method of calibrating is as follows:

1. Unscrew the upper lens of a 10× Huygenian eyepiece and insert the eyepiece micrometer disc, with engraved side facing down.

2. Place the stage graticule slide on the stage of the microscope and with the required objective in place, bring the scale into focus. Both the eyepiece scale and the calibration scale should be focused clearly. If required, unscrew slightly the top of the eyepiece lens to bring the eyepiece scale into sharp focus with the calibration scale of the stage graticule.

3. Adjust the field until the 0 line of the eyepiece scale aligns exactly with the 0 line of the calibration scale.

4. Look along the scales and note where a division of the eyepiece scale aligns exactly with a division of the calibration scale.

5. Measure the distance between the 0 point and where the alignment occurs. The measurements of the calibration scale (as described under *Required*) are 0.1 mm to 2.0 mm. Each small subdividion measures 0.01 mm.

6. Count the number of divisions of the eyepiece scale covered between the 0 point and where the alignment occurs.

7. Calculate the measurement of 1 of the divisions of the eyepiece scale, in μm.

Example (as shown in Fig. 4.8)

Distance measured = 0.2 mm
Number of divisions = 27

1 division measures: $\dfrac{0.2}{27} = 0.0074$ mm

To convert mm to μm: $0.0074 \times 1000 = 7.4 \ \mu$m

8. Make tables giving the measurements for 1 to 50 eyepiece divisions.

Repeat the calibration and calculations for each objective.

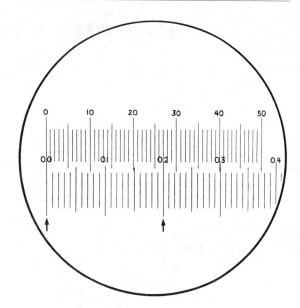

Fig. 4.8 Calibrating an eyepiece micrometer. Top scale is that of the eyepiece micrometer. Lower scale is that of the stage graticule.
From Melvin and Brooke 1969. Courtesy of US Dept of the Air Force and Army.

Measuring an object, e.g. cyst using a calibrated eyepiece micrometer

With the eyepiece micrometer scale and the cyst sharply focused, position the cyst along the scale and count the divisions covered. Refer to the previously prepared table for the objective being used to obtain the measurement for the number of divisions counted. This will give the size of the cyst in μm.

Recommended Reading

Bradbury, S. *An Introduction to the Optical Microscope*, Royal Microscopical Society Handbook 01. Oxford University Press, 1984.

Hartley, W. G. *Hartley's Microscopy*, Senecio Publishing Company Ltd, 1979.

SECTION II

ANATOMY AND PHYSIOLOGY

Organization and Framework of the Human Body

5:1 BASIC STRUCTURE AND ORGANIZATION OF THE HUMAN BODY

The human body is made up of a large number of cells which are the basic units of all living matter. Different kinds of cells are bound together to form special tissues and these specialized tissues working together form the organs of the body. A number of organs may work together as a system with a particular function. The different systems of the body work closely together. The study of the structure and arrangement of organs in the body is called anatomy and the study of how they function is called physiology.

Systems of the Body	*Organs*	*Function*
Skeletal	Bones Joints Muscles	• To provide a framework to support the body and enable it to move.
Respiratory	Lungs Nose Air passages (trachea, bronchi and bronchioles) Respiratory muscles	• To take in air containing oxygen for aerobic cell metabolism. • To expel air containing carbon dioxide, the main end product of metabolism.
Circulatory	Heart Blood vessels Lymphatics	• To provide tissue cells with oxygen and the substances and environment required for cellular activity. • To transport the waste products from the cells to the organs of excretion.
Digestive	Mouth and oesophagus Stomach Intestines Liver Pancreas	• To ingest and digest food so that nutrients can be absorbed and subsequently utilized by the body. • To excrete the waste matter which remains after digestion.
Urinary	Kidneys Ureters Bladder Urethra	• To filter out the waste substances from the blood and excrete them in the urine. • To reabsorb essential molecules. • To control the body's fluid and electrolyte balance. • To control acid-base balance.
Nervous	Brain Spinal cord Nerves Sense organs	• To co-ordinate the activities of the body in harmony with its environment.
Endocrine	Pituitary gland Thyroid gland Parathyroid glands Adrenal glands Sex glands (ovaries and testes) Endocrine glands in pancreas and kidneys	• To produce hormones which are chemical messengers released into the blood stream to regulate some of the body's activities.
Immune	Bone marrow Thymus Spleen Lymph nodes Mononuclear phagocytic network	• To defend the body against invasion by pathogens. • To remove toxins, damaged cells, and cellular debris. • To destroy tumour cells.
Reproductive	*Male*: Testes, prostate gland, seminal vesicles, penis *Female*: Ovaries, uterine tubes, uterus, cervix, vagina	• To produce new life.

5:2　CELL STRUCTURE AND PHYSIOLOGY

An animal cell which divides consists of:

- A central nucleus which controls the cell's activities. It is surrounded by a nuclear membrane.
- Cytoplasm which contains organized structures called organelles and substances necessary for the life of the cell. The cytoplasm is surrounded by a semi-permeable membrane which allows substances to pass through it selectively. This controls the concentration of different substances inside the cell.

Structure and function of the nucleus

The nucleus is important because it controls the activities of the cell, especially its reproduction. It contains the chromatin of the cell which is the material from which the chromosomes are formed when the cell divides (see 5:3). The chromatin is mainly composed of deoxyribonucleic acid (DNA), the molecules of which store the genetic information of the cell.

DNA

DNA is a large and complicated double stranded spiral (helix) molecule. It is composed of many small units called nucleotides, each of which contains:

— A sugar (deoxyribose)
— A phosphoric acid residue
— A nitrogenous base (adenine, guanine, thymine or cystosine)

The positioning of the nitrogenous bases in the double stranded molecule is shown in Fig. 5.2. Adenine (A) always pairs with thymine (T) and guanine (G) with cystosine (C). The information which the cell needs to make its various amino acids (organic acids from which proteins are built) is determined by the order in which the different bases are arranged along the strands of DNA.

The production instructions (genetic coding) stored in the DNA molecules are carried by messenger ribonucleic acid (m-RNA) to the 'factories' in the cytoplasm which make the proteins for the cell. The protein factories are called ribosomes. They are present in large numbers in living cells, either attached to the endoplasmic reticulum or present in small clusters (polyribosomes) in the cytoplasm. These sites of protein synthesis produce the polypeptide chains required by the cell.

RNA

RNA is similar in structure to DNA except that it generally consists of only one strand, contains ribose instead of deoxyribose and the base thymine is replaced by uracil (U). RNA is synthesized by an area within the nucleus called the nucleolus.

Strands of m-RNA are produced with base sets (each set consisting of 3 bases) which match those contained in the DNA molecule.

When a strand of m-RNA with its production instructions leaves the nucleus and enters the cytoplasm, a ribosome attaches to one end of it. Another type of RNA present in the cytoplasm called transfer RNA (t-RNA) then brings the correct amino acids to the ribosome for assembly. Each amino acid attaches to a particular t-RNA. The t-RNA with its attached amino acid links up with its corresponding base set along the strand of m-RNA (see Fig. 5.3).

The ribosome moves along the m-RNA joining together the different amino acids brought into position by the t-RNA. Several ribosomes can become connected to each strand of m-RNA so that a single m-RNA strand can produce a number of amino acid (polypeptide) chains. In this way highly complex proteins, which determine the nature and activity of the cell, are gradually built up.

Structure and function of cytoplasm organelles

The important organelles found in the cytoplasm of cells are as follows:

Mitochondria

Mitochondria are small bodies which are involved in cell respiration, i.e. a process of liberating energy from nutrients by oxidation. They are more plentiful in cells which require a great deal of energy and are often referred to as the powerhouses of the cell. Depending on the type of cell, the mitochondria may be evenly distributed or accumulated in selected sites in the cytoplasm.

Mitochondria contain all the enzymes required to convert nutrients and oxygen into energy in the form of a compound called adenosine triphosphate (ATP). This diffuses out of the mitochondria whenever it is needed to provide energy for cellular functions.

Endoplasmic reticulum

The endoplasmic reticulum (ER) is a complex network of membrane-bound canals and cavities which function as a kind of circulatory system to transfer materials through the cell. It is continuous with the outer wall of the nuclear membrane. Parts of the lining of the canals are coated with ribosomes. The parts of the membrane which are free from ribosomes (smooth ER) are thought in some cells to synthesize fats and similar substances.

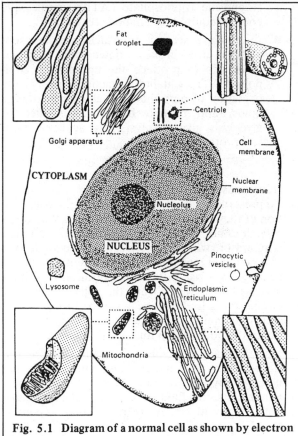

Fig. 5.1 Diagram of a normal cell as shown by electron microscopy.

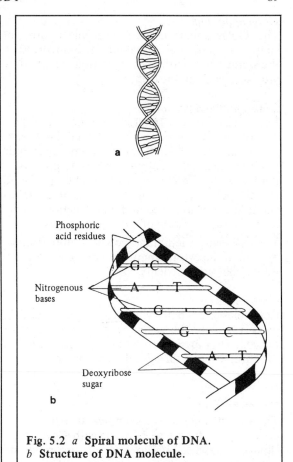

**Fig. 5.2 *a* Spiral molecule of DNA.
b Structure of DNA molecule.**

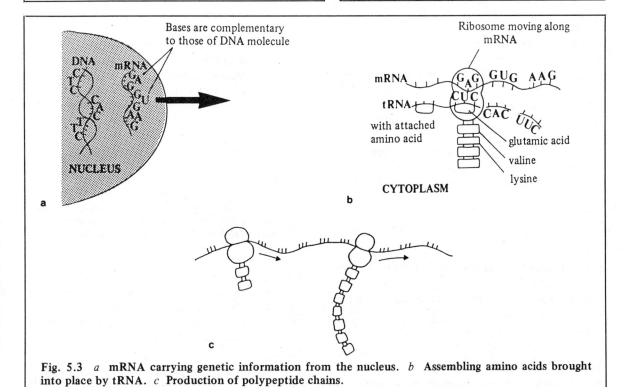

Fig. 5.3 *a* mRNA carrying genetic information from the nucleus. *b* Assembling amino acids brought into place by tRNA. *c* Production of polypeptide chains.

Acknowledgement: Fig. 5.1 Reproduced from Introduction to Medical Laboratory Technology, courtesy of Butterworth.

Golgi apparatus

The Golgi apparatus is a specialized area of smooth endoplasmic reticulum. It is involved in the storage and synthesis of secretions before they are excreted from the cell.

Lysosomes and vacuoles

Lysosomes are very small membrane-bound parcels of enzymes used in the intracellular breakdown of particles. They contain hydrolytic enzymes including acid phosphatases, proteases, nucleases, and lipases. Many lysosomes are found in cells such as macrophages and neutrophils where they are involved in the destruction of bacteria and the digestion of nutrient particles.

Vacuoles are membrane-bound compartments present in the cytoplasm of the cell. They contain water, salts and nutrients.

Centrioles

Centrioles are small cylindrical bodies found in pairs lying near the nucleus in the centrosome of the cell. They are important in the organization of the chromosomes during cell division (see 5:3).

Cell membrane

The cell membrane is a complex structure composed of a double layer of protein with a layer of fat (lipid) in between. It allows water to pass in and out of the cell and has the ability to absorb selectively certain molecules from the surrounding environment and to release certain products into it. This is brought about either by an active transport mechanism or by differences in the osmotic pressures of the fluids on each side of the membrane.

The cell membrane is also involved in the joining together of cells and their recognition by other cells.

Living cells are bound together for support and strength by what are called intracellular substances. These include collagen, elastic fibres, and reticular fibres.

5:3 METABOLISM AND MULTIPLICATION OF LIVING CELLS

Metabolism is the collective term used to describe the many chemical reactions which take place in the body.

Metabolic activity includes:

- Anabolic reactions, in which the essential constituents of cells are built-up (synthesized), e.g. the synthesis of protein from amino acids.

Adenosine triphosphate (ATP) supplies the energy required for anabolic reactions.

- Catabolic reactions, in which complex substances are broken down into simpler molecules to produce the energy-rich compound ATP. Catabolic reactions involve the oxidation of nutrients such as carbohydrates, lipids, and protein by processes such as glycolysis, glycogenolysis, fatty acid oxidation, and proteolysis.

Homeostasis

To preserve health it is essential that the composition of the medium in and surrounding the body's cells does not vary greatly. For example, a fall in temperature will slow down cellular metabolism, a change in pH may interfere with essential enzyme activity, or a rise in the concentration of solutes may withdraw water from the cells by osmosis. Homeostasis is the name given to the processes which maintain the chemical and physical properties of the body within functional ranges.

Many organs are involved in maintaining a constant internal environment. The skin assists in regulating body temperature, the kidneys are important in regulating fluid and electrolyte balance, and both lungs and kidneys work together to control the acid base-balance in the body.

Multiplication of cells

The multiplication of cells is essential for growth and for replacing damaged and worn out cells. The orderly process by which cells divide is called mitosis. In mitosis two new cells are produced, each having 46 chromosomes which contain genes identical to that of the original cell. It is a continuous process in which the following phases (stages) can be recognized:

Interphase

This is a resting stage during which there is an increase in DNA, RNA, and protein in preparation for cell division. When the nuclear material in the cell has doubled (replicated), cell division can begin.

Prophase

The nuclear chromatin becomes concentrated to form the chromosomes. Each pair of chromosomes consists of two identical chromatids (strands) attached at one point called the centromere.

The two centrioles separate and move to opposite ends of the cell joined by protein fibres called the mitotic, or achromatic, spindle. This is an important step in cell division because without the formation of the mitotic spindle, division cannot take place. At the end of prophase the nuclear membrane and nucleolus have disappeared.

Metaphase
During this stage the chromosomes migrate to the centre of the cell and arrange themselves in a line along the mitotic spindle. Each chromosome divides longitudinally.

Anaphase
This is a short phase in which the centromeres separate and the two chromatids are pulled apart towards opposite ends of the cell by the spindle fibres. At the end of anaphase the cell contains two sets of identical chromosomes.

Telophase
The chromosomes become thread-like and less distinct until they eventually become a mass of chromatin. A nucleolus appears. A nuclear membrane forms around each set of chromosomes and the cytoplasm then divides to give two independent cells which are identical one with another and with the parent cell from which they were formed.

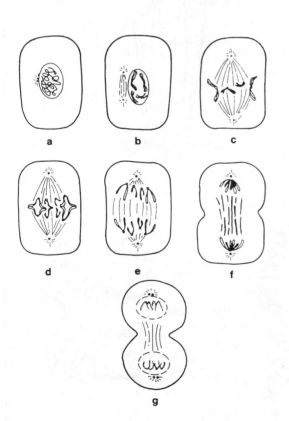

Fig. 5.4 Process of mitosis. *a* Early prophase, *b* later prophase, *c* metaphase, *d e f* anaphase, *g* telophase.
Reproduced from Introduction to Medical Laboratory Technology. Courtesy of Butterworth.

Note: A further description of the structure of chromosomes and of the inheritance of genetic material is given in Chapter 10.

5:4 SKELETAL SYSTEM

The skeletal system forms the supporting framework of the body.

It consists of:

- Bones
- Joints
- Muscles

The main functions of the skeletal system are as follows:

— To support the weight of the body.

— To protect the organs of the body such as the brain, heart, and lungs.

— To give movement to the body. Bones and joints act as levers for movement. Muscles are attached to the bones by way of tendons.

— To store calcium and release it when required. When the level of calcium in the blood falls, calcium is released from bone tissue into the plasma under the influence of parathyroid hormone.

— To manufacture erythrocytes, platelets, monocytes, and granulocytic leucocytes in the red marrow of the bones. The formation of blood cells in bone marrow is called haemopoiesis and is described in 11:2.

Bone tissue
Bone is a connective tissue produced by osteoblast cells. It consists of protein in which calcium salts (mainly calcium phosphate in complex crystal form) have been deposited to give it strength.

Vitamin D is essential for the adequate absorption and utilization of calcium in the body. A lack of vitamin D results in a failure to lay down calcium salts in bone (mineralization). This causes the bones to be soft and unable to support the weight of the body. In children this results in the disease rickets in which the legs are bent. In adults the condition is called osteomalacia and often causes bone pain or bone fractures.

Calcium is also required for the normal activity of muscle and therefore in rickets and osteomalacia there is often muscle weakness.

The bones of a healthy young person are flexible and strong. It has been shown that the density of bone declines in all people from the age of about forty. As a result the bones gradually become more brittle and fracture more easily. This condition is

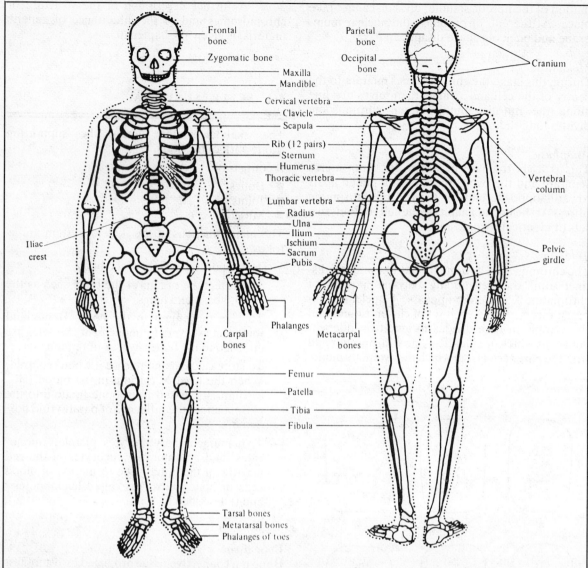

Fig. 5.5 Bones of the skeleton.

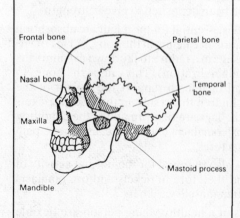

Side view of the skull.
Courtesy of St John Ambulance Association.

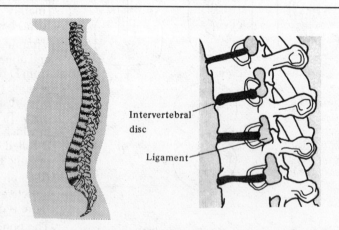

Left **Side view of the vertebral column.** *Right* **Close-up view showing the arrangement of vertebrae.**
Courtesy of St John Ambulance Association.

known as osteoporosis. It can be differentiated from osteomalacia by examining the bone tissue microscopically.The structure of osteoporotic bone is normal but less dense whereas in osteomalacia (or rickets) there is reduced mineralization of bone.

Bones of the skeleton

The bones of the skeleton are shown in Fig. 5.5 and consist of:

☐ Bones of the skull
☐ Vertebral column, or spine
☐ Ribs and the sternum
☐ Bones of the upper limbs and shoulder
☐ Bones of the lower limbs and pelvic girdle

Different types of bone

The bones of the skeleton are of four different types:

— Long bones, such as the tibia and femur.
— Short bones, such as the carpals and tarsals.
— Irregular bones, such as are found in the vertebral column.
— Flat bones, such as the iliac bones and skull bones.

Skull

The purpose of the skull (cranium) is to protect the brain. The different bones of the cranium are shown in Fig. 5.5. The teeth are found in the upper jaw (maxilla) and the lower jaw (mandible).

Vertebral column

The vertebral column consists of 33 separate bones. These surround and protect the spinal cord which lies in the vertebral canal (see also 9:1). Between each vertebra there is a disc of cartilage and ligaments which allows slight movement between the bones.

The ligaments, discs, and muscles support the backbone giving it strength to carry the body in the upright position.

Ribs and sternum

The ribs and the sternum (breastbone) form a cage which protects the lungs and the heart. When diagnosing blood cell disorders, the upper sternum is often the site from which bone marrow is aspirated for examination. The other site which may be selected for bone marrow aspiration is the iliac crest (see Fig. 5.5).

Joints

The movement of the bones of the skeleton occurs at joints and is brought about by muscles.

Different types of joint

Joints may be of three kinds:

— Immovable joints (sutures), such as are found between the bones of the skull.
— Slightly movable joints (cartilaginous joints), such as are found between two vertebrae or a rib and a vertebra.
— Freely movable joints (synovial joints), such as are found at the knee, elbow, shoulder, or hip.

The range of movement possible in these joints depends on the shape of the bones and on the ligaments and muscles holding the joints together. The knee and elbow are what are called hinge joints which means that movement is possible in only one plane. The shoulder and hip joints are of the ball and socket type enabling movement to be made in several directions.

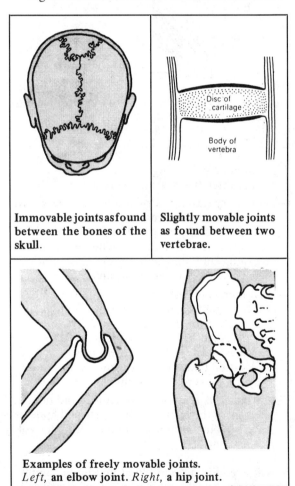

Immovable joints as found between the bones of the skull.

Slightly movable joints as found between two vertebrae.

Disc of cartilage

Body of vertebra

Examples of freely movable joints.
Left, an elbow joint. *Right,* a hip joint.

Muscles

Muscles are made of bundles of fibres which can contract, pulling together the bones to which they are attached as illustrated in Fig. 5.6. The muscles are covered in fibrous tissue and joined to the bone by a tendon. In a well-nourished person, muscle tissue makes up the major part of the soft tissue of the body.

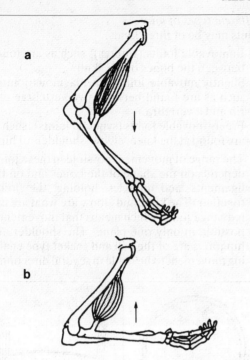

Fig. 5.6   Biceps muscle (voluntary) of the arm.
a Relaxed, *b* Contracted.
Courtesy of St John   Ambulance Association.

Types of muscle

There are three types of muscle tissue:

— Voluntary (striped, or striated) muscle which contracts and produces movements in response to conscious efforts of will, e.g. muscles of the head, trunk, arms and legs. The muscle fibres are long and thin and show cross-striations when examined microscopically.

— Involuntary (unstriped, or smooth) muscle which produces movements without a conscious effort of the will, e.g. muscles found in the digestive tract, air passages, bladder, and blood vessels. The muscle fibres are shorter and fatter than voluntary muscle fibres and they have no cross-striations.

— Cardiac (heart) muscle which is found only in the wall of the heart. It has the striped appearance of voluntary muscle but is not under voluntary control.

Muscles require a good blood and nerve supply. The energy which muscles need to contract is mainly supplied by the breakdown and oxidation of glucose from muscle glycogen. An additional source of energy for muscle contraction is creatine which combines with phosphorus in the muscle tissue to form the energy-rich compound phosphocreatinine. Creatinine is a breakdown product of creatine metabolism and is excreted by the kidneys.

Recommended Reading

The following publications are recommended as reference books for the entire Anatomy and Physiology Section:

Govan, A. T., Macfarlane, P., Callander, R. *Pathology Illustrated*, Churchill Livingstone, 2nd edition, 1986. International Student edition priced £8.25. Highly recommended.

Solomon, E. P., Davis, P. W. *Human Anatomy and Physiology*. Holt-Saunders, 1983. Available from medical bookshops and Holt Saunders Ltd, 1 St Anne's Road, Eastbourne, East Sussex BN21 3UN, UK. Paperback edition priced £12.95. This is an excellent 800 page book, well illustrated in full colour.

Ross, J. R. W., Marks, K. *Balliéres Anatomy Illustrated*, 1986. Available from medical bookshops and Holt Saunders Ltd, 1 St Anne's Road, Eastbourne, East Sussex, BN21 3UN, UK, priced £4.15. Compact 64 page book having 16 pages of colour illustrations.

Wilson, K. J. W. *Ross and Wilson: Foundations of Anatomy and Physiology*, Churchill Livingstone, 5th edition,1981. Available from medical bookshops and Longman Group Ltd,Pinnacles, Fourth Avenue, Harlow, Essex CM19 5AA, UK, ELBS price £3.50. A 291 page book, well illustrated in colour and black and white.

Akinsanya, J. A. *Human Biology*. Macmillan International College Editions, 1980. Copies available from medical bookshops and Macmillan Press Ltd, Houndmills, Basingstoke, Hampshire RG21 2XS, UK, priced £5.95. A 248 page book, applicable to developing countries and well illustrated in black and white.

Paterson, C. R. *Essentials of Human Biochemistry*, Pitman/Longman, 1983. Copies available from medical bookshops and Longman Group Ltd, Fourth Avenue, Harlow, Essex CM19 5AA, UK, priced £12.50. A 275 page book, applicable to developing countries and well illustrated in black and white.

Winwood, R. S., Smith, J. L. *Sears' Anatomy and Physiology for Nurses*, Edward Arnold, 6th edition, 1985. Copies available from Medical bookshops and Edward Arnold Ltd, PO Box 34, Woodlands Park Avenue, Woodlands Park, Maidenhead, Berkshire SL6 5BS, UK, ELBS price £2.95. Up to date book of 310 pages with some illustrations in colour.

6 Respiratory and Circulatory Systems

6:1 BASIC STRUCTURE OF THE RESPIRATORY SYSTEM

The organs which make up the respiratory system include:

- Nose
- Pharynx
- Air passages, i.e. trachea, bronchi and bronchioles
- Lungs

Lungs
The lungs are covered by two thin sheets of tissue called the pleurae. The inner, or visceral, pleura is a serous membrane which closely covers the lung.

The outer, or parietal, pleura lines the thoracic cavity. The two layers are continuous with each other at the root, or hilus, of the lung.

In health a small amount of fluid separates the two pleurae so that during normal breathing the two pleurae slide smoothly over each other. In some diseases, however, the volume of this fluid can increase, e.g. in pneumonia, tuberculosis, and lung cancer. Such a collection of fluid is called a pleural effusion. A pleural effusion can also form in illnesses in which the level of protein in the blood is low, e.g. severe malnutrition and the nephrotic syndrome. If the amount of fluid is large it can cause difficulty in breathing (dyspnoea).

The basic structure of the respiratory system is shown in Fig.6.1.

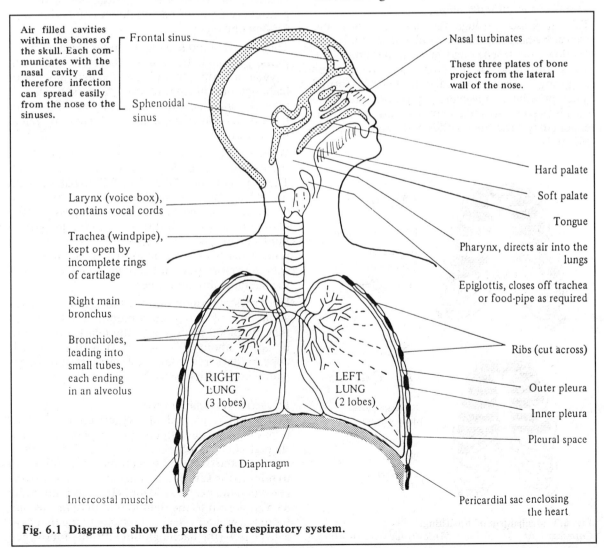

Air filled cavities within the bones of the skull. Each communicates with the nasal cavity and therefore infection can spread easily from the nose to the sinuses.

Frontal sinus

Sphenoidal sinus

Nasal turbinates

These three plates of bone project from the lateral wall of the nose.

Hard palate

Soft palate

Tongue

Larynx (voice box), contains vocal cords

Trachea (windpipe), kept open by incomplete rings of cartilage

Right main bronchus

Bronchioles, leading into small tubes, each ending in an alveolus

RIGHT LUNG (3 lobes)

LEFT LUNG (2 lobes)

Pharynx, directs air into the lungs

Epiglottis, closes off trachea or food-pipe as required

Ribs (cut across)

Outer pleura

Inner pleura

Pleural space

Diaphragm

Intercostal muscle

Pericardial sac enclosing the heart

Fig. 6.1 Diagram to show the parts of the respiratory system.

6:2   FUNCTIONING OF THE RESPIRATORY SYSTEM

The cells of the human body use oxygen during the process of forming energy from carbohydrates, protein, and fat. Carbon dioxide is produced as a waste product of this process. It is the function of the respiratory system to transfer oxygen from the atmosphere into the blood for transport to the cells and at the same time to expel the waste carbon dioxide.

Mechanism of breathing

The lungs and the chest wall are elastic structures. During inspiration (breathing in), the diaphragm contracts (flattens) and moves downwards and the intercostal muscles contract moving the rib cage upwards to make the thoracic cavity wider and greater in depth from front to back. These movements increase the volume of the thoracic cavity and the sponge-like tissue of the lungs expands to fill it. This draws air into the lungs.

The air passes through the nasal passages and pharynx where it is warmed and moistened. It passes down the trachea and bronchi and enters the lungs. Inspiration is therefore an active process requiring muscular contraction. During normal quiet breathing, however, expiration (breathing out) is passive. At the end of inspiration the air is expelled because the muscles and lungs relax (see Fig. 6.2).

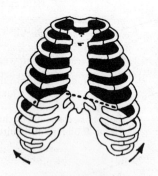

Air In

Rib cage moves up.

Diaphragm moves downwards.

Lungs expand.

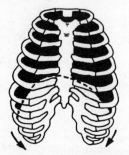

Air Out

Rib cage moves downwards.

Diaphragm moves upwards.

Lungs relax.

Fig. 6.2 Mechanism of breathing.
Courtesy of St John Ambulance Association.

The rate of breathing is controlled by the respiratory centre in the medulla of the brain and by stretch receptors in the lung as well as by voluntary control. At rest, a normal person breathes 12-15 times every minute. Approximately 500 ml of air are inspired and expired with each breath.

Uptake and release of oxygen in the lungs and tissues

The lungs are made up of millions of very small air pockets called alveoli. The walls of the alveoli are very thin and surrounded by blood vessels which means that the air in the alveoli is in very close contact with the blood.

Oxygen is transported in the blood by haemoglobin (Hb), an iron-containing protein found in the red cells. Haemoglobin takes up oxygen when the partial pressure of oxygen (pO_2) in the blood is high and releases oxygen when the pO_2 is low. When the blood is in the lungs therefore, oxygen rapidly combines with haemoglobin in the red cells to form oxyhaemoglobin (see Fig. 6.3). The blood becomes almost fully (97%) saturated with oxygen, every gram of haemoglobin combining with 1.34 ml of oxygen.

The arterial blood leaving the lungs to set off on its journey through the tissues is therefore laden with oxygen providing there is an adequate amount of haemoglobin in the blood. A person who is severely anaemic (low haemoglobin) will suffer from what is called hypoxia (insufficient oxygen in the tissues).

When the blood reaches the tissue cells the pO_2 in the tissues is much lower than that in the blood. The pO_2 in the blood therefore falls to balance with the pO_2 in the tissues. This causes the oxygen to dissociate from the haemoglobin and pass into the plasma from where it diffuses into the interstitial fluid and into the tissue cells. If the oxygen tension is particularly low, e.g. in muscle tissues following exercise, more oxygen becomes dissociated from the haemoglobin molecules.

Under resting conditions, the blood normally loses about 30% of its oxygen content in the tissues, so that the blood returning to the heart, i.e. venous blood, is about 70% saturated with oxygen. It appears dark red compared with arterial oxygenated blood which is bright red in colour.

Oxygen dissociation curve

If a graph is plotted of oxygen uptake and its release against the different partial pressures, an S-shaped curve is obtained (see Fig. 6.4). This is known as the oxygen dissociation curve. It is usual to refer to the saturation of haemoglobin with oxygen when the pO_2 is at 50 mm Hg. This is normally 83.5%. A shift to the right in the curve means that there is a greater release of oxygen to the tissues at a given pO_2 (the haemoglobin's affinity for oxygen

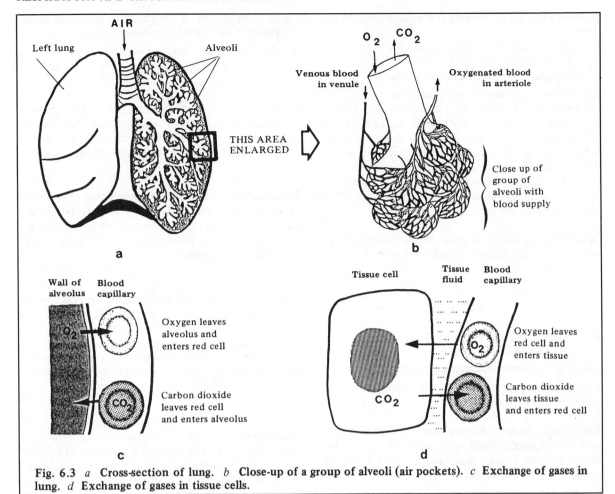

Fig. 6.3 *a* **Cross-section of lung.** *b* **Close-up of a group of alveoli (air pockets).** *c* **Exchange of gases in lung.** *d* **Exchange of gases in tissue cells.**

is reduced). A shift to the left in the curve means that less oxygen is released to the tissues at a given pO_2 (the haemoglobin's affinity for oxygen is increased).

In tropical countries, sickle cell disease is an important condition which produces a shift to the right in the oxygen dissociation curve. In sickle cell disease an abnormal haemoglobin (Hb) called Hb S is found in the red cells. The shift to the right which occurs in sickle cell disease is due to the red cells containing increased amounts of 2,3 diphosphoglycerate (2,3 DPG) which causes the abnormal haemoglobin to release more of its oxygen at a given pO_2. This is important because a person with sickle cell disease may be well oxygenated even though the level of his or her haemoglobin is low. This fact should always be considered when deciding whether to give a sickle cell patient a blood transfusion.

Affect of temperature and pH on the O_2 dissociation curve
Temperature and pH also affect the oxygen dissociation curve. There is a shift to the right in the curve when the temperature is increased and a left shift when the temperature of the blood is decreased.

A fall in pH moves the curve to the right whereas a rise in blood pH shifts the curve to the left. When the pH is low due to dissolved carbon dioxide, it assists the release of oxygen in the tissues and helps the take-up of oxygen in the lungs. The influence of pH on the oxygen dissociation curve is known as the Bohr effect. Because of the S-shape of the curve it can be seen that changes in the flat part of the curve have only a small effect but when the steep part of the curve is reached, a small change in one axis has a marked effect.

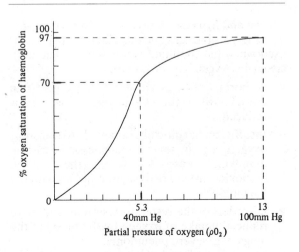

Fig. 6.4 **Haemoglobin oxygen dissociation curve.**

Transfer of carbon dioxide from the tissues to the lungs

An equally important function of the respiratory system is to expel the waste carbon dioxide (CO_2) that is produced in the cells of the body.

As the blood passes through the tissues, there is a transfer of CO_2 from the tissues into the blood. The partial pressure of carbon dioxide (pCO_2) in the blood when it leaves the tissues and reaches the lungs is about 15 mm Hg higher than that in the lungs. With the balance of partial pressures there is a transfer of CO_2 from the blood into the alveolar air in the lungs. From the alveoli, the carbon dioxide leaves the body in the expired air.

Note: The exchange of gases in the lungs and tissues is shown diagrammatically in Fig. 6.3).

6:3   TERMS USED IN RESPIRATORY MEDICINE

The following are some of the terms used in respiratory medicine:

Respiratory failure: A condition in which the normal pressures of oxygen and carbon dioxide in the blood are no longer maintained. Two types of respiratory failure occur:

Type I
The pO_2 in the arterial blood is low and the pCO_2 is normal or low, e.g. in asthma or pneumonia.

Type II
The pO_2 in the arterial blood is low but the pCO_2 is high. This occurs when there is paralysis of the respiratory muscles, e.g. in poliomyelitis or reduced activity of the respiratory centre in the medulla as may occur when taking narcotic drugs.

Anoxia and hypoxia: A severe shortage of oxygen in the tissues is called anoxia. The term hypoxia is used when the condition is less severe. The deficiency in oxygen may be due to:

- A shortage of oxygen in air inhaled, e.g. at high altitudes when the pO_2 in the atmosphere is reduced.
- Insufficient haemoglobin available to transport oxygen, e.g. in severe anaemia or in carbon monoxide poisoning when the carbon monoxide instead of oxygen combines with the haemoglobin.
- Disorders of the respiratory system leading to reduced uptake of oxygen by the blood in the lungs, e.g. severe pneumonia.
- Disorders of the cardiovascular system leading

to a reduction of the rate at which the blood passes from the lungs to the tissues.

- A failure of the cells to take up oxygen from the blood, e.g. in cyanide poisoning of the cells.

Cyanosis: The bluish colour seen in the mucous membranes and skin, especially in the lips, of hypoxic patients. It is due to excessive amounts of reduced haemoglobin in the skin capillaries.

Pneumothorax: A condition in which air is present between the visceral pleura and parietal pleura (the pleural cavity). It causes the lung to collapse. Air can enter the pleural cavity following a stab wound or rib fracture.

Empyema: The presence of pus (purulent effusion) in the pleural cavity as may occur with severe bacterial pneumonia or tuberculosis.

Note: The laboratory examination of pleural fluid and the tests used to differentiate exudates (inflammatory fluids) from transudates (non-inflammatory fluids), are described in 38:14 in Volume II of the manual.

Pneumonia: The filling of the lung alveoli with infected matter. The commonest causes of inflammation of the lung include infection with *Streptococcus pneumoniae* (pneumococci), *Haemophilus influenzae*, *Mycoplasma pneumoniae* and respiratory viruses. Pneumonia is a common cause of death in the elderly and sick.

In lobar pneumonia, the infection generally fills one or more lobes of the lung. In bronchopneumonia the infection is scattered throughout the lungs.

Asthma: A condition in which there are episodes of breathlessness due to severe narrowing of the air passages (bronchoconstriction) with swelling of the cells lining the air passages. Allergens (substances that cause allergies) are often the cause of asthma such as pollen, mite-containing dust, feathers, fungal spores, etc. The condition is often made worse by stress, smoke, or respiratory tract infections.

Bronchitis: Inflammation of the mucous membrane of the bronchi. This is characterized by the production of sputum and may be acute or chronic.

Pulmonary tuberculosis: This is caused by infection with *Mycobacterium tuberculosis* (tubercle bacillus). The disease results in the formation of small nodules (tubercles) in the lungs, each consisting of a mass of epithelioid cells surrounded by lymphocytes and fibroblasts. The enlargement and joining together of these tubercles cause widespread destruction of lung tissue with the production of highly infective sputum.

Lung cancer: A malignant tumour which may originate in the lung (primary lung cancer) or in other organs and spread to the lung (secondaries). The malignant cells may be found in the sputum. It has been proved that cigarette smoking greatly increases the risk of developing primary lung cancer.

URTI: An abbreviation meaning upper respiratory tract infection. It is often confused with UTI which means urinary tract infection (ideally, abbreviations should not be used even though their use saves space on laboratory forms).

PUO: An abbreviation meaning pyrexia (fever) of unknown origin.

6:4 BASIC STRUCTURE OF THE CIRCULATORY SYSTEM

The circulatory system, also called the cardiovascular system, consists of:

- The heart
- Network of vessels through which the heart continuously pumps blood

Heart
The heart is a muscular organ situated in the thorax, extending approximately from the third rib to about the sixth rib, just to the left of the midline. It is said to have an apex and a base. The heart is divided into two halves by a septum. Each half is further sub-divided into two chambers called the atria (singular atrium) and the ventricles (singular ventricle). The movement of blood through the chambers of the heart is controlled by the tricuspid valve and the mitral valve as shown in Fig. 6.5.

The heart is enclosed in a strong fibrous sac called the fibrous pericardium. This layer is continuous above and behind with the outer coats of the great vessels which enter and leave the heart, i.e. aorta, pulmonary arteries, superior vena cava, and pulmonary veins.

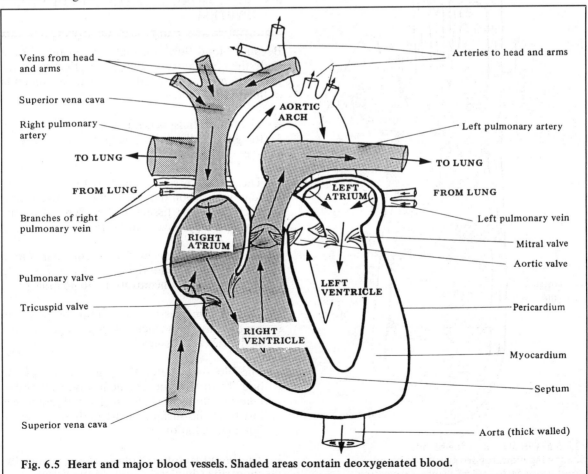

Fig. 6.5 Heart and major blood vessels. Shaded areas contain deoxygenated blood.

Within the fibrous sac lies the serous pericardium (see Fig. 6.5). The inner layer of serous pericardium which closely covers the heart is known as the visceral layer. The outer layer which lines the fibrous sac is known as the parietal layer. These two layers are continuous with each other and the space between them normally contains a small amount of fluid to prevent friction during the movement of the heart as it beats.

In a number of conditions, usually associated with a general disorder or with pulmonary disease, the pericardial linings can become inflamed. This is known as pericarditis. Common causes include tuberculosis, rheumatic fever, and viral infections especially coxsackie B virus. Pericarditis can also be caused by myocardial infarction and as a complication of bacterial infection. In response to inflammation the amount of pericardial fluid can increase. This is called a pericardial effusion and if the volume is large or it accumulates rapidly it can prevent the heart working efficiently.

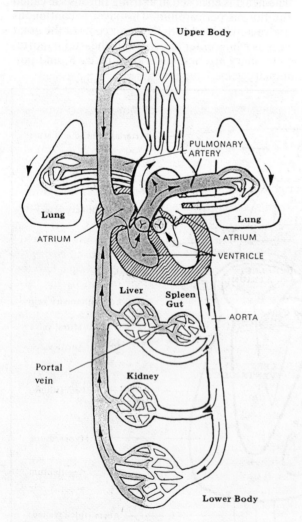

Fig. 6.6 Circulation of the blood.
Shadowing indicates deoxygenated blood.
Courtesy of St John Ambulance Association.

Blood vessels
The blood vessels which make up the cardiovascular system consist of:

☐ Arteries, which are thick-walled and carry the oxygenated (arterial) blood away from the heart.

☐ Arterioles, which are the smaller vessels into which the arteries lead.

☐ Capillaries, which are the smallest blood vessels. These form a network through all the organs and tissues of the body. As the blood circulates in the capillaries through the organs and tissues, oxygen and nutrients are removed from it.

☐ Venules, which are the small vessels that collect the venous blood from the capillaries.

☐ Veins, which are the thin-walled vessels containing valves that collect the venous blood from the venules and return it to the heart.

6:5 FUNCTIONING OF THE CIRCULATORY SYSTEM

Because blood flows through every organ in the body the circulatory system is an effective transport system. It is involved in every major function of the body as follows:

— The blood transports nutrients (absorbed from the gut) to all parts of the body for use or storage.

— The blood carries oxygen to the tissues and removes carbon dioxide and other waste products from the tissues to be excreted by the lungs, kidneys, liver, and skin.

— The blood contains buffer systems to maintain the pH of the blood between pH 7.37-7.45 (hydrogen ion concentration, 36-44 mol/l).

— The osmotic pressure of proteins in the blood controls the movement of water between the capillaries and tissues.

— The blood regulates the temperature of the body by distributing the heat produced by cellular metabolism. Heat which is not required is lost from the surface of the body by evaporation and radiation.

— The blood transports the hormones from the endocrine (ductless) glands to the tissues.

Volume of blood in the circulatory system

The heart and blood vessels form a closed system within the body. The same amount of blood that is pumped out of the heart returns to it. There are 5 to 6 litres (about 10 pints) of blood in the circulatory system of an adult and about 300 ml in the system of a newborn baby.

Conducting system of the heart and cardiac cycle

A specialized cluster of cells in the right atrium of the heart is able to discharge a regular electrical impulse. These cells make up what is called the sino-atrial node (SA node) which constitutes the normal cardiac pacemaker. From the SA node the electrical impulse passes through the atrial muscles to reach another cluster of cells called the atrio-ventricular node (AV node). From the AV node the impulse passes down a bundle of fibres to be carried to the ventricular muscle. This orderly progression of the electrical impulse causes the heart to beat in an organised manner. The atrial impulse causes atrial contraction and shortly afterwards the impulse passing through the ventricles causes ventricular contraction.

In certain diseases e.g. coronary artery disease the heart's conducting system can be damaged. As a result, either the impulses may not be formed normally by the SA node or their passage down the conducting system may be delayed or prevented. The heart may then beat too slowly to work efficiently and an artificial pacemaker may be used to restore a more normal heart rate.

At rest the heart of a healthy person beats about 60-80 times/minute. The pumping action is brought about by the contraction of the myocardium (heart muscle) which pushes blood out into the arteries. The phase of contraction is called systole. This is followed immediately by a period of rest when the heart relaxes and blood is sucked into the right and left atria from the superior and inferior vena cavae and pulmonary veins (see Fig. 6.5). The phase of relaxation is called diastole.

The blood in the right atrium passes through the tricuspid valve into the right ventricle while at the same time blood in the left atrium passes through the mitral valve into the left ventricle.

The ventricles then contract, the atrio-ventricular valves close, and the blood is squeezed out from the left ventricle through the aortic valve into the aorta and from the right ventricle through the pulmonary valve into the pulmonary artery. The aorta is the main artery of the general (systemic) circulation.

In the pulmonary (lung) circulation, carbon dioxide is given up and oxygen taken up. The oxygenated blood returns to the left side of the heart and is pumped into the aorta. A diagram of the circulation of the blood through the heart is shown in Fig. 6.6.

Note: The pulmonary vein from the lung contains arterial blood and the pulmonary artery contains venous blood. All other veins in the body contain venous blood, i.e. deoxygenated blood from the tissues and all other arteries in the body contain arterial blood, i.e. oxygenated blood going to the tissues.

6:6   BLOOD PRESSURE

The blood pressure is the force which circulates the blood around the body. It is dependant on the amount of blood pumped out by the heart (cardiac output) and the resistance produced by the arterioles (peripheral resistance).

Blood pressure = Cardiac output × Peripheral resistance

Cardiac output itself depends on the volume of blood which the heart pumps out with each beat (stroke volume) and the rate at which the heart is beating (heart rate).

Cardiac output = Stroke volume × Heart rate

Low blood pressure

It is important that the blood pressure should be maintained within fairly narrow limits. If it falls then the circulation of blood to the brain and other vital organs e.g. kidneys, will be reduced and less oxygen and nutrients will reach them.

A low blood pressure (hypotension) may be due to a low stroke volume when the volume of circulating blood is reduced. Low blood pressure due to low circulating volume may be caused by the following:

Loss of fluid as in: — severe diarrhoea
                       — severe sweating in fever
                       — burns

Loss of blood as in: — haemorrhage during pregnancy or childbirth
                       — severe injuries
                       — surgery

In these situations it is important to maintain the blood pressure by replacing the lost fluid with blood or electrolyte solutions as appropriate (e.g. oral rehydration fluid in diarrhoea).

Raised blood pressure

A persistently raised blood pressure (hypertension) is usually associated with increased peripheral resistance. It damages the vessels in the brain (cerebral vessels) and kidneys (renal vessels) and increases the work of the heart. It can result in haemorrhage or thrombosis of the damaged cerebral vessels causing a stroke ('cerebrovascular accident').Depending on the site of haemorrhage or thrombosis, the patient may suffer paralysis on one side of the body, visual problems, or difficulty with speech. Damage to renal vessels over a period of time may cause impairment of kidney function.

Because of the extra work of the heart, hypertension is a cause of cardiac failure (see also 6:7).

Measurement of blood pressure
The blood pressure is measured using an instrument called a sphygmomanometer. It is recorded in millimetres of mercury (mm Hg) with 0 mm Hg on the sphygmomanometer scale representing atmospheric pressure, i.e. 760 mm Hg.

SI Units
Although the unit of pressure in SI units is correctly the kilopascal (1 kPa = 7.5 mm Hg), blood pressures and blood gases tend to be still recorded in mm Hg because instruments are calibrated in millimetres of mercury and because there are many clinical uses for figures in the traditional units.

It is usual to take the blood pressure by measuring the pressure exerted by the blood on the wall of the brachial artery (see Fig. 6.7).

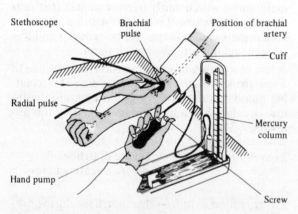

Fig. 6.7 **Measuring blood pressure using a sphygmomanometer.**

Method
1. Wrap the cuff of a sphygmomanometer around the upper arm as shown in Fig. 6.7. The cuff must be smooth with the rubber against the inside of the upper arm and the rubber tube with its valve to the front.

2. Connect the tubing from the mercury manometer to the cuff.

3. Tighten the screw of the rubber bulb (hand pump), see Fig. 6.7.

4. Locate the pulse of the brachial artery, medial to the middle of the elbow below the cuff.

5. Feel the radial pulse. Inflate the cuff until the radial pulse can no longer be felt and then increase the pressure a little more.

6. Place the end of a stethoscope over the place where the brachial artery pulse was felt.

7. Slowly loosen the screw of the pump to allow the air to escape from the cuff, listening for a tapping sound (pulse beat) through the stethoscope. Note the height of the mercury column at the point when the pulse beat is heard. This is the *systolic blood pressure* (the pressure in the arteries when the heart is contracted).

8. Let out more air listening as the sounds first become louder and then suddenly quieter (muffled). Note the height of the mercury column at the point when the sounds become quieter again.

9. Continue to let the pressure fall listening for the sounds to disappear. It is now internationally agreed that the point at which the sounds disappear should be taken as the *diastolic blood pressure*.
   Note: In the past, the level at which the sounds become muffled was considered the diastolic pressure. Ideally therefore, to avoid any possible confusion both figures should be recorded.

10. Continue to allow the air to escape making sure the sounds do not return. Occasionally there is a silent gap and unless listening is continued a false high diastolic pressure may be recorded.

11. Record the blood pressure (BP) in millimetres of mercury (mm Hg) as follows:

    Systolic BP/Diastolic BP
    or ideally,
    Systolic BP/Level of muffling/Level of disappearance.

The blood pressure of most adults at rest varies from 95/55 to 140/90. In many cultures, though not all, blood pressure increases with age.

Important: A laboratory worker who must perform blood pressure measurements, for example before collecting blood from a blood donor, must first receive sufficient practical training from an experienced person.

6:7 TERMS USED IN CARDIAC MEDICINE

Angina: The pain arising in the heart when its blood supply is inadequate for its activity.

Atherosclerosis: A disorder in which fatty material is deposited in the lining of blood vessels. It has been shown that smoking increases the chance of developing atherosclerotic disease, especially in the coronary arteries and arteries supplying the legs.

'Blue baby': This term is used to describe a newborn baby which is cyanosed (see also 6:3). It is due to a congenital defect of the heart or blood vessels causing a mixing of venous blood with arterial blood. This mixed blood cannot become fully oxygenated.

Brachycardia: An abnormally low heart rate i.e. less than 60 beats per minute for an adult or less than 120 beats per minute for a foetus.

Cardiac arrest: The stopping of the heartbeat. If the heart muscle stops beating completely this is referred to as asystole and, if it stops beating but quivers without pumping blood, this is termed ventricular fibrillation. Following a cardiac arrest, if emergency cardiac massage is applied and the heart beat restarted within a few minutes there is little risk of permanent brain damage occurring. The commonest cause of cardiac arrest is myocardial infarction (see later text).

Cardiac (heart) failure: This term is used when the heart is unable to transfer sufficient blood from the venous side to the arterial side. In left ventricular failure (LVF), the blood is not transferred adequately from the pulmonary veins through the left side of the heart to the aorta. This results in a build-up of pressure in the pulmonary veins which is transmitted back to the pulmonary artery and capillaries. This increase in pressure leads to fluid collecting in the lungs (pulmonary oedema). LVF is associated with hypertension, coronary artery disease, or disease of the aortic valve.

In right ventricular failure (RVF), the right ventricle fails to transfer blood adequately from the great veins through to the pulmonary artery. It causes an increase in venous pressure leading to generalized oedema. RVF is commonly caused by mitral valve stenosis, pulmonary embolism, or pulmonary hypertension. Often, however, combined failure occurs because the heart functions as a whole.

Electrocardiogram (ECG): A recording in graph form made by an electrocardiograph machine of the electrical current produced by the heart's contraction. The electrical charges, known as waves and complexes which occur throughout the cardiac cycle are recorded. The P wave corresponds to atrial systole and the QRST complex (series of waves) corresponds to the ventricular systole. In heart disease the ECG shows characteristic changes in the duration of the waves and complexes.

Endocarditis: Inflammation of the endocardium which is the lining membrane of the heart cavities and its valves. It may be caused by bacteria (bacterial endocarditis), particularly staphylococcal and streptococcal organisms, fungi, or rickettsial organisms such as *Coxiella burnetti* (Q fever endocarditis). Bacterial endocarditis is confirmed by blood culture.

Heart murmurs: These are abnormal sounds which can be heard in addition to the normal heart sounds when blood flow becomes excessively turbulent. This may occur because a normal amount of blood is flowing through an abnormal or damaged valve e.g. in rheumatic fever, or because an increased volume of blood is flowing through normal valves e.g. severe anaemia, fever, or pregnancy. Heart murmurs can also be heard when there are abnormal communications between the right and left side of the heart, e.g. congenital heart defects.

Ischaemic heart disease: A condition in which there is an inadequate blood supply to the heart muscle (myocardium) to provide oxygen and nutrients for its activity during rest and exercise. Most commonly this problem is caused by an abnormal narrowing of the coronary arteries by a pathological process called atherosclerosis (see previous text).

Myocardial infarction ('heart attack' or 'coronary'): The death of an area of cardiac muscle caused by an obstruction to its blood supply. This is usually the result of a blood clot forming on top of an area of atherosclerosis in coronary artery disease.

Myocarditis: A condition in which the myocardium which is the muscle tissue of the heart becomes inflamed. Acute myocarditis is usually a result of the toxic effects of infections such as typhoid fever, scrub typhus fever, meningitis, diphtheria, or pneumonia. It is also associated with chronic Chagas' disease and certain viral infections.

Tachycardia: An excessively raised heart-rate.

Recommended Reading

See books listed at the end of Chapter 5.

7

Urinary System

7:1 STRUCTURE OF THE URINARY SYSTEM

The urinary system consists of:

■ A pair of kidneys situated against the back muscles on each side of the vertebral column beneath the diaphragm.

■ A pair of ureters which link the kidneys to the bladder.

■ The bladder which is a muscular bag into which the ureters drain. It stores and excretes the urine.

■ The urethra which is a tube (longer in the male than the female) leading from the bladder through which the urine passes during urination.

Kidneys
The kidneys are flattened, bean-shaped, capsulated organs divided into an outer region called the cortex and an inner area called the medulla. The medulla is subdivided into triangular shaped regions called the medullary pyramids directed towards the pelvis of the kidney (see Fig. 7.2). The cortex and medullary pyramids are composed of a million or more small filtration units called nephrons.

The filtration part of each nephron lies in the cortex of the kidney and consists of a cup-shaped structure called a Bowman's capsule which surrounds a mass of capillaries known as the glomerulus (see Fig. 7.3). Each Bowman's capsule leads into a tubule which has a complicated course within the kidney before reaching the renal pelvis, as shown in Fig. 7.3.

Each kidney is supplied with oxygenated blood through the renal artery (a branch of the dorsal aorta). This divides forming interlobular arteries and a network of arterioles. Blood leaves each kidney by way of the renal vein which drains the venules from the capillary bed.

The urine formed in the nephrons is collected by a system of ducts which drain into the ureters.

7:2 FUNCTIONING OF THE URINARY SYSTEM

The main functions of the urinary system are as follows:

— To regulate the water content of the body.

— To maintain the correct electrolyte balance in the body.

— To maintain the reaction of the blood between pH 7.37-7.45 by excreting surplus acids and alkalis.

— To excrete the waste products of metabolism including urea, creatinine, uric acid, and also drug metabolites.

— To produce erythropoietin, a substance made by the kidneys which is necessary for the normal production of red cells in the bone marrow.

— To produce renin which assists the secretion of the hormone aldosterone and causes the constriction of arterioles.

— To reabsorb filtered compounds of value to the body such as glucose and amino acids.

Functioning of a nephron
Blood enters the glomerulus through the afferent arteriole and leaves through the efferent arteriole (see Fig. 7.3). The wall of the capillaries within the glomerulus and the wall of the Bowman's capsule act as semi-permeable membranes. This means that they let some molecules pass through while keeping others within the capillary lumen. Because the efferent arteriole is able to constrict, the pressure in the glomerulus is higher than that in the capsule and this results in water, glucose, electrolytes, amino acids, and the waste products of metabolism (urea, creatinine and uric acid) passing from the blood into the Bowman's capsule.

The water and substances filtered from the blood, known as the glomerular filtrate, pass from the Bowman's capsule into the renal tubule. As the filtrate passes through the tubule, the tubular cells reabsorb those substances which the body requires such as amino acids, glucose, and electrolytes. These pass into the blood in the capillary network which surrounds the renal tubule and eventually re-enter the blood stream by way of the renal vein and inferior vena cava.

Water reabsorption and ADH production
About 85% of the water filtered by the glomerulus is reabsorbed by the proximal tubules. The remainder passes through the loop of Henlé where a little is reabsorbed. In the distal convoluted tubule and collecting duct, the amount of water reabsorbed depends on the body's needs. If the plasma is concentrated as occurs for example in dehydration, the posterior pituitary gland produces antidiuretic hormone (ADH). This makes the collecting ducts permeable to water which then

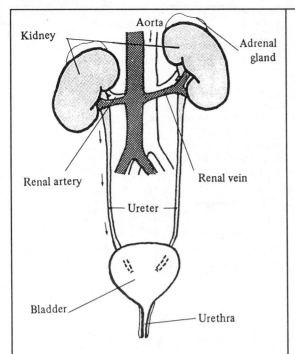

Fig. 7.1 Renal system consisting of kidneys, ureters, bladder and urethra.

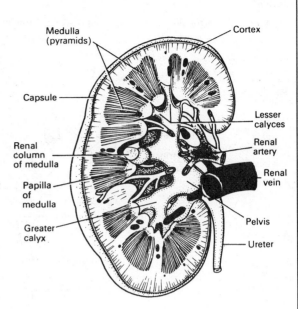

Fig. 7.2 Section through a kidney. *Reproduced from Foundations of Anatomy and Physiology.*

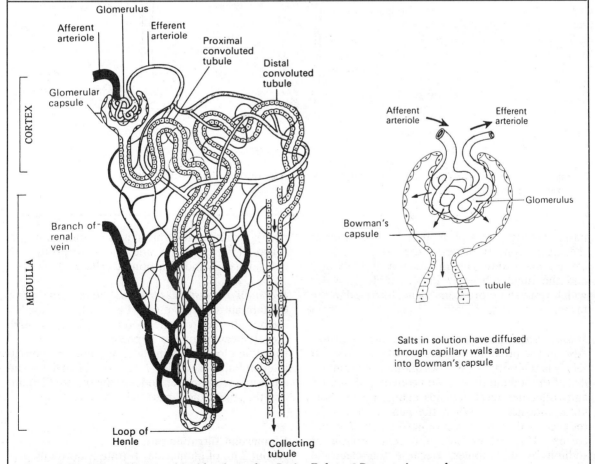

Fig. 7.3 *Left* **A nephron and its blood supply.** *Right* **Enlarged Bowman's capsule.**
Reproduced from Foundations of Anatomy and Physiology. Courtesy of Churchill Livingstone.

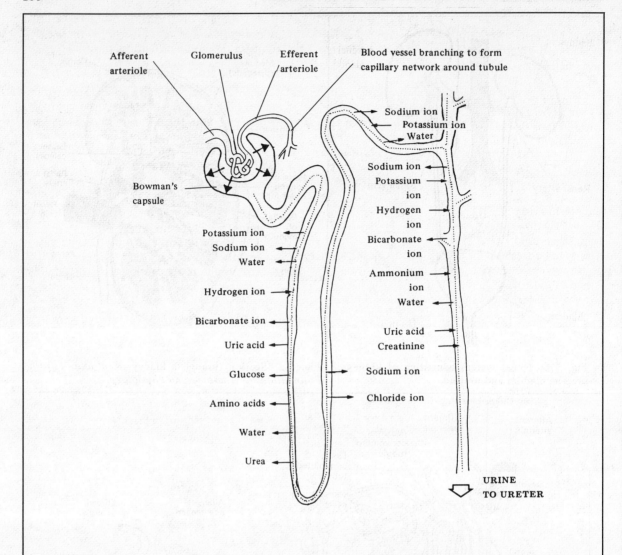

Fig. 7.4 Diagram to show tubular reabsorption and secretion and the passive transfer of water from the glomerular filtrate.

passes through the wall of the tubule to re-enter the circulation. If however the body needs to excrete more water, the production of ADH falls and the tubules become impermeable to water which results in more water being excreted in the urine.

Sodium reabsorption and alderosterone production
Also in the proximal tubules most of the sodium (Na^+) is reabsorbed. Reabsorption of the remainder of the sodium in the distal convoluted tubules and collecting ducts depends mainly on the hormone aldosterone. When the plasma volume is reduced, aldosterone is produced by the adrenal cortex. This causes increased reabsorption of sodium by the tubules. Because the electrical charge of the ions retained and excreted must be kept balanced in the body (electrostatic equilib-

rium), sodium reabsorption is associated with hydrogen (H^+) excretion and the reabsorption of chloride (Cl^-) and bicarbonate (HCO_3^-).

Secretion of substances from the blood into urine
Certain substances, e.g. drugs such as penicillin are not filtered from the blood as it passes through the glomerulus of the nephrons but are cleared from the blood by being secreted into the convoluted tubules (see Fig. 7.4). Hydrogen ions and ammonia are also secreted into the filtrate to maintain the correct acid-base balance in the body.

Glomerular filtration rate
About 2 ml of glomerular filtrate is normally produced per second (sec). This is known as the glomerular filtration rate (GFR).

The glomerular filtration rate can be calculated by measuring urine excretion and the plasma level of a substance which is freely filtered by the glomeruli and neither secreted nor reabsorbed by the tubules. Creatinine partly fulfils these criteria. There is some tubular secretion and probably a little tubular reabsorption but creatinine clearance (degree to which creatinine is removed from the body by excretion in the urine) is a good guide to glomerular filtration rate, and gives results around 2 ml/sec. Creatinine clearance is therefore often used as a test of kidney function. When the filtration rate is low the concentration of creatinine in the plasma rises.

Renal threshold

The renal threshold of a substance refers to its highest concentration in the blood before it is found in the urine. A substance such as glucose is a high renal threshold substance because it is completely absorbed from the filtrate and is only found in the urine when the blood glucose level is markedly raised as for example in diabetes mellitus. Urea and creatinine, however, are low threshold substances because very little, if any, of these substances is reabsorbed. They are always present in the urine independent of their blood levels.

7:3   URINE

As has been explained in 7:2, the production and composition of urine depends on glomerular filtration, tubular reabsorption, and tubular secretion.

The volume of urine excreted daily depends on fluid intake, diet, climate, and other physiological factors. It is usually between 1-2 litres per 24 hours.

Normal appearance and composition of urine

Normal freshly passed urine is clear and pale to dark yellow in colour whereas a dilute urine appears pale in colour and a concentrated one has a dark yellow appearance. The yellow colour is due to the pigments urochrome, urobilin, and porphyrins.

When normal urine has been allowed to stand for some time, a white phosphate deposit may form if the urine is alkaline (dissolved by adding a drop of acetic acid) or a pink uric acid deposit may form if the urine is highly acidic or concentrated (disappears on warming). A 'mucus' cloud may also form if normal urine is left to stand.

Composition

The composition of the urine is greatly dependent on diet and the metabolic activities of the body's cells. In health, urine usually contains the following:

- Water, making up about 95% of the urine. The amount of water reabsorbed by the kidney tubules and collecting ducts depends on the fluid balance in the body (see 7:2 and 29:1).

- Electrolytes, including sodium, potassium, magnesium, chloride, and bicarbonate. The concentration of the different ions in the urine is dependent on the degree of tubular reabsorption and secretion required to maintain electrostatic equilibrium (see 7:2).

- The waste products of metabolism, including:
  - Urea formed from the metabolism of proteins.
  - Uric acid formed mainly from purine metabolism.
  - Creatinine produced from the metabolism of creatine in skeletal muscle.

- Surplus acids and alkalis to maintain the acid-base balance in the body (see 29:1). The acids are usually excreted in buffered form as dihydrogen phosphate and ammonium ions and the surplus alkalis as bicarbonate and monohydrogen phosphate.

  The normal reaction of freshly passed urine is slightly acid, around pH 6.0.

Urine changes in disease

Some of the changes which can occur in the volume, appearance, odour, constituents and mass density (specific gravity) of urine in disease are as follows:

Volume changes

An increase in the volume of urine is called polyuria. It occurs in diabetes mellitus due to an increase in the osmolality of the filtrate preventing the normal reabsorption of water (osmotic diuresis). Polyuria also occurs when the secretion of the antidiuretic hormone (ADH) is reduced as for example in diabetes insipidus.

A decrease in the volume of urine excreted is called oliguria. It occurs when the renal blood flow and, or, glomerular filtration rate are reduced. One of the causes of a reduced renal blood flow is low blood pressure (hypotension) caused for example by severe dehydration or cardiac failure. A fall in glomerular filtration rate occurs in acute glomerulonephritis (inflammation of the kidney glomeruli) and also in the early stages of acute tubular necrosis.

If severe oliguria progresses to a complete cessation of urine flow, this is called anuria and is usually due to severe damage to the renal tubules (acute tubular necrosis). Acute tubular necrosis may follow any of the conditions which cause severe hypotension or may be due to a direct toxic effect on the tubules by drugs or following an incompatible blood transfusion.

Appearance changes
The appearance of urine may be altered in many conditions including:

- □ Urinary tract infections in which the urine appears cloudy because it contains pus cells and bacteria.

- □ Urinary schistosomiasis in which the urine often appears red and cloudy because it contains blood (haematuria).

- □ Blackwater fever and other conditions causing intravascular haemolysis in which the urine appears brown and cloudy because it contains free haemoglobin (haemoglobinuria).

- □ Jaundice in which the urine may appear yellow-brown or green-brown because it contains bile pigments or increased amounts of urobilin (oxidized urobilinogen).

- □ Bancroftian filariasis in which the urine may appear milky-white because it contains chyle.

Composition changes
Abnormal chemical constituents in urine include:

- □ Glucose (glycosuria), which may be found in the urine of diabetics and occasionally in some healthy individuals.

- □ Ketones (ketonuria), which can be found in the urine of untreated diabetics or persons suffering from starvation.

- □ Protein (proteinuria), which can be found in the urine of persons with urinary schistosomiasis, urinary tract infections, nephrotic syndrome, renal diseases such as pyelonephritis and glomerulonephritis, and renal tuberculosis. It may also be found in urine from pregnant women and sometimes from healthy young individuals.

- □ Bilirubin (bilirubinuria), which can be found in the urine of persons with hepatocellular jaundice or cholestatic (obstructive) jaundice.

- □ Urobilinogen (in increased amounts), which can be found in the urine of those with conditions causing abnormal haemolysis.

- □ Galactose which is found in the urine of persons with the rare congenital metabolic disorder called galactosaemia. In this disease, the enzyme which converts galactose to glucose in the liver is lacking.

Note: The microscopical examination of urine for cells, casts, crystals, and parasites is described in the microbiology section in Volume II of the Manual.

Relative mass density (specific gravity) changes
The normal mass density (specific gravity) of urine varies from 1.002-1.025 depending on the state of hydration of the person and the time of day. It is highest at the beginning of the day. Normal mass density is mainly proportional to the urea and sodium concentrations in the urine.

Methods of measuring the concentration of urine using a urinometer, weighing technique, or specific gravity strip test are described in 28:5.

In renal failure, the ability of the kidneys to concentrate and dilute urine is reduced. Normal concentrating power can be assumed if the mass density of a urine sample reaches 1.018 or over.

Unusually high mass density measurements may be found when the urine contains glucose, protein, or other heavy particles (see also 28:5).

7:4   TERMS USED TO DESCRIBE DISORDERS OF THE URINARY SYSTEM

Anuria: Cessation of the flow of urine due to a failure of the kidneys to produce urine.

Cystitis: Inflammation of the urinary bladder, usually caused by bacteria (see also *Urinary Tract Infection*). It is often accompanied by frequency and a burning sensation when passing urine. The condition may be acute or chronic. Cystitis is more common in women than men.

Diuretic: A drug that is used to increase the volume of urine produced by increasing the excretion of salts (mainly sodium) and water in the urine. A diuretic is commonly used to reduce oedema due to salt and water retention as may occur in diseases of the kidneys, heart, lungs or liver. It is also used with other drugs in treating high blood pressure (hypertension). Potassium deficiency is associated with some diuretics and this is corrected by giving the patient drugs containing potassium.

Frequency: Frequent passing of small amounts of urine as may occur in urinary tract infections (see also *Polyuria*).

Glomerulonephritis: Inflammation   of   the glomeruli of the kidneys.

Acute glomerulonephritis (acute nephritis)
This is usually caused by an abnormal allergic response following infection with beta-haemolytic streptococci and sometimes with *Plasmodium malariae*, *Schistosoma* species, *Mycobacterium leprae*, or viruses such as Epstein-Barr virus. It may also occur as a complication of infective

endocarditis. Immune complexes are deposited in the capillary wall of the glomerulus which cause inflammation, leading to damage of the kidney tubules. There is usually oedema caused by fluid retention. The urine is concentrated and contains red cells, protein, and granular casts. Most patients recover from acute glomerulonephritis with a return to normal kidney function.

Chronic glomerulonephritis
Occasionally acute glomerulonephritis progresses to chronic glomerulonephritis with hypertension. Chronic glomerulonephritis leads to renal failure. The nephrotic syndrome (see later text) may also progress to chronic glomerulonephritis.

Nephrotic syndrome: A condition in which protein leaks through the damaged walls of glomeruli and is excreted in large amounts in the urine. Loss of protein leads to reduced levels of albumin in the blood which results in oedema. The nephrotic syndrome is found in glomerulonephritis associated with permeability of the glomerular basement membrane, infection with *Plasmodium malariae*, diabetic nephropathy, systemic lupus erythematosus, and following treatment with certain drugs.

Oliguria: Insufficient production of urine usually in association with a reduced renal blood flow and reduced rate of glomerular filtration (see also 7:3).

Polyuria: Increase in the volume of urine output (see also 7:3).

Pyelitis: Inflammation of the pelvis of the kidney, usually caused by a bacterial infection.

Pyelonephritis: Inflammation of the parenchyma and pelvis of the kidney usually caused by bacterial infection (see also *Urinary Tract Infection*).The disease may be acute or chronic.

Pyuria: Presence of pus cells in the urine due to inflammation of the urinary tract, usually in response to a bacterial infection. Persistent pyuria with a sterile routine urine culture is suggestive of renal tuberculosis.

Renal calculus: Presence of a stone (or stones) in the urinary tract. Renal stones are often composed of calcium oxalate and the repeated finding of calcium oxalate crystals in *fresh* urine specimens is suggestive of renal calculus.

The term renal colic is used to describe the severe pain which is caused when a stone passes down the ureter or other urinary duct.

Renal failure: Failure of the kidneys to produce urine in the normal way. Such failure may be the result of glomerulonephritis or other disease of the kidneys, circulatory failure, or to conditions in which the flow of urine is obstructed. Certain toxins and drugs can also cause renal failure.

Renal failure leads to uraemia (see later text), water and electrolyte imbalance, and the accumulation in the body of toxic products of metabolism. It is usually accompanied by hypertension.

Retention: Inability to pass urine which is in the bladder. The condition may be chronic or acute.Among the causes of retention are enlargement of the prostate gland and urethral obstruction. Retention causes stasis and a rise in pressure within the urinary tract which can lead to infection, stone formation, and renal failure.

Urinary tract infection (UTI): When the kidneys are infected the term pyelonephritis is used and when the bladder is infected the term cystitis is used. Infection of the urethra is called urethritis.

Urinary tract infection, especially cystitis, is commoner in women than men and is probably due to the shorter urethra with the urethral opening being closer to the rectum in women. The commonest pathogen is *Escherichia coli* (normal commensal of the gut) which is a Gram negative motile bacillus. Infection produces an acid urine. Other pathogens which cause urinary infections include *Proteus* species (produce an alkaline urine), *Pseudomonas aeruginosa*, and *Staphylococcus* species. A common cause of urethritis is *Neisseria gonorrhoeae*.

Conditions which predispose to urinary tract infection include renal calculus, stricture or prostatic disease, incomplete emptying of the bladder, catheterisation of the bladder, and diabetes.

In bacterial urinary tract infection, the urine contains significant numbers of bacteria, pus cells and usually protein.In acute infections, red cells may also be found.

Uraemia: Accumulation of an excessive amount of urea and other nitrogenous waste products in the blood due to renal failure.

In uraemia there is a marked increase in the concentrations of urea and creatinine in the blood. Metabolic acidosis develops and there is polyuria with inabiity to dilute or concentrate urine normally. Burr cells may be seen in the peripheral blood film.

Recommended Reading
See books listed at the end of Chapter 5.

Digestive System
Nutrition and Metabolism

8:1 DIGESTIVE SYSTEM

Food of the correct type and in adequate amount is essential for life. It provides the body with energy to perform its essential functions and the substances it needs for its growth, repair, and protection. Before food can be used by the body it needs to be digested and the required nutrients absorbed. Unwanted food is excreted from the body as faeces.

Digestion

Digestion is the mechanical and chemical splitting of large complex foods into smaller simpler substances that can be absorbed and assimilated by the body. The chemical breaking down of the food is performed by enzymes which are secreted in the digestive juices of the mouth, stomach, pancreas, liver, and small intestine.

The main classes of food ingested and digested are as follows:

☐ Carbohydrates (starches and sugars) which are digested to simple sugars, the most important being glucose. Most of the body's energy is obtained from glucose.

☐ Fats which are digested to fatty acids and glycerol and also provide the body with energy and heat.

☐ Proteins which are digested to amino acids which are the building blocks used by the body to make its cells, enzymes, antibodies, hormones and other secretions.

Note: The types of food which contain carbohydrates, fats and proteins are listed in 8:3. The metabolism of these foods is described in 8:4.

Digestive tract

The digestive tract is a muscular tube measuring just over 9 metres long in an adult. Parts of it are modified to carry out special functions.

The different parts of the digestive tract are as follows:

- Mouth
- Oesophagus
- Stomach
- Small intestine
- Large intestine
- Anus

Mouth

Digestion starts in the mouth where the lips, cheeks, muscles, and teeth are involved in the mastication (chewing) of food. The food is moistened by saliva which is secreted by three pairs of salivary glands (parotid, submandibular, and sublingual).

Saliva consists of water, mucin, and mineral salts and contains the enzyme ptyalin (alpha-amylase) which is identical with pancreatic amylase. Ptyalin begins the digestion of cooked starches to maltose. Mucin lubricates the food.

Saliva keeps the mouth and teeth clean and may also have some antibacterial action. It is also necessary for speech.

Oesophagus

The oesophagus extends from the pharynx at the back of the mouth to the stomach (see Fig. 8.1). Food is moved along the oesophagus to the stomach by what is called peristalsis, i.e. movement of the contents of the oesophagus by contraction and relaxing of its muscular wall.

Stomach

The stomach is a strong muscular bag which is situated just under the diaphragm. The upper part of the stomach is called the fundus, the central part is called the body and the lower part is called the pylorus. The part closest to the oesophagus is called the cardia. The pyloric sphincter muscle controls the passage of food from the stomach into the duodenum.

In the stomach the food is mixed with gastric juice which is secreted by the gastric mucosa (lining) of the stomach. The food remains in the stomach until a semi-fluid mass called chyme is produced. The chyme is slowly released into the duodenum at a rate the small intestine can digest and absorb.

Gastric juice contains:

☐ Hydrochloric acid which is secreted by the parietal (oxyntic) cells in the fundus and body of the stomach. The hydrochloric acid kills bacteria and activates the enzyme pepsinogen to pepsin. Hydrochloric acid secretion is stimulated by the hormone gastrin.

☐ Pepsin which is produced by cells in the fundus of the stomach. It digests protein into large peptides.

☐ Mucus which is secreted by glands in the cardiac and pyloric regions of the stomach. It lubricates the food and also lines the stomach to

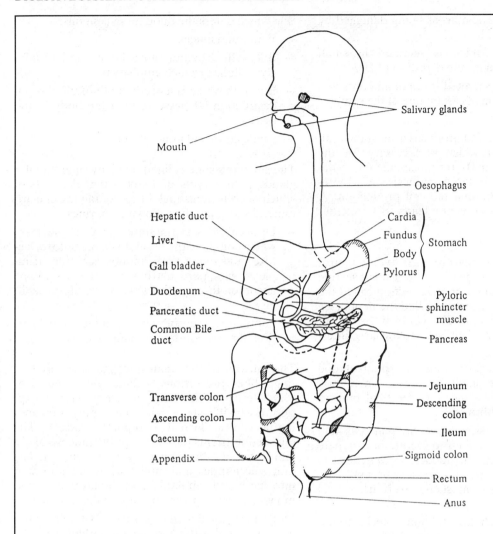

Fig. 8.1 *Upper* **Parts of the digestive tract.**

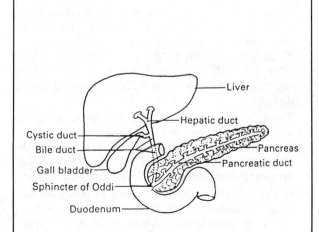

Fig. 8.1 *Lower* **Enlarged view of the liver, pancreas, gall bladder, and ducts.**

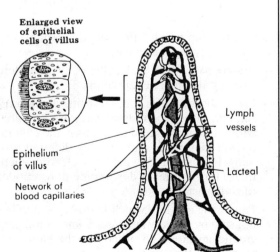

Fig. 8.2 Diagram of a villus showing lacteal, lymph vessels and blood supply.

prevent the gastric mucosa being damaged by hydrochloric acid.

☐ Gastric lipase which is secreted in small amounts and begins the digestion of fat.

☐ Renin which is secreted in small amounts and aids the digestion of casein, one of the proteins in milk.

The gastric mucosa also produces a substance called intrinsic factor which is necessary for the absorption of vitamin B_{12} (cyanocobalamin). Vitamin B_{12} is required for DNA synthesis and is therefore essential for normal red cell production. A deficiency of intrinsic factor leads to pernicious anaemia.

Small intestine

The small intestine measures just over 5 metres long in an adult. It is divided into a small section called the duodenum, a middle section called the jejunum and a lower section called the ileum (see Fig. 8.1). The ileocaecal valve controls the flow of material from the small intestine to the large intestine.

About 90% of the digestion and absorption of food takes place in the small intestine. When food enters the small intestine, the intestinal mucosa secretes two main hormones:

☐ Secretin which stimulates the pancreas and biliary tract epithelium to secrete bicarbonate which passes into the duodenum to neutralize the acid chyme. This is necessary because pancreatic enzymes act most effectively at a neutral pH.

☐ Pancreozymin-cholecystokinin which stimulates the pancreas to release fluid containing the enzymes required for continued digestion. It also causes the gall bladder to contract, releasing bile into the intestine at a time when fat has to be digested.

Pancreatic fluid which enters the duodenum contains the following substances:

— Bicarbonate which makes the pancreatic fluid strongly alkaline, i.e. about pH 8.

— Precursors of the enzymes trypsin, chymotrypsin, and carboxypeptidase. They are activated within the small intestine. Trypsin and chymotrypsin split whole and partially digested proteins into small polypeptides. Carboxypeptidase further breaks down some polypeptides to amino acids.

— Pancreatic amylase which hydrolyzes starches not split by salivary amylase. Some of the pancreatic amylase is absorbed into the blood and excreted in the urine.

— Pancreatic lipase which hydrolyzes neutral fats (triglycerides) into monoglycerides and fatty acids.

Bile which enters the duodenum contains:

— Water and mucus.

— Bile salts (sodium taurocholate and sodium glycocholate) which emulsify fats.

— Bilirubin which is a product of normal red cell destruction. It passes out of the body in the faeces.

— Cholesterol and mineral salts.

The small intestine is lined by many small tubular glands called crypts of Lieberkuhn, the cells of which secrete intestinal juice containing mucus, mineral salts, and the following enzymes:

— Disaccharidases (maltase, lactase, sucrase) which complete the breakdown of maltose, lactose, and sucrose into monosaccharides (simpler sugars, particularly glucose) which can be absorbed through the walls of the blood capillaries.

— Peptidases (erepsin) which complete the digestion of polypeptides into amino acids.

The mucosa of the small intestine is covered by finger-like projections called villi (see Fig. 8.2). These provide a large surface area for absorption. Each villus has a rich blood supply surrounding a central lacteal (lymphatic vessel). The digested nutrients pass through the mucosa of the villi by passive diffusion and active transport. The monosaccharides and amino acids are absorbed into the blood capillaries and the fatty acids and monoglycerides are absorbed into the lacteals.

Other nutritional materials such as vitamins, mineral salts, and water, are also absorbed from the small intestine into the blood stream.

Large intestine

The large intestine measures about 1.5 metres long in an adult. It is divided into the caecum which leads into the colon (ascending, transverse, descending), sigmoid colon, rectum, and anus.
A small blind-ended tube called the appendix is attached to the caecum. It has no known role in digestion and can become inflamed causing appendicitis.

The main functions of the large intestine are to absorb water from the remaining chyme and to store the waste solidified matter (faeces). The absorption of glucose, some electrolytes, and drugs also continues in the large intestine.

In the caecum, cellulose is broken down by bacteria. Vitamins B_{12}, D, K, thiamin, and riboflavin are synthesised in the large intestine by bacteria.

The elimination of the waste matter is carried out by the muscular action of the rectum. Two sphincter muscles control the excretion of faeces through the anus.

8:2 METABOLISM OF CARBOHYDRATES, FATS, AND PROTEIN

The process of metabolism is made up of:

■ Anabolic reactions in which absorbed nutrients are built up into the compounds the body needs for its structure and physiology.

■ Catabolic reactions in which complex substances are broken down to simpler forms with the release of energy for cellular activity.

Body's energy requirements

The energy requirements of a person depend on the age, size, and metabolic rate of the individual. The metabolic rate is partly controlled by thyroid gland hormones and is affected by temperature and a person's activity. What is called the basal metabolic rate refers to the heat and energy required to maintain cellular functions when the body is at rest.

The unit used for measuring heat and energy has in the past been the Calorie (C).

A Calorie is defined as the amount of heat required to raise the temperature of 1 litre (1 kg) of water by 1 °C. The subunit of the Calorie is also called a calorie (c). There are 1 000 calories in 1 Calorie.

The SI unit for measuring energy is called the joule (J). Heat and energy production is expressed in kilojoules per hour or kilojoules per day. The correlation between Calories and joules is as follows:

1 Calorie = 4.2 kilojoules (kJ)

The estimated energy values of foods that can be metabolised to produce heat and energy are as follows:

— 1 gram of fat gives 38 kJ (9 Calories)
— 1 gram of carbohydrate gives 17 kJ (4 Calories)
— 1 gram of protein gives 17 kJ (4 Calories)

An individual's intake of calorie-producing nutrients can be considered adequate if the person is maintaining his or her correct weight.

Metabolism of carbohydrates

Carbohydrates contain carbon, hydrogen, and oxygen and are used by the body as sources of heat and energy.

The main end-product of carbohydrate digestion is the monosaccharide GLUCOSE. Small amounts of fructose and galactose are also produced.

The main sources of carbohydrates in the diet are listed in 8:3.

Classification of carbohydrates

There are three main groups of carbohydrates:

— Monosaccharides, which are simple sugars that can be absorbed directly from the intestine, e.g. glucose, fructose, galactose (hexoses), and the plant sugars including ribose, xylose, and arabinose (pentoses).

— Disaccharides, which on hydrolysis give two molecules of monosaccharides. Examples include sucrose (cane sugar), lactose, and maltose. Each sugar is hydrolyzed by its own specific enzyme, i.e. sucrase, lactase, and maltase.

— Polysaccharides, which on digestion or hydrolysis give many molecules of monosaccharides. Examples include starch and glycogen.

Carbohydrate metabolism begins with the absorption of glucose from the small intestine into the blood stream. The glucose is transported to the liver and depending on the body's needs it is used or stored as follows:

□ It is used to maintain a correct level of glucose in the blood. From the blood, glucose is taken up by the tissues. In tissue cells, the glucose is converted to pyruvate by glycolysis and oxidized to produce energy and heat for cellular activities (aerobic pathway). The energy-rich compound adenosine triphosphate (ATP) is formed from energy released in this way. ATP is a direct source of energy for cells.

Aerobic pathway

$$\text{Glucose} \xrightarrow{\text{Glycolysis}} \text{Pyruvate} \xrightarrow{\text{Oxidation}} \begin{array}{l}\text{ENERGY}\\\text{HEAT}\\CO_2 + H_2O\end{array}$$

If the demand for energy exceeds the oxygen available, e.g. energy required for extra muscular activity, pyruvate can be reduced to lactate with the release of energy (anaerobic pathway). This way of producing energy can be maintained for only a limited period.

□ Glucose not required for the body's immediate energy needs is converted to the complex sugar glycogen and stored in the liver and muscles, a process known as glycogenesis.

$$\text{Glucose} \xrightarrow{\text{Glycogenesis}} \text{GLYCOGEN}$$

When glucose is required to maintain the blood glucose level, liver glycogen is converted back to glucose, a process known as glycogenolysis. Muscle glycogen provides the glucose required for muscular activity (converted to lactate by anaerobic glycolysis).

□ Glucose which exceeds both the body's immediate needs and the body's glycogen storage capacity is oxidized to fatty acids and stored as fat in the tissues.

$$\text{Glucose} \xrightarrow{\text{Oxidized}} \text{Fatty acids} \longrightarrow \text{FAT}$$

Note: When required, glucose can be formed from fats and protein. The production of glucose from

non-carbohydrate sources is called gluconeogenesis.

Control of carbohydrate metabolism

Insulin is the most important hormone that regulates the amount of glucose in the blood, the rate at
which glucose is taken up by the tissues, and the
conversion of glucose to glycogen.

Insulin is made and secreted by the beta-islet cells
of the pancreas. It is the only hormone capable of
reducing the concentration of glucose in the blood.
Its secretion is stimulated by a rise in the blood glucose level and directly or indirectly by gastrointestinal hormones, certain sugars, fatty acids, caffeine, and other substances.

An absolute or relative deficiency of insulin, as
occurs in diabetes mellitus (see later text), causes a
rise in blood glucose, depression of glucose
metabolism in the tissues, an increase in the breakdown of liver glycogen to glucose, and the stimulation of gluconeogenesis.

Other hormones and substances involved in carbohydrate metabolism

— Glucagon, a polypeptide which is synthesised in the
  pancreas and gut. It increases glycogenolysis in the
  liver and stimulates gluconeogenesis.

— Adrenaline, a hormone which is produced in the
  adrenal medulla. It increases glycogenolysis and
  inhibits the uptake of glucose by the tissues.

— Growth hormone which is synthesised in the anterior
  pituitary gland. It blocks the uptake of glucose by muscle and assists in the gluconeogenesis of fat.

— Corticosteroid hormones, e.g. hydrocortisone (cortisol) which are produced by the adrenal cortex. These
  hormones are major insulin antagonists, inhibiting
  carbohydrate utilization by tissues and promoting the
  use of protein instead of carbohydrate for the production of heat and energy.

— Thyroxine, which is produced by the thyroid gland. Its
  effect on glucose metabolism is complex because it
  influences and speeds up many metabolic processes
  in the body as well as increasing the sensitivity of
  many tissues to the effects of catecholamines (noradrenaline and adrenaline).

Diabetes mellitus

Diabetes mellitus is defined as a state of chronic
hyperglycaemia, i.e. an excessive concentration of
glucose in the blood. There are several clinical
forms arising from a variety of pathogenic
mechanisms brought about by genetic,
immunological, and environmental factors (see
also 31:1). The different forms of diabetes can be
grouped under the headings:

☐ Primary (idiopathic) diabetes
☐ Secondary diabetes
☐ Other abnormalities of glucose tolerance

Primary diabetes, caused by:

— Inability of the pancreas to produce sufficient
  insulin (from the earliest stages of the disease).
— Substances in the blood which inhibit or interfere with the action of insulin.
— Production of an abnormal form of insulin.

Types of primary diabetes

There are two main types of primary diabetes:

Insulin dependent diabetes mellitus (IDDM): This is an
acute severe form of diabetes in which insulin is lacking
following the destruction of islet cells in the pancreas possibly by viruses, production of autoimmune antibodies
which damage islet cells and, or, genetic factors. Individuals with certain human leucocyte antigens (HLA) have
been shown to carry a particularly high risk of developing
this form of diabetes.

Non-insulin dependent diabetes mellitus (NIDDM):
Patients are divided into two groups, i.e. obese (fat) and
non-obese. The disease is usually less acute than IDDM
and insulin is not usually essential in treatment. There
does not appear to be an association between NIDDM and
the HLA system or the development of autoimmune
antibodies, but a genetic association does exist.

Secondary diabetes, caused as a result of:

— Pancreatic diseases such as pancreatitis (inflammation of the pancreas) in which insulin
  secretion is reduced.
— Endocrine disorders in which there is an abnormal secretion of hormones that make the action
  of insulin ineffective, e.g. Cushing's syndrome,
  acromegaly, and phaeochromocytoma.
— Drugs that interfere with carbohydrate
  metabolism, e.g. beta-blockers, corticosteroids, oestrogen-containing oral contraceptives, and thiazide diuretics.
— Occasionally genetic disorders such as Down's
  syndrome or Turner's syndrome.

Other abnormalities of glucose tolerance, which
include persons in whom abnormalities of glucose
tolerance may be found often only temporarily or
who are recognized as having an increased risk of
developing diabetes mellitus.

The abnormalities can be grouped as follows:

— Gestational (pregnancy) diabetes mellitus.
— Impaired glucose tolerance which can be
  described as an intermediate state of glucose
  tolerance (i.e. between diabetes mellitus and
  normality) which is asymptomatic and requires
  no treatment.
— Previous abnormality of glucose tolerance.
— Potential abnormality of glucose tolerance.

Metabolism of fats

Fat, being mostly composed of carbon and hydrogen, supplies energy to the body in a concentrated
form. It also carries the fat-soluble vitamins A, D,

and K. Fat is stored under the skin and acts as a shock-absorber. It also surrounds and protects certain organs of the body such as the kidneys. High concentrations of fat are found in nervous tissue.

The end-products of the digestion of fats are FATTY ACIDS and GLYCEROL.

Classification of fats (lipids)

Fat is a substance that contains one or more fatty acids. A fatty acid is an organic acid having a long hydrocarbon chain and an even number of carbon chains. Some fatty acids can be made in the body while others must be obtained in the diet, i.e. essential fatty acids.

The term lipids is used to describe fats and fat-like substances which include:

— Triglycerides (neutral fat), which are compounds of glycerol and three fatty acids. They are the main form of ingested fat and are digested in the small intestine to monoglycerides, fatty acids and glycerol.

— Phospholipids, which are esters of glycerol with fatty acid residues and a phosphoric acid group to which an organic base is attached. They are synthesised in the liver and in the mucosa of the small intestine and are important constituents of nerve cells.

— Cholesterol, which is not a lipid but belongs to the group of high molecular weight solid alcohols called sterols (steroid alcohols). These substances are grouped with the glycerides because they are insoluble in water and soluble in fat solvents.

Cholesterol is found in animal fats e.g. meat and eggs. It is absorbed into the lymphatic system in the presence of bile salts ('chole' means bile). It can also be synthesised in the body, mainly by the liver and intestinal mucosa. About 70-75% of plasma cholesterol exists in chemical combination (esterified) with fatty acids and protein and the remainder as 'free' cholesterol bound to proteins. It is used by the adrenal cortex, ovaries, and testes to produce steroid hormones.

Note: Proteins which transport triglycerides, phospholipids and cholesterol in the plasma are called lipoproteins.

After absorption into the cells of the intestinal mucosa, free fatty acids and glycerides are reconverted to triglycerides. The triglycerides, together with cholesterol, phospholipid and a small, but very important amount of protein, form the small lipoprotein particles called chylomicrons. These pass into the lacteals of the lymphatic system, and eventually into the blood stream. They are transported to fat storage depots (adipose tissue), liver, and muscles. When required for heat and energy, tissue lipase breaks down fat into glycerol and fatty acids. The fatty acids are then oxidized to acetyl co-A which enters the energy producing tricarboxylic acid cycle (see later text). The glycerol is oxidized or converted to glycogen.

Ketones

When more acetyl co-A molecules are produced than there are oxaloacetate molecules being formed in the tricarboxylic acid cycle, the excess acetyl co-A molecules form acetoacetate. Most of this is reduced to beta-hydroxybutyric acid and some is decarboxylated to acetone. Acetoacetate, beta-hydroxybutyric acid, and acetone are collectively termed ketone bodies, or simply ketones. Normal amounts of ketones are expired in the air and excreted in trace amounts in the urine.

In diabetes mellitus and also in starvation, insufficient glucose reaches the body's cells which leads to an increased breakdown of fats to provide the energy requirements for cellular activity. This results in excess acetyl co-A molecules being formed and an increase in the production of ketones with their excretion in the urine. If left untreated, the build up of ketones in the blood causes a state of ketosis which can lead to coma and death.

Control of fat metabolism

The storage and oxidation of fat are mainly under the control of the endocrine system. Insulin, growth hormone, adrenaline, glucagon, and thiamine are among the hormones involved in fat metabolism.

Metabolism of protein

Protein forms an essential part of every living cell and is therefore needed for growth and the production of new cells. It is used in the synthesis of enzymes, hormones, antibodies, and other substances which are required for the healthy functioning and development of the body and its protection (see also 8:3 and 8:4).

The end-products of protein digestion are AMINO ACIDS. They are composed of atoms of nitrogen, carbon, hydrogen, oxygen, and sulphur.

More than 20 different amino acids are used by the body to make its various proteins. Eight of these are called essential amino acids because they are not normally made by the body and must therefore be present in the diet.

Classification of amino acids

The essential amino acids are as follows:

Isoleucine	Phenylalanine
Leucine	Threonine
Lysine	Tryptophan
Methionine	Valine

The remaining amino acids can be synthesised in the liver from amino groups and simple carbon compounds. They include:

Alanine	Glutamine
Arginine	Glycine
Asparagine	Histidine
Aspartic acid	Proline
Cysteine	Serine
Glutamic acid	Tyrosine

The way in which the body makes its various proteins by joining together the different amino acids to form chains is described in 5:2. A chain made up of amino acids joined by peptide links is called a polypeptide chain.

Simple and conjugated proteins

The simple proteins found in the blood include albumin and fibrinogen.

Protein is also found in the body joined (conjugated) to other substances. Examples of conjugated proteins include:

— Haemoglobin, consisting of haem joined to protein.
— Lipoprotein, made up of lipid (fat) and protein.
— Nucleoprotein, formed from the joining of nucleic acids to protein.
— Glycoprotein, consisting of carbohydrate conjugated to protein.

After absorption, amino acids are transported in the blood to the liver and to the cells of the body. In the tissues, amino acids are used to build the specific proteins required by the different types of cell.

Amino acids (derived from ingested protein or from protein recovered from dead cells and secretions) that are not needed for tissue growth or repair are metabolized and converted to carbohydrate or fat, or oxidized in the tricarboxylic acid cycle (see later text) to produce heat and energy.

Normally protein provides about 5-10% of the energy requirements of the body. An increase in the oxidation of protein occurs when the body's energy requirements are not met from carbohydrate metabolism as for example in diabetes mellitus and starvation.

The breakdown of excess amino acids occurs in the liver. The nitrogen-containing amino groups are removed from the amino acids by a process called deamination. During deamination, ammonia is produced which is toxic to the body. It is expelled from the body by being converted into urea which is transported in the blood to the kidneys where it is removed and excreted in the urine. The carbon residues of amino acids are oxidized to produce energy or converted to carbohydrate or fat.

Unlike carbohydrates and fats, protein cannot be stored in appreciable amounts in the tissues. An adequate sustained intake of protein is therefore essential to avoid protein deficiency (see also 8:4).

Control of protein metabolism

The metabolism of protein is influenced by hormones. Protein anabolism (synthesis of various proteins) is controlled mainly by growth hormone and androgen hormones and protein catabolism (breakdown) is regulated by glucocorticoids and adrenocorticotrophic hormone.

Tricarboxylic acid (Krebs') cycle

The tricarboxylic acid cycle, also known as the Krebs' citrate cycle, is a sequence of enzyme controlled reactions in which acetyl co-A from the metabolism of foodstuffs is converted to carbon dioxide and water with the release of energy. It takes place in the mitochondria of the body's cells in the presence of oxygen. It is the final common pathway in the oxidative catabolism of proteins, fats, and carbohydrates.

Acetyl co-A molecules enter the cycle and condense with oxaloacetate which is produced in the cycle. One molecule of oxaloacetate reacts with one molecule of acetyl co-A. There then follows a series of oxidative reactions in which the condensed acetyl co-A is converted to carbon dioxide and hydrogen atoms. The hydrogen atoms eventually react with oxygen to form water.

The energy released at each stage of the chain is used to generate molecules of adenosine triphosphate (ATP) which are the direct sources of energy for tissue cells. When required for cellular activity, the energy stored in ATP is rapidly released.

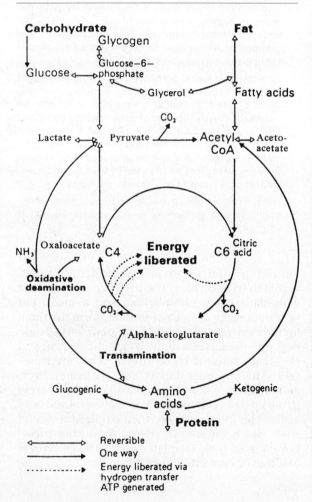

Fig. 8.3 Tricarboxylic acid cycle. *From Principles of Medicine. Courtesy of Oxford University Press.*

8:3 NUTRITION AND DEFICIENCY DISORDERS

An intake of essential nutrients and water is required to sustain life and to keep the different systems of the body functioning well and in harmony.

The following are required:

- Carbohydrates and fats
- Protein
- Fibre
- Iron
- Iodine
- Other mineral salts
- Vitamins

Water is required to maintain the correct fluid balance in the body, to assist in the transport of nutrients and the exchange of substances between cells, and to help in the excretion of waste products. Water is made available to the body not only in fluid drinks and water-containing foods but also from cellular respiration.

Carbohydrates and fats

As previously explained, carbohydrates and fats are the body's main sources of energy and heat. Fat provides the body with energy in a particularly concentrated form. It also helps to protect vital organs, acting as an insulating layer and when required, as a shock absorber.

Sources of carbohydrate in the diet

Sugar	Millet
Cereals e.g. wheat, rice, maize	Tubers and roots e.g. potatoes, yams
Bread	Bananas and plantains
	Sorghum

Sources of fat in the diet

Vegetable oils	Cheese
Groundnuts	Meat
Milk	Fish e.g. sardines, herring
Margarine and butter	
Coconut	Maize and sorghum

Starvation and ketosis

In starvation, the body has less carbohydrate available for metabolism and has to metabolize its fat stores. A similar state occurs in untreated diabetes when the body is unable to use glucose because of a relative lack of insulin. In these conditions more acetyl co-A is produced than there are oxaloacetate molecules with which it can combine. Ketone bodies are therefore formed and because these molecules are acidic, the person can develop a metabolic acidosis (see also 8:2).

Marasmus

This condition is caused by a diet that is extremely low in both calories and protein (see later text).

Protein

Protein is required by the body to make and repair its tissues. It is also needed to synthesise the enzymes, blood clotting factors, hormones and other secretions it needs for its metabolic activities, make antibodies, help to maintain a correct fluid balance, and provide about 10% of the body's energy requirements.

Sources of protein in the diet

Meat	Groundnuts
Fish	Peas and beans
Eggs	Lentils
Milk and yoghourt	Soya bean
Cheese	Dahl
Edible locusts, ants, and grass hoppers	Sorghum

Protein energy malnutrition

Protein energy malnutrition (PEM) occurs in two forms:

— Kwashiorkor
— Marasmus

Kwashiorkor: This condition is most common during the second year of life and occurs when a child receives an unbalanced diet which is very low in protein but relatively adequate in calories. It is more likely to occur when a mother has another baby and the child is no longer able to receive any breast milk.

Importance of breast-feeding a baby

Breast milk contains antibodies and other protective substances. It is a very nutritious food and is enough on its own for a baby's needs until the infant is about four months old. After this, breast milk is not enough and other food must be added to a baby's diet to provide extra calories and protein, as well as vitamins and minerals. If this is not done a child will not grow and develop normally and will suffer from protein-energy malnutrition (PEM).

Infections such as measles, whooping cough, tuberculosis, or infective diarrhoea can also predispose to kwashiorkor because of a child's extra need for protein.

Children with kwashiorkor are miserable, whining and apathetic. They have swelling of the legs, face and body, and their hair may become straight, thin, and change in colour becoming light brown, red-brown, blond, or grey. The skin becomes rough, flaky, and sore. The child is often anaemic and the level of albumin in the blood is reduced. A child with kwashiorkor is shown in Plate 8.1.

Marasmus: This results when the intake of both protein and calories is very low. There are two forms of the condition, early and late marasmus. Early marasmus occurs in the first year of life when a child is weaned on to an inadequate diet. It may also occur during times of famine when a mother has inadequate breast milk. Late marasmus is usually seen in toddlers when their energy requirement is high and their diet does not provide adequate calories.

Children with marasmus show growth retardation. They have wasted muscles, no subcutaneous fat and are very underweight. They are likely to have infections. In malnourished children, diarrhoea tends to occur more frequently and is of longer duration. Such children are more likely to die from severe dysentery. A child with marasmus is shown in Plate 8.2.

If a child has severe kwashiorkor or marasmus, it is easy to diagnose but many children in developing countries suffer from mild malnutrition of protein and calories and these children are also in need of dietary help.

Children with PEM need to be supplied with an adequate diet of protein, calories, vitamins, and minerals. Any associated infections must be treated and the family supported. It is important that a malnourished child receives frequent small meals because the stomach and bowel will only be able to absorb a little at a time. If the child is still breast-feeding then it is important that the mother should also receive a good diet and that the child should be fed often.

In some societies, female children are more likely to suffer from PEM as any available food is often given to the male children. This situation will only change as education improves and attitudes alter, but until then it is important to see that female children receive extra dietary help whenever necessary.

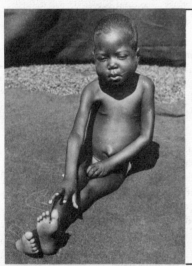

Plate 8.1 Child with kwashiorkor.
Courtesy of David Morley, FAO photograph.

Right
Foods which can help to prevent kwashiorkor.

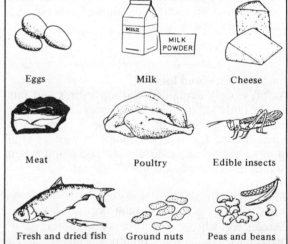

Eggs   Milk   Cheese

Meat   Poultry   Edible insects

Fresh and dried fish   Ground nuts   Peas and beans

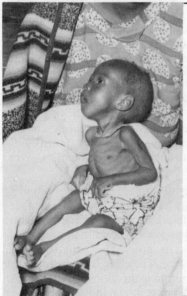

Plate 8.2 Young child with marasmus.
Courtesy of David Morley. Kenya Information Office photograph.

Right
Foods which can help to prevent marasmus.

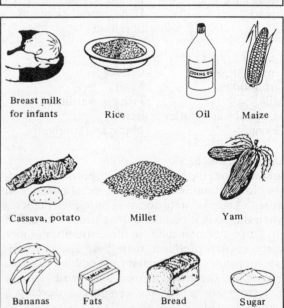

Breast milk for infants   Rice   Oil   Maize

Cassava, potato   Millet   Yam

Bananas   Fats   Bread   Sugar

Iron

Iron is essential for the synthesis of haemoglobin which is the iron (haem) -containing protein found in red cells. Haemoglobin is responsible for transporting oxygen to the tissues and removing waste carbon dioxide from the cells. When examined microscopically, iron deficient red cells appear small and poorly filled with haemoglobin, i.e. microcytic hypochromic cells.

Sources of iron in the diet

Meat and meat products	Quinca
Fish	Red palmoil
Spinach and other	Citrus fruits
green vegetables	Mango
Whole grain cereals	Pineapple
Peas and beans	Guava
Groundnuts	Egg yolk
Certain berries	Alfalfa shoots

Unfortunately the iron in plant foods is less easily absorbed than that present in diets containing mainly animal protein. Vitamin C (ascorbic acid) increases the absorption of iron and therefore can help to prevent iron deficiency in people having a strictly vegetarian diet.

Iron deficiency anaemia

Iron deficiency is probably the commonest cause of anaemia in the world, particularly in infants and growing children and in pregnant women. At these times the body has a greater need for iron.

In developing countries, people are more likely to suffer from iron deficiency because of an inadequate intake of absorbable iron in their diet and also because of parasitic infections which cause blood loss such as hookworm infection and schistosomiasis.

Iodine

Iodine in small amounts is required for the correct functioning of the thyroid gland and the production of the hormones thyroxine and triiodothyronine. These thyroid gland hormones are essential for normal mental and physical development. Their other important functions include the maintenance of healthy skin and hair, control of oxygen use in the body, regulation of heat production, and stimulation of carbohydrate absorption.

Sources of iodine in the diet

Salt water fish
Shellfish and other seafood
Iodized salt

Goitre

A deficiency of iodine causes enlargement of the thyroid gland, i.e. goitre.

In some parts of the world goitre is associated with the eating of cassava as a staple food. This is because large amounts of hydrocyanic acid (cyanide) are present in the tuber and fresh leaves of the cassava plant. Although washing, soaking and boiling can remove most of the cyanide, traces of the chemical usually remain. When ingested, the cyanide is converted to thiocyanate which interferes with the metabolism of the thyroid gland. This, when combined with a barely adequate intake of iodine, can lead to goitre.

During pregnancy, thiocyanates are able to cross the placenta which leads to infants being born with cretinism (syndrome of dwarfism and mental retardation due to lack of thyroid hormone from birth).

Mineral salts

Besides iron and iodine, the body also requires other minerals such as calcium, phosphate, sodium, and potassium.

Calcium is required for the synthesis of teeth and bones and is important in the contraction of muscles and coagulation of blood. It is found mainly in milk, cheese, eggs, and fresh green vegetables.

Phosphate is also an important constituent of bone and teeth and helps to maintain the normal fluid balance in the body. It is found in oatmeal, cheese, and meat such as liver and kidney.

The important roles of sodium and potassium in the body are described in Chapter 29.

Vitamins

An adequate supply of various vitamins is required to enable the body to grow and perform its various metabolic functions. Vitamins are co-factors for enzyme activity.

Classification of vitamins

Vitamins are divided into those that are fat soluble and those that are water soluble.

Fat soluble vitamins
Vitamin A
Vitamin D (calciferol)
Vitamin E
Vitamin K

Water soluble vitamins
Vitamin B complex: i.e. thiamin (B_1), niacin, riboflavin, pyridoxine, cyanocobalamin (B_{12}), folate, pantothenic acid and biotin.
Vitamin C

The functions and common dietary sources of the important vitamins, and the disorders which arise due to vitamin deficiencies are summarized in Chart 8.1.

Chart 8.1 Functions and Dietary Sources of Important Vitamins and Vitamin Deficiency Disorders

Vitamin	Functions	Dietary Sources	Deficiency Disorders
Vitamin A	□ Necessary for the eye to respond to light. □ Assists in the normal functioning of sweat, lacrimal and salivary glands.	Green leafy vegetables, carrots, mango, papaya, milk, dairy products, egg yolks, red palm oil, cod liver oil. Breast milk after birth (colostrum) is rich in Vitamin A.	● Xerophthalmia, causing dryness of the whites of the eyes, poor vision in dim light (night blindness), and corneal opacity leading to blindness *Note*: Vitamin A deficiency is one of the principal deficiency disorders in the world.
Vitamin D	□ Required for normal mineralization of bone. □ Strengthens muscles.	Milk, egg yolks, cheese, butter, cabbage, and oily fish. Also produced in the body by the action of sunlight on the skin.	● Softening of bones causing: – Rickets in children. – Osteomalacia in adults. *Note*: The need for Vitamin D is high in young children and pregnant women. Adequate exposure to sunlight should be encouraged.
Vitamin K	□ Required for the synthesis of prothrombin and therefore essential for normal blood clotting.	Green leafy vegetables. Also synthesised in the colon by bacteria.	Deficiency is rare except in newborns and following prolonged antibiotic treatment.
Vitamin B complex: – Thiamin (B₁)	□ Necessary for the normal metabolism of carbohydrates. □ Required for the normal functioning of the nervous system.	Husks of rice and other whole grain cereals, yeast, peas, beans, and other pulses. *Note*: Thiamin is present mainly in the outer layers of grain. After boiling, up to 85% of the vitamin is contained in the boiled water.	● Cardiac (wet) beri-beri leading to cardiac failure and oedema. ● Neurological (dry) beri-beri with numbness, tingling and weakness of the limbs. Paralysis may occur. ● Infantile beri-beri with vomiting, diarrhoea, hoarse voice, and paralysis of cranial nerves. Cardiac failure and convulsions may occur.
– Niacin	□ Needed for normal carbohydrate and fat metabolism. □ Necessary for correct functioning of the digestive and nervous systems.	Groundnuts, fish, yeast, wheat (outer grain), rice, pulses, and millets.	● Pellagra, causing dermatitis, diarrhoea, nerve damage and spinal cord changes, mental confusion, numbness of the limbs, unsteady walking, and anaemia. *Note*: Common when maize or sorghum is the staple diet.

Vitamin	Functions	Dietary Sources	Deficiency Disorders
– Riboflavin	□ Necessary for growth and catabolism in all tissues.	Beans, peas, green leafy vegetables, eggs, liver, oil-seeds, whole-meal flour. Note: As with other B vitamins, riboflavin is lost in the milling process of cereals or in water used for cooking.	• Sore inflamed tongue, soreness and cracking at the corner of the mouth, and dermatitis especially of the nose. The skin becomes rough and greasy. Note: Often found with other vitamin B deficiencies.
– Pyridoxine (B_6)	□ Essential for normal amino acid metabolism. □ Needed for the normal use of iron in the bone marrow.	Vegetables, liver, cereals (especially outer layers of grain).	A primary nutritional deficiency is rare, but can occur with other vitamin deficiences. • Causes sore tongue and mouth and iron deficiency anaemia. • Peripheral nerve damage can occur in pyridoxine deficient persons receiving antituberculosis drugs (isoniazid).
– Cyanocobalamin (B_{12}) – Folate	□ Required for DNA synthesis and therefore essential for normal red cell production and other metabolic processes.	Vitamin B_{12} is found in meat, eggs, milk and fish. Note: Before B_{12} can be absorbed it must first combine with intrinsic factor secreted by cells in the stomach wall. Folate is found in green leafy vegetables, lentils and milk (cow's).	• B_{12} or folate deficiency causes megaloblastic anaemia. There may also be inflammation of the tongue and pigmentation of exposed parts of the finger joints. • B_{12} deficiency can also cause degeneration of the spinal cord and nerves, leading to paralysis. Note: There is an increased need for folate in pregnancy, lactation, and in the early years of life.
Vitamin C	□ Needed for making collagen. □ Gives strength to the walls of blood capillaries. □ Necessary for normal red cell production. □ Required for healthy bones and teeth.	Citrus fruits e.g. oranges, green leafy vegetables, tomatoes, Indian gooseberry, blackcurrants, bananas, potatoes (when cooked in their skin). red and green peppers.	• Scurvy, causing bleeding from gums and around hair follicles, easy bruising, slowness in healing, generalized weakness, and fatigue. Infantile scurvy commonly affects babies about 6-8 months after weaning (breast milk contains vitamin C).

Fibre (roughage)

This is insoluble material which includes a mixture of substances that are relatively resistant to digestion such as bran, pectins, cellulose, and vegetable fibres. It is considered to be an important part of a balanced healthy diet, possibly helping to prevent intestinal and vascular disorders, obesity and diabetes mellitus. Foods with a high fibre content include wholemeal cereals and flour, root vegetables, nuts, and fruit.

8:4 THE LIVER

The liver is a lobed organ lying in the upper right side of the abdomen beneath the diaphragm. It is the largest single organ in the body and chemically the most active.

Blood supply of the liver

The liver has a rich blood supply, with oxygenated blood reaching it through the hepatic artery which is a branch of the aorta. In the liver the hepatic artery divides into hepatic arterioles which branch into smaller tubes called sinusoids which supply the liver cells.

The hepatic portal circulation consists of the portal vein and its tributaries. Blood draining from the stomach, intestinal tract, spleen, pancreas, and gall bladder enters the liver through the portal vein (see Fig. 8.4). This blood carries the digested nutrients to the liver cells through a network of portal venules and venous sinusoids.

Both the venous and arteriolar sinusoids drain into a central vein which leads through larger veins into the hepatic vein. The deoxygenated blood is returned to the heart by way of the inferior vena cava into which the hepatic vein drains (see Fig. 8.4).

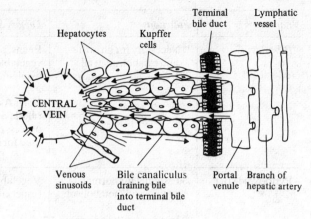

Fig. 8.5 Section of a liver lobule.
Reproduced in part from the Study Guide 851, with the permission of the US Army, Fort Sam Houston, Texas, USA.

Structure of the liver

The liver is divided into many small roughly circular units called lobules. Each lobule consists of rows of cells (hepatocytes) radiating from a central vein (see Fig. 8.5). The hepatocytes are supplied with arterial blood through an hepatic arteriole and arterial sinusoids, and with blood from the portal vein through a portal venule and venous sinusoids.

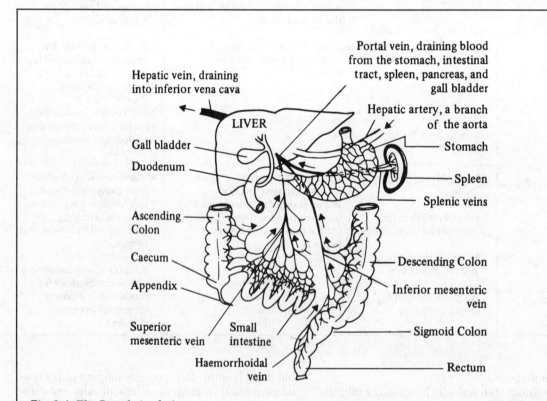

Fig. 8.4 The Portal circulation.
Reproduced in part from the Study Guide 851, with the permission of the US Army. Fort Sam Houston, Texas, USA.

The venous sinusoids are lined with phagocytic cells called Kupffer cells which remove bacteria (of intestinal origin) and other foreign bodies from the blood before it enters the systemic circulation. About 20% of the hepatic cell mass is composed of phagocytic cells.

Running between the rows of hepatocytes are small channels called canaliculi which collect the bile made by the hepatocytes. These bile canaliculi drain into terminal bile ducts which lead, by way of larger interlobular bile ducts, into the main hepatic duct which drains into the gall bladder.

Functions of the liver

— To manufacture and secrete bile. Bile is a yellow-green coloured fluid which contains cholesterol, a small amount of bilirubin, and bile salts, (cholic acid and chenodeoxycholic acid, conjugated with glycine and taurine). The bile is transported through the hepatic ducts to the gall bladder where it is stored, concentrated, and released into the duodenum where it is essential for the adequate absorption of fats and of vitamin K. Bacterial reduction produces the bile salts deoxycholic acid and lithocholic acid.

Much of the bile secreted into the intestine is reabsorbed into the hepatic portal circulation, recycled in the liver, and re-excreted in the bile. Only a small amount of bile is normally excreted in the faeces.

— To conjugate bilirubin in the hepatocytes and excrete it in the bile (see later text).

— To store glycogen and when required to convert it to glucose (glycogenolysis) to maintain the blood glucose level.

If the liver has used up all its glycogen stores and the blood glucose level is below normal, the liver is able to convert protein and fat into glucose (gluconeogenesis).

— To manufacture the plasma proteins fibrinogen, albumin, and globulin (except gamma globulin).

The liver also produces transport proteins such as transferrin which binds and transports iron, and haptoglobin which combines with free haemoglobin.

Alpha fetoprotein is normally produced by the liver only before birth.

— To synthesise blood clotting factors including prothrombin, and factors V, VII, IX, X, XI, and XII. Vitamin K is required for the synthesis of prothrombin and factors VII, IX, and X.

— To detoxicate (detoxify) the ammonia released from amino acid deamination by converting it to urea for excretion by the kidneys. The liver is also involved in the oxidation, reduction, hydrolysis, or conjugation of other metabolic products, drugs, hormones, and alcohol.

The prolonged intake of alcohol can seriously damage liver cells, causing cirrhosis of the liver.

— To store iron, vitamin A, and vitamin B_{12}. Metabolic reactions involving vitamin D, thiamin, and niacin are also carried out in the liver.

— To assist in the removal of worn out blood cells and microorganisms from the blood. The Kupffer cells form part of the mononuclear phagocytic defence (reticuloendothelial system) of the body as explained in Chapter 11.

Metabolism of bilirubin

Bilirubin is mainly formed from the breakdown of haemoglobin in the cells of the liver, spleen, and bone marrow. A small amount is produced from the breakdown of haem-containing proteins such as myoglobin (oxygen-transporting muscle protein), and the enzymes catalase, cytochromes, and peroxidases.

The haem (iron porphyrin) of the haemoglobin molecule is first separated from the globin and the porphyrin part is converted to biliverdin which is then reduced to bilirubin. This bilirubin is referred to as unconjugated (indirect) bilirubin. It is not soluble in water and cannot be excreted in the urine. It is bound to albumin and transported in the blood to the liver.

In the liver cells, the enzyme glucuronosyltransferase joins (conjugates) glucuronic acid to bilirubin forming bilirubin glucuronides (mainly diglucuronide). This bilirubin is known as conjugated (direct) bilirubin. It is water-soluble and non-toxic.

Glucuronosyltransferase

This enzyme becomes fully active about 3 weeks after birth. A rise in plasma bilirubin may therefore occur during the first week of life, resulting in 'physiological jaundice' of the newborn, especially in an infant born prematurely (see also 30:2).

Conjugated bilirubin passes into the bile canaliculi, through the bile duct, and into the intestine. In the terminal ileum and colon, the conjugated bilirubin is deconjugated and reduced by bacteria to various pigments and colourless chromogens (urobilinogen), most of which are excreted in the faeces. One of the urobilinogen chromogens excreted in the faeces is stercobilinogen.

Some of the urobilinogen from the intestine is absorbed into the portal circulation and reaches the liver where it re-enters the intestine in the bile and is excreted in the faeces. A small amount of this reabsorbed urobilinogen is carried in the blood through the liver and transported to the kidneys where it is excreted in the urine.

Urobilinogen is rapidly oxidized to the coloured pigment urobilin (stercobilinogen to stercobilin). A diagram illustrating normal bilirubin

metabolism is shown in Fig. 8.6.

The normal level of total bilirubin (unconjugated and conjugated) in the blood of an adult is usually 3-17 μmol/1 (0.2-0.9 mg%). When the plasma bilirubin reaches around 34 μmol/l (2 mg%) a person will become jaundiced, with the skin and particularly the white part of the eyes appearing yellow-coloured. The causes of jaundice and the tests used to investigate liver disorders are described in Chapter 30.

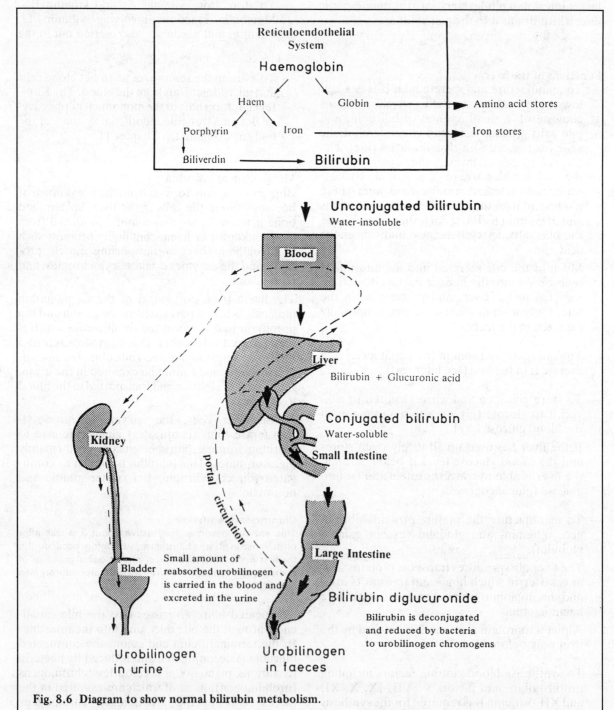

Fig. 8.6 Diagram to show normal bilirubin metabolism.

8:5 TERMS USED IN GASTROINTESTINAL MEDICINE AND LIVER DISORDERS

Cholangitis: An inflammation of the bile ducts.

Cholecystitis: Inflammation of the gall bladder. Acute cholecystitis is usually caused by a gallstone obstructing the neck or cystic duct of the gall bladder (cholecystolithiasis).

Cirrhosis of the liver: Refers to the destruction of liver cells and their replacement by fatty or fibrous tissue (fibrosis). Cirrhosis of the liver can be caused by viruses, toxins, and parasites such as *Schistosoma japonicum* and *Schistosoma mansoni*. It is also associated with heavy alcohol drinking. Cirrhosis may cause obstruction of the circulation through the portal vein with associated haematemesis and bleeding from the varicose veins in the rectum. In advanced liver cirrhosis, there is a build-up of fluid in the abdomen (ascites) and jaundice develops as more liver cells are damaged. The spleen also becomes enlarged.

Gastrectomy: Surgical removal of the whole stomach (total gastrectomy) or acid-pepsin producing part of the stomach (partial gastrectomy). This may be done to remove a malignant growth or as treatment for a peptic ulcer. Because of the changes in gastric emptying and the loss of production of acid and intrinsic factor, gastrectomy patients may develop malabsorption and anaemia, sometimes many years after surgery.

Haematemesis: Vomiting of blood, often as a result of a bleeding gastric or duodenal ulcer, or to increased pressure in the portal vein causing bleeding from dilated veins (varices) at the lower end of the oesophagus and upper part of the stomach. Following bleeding in the gastrointestinal tract, the occult blood test is positive (see 30:12).

Haemoptysis: Coughing up sputum containing blood. It must be distinguished from haematemesis. Haemoptysis is associated with advanced pulmonary tuberculosis and severe paragonimiasis.

Hepatoma: A malignant tumour of the liver. A common cause of hepatocellular carcinoma in tropical countries is the eating of foods contaminated with aflatoxin, a toxic metabolite produced by certain moulds that grow on groundnuts and grains stored under damp conditions.
Testing the serum for alpha fetoprotein may be a helpful investigation in diagnosing hepatoma, but it is not always positive.

Hiatus hernia: A hernia is the projecting of an organ or part of an organ through the containing wall of its cavity. A hiatus hernia is the projecting of part of the stomach into the chest cavity through a weak point in the muscular wall of the diaphragm (usually where the oesophagus passes through the diaphragm).

Melaena: The passing of black faeces which contain digested blood. It usually occurs following serious bleeding in the upper gastrointestinal tract. Faeces from a person taking iron tablets will also appear black. Dark streaks may also be seen in haemolytic diseases.

Paralytic ileus: A condition in which there is a failure of the intestinal muscles to move the food along the bowel. It leads to intestinal obstruction and electrolyte and fluid imbalance.

Pyloric stenosis: A condition in which the pylorus of the stomach is obstructed. In adults it is often due to cancer or caused by scarring from a long-standing duodenal ulcer. In babies it is caused by a congenital defect and is corrected by surgery.

Sprue: A condition associated with diarrhoea and weight loss. The faeces are pale and frothy because they contain an abnormally high fat content (steatorrhoea). The cause of the disease is not known but may be partly due to a result of bowel infection. In sprue the bowel is unable to absorb nutrients in the normal way and therefore there is often a deficiency of essential vitamins especially folate, and also of electrolytes, iron, and calcium. Sprue occurs mainly in Asia and parts of South America. It is rare in Africa.

Ulcerative colitis: A condition in which the mucosa and submucosa of the colon become inflamed (ulcerated), causing pain, diarrhoea, and often rectal bleeding.

Vagotomy: Surgical cutting of the vagus nerve to reduce acid production by the stomach. This operation is sometimes carried out to treat duodenal ulceration.

Recommended Reading

See the books listed at the end of Chapter 5 and also:

Brown, J and R. *Finding the Causes of Child Malnutrition*, Centre pour le promotion de la santé, 1985. Available from Teaching Aids at Low Cost (TALC), PO Box 49, St Albans, Herts, AL1 4AX, UK priced £1.00.

Cameron and Hofvander. *Manual on Feeding Infants and Young Children*, Oxford University Press, 1981. Available from Teaching Aids at Low Cost (see above for address), priced £2.00.

Hampton, J. *Happy Healthy Children*, Macmillan Publishing Ltd, 1985. Available from Teaching Aids at Low Cost (see above for address), priced £1.25.

Ritchie, J. *Nutrition and Families*, Macmillan Publishing Ltd, 1983. Available from Teaching Aids at Low Cost (see above for address), priced £2.95.

9

Nervous System and Sense Organs
Endocrine System

9:1   NERVOUS SYSTEM

The nervous system (together with the endocrine system) controls and coordinates the functioning of the body. It provides the mechanism by which an individual can respond to changes in their internal and external environment.

Every activity involving the nervous system includes:

— A sensory function which detects, or senses, change and harmful stimuli.

— An interpretive function which interprets sensory stimuli and organizes appropriate action.

— A motor function which carries out the appropriate action.

The nervous system is divided into:

■ A central nervous system which is composed of:

— The brain
— Spinal cord

The brain and spinal cord carry out the interpretive and organizing roles of the nervous system.

■ A peripheral nervous system which is composed of:

— Cranial nerves (12 pairs)
— Spinal nerves (31 pairs)

The peripheral nerves carry out the sensory and motor functions of the nervous system. They also carry the nerve fibres of what is called the autonomic nervous system. This is the area of the nervous system which regulates the body's autonomic, or involuntary, functions (explained in later text).

Nerves

A nerve is a bundle of separate cells called neurones. As shown in Fig. 9.1, each neurone consists of a cell body, a number of short thread-like extensions called dendrites, and one larger fibre called an axon. The axon of most nerves is surrounded by a fatty substance called myelin (myelin sheath).

Neurones receive, transmit, and pass on information. They respond to stimuli by conducting impulses. The dendrites conduct impulses into the cell body and the axon conducts impulses away from the cell body.

Note: The central nervous system and peripheral nervous system are not separate systems but form part of the same nervous system. They are completely dependant on each other for efficient activity.

Central nervous system

The brain is protected by the cranium (skull), and the spinal cord by the vertebral column.

The brain and spinal cord are covered by three membranes called the meninges which consist of:

— An outer protective membrane called the dura mater.
— A middle membrane called the arachnoid mater.
— An inner membrane called the pia mater.

Between the arachnoid mater and the pia mater there is a space called the subarachnoid space. This is filled with a fluid called cerebrospinal fluid which acts as a shock absorber and also as a circulatory system for the brain and spinal cord. The composition and laboratory investigation of this fluid in meningitis and other diseases involving the central nervous system are described in 9:2.

Brain

The brain is the central control centre for all nervous activity in the body. The main parts of the brain are as follows:

☐ Cerebrum: This is the largest part of the brain. It is made up of a mass of white nerve fibres covered by a folded (convoluted) grey layer called the cerebral cortex. A groove extending from front to back divides the cerebrum into two similar halves, or hemispheres. The right hemisphere coordinates activity on the left side of the body and the left hemisphere coordinates activity on the right side of the body. The work of the different areas of the cerebrum is shown in Fig. 9.3.

☐ Cerebellum: This part of the brain lies below and behind the cerebrum and is divided into two lobes. It coordinates muscular activity, posture, and balance in the body.

☐ Pons varolii: This is situated at the base of the brain in front of the cerebellum. It connects the various lobes of the brain. The groups of cells within it act as relay stations.

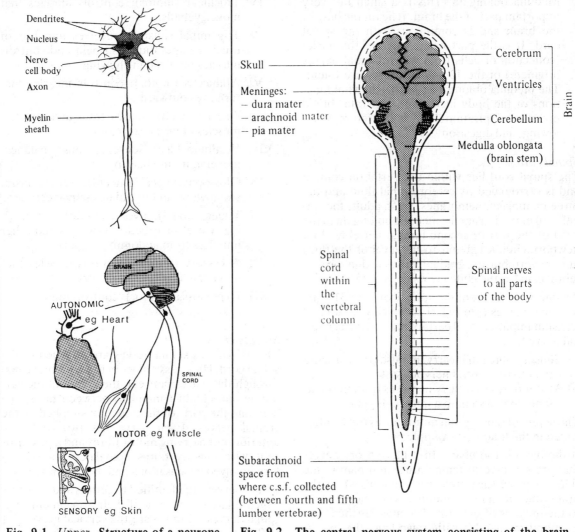

Fig. 9.1 *Upper* Structure of a neurone. *Lower* Relationship between the autonomic, motor, and sensory activities.

Fig. 9.2 The central nervous system consisting of the brain, spinal cord, and spinal nerves. In the diagram only the nerves on one half of the spinal cord are shown.

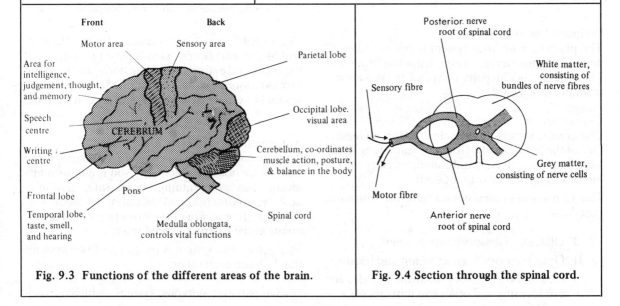

Fig. 9.3 Functions of the different areas of the brain.

Fig. 9.4 Section through the spinal cord.

□ Medulla oblongata: This is a small but very important part of the brain. It lies at the base of the brain and is continuous with the spinal cord. It is the part where most of the nuclei (collection of cells from which cranial nerves originate) of the 12 cranial nerves are found. The medulla oblongata controls the vital functions of the body including heart rate, blood pressure, respiration, body temperature, swallowing, and digestion.

Spinal cord
The spinal cord lies within the vertebral column and is surrounded by cerebrospinal fluid and the three meningeal membranes. In an adult, the spinal cord extends from the medulla oblongata to the level of the first or second lumbar vertebra. In a newborn child it extends to the level of the third lumbar vertebra and gradually rises within the vertebral canal as the child grows.

Arising laterally from the spinal cord are 31 pairs of spinal nerves (see Fig. 9.2) which pick up and transmit impulses to all parts of the body. Each spinal nerve has:

— Sensory fibres that carry impulses from a sense organ to the central nervous system.
— Motor fibres that carry impulses from the central nervous system to a muscle or gland.

The action of sensory and motor fibres can be illustrated in the following example:

If the hand is too near a fire, the sensory nerves that are sensitive to temperature and pain in the skin relay messages (electrical impulses) to the brain which then relays impulses via a motor nerve to the muscles of the arm. The muscles then contract and the hand is withdrawn from the fire. A cross-section through the spinal cord is shown in Fig. 9.4.

Peripheral nervous system
The peripheral nervous system is composed of 12 pairs of cranial nerves arising from the brain and brain stem, and 31 pairs of spinal nerves arising from the spinal cord.

Cranial nerves
The cranial nerves are attached to the undersurface of the brain, mostly from the brain stem. They have numbers I to XII, and contain sensory fibres, motor fibres, or a mixture of both.

The 12 pairs of cranial nerves have the following functions:

   I Olfactory (sensory): senses smell.

  II Optic (sensory): senses vision and balance.

 III Oculomotor (motor): controls muscles for eye focusing and other eye movements.

 IV Trochlear (motor): controls muscles that move eyeballs.

  V Trigeminal (mixed): receives impulses of touch, temperature and pain and controls muscles involved in chewing.

 VI Abducens (motor): controls muscles that turn eyes outwards.

 VII Facial (mixed): senses taste and controls muscles of facial expression.

VIII Vestibulochlear (sensory): senses balance, movement, and hearing.

 IX Glossopharyngeal (mixed): senses taste, swallowing, and stimulates saliva secretion.

  X Vagus (mixed): involved in taste, swallowing, voice, heartbeat, peristalsis and other impulses from abdominal organs.

 XI Accessory (motor): controls muscles that move the head and shoulders.

 XII Hypoglossal (motor): controls muscles that move the tongue.

Spinal nerves
The 31 pairs of spinal nerves are attached to the spinal cord. They pass out from the vertebral canal through the spaces between the arches of the vertebrae and conduct impulses between the spinal cord and the parts of the body not supplied by the cranial nerves. Each nerve has two roots, an anterior root carrying motor fibres and a posterior root with sensory fibres. Spinal nerves are therefore involved in sensations and movements.

Spinal nerves are identified by letters and numbers which relate to the area of their attachment, e.g. spinal nerves C1 to C8 are the cervical nerves, T1 to T12 the thoracic nerves, L1 to L5 the lumbar nerves, S1 to S5 the sacral nerves and C0 the one coccygeal nerve. The many branches of the spinal nerves have names which can be found in anatomy textbooks.

The spinal nerves have voluntary (under the control of the will) fibres extending to the muscles of the trunk and extremities of the body, and involuntary (autonomic) fibres extending to the gastrointestinal tract, urinary system, and cardiac system.

Autonomic nervous system
The autonomic nervous system regulates those bodily functions of which a person is not normally aware such as breathing, heart rate, glandular activity, contraction and dilatation of blood vessels, variation in size of the eye's pupil, and movements in the gastrointestinal tract.

The autonomic system is made up of two systems that balance each other:

□ Sympathetic nervous system, which is concerned with maintaining the body's systems when a person is alert, exercising, or in danger. It controls the emotions such as fear or excitement, causing the heart to beat faster, the blood pressure to rise and breathing to deepen or quicken.

The system consists of collections of nerve cells (ganglia) mediated by noradrenaline at the nerve endings and acetylcholine as the chemical transmitter at the ganglia.

☐ The parasympathetic nervous system predominates when the body is resting. It consists of ganglia in the midbrain, medulla oblongata, and sacral region.

The relationship between the sympathetic and parasympathetic parts of the autonomic system can be summarized as follows:

Sympathetic System	Parasympathetic System
● Quickens the action of the heart.	● Slows the action of the heart.
● Dilates air passages.	● Contracts air passages.
● Contracts the blood vessels of the skin and gut so that more blood flows to the muscles where it is needed.	● Dilates the blood vessels of the gut where the blood is needed for digestion. Blood flow to muscles is reduced.
● Decreases gut movements.	● Increases gut movements.
● Decreases secretions of most glands except sweat glands.	● Increases secretions of most glands except sweat glands.
● Increases sweating.	● Decreases sweating.
● Prevents emptying of the bladder and bowels.	● Allows emptying of the bladder and bowels.
● Dilates the pupil of the eye.	● Constricts the pupil of the eye.
● Adjusts ciliary muscles so that the eyes are able to see distant objects.	● Contracts ciliary muscles so that the eyes are able to see near objects.

9:2   CEREBROSPINAL FLUID (CSF)

Deep within each cerebral hemisphere lies a large, irregularly shaped chamber called the lateral ventricle. This is filled with a fluid called cerebrospinal fluid (c.s.f.). The fluid passes into a third ventricle before flowing down the cerebral aquaduct into a fourth ventricle which lies between the pons and cerebellum of the brain. From the fourth ventricle the c.s.f. passes down the small central canal of the spinal cord and through openings into the subarachnoid space.

The c.s.f. is made continuously by small collections of blood vessels (choroid plexuses) which line the ventricular cavities. In an adult about 250-750 ml of c.s.f. are produced daily and about 120-125 ml fill the subarachnoid space. Small vessels in the subarachnoid space called arachnoid villi reabsorb the c.s.f. into the blood stream. In health there is therefore a constant circulation of c.s.f. within the ventricular system and subarachnoid space.

Cerebrospinal fluid has a composition similar to plasma except that it contains less protein, more chloride, and less glucose.

Functions of c.s.f.
— To provide a fluid cushion to protect the brain and spinal cord from mechanical injury caused by any sudden movement of the body.
— To carry nutrients to the brain and spinal cord and remove waste substances.
— To maintain a constant pressure inside the head and around the spinal cord.

Laboratory testing of c.s.f.
Requests for laboratory testing of c.s.f. are usually made when meningitis (inflammation of the meninges) is suspected or any other disease which produces changes in the c.s.f.

Cerebrospinal fluid for laboratory investigations is usually obtained by lumbar puncture (spinal tap), or occasionaly from infants by ventricular puncture. The procedure should be carried out by a medical officer.

Lumbar puncture site
The spinal cord in an adult ends at the first or second lumbar vertebra but the arachnoid space continues to the sacral region. A sample of c.s.f. can therefore be taken safely between the third and fourth or fourth and fifth vertebra (see Fig. 9.2).

Note: The collection of c.s.f. for bacteriological and parasitological investigations is described in 38:12 in Volume II of the Manual.

Investigations
The laboratory testing of c.s.f. usually includes:

☐ Describing the appearance of the c.s.f.

A normal c.s.f. appears clear and colourless. A purulent or markedly cloudy c.s.f. is associated with meningitis caused by pyogenic bacteria such as *Neisseria meningitidis*, *Streptococcus pneumoniae*, and *Haemophilus influenzae*. A c.s.f. appears cloudy when it contains over about 200 white cells × 10^6/l. A slightly cloudy c.s.f. may be seen in tuberculous and viral meningitis and trypanosomiasis meningoencephalitis.

When blood is present in c.s.f., this is often the result of a traumatic lumbar puncture. Pathological causes of blood in c.s.f. include a recent subarachnoid haemorrhage and meningoencephalitis caused by pathogenic amoebae such as *Naegleria* species. Biochemical tests should not be performed if the c.s.f. is blood stained (smears for pathogens and culturing should be carried out).

A c.s.f. which is yellow-coloured (xanthrochromic) due to the breakdown of haemoglobin, is associated with an earlier subarachnoid haemorrhage, cerebral tumour, or jaundice.

Spontaneous clotting of c.s.f. occurs when there is an excess of fibrinogen in the fluid, e.g. in meningitis. In tuberculous meningitis, a small skin (pellicle) may form on the surface of the c.s.f.

□ A total and differential white cell count.

Normal c.s.f. may contain up to 5 lymphocytes × 10^6/l (5/mm^3). A raised white cell count is found in meningitis, meningoencephalitis and neurosyphilis. In pyogenic meningitis, the cells are mostly neutrophils (pus cells). In tuberculous, viral, and leptospiral meningitis, trypanosomiasis meningoencephalitis, and neurosyphilis, the cells are mostly lymphocytes and other mononuclear cells.

□ Mesurement of total protein.

Normal c.s.f. contains 0.15-0.40 g/l of protein (slightly lower in ventricular c.s.f.). A raised c.s.f. total protein is found in all forms of meningitis, meningoencephalitis, neurosyphilis, brain tumours, subarachnoid haemorrhage, cerebral injury, spinal cord compression, poliomyelitis, Guillain-Barré syndrome (often the only c.s.f. abnormality) and polyneuritis.

□ Measurement of glucose.

Normal c.s.f. contains 2.5-4.0 mmol/l glucose depending on the blood glucose (usually about two thirds of the blood glucose). A markedly reduced c.s.f. glucose is found in pyogenic meningitis. In viral meningitis, the c.s.f. glucose may be low or normal and in tuberculous meningitis it is reduced.

□ Microscopical examination of unstained and stained preparations for bacteria (e.g. meningococci, pneumococci, *H. influenzae*, *M. tuberculosis*), parasites such as trypanosomes and amoebae, and fungi such as *Cryptococcus neoformans*.

□ Culturing when this is indicated from the results of the cell count, biochemical tests, and smears.

Note: Details of the cell count, microscopical examination, and culturing of c.s.f. can be found in 38:12 in Volume II of the Manual.

Summary of the characteristics of normal c.s.f.
Hydrostatic pressure   ....   About 120 mm Hg
Appearance   ....   Clear and colourless
Reaction   ....   pH 7.4-7.6
Relative density 1.005-1.008
Total protein   ....   0.15-0.40 g/l (15-40 mg%)
                Slightly lower in ventricular c.s.f.
Glucose   ....   2.5-4.0 mmol/l (45-72 mg%)
                About two thirds of the blood glucose
Cells   ....   Up to 5 cells × 10^6/l (5/mm^3)

9:3   SPECIAL SENSES OF THE BODY

The five special senses of the body are as follows:
■ Sight
■ Hearing
■ Smell
■ Taste
■ Touch

Sight
The organ of sight is the eye. Reflected light enters the eye through a small hole in the coloured muscular ring (iris) of the eye called the pupil (see Fig. 9.5). The light is focused by the lens onto a light-sensitive area of the eye called the retina. The receptor cones and rods of the retina convert this light energy into nerve impulses which are conveyed in the optic nerve to the brain where they produce the sensation of sight.

The size of the pupil is automatically adjusted to control the amount of light entering the eye. The lens has the power of accommodation, i.e. it can become thinner to focus rays of light from distant objects and thicker to focus light from very near objects. The thickness of the lens is altered by ciliary muscles.

The eyes are protected and kept clean by the reflex action of blinking accompanied by a 'washing' of the eye surface with protective fluid produced from tear glands in the eyelids.

The parts of the eye are shown in Fig. 9.5.

Major causes of blindness in tropical countries
In tropical and developing countries, eye diseases are common.The main causes of serious eye diseases and loss of vision are xerophthalmia caused

by severe vitamin A deficiency, onchocerciasis (river blindness) caused by the filarial worm *Onchocerca volvulus*, and trachoma caused by an easily spread small bacterium called *Chlamydia trachomatis*. Poverty, malnutrition, overcrowding, poor personal hygiene, inadequate and unsafe water supplies, and lack of basic medical care in rural areas, contribute to the high incidence of blindness found in developing countries.

Short-sightedness and long-sightedness

In the normal eye, parallel light rays are brought to a focus on the retina with the accommodation relaxed. This enables a person to see clearly objects near to the eye and some distance from it.

A short-sighted person is able to see clearly only those objects that are near to the eye because

parallel light rays are brought to a focus in front of the retina instead of on it. Objects further than about 6 metres from the eye are blurred and cannot be made sharp by accommodation. The medical term for short-sightedness is myopia. It is corrected by wearing spectacles with concave lenses (see Fig. 9.6a).

A long-sighted person is unable to see clearly objects that are near to the eye because parallel light rays are brought to a focus behind the retina when accommodation is relaxed. Objects closer than 6 metres from the eye appear blurred and objects further than six metres may be made sharp with an effort of accommodation. The medical term for long-sightedness is hypermetropia. It is corrected by wearing spectacles with convex lenses (see Fig. 9.6b).

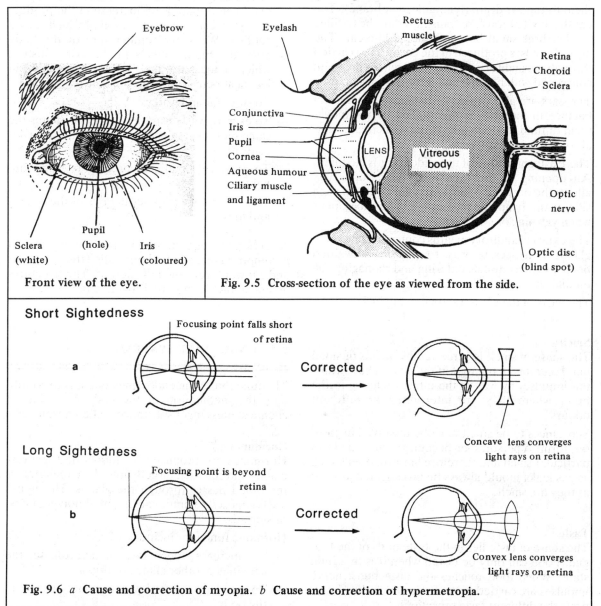

Front view of the eye.

Fig. 9.5 Cross-section of the eye as viewed from the side.

Fig. 9.6 *a* Cause and correction of myopia. *b* Cause and correction of hypermetropia.

Colour blindness

This refers to conditions in which colours are confused with one another. The most common type of colour blindness is red-blindness in which a person is unable to distinguish between red and green. It is usually due to an inherited defect in the functioning of the light sensitive cells of the retina which are responsible for colour perception.

The microscopical examination of stained specimens requires normal colour vision. Before beginning work in a medical laboratory, trainees should therefore have their colour vision tested.

Hearing

The organ of hearing is the ear. Sound is produced by vibration. The outer ear (see Fig. 9.7) collects the sound wave vibrations from the air and directs them to the ear drum (tympanic membrane). The ear drum vibrations are transmitted to the cochlea by the three small bones of the middle ear. The nerve impulses produced in the cochlea are carried through the auditory nerve to the areas of the brain concerned with hearing and interpreting sounds.

The ears are also organs of balance. The correct balance in the body is maintained by the movement of fluid (endolymph) in the semicircular canals of the inner ear (see Fig. 9.7).

The Eustachian tube of the middle ear is air-filled. An opening of the tube into the nasopharynx allows the pressure of air to remain equal on each side of the tympanic membrane. The tube opens when yawning or swallowing.

The external auditory meatus contains many small glands that secrete wax to prevent unwanted bodies such as insects entering and damaging the middle and inner ear.

The parts of the ear are shown in Fig. 9.7.

Smell

The sense of smell is perceived by means of small hair receptors in the roof of the nose. These transmit impulses by way of the olfactory nerve to the brain where they are interpreted as different odours.

Substances to be smelt must be dissolved in gaseous form. A person soon becomes accustomed to a particular smell and therefore harmful smells such as gas leaks should always be investigated as soon as they are smelt.

Taste

The sense of taste lies in the taste buds of the tongue. Food can only be tasted when it is in a fluid state. When food touches the taste buds, nerve impulses are carried to the brain which then interprets the different taste sensations.

There are four basic tastes: sweet, sour, salty, and bitter.

Touch

Receptors of touch are embedded in the skin. When pain, temperature change, or another stimulus is sensed by the receptors, nerve impulses are sent to the brain which interprets the different sensations.

Besides being an organ of touch the skin has the following functions:

— To provide the body with a waterproof covering, preventing the loss or absorption of fluid.

— To protect the body from infective organisms.

— To regulate the body temperature, by varying the blood flow through the skin and the amount of sweating from the skin. When the body is overheated there is an increase in the production of sweat, the evaporation of which causes cooling. When the temperature of the body falls, the blood vessels in the skin constrict which reduces the flow of blood, resulting in less heat being lost from the body.

— To store fat and water.

— To excrete waste products. Sweat contains the same inorganic salts as blood but in lower concentrations.

— To produce vitamin D precursors from sunlight.

— To grow nails to protect the tips of the fingers and toes.

A section through the skin is shown in Fig. 9.8. It is composed of an upper layer called the epidermis and a lower layer called the dermis. The structures arising in the dermis are illustrated in Fig. 9.8.

9:4 ENDOCRINE SYSTEM

The function of the endocrine system is to coordinate the metabolism of the body by means of chemical messenger substances called hormones.

Hormones

Hormones are produced by endocrine (ductless) glands and released directly into the circulation as the blood passes through the glands. Hormones are composed of amino acids, small polypeptides, or steroids.

Hormone functions include:

— To increase, decrease, or coordinate the activities of other glands or organs.

— To speed up or slow down the metabolic rate in the body.

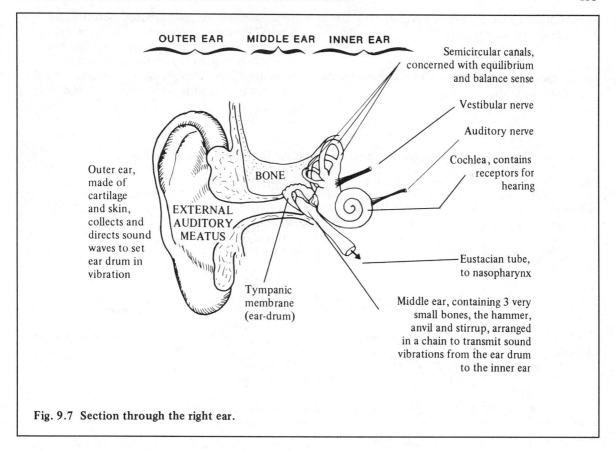

Fig. 9.7 Section through the right ear.

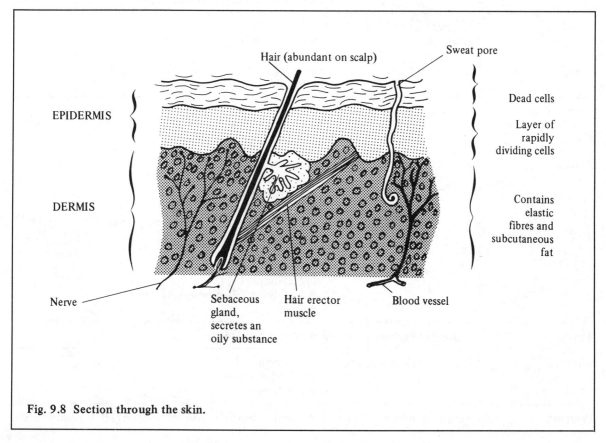

Fig. 9.8 Section through the skin.

— To influence the growth or development of the body or certain parts of it.

— To maintain homeostasis, i.e. a stable state within the body.

Serious physical and mental disturbances may result if hormones are secreted in too small or too large amounts due to the abnormal functioning of an endocrine gland. A balanced activity of hormone functions is necessary to maintain controlled cell growth and normal metabolism in the body.

Chart 9.2 Endocrine Glands and the Hormones they Secrete

Gland	Position in Body	Hormones Secreted
Adrenals	Lying above each kidney	Cortex region: • Aldosterone • Cortisol and other corticosteroids • Androgens Medulla region: • Adrenaline ⎤ ⎬ Catecholamines • Noradrenaline ⎦
Gonads: Ovaries	Lateral wall of female pelvis	• Oestrogens • Progestogens
Testes	Suspended under penis	• Androgens (testosterone)
Kidney	Posterior abdominal wall	• Renin • Renal erythropoietic factor (erythropoietin)
Pancreas	In abdomen behind stomach	*Alpha* cells: • Glucagon *Beta* cells: • Insulin
Parathyroids	Behind thyroid	• Parathormone (PTH)
Pineal	Brain	• Melatonin
Pituitary	Base of brain, behind the optic nerve	Anterior part: • Growth hormone (GH) • Thyrotrophin (TSH) • Corticotrophin (ACTH) • Follicle stimulating hormone (FSH) • Luteinising hormone (LH) • Prolactin Posterior part: • Antidiuretic hormone (ADH) • Oxytocin
Thymus	Behind upper sternum	• Probably thymosin
Thyroid	Base of neck on each side of trachea	• Thyroxine • Triiodotyrosine • Calcitonin
Placenta	Pregnant uterus	• Human chorionic gonadotrophin (HCG) and others

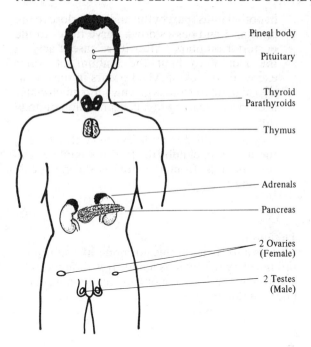

Fig. 9.9 The endocrine glands.

Pineal body
Pituitary
Thyroid
Parathyroids
Thymus
Adrenals
Pancreas
2 Ovaries (Female)
2 Testes (Male)

Adrenal hormones
- Aldosterone promotes reabsorption of sodium ions in the kidney tubules, resulting in a decrease in the reabsorption of potassium or hydrogen ions and an increase in the reabsorption of chloride and water.

- Cortisol and its related hormones are concerned with resistance to stress. These hormones mobilize fats and amino acids from the cells and release them into the blood stream to be transported to the liver for conversion into glucose.

  Cortisol is also involved in anti-allergic and anti-inflammatory processes and has some aldosterone-like activity, causing the retention of salt and water.

  Corticosteroids are used medically in the treatment of inflammatory conditions such as arthritis or allergic diseases such as asthma. The drugs have many side effects including the reactivation of tuberculosis, peptic ulceration, and delayed wound healing.

- About 80% of the catecholamines produced by the adrenal medulla is adrenaline and the remaining 20% is noradrenaline.

  Adrenaline increases the heart rate and the force of each heart beat. It dilates the blood vessels in skeletal muscle. In the liver, it increases the breakdown of glycogen causing a rise in the level of glucose in the blood. In the lungs it causes dilatation of the air passages.

Adrenaline is partly responsible for the symptoms of anxiety, increased rate of breathing, shaking (tremor) of the fingers, and increased alertness.

Noradrenaline has many similar actions to adrenaline but causes predominantly the vasoconstriction of blood vessels.

Gonadal hormones
A description of the functions of gonadal hormones is included in Chapter 10.

Kidney
In specialized cells of the efferent arteriole near the glomerulus, the kidney produces an enzyme called renin in response to stress. It reacts with a substrate from the liver to produce angiotensin which causes the constriction of blood vessels, leading to an increase in blood pressure. Angiotensin also stimulates the adrenal cortex to produce aldosterone.

The production of red blood cells is called erythropoiesis. The kidney produces the hormone erythrogen (renal erythropoietic factor) which acts on a plasma protein to form erythropoietin. This stimulates erythropoiesis, especially when the amount of oxygen reaching the tissues is reduced.

Pancreatic hormones
Although the pancreas has a duct and therefore functions as an exocrine gland (in the digestive system), it is also an endocrine gland. Its *alpha* islet cells secrete glucagon and its *beta* cells secrete insulin.

- Glucagon breaks down glycogen to glucose in the liver, leading to a rise in blood glucose.

- Insulin, together with other substances, regulates carbohydrate and fat metabolism. It regulates the level of glucose in the blood and causes the transfer of glucose from the blood to the cells for conversion into glucose 6-phosphate. Lack of insulin causes diabetes mellitus in which there is an excess of glucose in the blood.

Parathyroid hormone
Parathyroid hormone (parathormone, or PTH) acts to raise plasma calcium levels and also to decrease plasma phosphate concentration. When the level of calcium in the blood falls, parathormone is released from the parathyroid glands. In the kidneys it increases calcium reabsorption and

phosphate excretion. It also causes the removal of calcium from bone.

Oversecretion of parathormone (hyperparathyroidism) causes a raised level of calcium in the blood (hypercalcaemia). This can cause tiredness, kidney stones, peptic ulceration and in severe cases, bone pain.

Undersecretion of parathyroid hormone (hypoparathyroidism) may follow surgery to the neck (e.g. thyroid surgery) when the parathyroid glands may be removed unintentionally. This causes a low serum calcium. Because calcium is required for the normal activity of muscles and nerves, a low serum calcium causes increased excitability of these tissues. This causes tingling and cramps. Mild hypocalcaemia may over months to years cause cataracts and psychiatric illness.

Melatonin
Very little is known about this hormone. It appears to have an inhibitory effect on the ovary and may influence the menstrual cycle.

Pituitary hormones
Anterior pituitary
The anterior lobe of the pituitary produces many hormones which exert control over other endocrine glands. These are as follows:

☐ Growth hormone (GH) which regulates the growth of the body. In children, a deficiency of this hormone leads to dwarfism and an oversecretion leads to gigantism. In adults, excess growth hormone causes acromegaly which is characterized by a thickening of the skin and increase in the size of the hands, feet, and lower jaw.

☐ Thyrotrophin (TSH) which stimulates the thyroid gland to produce and secrete the thyroid hormones thyroxine and triiodotyrosine.

☐ Corticotrophin (adrenocorticotrophic hormone, ACTH) which stimulates the adrenal cortex to produce and release corticosteroid.

☐ Follicle stimulating hormone (FSH) and luteinising hormone (LH), which are described in Chapter 10.

☐ Prolactin, which after delivery, stimulates the breasts to produce milk and then maintains lactation.

Posterior pituitary
The posterior pituitary produces the following hormones:

☐ Antidiuretic hormone (ADH), also known as vasopressin, which is produced in the hypothalamus (part of the midbrain close to the pituitary) and passes down nerve fibres to the posterior pituitary. After its release it acts on the kidney to limit the amount of water excreted. A lack of ADH occurs in the condition diabetes insipidus in which too much water is excreted, leading to a concentration of body fluids.

☐ Oxytocin, which stimulates the contraction of the uterus in childbirth. It also stimulates the flow of milk from the breasts during breast feeding.

Thymosin
Little is known about this hormone-like substance produced by the thymus gland. It is thought to be involved in the development and functioning of the body's immune system.

Thyroid hormones
The thyroid gland produces two main hormones containing iodine, i.e. thyroxine and triidotyrosine. These hormones speed up metabolism, quicken the heart rate, use up fat stores, and increase the activity of the gastrointestinal tract.

If iodine is lacking in the diet the thyroid gland may swell. An enlarged thyroid gland is called a goitre, and when a lack of iodine is the cause it is called iodine deficiency goitre.

Thyroid hormone is essential during the growth of a foetus and for the normal development of the brain. Underactivity of the thyroid gland during this stage results in cretinism, a condition characterized by mental as well as physical retardation. If the deficiency is not corrected by giving oral thyroxine within a few weeks of birth, irreversible damage occurs.

In an adult, underactivity of the thyroid gland causes increase in weight with reduced mental and physical activity. This condition is called myxoedema and is also treated with oral thyroxine.

Overactivity of the thyroid gland is called thyrotoxicosis. A person with thyrotoxicosis has a big appetite but loses weight because of the increase in metabolic rate. The person may also have a goitre. Thyrotoxicosis may be treated medically or surgically.

Calcitonin is also secreted by the thyroid. It is secreted in response to a high calcium level. In a healthy person there is continual breakdown of bone tissue and a building of new bone by osteoblasts. When these activities are balanced the level of calcium in the blood remains normal. If, however, the level of calcium rises, calcitonin is released by the thyroid gland to bring down the calcium level.

Placental hormones

In pregnancy, the placenta acts as an endocrine gland. It produces many hormones, including human chorionic gonadotrophin (HCG) which may be found in blood and urine, and is the basis of the pregnancy test. Measurement of HCG is also used in the diagnosis of certain tumours and in monitoring their response to treatment.

9:5 TERMS USED TO DESCRIBE DISORDERS OF THE NERVOUS AND ENDOCRINE SYSTEMS

The following are some of the terms used to describe disorders associated with the nervous system, sense organs, and the endocrine system:

Addison's disease: A condition in which the secretion of the hormones aldosterone and cortisol is deficient due to a wasting or destruction of the adrenal gland. This can occur as a complication of tuberculosis.

The lack of these hormones leads to a loss of sodium and water from the body, muscular weakness, nausea and vomiting, hypotension, and low blood glucose levels. The skin becomes pigmented.

Cataract: A cloudiness (opacity) in the lens of the eye causing blurred vision which may lead to blindness. The cataract can be removed surgically. The eyes of elderly people are often affected or a cataract may develop in association with diabetes mellitus or following eye injury.

Conjunctivitis: This refers to inflammation of the conjunctiva of the eye (see Fig. 9.5). A severe form of conjunctivitis can affect babies born of mothers with gonorrhoea. If untreated it can lead to blindness.

Cushing's syndrome: A condition in which there are symptoms and signs of excess corticosteroid levels in the body. There are a number of causes including:
— Steroid therapy by doctors.
— Pituitary tumours producing ACTH, causing increased steroid production by the adrenal.
— Tumours of the adrenal producing excess steroid.

Patients with Cushing's syndrome lose potassium from the body, resulting in a low serum potassium level. They tend to be obese with a raised blood pressure and may have high blood sugar levels.

Cutaneous: Referring to the skin. The term subcutaneous refers to the fibrous and fatty tissue beneath the skin.

Encephalitis: An acute inflammation of the brain often caused by infection with mosquito or tick-borne viruses.

Another cause of encephalitis is African trypanosomiasis. Because the trypanosomes cause inflammation of both the brain and meninges, the term meningoencephalitis is usually used.

Epilepsy: A brain disorder in which there is intermittent abnormalities of cerebral function, usually associated with disturbance of consciousness and accompanied by sudden excessive electrical discharge of cerebral neurones.

The clinical signs vary depending on the site of the electrical activity. There may be twitching of the limbs with unconsciousness (grand mal), or twitching of a single limb or part of the body sometimes with normal consciousness (partial or focal fit). When the electrical activity is in the temporal lobe, the patient may only be aware of strange sensations, a strange taste in the mouth or unpleasant smell. In children, there may be only a very brief loss of awareness lasting only a few seconds (petit mal).

Glaucoma: A condition in which the pressure of the aqueous humour fluid of the eye (intra-ocular pressure) is increased due to more fluid being produced than can be reabsorbed. Unless corrected, glaucoma can lead to degeneration of the optic nerve with permanent damage to sight.

Hydrocephalus ('water on the brain'): An excessive accumulation of cerebrospinal fluid within the ventricles of the brain due to an obstruction in the ventricular system or subarachnoid space. This prevents the normal flow of cerebrospinal fluid and its reabsorption by the arachnoid villi.

Hydrocephalus may be present at birth because of an abnormality in the structure of the brain or it may occasionally occur as a complication of meningitis or subarachnoid haemorrhage.

Meningitis: Inflammation of the meninges, usually due to a bacterial or viral infection.

Muscular dystrophy: A term used to describe a group of hereditary conditions associated with muscle wasting. Most of the disorders are progressive, leading to increasing disability as the muscles become weaker and non-functional.

Degeneration of the muscles does not involve the central nervous system. The wasting is caused by the replacement of muscle protein with fatty tissue.

Neuropathy: A disorder of function of peripheral nerves. It may affect only a single nerve (mononeuropathy) or many nerves may be affected (polyneuropathy). Sensory, motor or both types of activity may be involved. The patient often has a tingling or numbness, weakness in the area supplied by the affected nerves, and sometimes also severe pain.

Polyneuropathy can be caused by malnutrition especially vitamin B deficiency, viral infections, damage by some metals and chemicals, diabetes, or alcohol intake.

Palsy: Another term meaning paralysis, weakness, or disorder of movement. Facial (Bell's) palsy is paralysis of the muscles of one side of the face. Cerebral palsy is a disorder of coordination of movement and is usually caused by damage to the brain during or immediately after birth. The child may have paralysis or uncontrolled movements of part or all of the body.

Paralysis: A complete or partial loss of power of any part of the body following damage to its nerve supply. It may be caused by a disease or injury to the brain, spinal cord, or peripheral nerves.

The term paraplegia is used when the paralysis involves the legs and the organs in the lower part of the body. It is usually caused by damage to the spinal cord.

Poliomyelitis: A viral infection of the motor neurones of the central nervous system. Infection may or may not result in paralysis. Prevention of the disease is by vaccination using inactivated poliomyelitis virus.

Shingles (herpes zoster): Herpes virus infection which causes severe pain along the distribution of a nerve often in the face, chest, or abdomen, followed by blistering of the skin. The same virus can cause chickenpox in children.

Stroke: A disorder of function of the brain due to impairment of part of its blood supply. This may be due to clotting of blood within a cerebral vessel (cerebral thrombosis), bleeding into the brain (cerebral haemorrhage) or obstruction of a vessel by a clot which has come from elsewhere in the circulation.

Cerebral thrombosis and haemorrhage occur more commonly in people with high blood pressure. Cerebral thrombosis may occur as a complication of severe dehydration. A cerebral embolus may originate from a valve which has been damaged by rheumatic fever.

If the blood supply to the area of the brain which normally controls the movements of the arm and leg is affected, the patient will have weakness on the opposite side of the body (hemiplegia).

Sometimes a vessel at the base of the brain may bleed into the subarachnoid space (subarachnoid haemorrhage). This can cause severe headache and sometimes loss of consciousness or hemiplegia.

Trachoma: An infectious disease caused by *Chlamydia trachomatis* in which the eyelids become inflamed. If left untreated the conjunctiva becomes scarred and irritates the cornea of the eye which can cause permanent damage to the cornea and eventual blindness. The infection can be easily treated with antibiotics.

Urticaria: A skin rash, usually allergic in type in which histamine is activated and released.

An urticarial reaction may occur following a blood transfusion if the donor blood contains protein substances to which the recipient is allergic. Other more common causes of urticaria are drugs, chemicals, and certain foods.

Vertigo: A severe dizziness in which the person or his or her surroundings appear to rotate. It is often associated with severe nausea or vomiting. Disorders of the inner ear, vestibular nerve, or brain stem are also associated with vertigo. Streptomycin, a drug used in the treatment of tuberculosis can damage the balance organs of the inner ear if given in too high a dosage.

Recommended Reading

See books listed at the end of Chapter 5.

10 Basic Genetics and the Reproductive System

10:1 BASIC GENETICS

Reproduction is the process by which a new life is produced following the fertilization of a female reproductive cell called an ovum by a male reproductive cell called a sperm.

Genetics is the study of the way in which the different mental or physical characteristics are passed on (inherited) from parents to children. A child receives half its genetic material from one parent and half from the other parent.

Autosomes and sex chromosomes

As explained in 5:2, the genetic information required for cell replication is stored in the DNA molecules of chromosomes.

Human cells contain a total of 23 pairs of chromosomes (diploid number). Twenty-two of these determine the characteristics of body cells and are called autosomes. The chromosomes of each autosome pair are homologous, i.e. they are similar in size and shape (see Fig. 10.1b).

The remaining two chromosomes determine the sex of an individual and are called sex chromosomes. They are referred to as the X and Y sex chromosomes (see Fig. 10.1c). A female has two X chromosomes (XX), and a male has one X and one Y chromosome (XY). In female cells, only one of the X chromosomes is active, the other is non-functional. In the male the X chromosome is always active.

Meiosis

During the development of male and female reproductive cells a special type of cell division occurs called meiosis. This reduces the number of chromosomes in the sperm or ovum to half the number (haploid number) found in normal body cells. Each sperm will therefore contain 22 autosomes and an X or Y chromosome, and an ovum will contain 22 autosomes and an X chromosome. When the ovum is fertilized by the sperm, the zygote which results contains the full diploid number of chromosomes (46).

The sex of a baby is therefore determined by the sperm. If an X-bearing sperm fertilizes an ovum, the sex of the baby will be female (XX). If however a Y-bearing sperm fertilizes the ovum, the sex will be male (XY) as shown in Fig. 10.2.

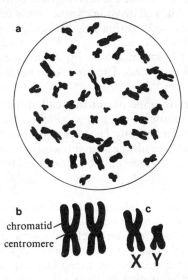

chromatid
centromere

X Y

Fig. 10.1 *a* Microscopical preparation of human chromosomes. *b* Pair of autosomes. *c* Sex chromosomes.

Before fertilization
Sperm: 22 autosomes and X or Y sex chromosome
Ovum: 22 autosomes and X sex chromosome

After fertilization
Zygote: 44 autosomes and *either* XX sex chromosomes (female)
or XY sex chromosomes (male)

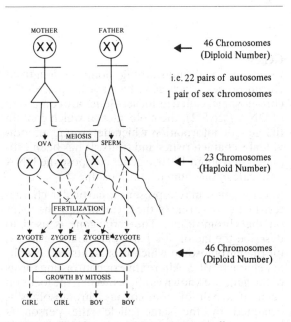

MOTHER   FATHER

XX   XY

46 Chromosomes
(Diploid Number)

i.e. 22 pairs of autosomes
1 pair of sex chromosomes

OVA   MEIOSIS   SPERM

X X   X Y

23 Chromosomes
(Haploid Number)

FERTILIZATION

ZYGOTE ZYGOTE ZYGOTE ZYGOTE

XX XX XY XY

46 Chromosomes
(Diploid Number)

GROWTH BY MITOSIS

GIRL GIRL BOY BOY

Fig. 10.2 Fertilization of reproductive cells.

Structure and karyotyping of chromosomes

As the cells of the body grow and divide so the chromosomes within each cell must divide. As discussed above, the cell division which occurs during the development of the reproductive cells is called meiosis. The cell division of other body cells is called mitosis and during this process the chromosomes divide in such a way as to maintain the full number (diploid number, 46) of chromosomes in each cell produced. The process of mitosis is fully described in 5:3.

At a certain stage of mitosis (called metaphase), the chromosomes when viewed under the microscope appear roughly H shaped as shown in Fig. 10.1. Two thread-like structures called chromatids are joined together at one point called the centromere.

In tissue culture laboratories, stained microscopical preparations can be made of the chromosomes contained in a person's cells. A photograph can then be taken of the chromosomes as seen under the microscope and the individual chromosomes arranged according to their size and shape into homologous pairs. This will show whether the structure and number of the chromosomes are normal. The process is referred to as karyotyping and is used to investigate disorders caused by chromosome abnormalities, such as Down's syndrome.

Chromosomes are classified into seven groups A to G, and numbered in pairs from 1 to 22, with the 23rd pair being the sex chromosomes. They decrease in size from chromosome pair 1, which are the largest, to pair 22 which are the smallest chromosomes. The X chromosome differs in size and shape from the Y sex chromosome (see Fig. 10.1c).

Genes

Genes are small units strung along the length of chromosomes. Each gene has its own place on a chromosome, called its locus. Genes are composed of DNA (see 5:2), the molecules of which contain the genetic information which determine an individual's characteristics and traits. It has been estimated that about 100 000 genes compose the DNA molecule of one human chromosome.

Several genes may represent a particular characteristic but only one of these can occupy the locus on the chromosome. The term gene is used to describe the factor at a particular point, or locus, on the chromosome which represents an hereditary characteristic. Alternative or contrasting forms of the gene are known as alleles. When the locus on each of a pair of homologous chromosomes is occupied by the same allele, the person is homozygous for the particular gene characteristic (homozygote). If, however, the alleles are different the person is said to be heterozygous for the particular gene characteristic (heterozygote).

Dominant and recessive genes

The genes inherited for any particular characteristic can be either dominant or recessive. A dominant gene will always show itself if it is present, whereas a recessive gene will only show itself if there is no dominant one, that is if both genes are recessive.

A dominant gene is therefore one which shows itself in the heterozygote and a recessive gene is one which is manifested only in the homozygote.

Autosomal and sex-linked disorders

If an inherited disease is caused by an abnormal (mutant) gene situated on an autosome (body chromosome), the disorder is referred to as autosomal. It may be either dominant or recessive. If, however, the mutant gene is located on one of the sex chromosomes (usually on the X chromosome), the disorder is said to be sex-linked. It may also be dominant or recessive.

Autosomal dominant disorders

With autosomal dominant disorders the presence of only one mutant gene is necessary for the trait to be manifested in the carrier. As shown in Fig. 10.3, when one parent carries a mutant gene, on average half the children will inherit the abnormal gene and these children will be clinically affected. Autosomal dominant disorders include haemoglobinopathies such as sickle cell disease, hereditary spherocytosis, and acute intermittent porphyria.

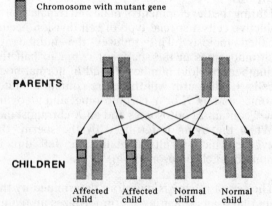

□ Chromosome with mutant gene

PARENTS

CHILDREN

Affected child   Affected child   Normal child   Normal child

Fig. 10.3 Inheritance of an autosomal dominant disorder.

Autosomal recessive disorders

With autosomal recessive disorders, the disease is only manifested in homozygotes (presence of two mutant genes). Only if a child receives the abnormal gene from both parents will it be clinically affected. On average only 1 in 4 children will be affected, but two in four will possess the abnormal gene and could pass it on to their children (see Fig. 10.4). People who possess the abnormal gene but are not clinically affected are called carriers.

Autosomal recessive disorders include cystic fibrosis, galactosaemia, and phenylketonuria. If the abnormal gene is rare in the population then it will be very uncommon for two people with the gene to meet and produce affected children. If, however, a family possesses the abnormal gene then any marriages between related people (consanguineous marriage) will be more likely to produce clinically affected children. Such marriages are now quite uncommon in western countries but in some parts of the world, particularly in rural communities, autosomal recessive disorders are more common because of consanguineous marriages.

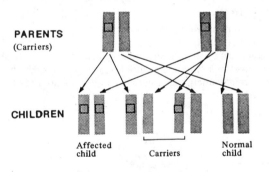

Fig. 10.4   Inheritance of an autosomal recessive disorder.

Sex linked disorders

Most of the known sex-linked disorders are carried on the X chromosome and of these, X-linked recessive conditions are the more common. As already discussed, a female has two X chromosomes (XX) but only one of them is active. Consequently a female with one X chromosome carrying a recessive disorder (heterozygote) is clinically unaffected. She is a carrier of the recessive condition. A homozygous female, however, will show the disorder. Males have only one X chromosome and this is always active. A male with an X chromosome carrying a recessive disorder is therefore always clinically affected.

The most important X linked recessive disorders include the blood disorders haemophilia and the red cell enzyme deficiency disease, glucose 6-phosphate dehydrogenase deficiency. In practice, therefore, these disorders usually affect males with women acting as carriers.

With regard to passing on a sex-linked recessive disorder two possibilities arise:

☐ If a female carrier marries a normal man, about half the sons born will suffer from the disorder and half the daughters will be carriers (see Fig. 10.5).

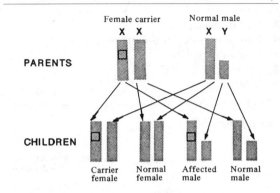

Fig. 10.5 Inheritance of a sex-linked recessive disorder when female carrier marries a normal male.

☐ If an affected male marries a normal woman, none of the sons will be affected but all the daughters will be carriers (see Fig. 10.6).

X linked dominant disorders are very rare. Because the mutant gene is dominant, both males and females who carry it will be clinically affected. On average half the children (sons or daughters) born to an affected mother marrying a normal male will inherit the gene. An affected father marrying a normal female will pass on the gene to all his daughters but all his sons will be normal.

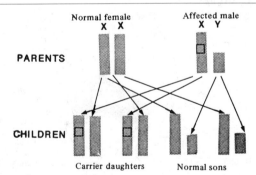

Fig. 10.6 Sex-linked recessive disorder with affected male.

Genotype and phenotype

The genetic composition for a particular inherited characteristic is called the genotype and its manifestation, or clinical effect, is called the phenotype. For example, in the genetics of blood groups, the gene for group B is dominant over the gene for group O. Therefore a person with blood group B (phenotype group B), may have a genotype BO having inherited a gene B from one parent and a gene O from another, or genotype BB having inherited a gene B from both parents.

10:2 FEMALE REPRODUCTIVE SYSTEM

The organs of reproduction in a female consist of:

External (genitalia)
- Collectively called the vulva

Internal
- Pair of ovaries
- Pair of uterine, or Fallopian, tubes
- Uterus (womb)
- Cervix
- Vagina

FRONT VIEW

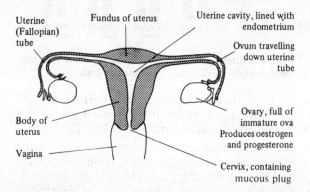

Fig. 10.7 Front view of female reproductive system.

SIDE VIEW

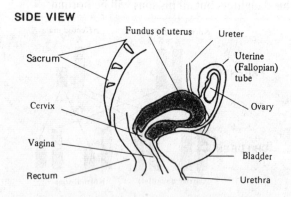

Fig. 10.8 Side view of female reproductive system.

The internal female organs of reproduction and their position in the body are shown diagrammatically in Fig. 10.7 and Fig. 10.8.

Functioning of the female reproductive system
Each month, from puberty to the menopause i.e. child-bearing years, an ovum matures in an ovary and is released into the uterine tube. The membrane in which the ovum matures is called an ovarian follicle and the hormone which regulates mat-

uration in the ovary is called the follicle stimulating hormone (FSH). This hormone is secreted by the pituitary gland. During maturation, the ovarian follicle produces the hormone oestrogen which enters the blood stream. One of the effects of this hormone is to cause an increase in the multiplication of the cells lining the uterus (endometrium).

After the release of the ovum (ovulation), the follicle from which the ovum ruptures develops into a structure called a corpus luteum. Under the influence of another gonadotrophic hormone secreted by the pituitary gland, called luteinising hormone (LH), the corpus luteum begins producing a hormone called progesterone. This causes further thickening of the endometrium and an increase in the secretion of mucus in preparation for fertilization and implantation. The production of oestrogen is also continued.

If the ovum is not fertilized the corpus luteum degenerates and progesterone production ceases. A reduction in the level of progesterone causes a breakdown of the glandular endometrium of the uterus and this together with the ovum tissue and blood is shed over 3-6 days of menstruation (see Fig. 10.9).

Days of menstrual cycle
The first day of menstruation is taken as Day 1 of the menstrual cycle. Ovulation takes place around day 14 and the next menstruation occurs on average after day 28. In different women, cycles vary in length from about 24 to 34 days.

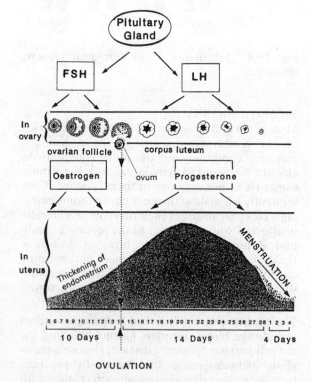

Fig. 10.9 Normal menstrual cycle.

If after ovulation, the ovum on its way to the uterus is fertilized by a sperm, the resulting zygote burrows into the thick endometrium of the uterus and starts to develop into an embryo. It produces the chorionic gonadotrophic hormone (HCG) which stops the degeneration of the corpus luteum. Progesterone continues to be secreted and this prevents menstruation occurring during the 40 weeks of pregnancy.

Fertilization by a sperm can only occur around the time of ovulation and therefore a woman is fertile for only a few days in each month.

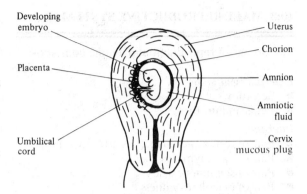

Fig. 10.10 The uterus and embryo early in pregnancy.

Development of a fertilized ovum

Fertilization usually takes place in the uterine tube so that by the time the zygote embeds in the uterus it is already composed of several cells (blastocyst). The embryo is surrounded by two membranes, an inner one called the amnion and an outer one called the chorion (see Fig. 10.10). The amnion secretes the amniotic fluid in which the baby develops. The term embryo is used to describe the developing fertilized ovum in its first 8 weeks of life. After 8 weeks and up until birth the term foetus is used.

The HCG secreted by the chorion can be found in the blood soon after conception. The high concentration of HCG in the blood following the formation of the chorion, leads to its excretion in urine. The pregnancy test is based on the detection of HCG, usually in the urine.

As the foetus grows it bulges into the uterine cavity. One area of the chorion is left in contact with the uterine wall to form the placenta (see Fig. 10.10). The umbilical cord connects the baby to the placenta. Through the umbilical cord, oxygen and nutrients are carried in the mother's blood to the baby and the waste products of metabolism from the baby are transferred into the mother's circulation for excretion.

By the fifth week of development the embryo's heart is pumping and by the fourth month all its organs are formed and functioning. By the seventh month the foetus reaches half the weight it will have at birth.

During pregnancy an adequate diet is essential for the mother so that she can provide her child with all the nutrients it requires and be fit to give birth and have sufficient milk to feed the baby when it is born. The mother's haemoglobin level should be measured during the pregnancy. Other antenatal tests are also required to make sure the pregnancy is progressing normally and that the mother does not have any disease or condition which could put the baby or herself at risk, e.g. syphilis (see also 10:5).

Childbirth

A baby is born by contractions of the muscles of the uterine wall and the bearing down action (labour) of the mother.

Three stages are recognized:

— Dilatation of the cervix, and the rupturing of the membranes with the release of amniotic fluid (see Fig. 10.11).

— The passage of the baby, normally head first, through the dilated cervix and out through the vagina.

— The detaching of the placenta from the uterine wall and its expulsion a short time after the birth.

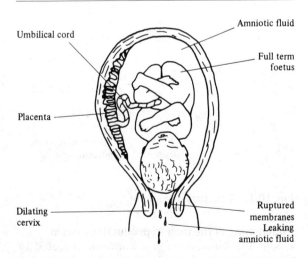

Fig. 10.11 The uterus and foetus at the onset of delivery.

Disorders associated with childbirth are described in 10:5.

10:3 MALE REPRODUCTIVE SYSTEM

The organs of reproduction in a male consist of:

External (genitalia)
- Scrotum
- Penis and urethra

Internal
- Pair of testes and ducts (vas efferentia)
- Pair of epididymides
- Pair of seminal vesicles
- Pair of ejaculatory ducts
- Prostate gland

The male organs of reproduction and their position in the body are shown diagrammatically in Fig. 10.12.

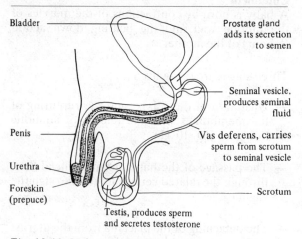

Fig. 10.12 Male reproductive organs.

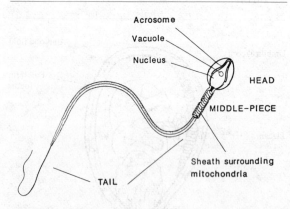

Fig. 10.13 Structure of a sperm.

Functioning of the male reproductive system
Under the stimulation of a hormone secreted by the pituitary gland, called interstitial cell stimulating hormone (ICSH), the cells of the testes produce the male sex hormone called testosterone. This hormone first appears at puberty and causes the development of the secondary male sex characteristics, such as deepening voice, increase in body hair, and development of muscles. The male reproductive cells are called sperm, or spermatozoa. They are formed in the testes which are situated in the scrotum. The production of sperm is regulated by the follicle stimulating hormone (FSH) which is also secreted by the pituitary gland.

Sexual intercourse
During sexual intercourse (coitus), sperm are released from the testes and pass through the epididymides, up the vas efferentia to the seminal vesicles. Fluid from the seminal vesicles and prostate gland is added to the sperm, to form semen. Under the stimulus of sexual emotion, blood fills the erectile tissue of the penis which causes its erection. Semen containing about 200 million motile sperm then passes down the urethra and is ejaculated from the penis into the vagina of the woman.

Semen (seminal fluid) is a viscous mucous fluid which contains fructose to help nourish the sperm and keep them active. The counting and examination of sperm in seminal fluid is described in 38:15 in Volume II of the Manual.

Fertilization
Following entry into the vagina, the sperm swim through the cervix into the uterus and uterine tubes in search of an ovum. Each sperm consists of a head (nucleus) and long tail with which it is propelled (see Fig. 10.13). When a sperm enters an ovum its tail breaks off and its nucleus fuses with the nucleus of the ovum to form a zygote.

The zygote contains all the genetic material required to determine the characteristics of the baby.

10:4 FAMILY PLANNING AND CONTRACEPTION

Each year the population of the world increases by about 70 million. Most people believe that it is very important to control this increase. At a more personal level it is of great benefit to a family's health and well-being if the number of children is planned and the mother is able to have a reasonable length of time between one pregnancy and the next.

There are a number of ways in which conception and pregnancy can be prevented. Some religious faiths do not support certain modern forms of contraception but accept natural methods. For example the Roman Catholic Church supports the use of the rhythm method but not the contraceptive pill. These subjects should, of course, be discussed between a couple and their religious leaders.

Rhythm method

Conception occurs only within about forty eight hours of ovulation, and ovulation takes place approximately fourteen days before the beginning of the next period (menstruation). Allowing for possible variation in the date of ovulation, there is a time between approximately the eleventh and sixteenth day of the menstrual cycle when a woman is likely to be fertile. If intercourse takes place at this time then pregnancy may result. The rhythm method of preventing pregnancy is based on limiting intercourse to those days in the menstrual cycle when fertilization is least likely to occur.

This method of avoiding unwanted pregnancies is however unreliable because it depends on the woman keeping an accurate record of her cycles and the time of ovulation can vary.

Coitus interruptus

This is the name given to the method in which, during sexual intercourse, the man withdraws the penis from the woman's vagina before sperm is released (ejaculation). Many couples would find this method difficult and likely to reduce their enjoyment of intercourse. Some release of sperm may also occur before complete ejaculation and therefore the method is often not effective.

Medical barriers to conception

Medical barriers to conception include:

— Male sheath (condom)
— Female cap (diaphragm)

Male sheath (condom)

This is a rubber sheath which fits over the erect penis and collects the semen at ejaculation to prevent it from entering the vagina. To be effective it must be placed on the penis before there is any possibility of leakage of sperm. The sheath may be made of thin rubber which is meant to be used only once or of stronger rubber which is washable. It is of course important before intercourse to be sure that the sheath contains no holes through which semen could leak.

Female cap (diaphragm)

This consists of a dome of soft rubber surrounded by a spring rim. There are different sizes and the cap is made to fit over the cervix across the upper vagina. Many women find it difficult to put in and take out and it is therefore not a popular method.

Note: Various chemicals are manufactured which kill sperm. They are not completely effective if used on their own and are therefore usually used together with a mechanical barrier.

Oral contraception (The 'pill')

The 'pill' is one of the most effective reversible methods of contraception and is used by over 50 million women around the world. There are many different types of contraceptive pill and most are aimed at preventing ovulation. Contraceptives contain synthetic oestrogen which suppresses the secretion of FSH and therefore prevents ovulation from occurring. Most also contain a progesterone which blocks the normal control of the menstrual cycle. They also have an effect on the lining of the uterus and on the mucus produced by the cervix which helps to increase their contraceptive effect.

The woman takes one pill every day for 21 days and then stops for 7 days for menstruation to occur. It is very important not to forget the pill or the contraceptive effect is reduced. Sometimes the 21 pills are packaged together with 7 days of iron or vitamin preparation so that the woman can continue to take one pill every day which may be easier to remember.

For most healthy young women the pill is a safe form of contraception and certain types of pill can be taken even if a woman is breast-feeding. Because the pill reduces the amount of blood lost during menstruation it can be an advantage to women who are anaemic. If a woman is taking other drugs, the dose of a contraceptive pill may have to be increased to maintain its contraceptive effect. This is necessary with some antibiotics, including rifampicin which may be used in the treatment of tuberculosis.

When first taking a contraceptive pill, a few women suffer from slight nausea, headache, and there may be an increase in weight or breast tenderness but these effects usually settle down over a few weeks as the body adapts to the new hormones. In a small number of women the pill causes a rise in blood pressure. Sometimes this returns to normal after changing to a pill containing a different amount of hormone, but occasionally the pill has to be stopped and a different form of contraception used.

One rare side effect of the pill is clotting of the blood in an artery or vein. This may occur in the leg veins (venous thrombosis), in the arteries of the brain causing a stroke, or even more rarely in the coronary arteries resulting in a heart attack. Although this is very rare, it is slightly more common in women who smoke, particularly if they are also over forty years of age. For this small group of women, a different form of contraception is usually more suitable.

Intra-uterine contraceptive device (IUCD)

It has been known for many years that a woman will not become pregnant if a 'foreign body' is inserted into the uterus. Many devices are now available and this method has many advantages. It is however very important to insert the IUCD under sterile conditions to prevent infection from reaching the uterus and uterine tubes. Once inserted the contraceptive effect begins immediately.

Some uterine bleeding is common after insertion and there may be a little bleeding between periods for a few months. Blood loss at menstruation is often a little more than before, but with newer devices this is rarely a problem. If serious infection occurs, antibiotic treatment is required and the IUCD may have to be removed. This should happen very rarely if correct sterile procedures are carried out when the device is inserted.

This method of contraception is particularly useful for a woman and her husband who already have a family and do not want any more children. The device can be left in the uterus for a number of years.

Sterilisation

Sterilisation can be carried out on a man or a woman when they have had children and do not want to have any more. The operation on the male is a very minor procedure and with newer techniques the female operation is also easier than it used to be.

Male sterilisation (vasectomy)

Local anaesthetic is used for this procedure. The vas deferens on each side is cut and tied to prevent sperm from reaching the penis during intercourse. Because the male hormones continue to be secreted, a man's virility is unchanged and he remains able to perform intercourse normally.

Female sterilisation

This operation may be carried out under general or local anaesthetic. Because the uterine tubes are much deeper within the body than the vas efferentia, it is not such a simple procedure but with modern equipment it is possible to do the operation through a very small cut in the abdominal wall. The Fallopian tubes are cut and tied to prevent the ovum from passing down the tube to the uterus.

10:5 TERMS ASSOCIATED WITH THE REPRODUCTIVE SYSTEM

The following are some of the terms associated with the reproductive system and disorders of inheritance:

Abortion: The spontaneous or artificially induced expulsion of an unborn baby (foetus) before the 28th week of pregnancy.

A complete abortion refers to the entire contents of the uterus being expelled, whereas an incomplete abortion is one in which part of the foetus or placenta remains in the uterus. A threatened abortion occurs when there is vaginal bleeding with the cervix remaining closed.

A septic abortion refers to the uterine infection which occurs after an abortion, usually as a result of an induced abortion being carried out in an unsterile way. It is a serious condition which can be fatal.

A spontaneous abortion (miscarriage) may be due to an abnormality in the implantation or development of an embryo. It may also occur due to severe malaria.

Antepartum haemorrhage (APH): Refers to vaginal bleeding after the 28th week of pregnancy. One of the commonest causes of haemorrhage occurring before the birth of a baby, is placenta previa (see below). APH is more correctly termed placental disruption.

Circumcision: The surgical removal of the foreskin (prepuce) of the penis. The operation may be required for medical reasons or it may be performed for religious and ethnic reasons.

Congenital: Existing at the time of birth. A congenital abnormality is one with which a child is born.

Dilatation and curettage (D and C): A surgical procedure involving the widening (dilatation) of the cervix and scraping of the wall of the uterus with a spoon-shaped instrument (curette).

The procedure is usually performed to remove the remaining products of conception following an incomplete abortion or to investigate a cervical or uterine disease. The scrapings (curettings) are usually processed in the histology laboratory and the cells examined microscopically for any abnormality.

Down's syndrome (mongolism): A congenital condition in which there is an abnormality associated with number 21 chromosome. It is usually caused by the 21 chromosome pair failing to separate during meiosis so that when fertilization of the ovum occurs the resulting zygote has three 21 chromosomes instead of the usual two. The child is then born with a total of 47 chromosomes in each cell.The condition may also be caused by what is caused translocation in which a large part of chromosome 21 breaks off and attaches to another nearby chromosome.

A child with Down's syndrome is mentally retarded, has a flat face with slanting and widely spaced eyes, malformed ears, and a broad neck which may be short.

Ectopic pregnancy: A pregnancy which does not take place in the uterus. It usually occurs when the fertilized ovum becomes lodged in one of the uterine tubes instead of passing down the tube into the uterus. After a few weeks (usually about the 6th week) the embryo ruptures out of the tube causing abdominal pain, haemorrhage, and shock.Immediate surgery is required to remove the ectopic pregnancy and arrest the bleeding.

Haemolytic disease of the newborn (erythroblastosis foetalis): A haemolytic condition caused by maternal antibody (Ig G) crossing the placenta and destroying the red cells of the baby. In tropical countries the commonest cause of haemolytic disease of the newborn (HDN) is an ABO incompatibility between the mother and baby (mother Group O, baby Group A or B). The baby is born jaundiced. Occasionally an exchange blood transfusion is required especially if the unconjugated bilirubin level rises to a dangerous level (see also 30:2).

Haemophilia: A sex-linked recessive blood disorder in which there is a lack of factor VIII, an essential blood clotting factor (haemophilia A). As explained in 10:1, the condition usually affects males with the abnormal recessive gene being carried and transmitted by females.

Haemophilia B (Christmas disease) is caused by a deficiency of clotting factor IX.

Both types of haemophilia result in abnormal bleeding as the blood is unable to clot in the normal way. The slightest injury may cause severe haemorrhaging into the tissues with subsequent discoloration of the skin (bruising).

Obstetrics: A branch of medicine which is concerned with pregnancy, childbirth (parturition), and the care of the mother and baby during the 6 to 8 weeks after birth (puerperium).

The term gynaecology refers to the study of the disorders of women especially those affecting the female reproductive system.

Philadelphia chromosome (Ph^1): This chromosome is found in a high proportion of the myelocytes in chronic myeloid leukaemia. It is an abnormal autosomal chromosome 22 in which about half of its substance is transferred (translocated) to another chromosome.

Placenta previa: A condition in which the fertilized egg becomes implanted in the lower part of the uterus instead of the upper segment, so that the placenta lies over the opening of the uterus. This may cause the placenta to become detached before or during delivery, resulting in severe bleeding. It is usually necessary to deliver the baby surgically through the abdomen (Caesarian section) to avoid haemorrhage and to prevent damage to the brain of the baby caused by lack of oxygen.

Postpartum haemorrhage (PPH): This refers to severe bleeding following the birth of a baby due to the uterus not contracting correctly after delivery. It may occur when the placenta has failed to separate properly (this is third stage haemorrhage) or when some placental fragments have remained within the uterus. It is more common in women who have had many children (multigravida) and can cause severe bleeding and death. Abnormally heavy bleeding more than 24 hours after delivery is called secondary PPH and may be due to infection.

Primigravida: A woman who is pregnant for the first time.

Retained placenta: Refers to when the placenta does not become detached from the uterus after childbirth. Normally the placenta is expelled within one hour of delivery.

During the third stage of labour, the uterus should be handled as little as possible to prevent abnormal contractions.A retained placenta may be caused by incorrect or over vigorous management at this stage of labour. If the placenta is not passed after about an hour it is necessary to remove it, sometimes by surgery. The longer the delay, the greater the chance of haemorrhage (see PPH).

Recommended Reading

See books listed at the end of Chapter 5.

11 Immune System

11:1 IMPORTANCE OF THE IMMUNE SYSTEM

Immunology is the study of how the body protects itself against invading pathogens and harmful cells or substances.

The basic functions of the immune system are to:

- Protect the body from the harmful effects of viral, bacterial, fungal, and parasitic pathogens and their toxins.
- Destroy abnormal cells which may form in the body such as cancer cells.
- Prevent the abnormal breakdown of the body's own tissues.

Recent advances in immunology

In recent years, research into the body's immune system combined with studies in genetics and biotechnology have contributed in a major way to an improved and integrated understanding of the causes of a wide range of diseases including:

— Infections
— Cancer and malignant diseases of the bone marrow and blood cells.
— Connective tissue diseases.
— Allergic reactions.
— Autoimmune diseases in which the body reacts against its own tissues.
— Immune deficiency disorders in which there is a deficiency of immune cells or other components of the immune system.
— Diseases that are associated with immunosuppression.

Such research is leading to a better control and treatment of many (now known to be) immune-related diseases. New and improved vaccines and drugs are also becoming available based on a greater understanding of the body's immune responses. Genetic engineering and biotechnology processes are being used to produce monoclonal (highly specific) antibody products. Monoclonal antibody reagents are also becoming available for the laboratory diagnosis of infectious diseases and the investigation of diseases arising from defects of the immune system.

Natural and acquired immunity

The body's immune mechanisms consist of:

Non-specific natural immunity
Specific acquired immunity

Non-specific immunity
This form of immunity includes:

- Mechanical barriers against invading microorganisms such as the skin, mucous membranes of the respiratory and genital tracts, hairs in the nasal tract, and lining cells of the intestinal tract.
- Chemical barriers which contain antibacterial substances. These barriers include gastric juices, sweat, saliva, tears, and human milk. Interferons produced by virus-infected cells are important in combating viral infections.
- Process of phagocytosis in which a cell called a phagocyte engulfs and destroys an invading organism, cellular debris, toxin or other foreign body. The phagocytic cells involved are neutrophils and macrophages. They are attracted to sites of infection by chemotactic substances such as bacterial products or damaged and dead tissues.
- Action of natural killer cells, i.e. non-specific, non-phagocytic cells which can damage virus-infected tissue cells and some types of tumour cell.
- Action of the body's natural microbial flora (bacteria normally found in certain parts of the body, e.g. mouth, intestinal tract, vagina) in preventing the establishment of pathogens by occupying attachment sites, competing for essential nutrients, or producing substances antagonistic to pathogenic bacteria.
- Genetic factors which influence how susceptible or resistant a person is to certain pathogens e.g. persons with sickle cell trait or glucose 6-phosphate dehydrogenase deficiency are resistant to severe infection with *Plasmodium falciparum*.

Specific immunity
In this form of immunity there is a specific immune reaction against a foreign antigen which may be an invading organism, harmful cell, or toxic substance.

Acquired immunity involves:

I   Humoral immune responses in which antibodies (immunoglobulins) are produced by antigen-stimulated immune cells called B lymphocytes. These antibodies circulate in the blood and react specifically against the antigen which caused their production.

II Cell-mediated immune responses in which sensitized (exposed to antigen) immune cells called T lymphocytes and macrophages directly attack intracellular pathogens, tumour cells, or other foreign tissues.

Acquired immunity is usually described as being active or passive.

Active
☐ In active acquired immunity, the cells of the immune system recognize a foreign antigen, react specifically with it to bring about its destruction or inactivation and record information about it. The recorded information provides a memory of the invading organism or other foreign antigen so that the next time it is met a more rapid response will occur.

Active immunity occurs:

— Naturally when the body is exposed to infection.

— Artificially when a person is stimulated to produce antibodies by being immunized or vaccinated against a particular disease.

Passive
☐ In passive acquired immunity, antibodies that have been formed in another person or animal are introduced into the body of a non-immune person and afford that person protection for a limited period.

Passive immunity occurs:

— Naturally, e.g. during pregnancy when antibodies cross the placenta or when antibodies are transferred in breast milk after birth. These antibodies protect a baby during the first few months of its life until it begins to make its own antibodies.

— Artificially, e.g. when a person receives an antitoxin or gammaglobulin in the treatment of diphtheria, tetanus or snake bite. Immunoglobin may also be used to help prevent viral diseases such as hepatitis, measles, or rabies or to prevent recurrent infections in persons with low antibody levels.

Components of the immune system
The immune system is composed of:

■ Immune cells which include B lymphocytes, T lymphocytes, and phagocytic macrophages and neutrophils.

■ Antibodies

■ Complement

■ Tissues involved in the production, storage, and function of immune cells, i.e. bone marrow, thymus gland, lymph nodes and lymphatic vessels, spleen, and other lymphoid tissue.

Note: The cells of the immune system, antibodies, and complement are described in 11:2 and the tissues associated with the immune system are described in 11:3.

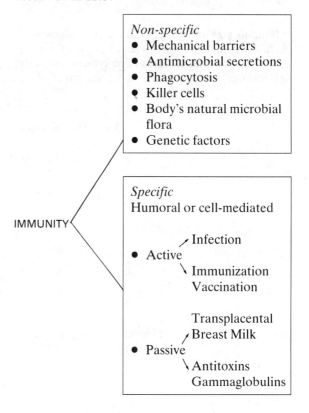

IMMUNITY

Non-specific
● Mechanical barriers
● Antimicrobial secretions
● Phagocytosis
● Killer cells
● Body's natural microbial flora
● Genetic factors

Specific
Humoral or cell-mediated

● Active
    ↗ Infection
    ↘ Immunization
      Vaccination

● Passive
    ↗ Transplacental
      Breast Milk
    ↘ Antitoxins
      Gammaglobulins

Note: Non-specific natural immunity and specific acquired immunity are more fully explained in Chapter 37 in Volume II of the Manual.

11:2 CELLS OF THE IMMUNE SYSTEM ANTIBODIES AND COMPLEMENT

All the cells of the immune system i.e. B lymphocytes, T lymphocytes, macrophages, eosinophils and neutrophils, are derived from a pluripotential stem cell which forms in an embryo during the first few weeks of life. This stem cell migrates from the embryo's liver to the bone marrow where it differentiates to produce lymphoid stem cells and what are called colony-forming units.

The lymphoid stem cells are the parent cells from which a person's different lymphocytes are derived. The colony-forming units produce mono-cytes (which become macrophages), neutrophils, eosinophils and the other blood cells as shown in Table 11.1.

B and T lymphocytes

B lymphocytes are so called because they were first associated with the Bursa (B) of Fabricius in the intestinal tract of the chicken. T lymphocytes are so called because they are derived from the thymus (T) gland.

B lymphocytes and antigen-antibody responses

A few weeks after birth, small B lymphocytes, each containing molecules of one type of antibody, are released into the blood and are carried to the lymph nodes, spleen, and lymphoid tissue in the intestinal tract and other parts of the body where they replicate. Each cell produces a series, or clone, of B cells containing identical antibody to itself. B lymphocytes circulate through the blood and lymphoid tissues. Normally 25-35% of small lymphocytes circulating in the blood are B lympho-cytes.

Further development (transformation) of a B lym-phocyte occurs when a foreign antigen (e.g. anti-gen molecules of a bacterial cell) is met which cor-responds to the antibody on the surface of the lym-phocyte. Attachment of antibody to antigen stimu-lates the B cell to replicate and produce more cells.

Table 11.1 Development of Haemopoietic Cells

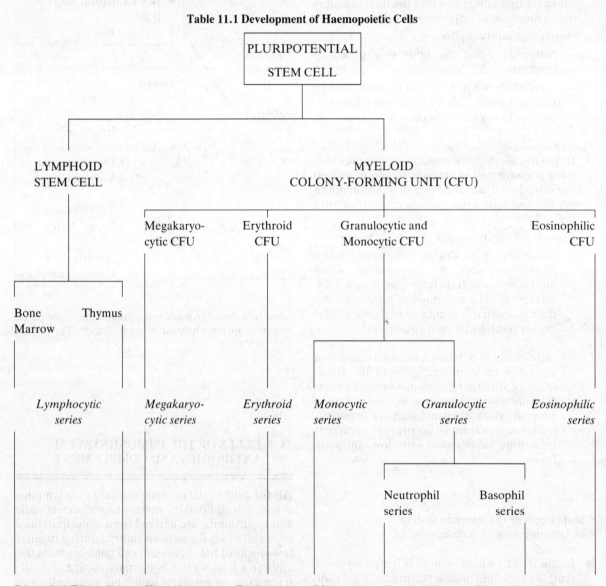

B lymphs* T lymphs*   Thrombocytes   Erythrocytes   Monocytes   Neutrophils   Basophils   Eosinophils
* *Note*: Small B and T lymphocytes become active and replicate in follicles in lymph nodes, spleen and other lymphoid tissues.

The clones of B cells produced in lymphoid tissue following antigen stimulation are:

☐ Plasma cells which manufacture and release large amounts of specific antibody into the blood to act against the invading foreign antigens.

☐ Memory cells which remain in the lymph nodes, ready to be rapidly transformed into antibody-producing plasma cells should the same antigen be met in the future.

Antigen-antibody reactions and the role of complement

B lymphocytes are involved in antibody, or humoral, immune responses against pyogenic bacteria and exotoxin-producing pathogens that multiply extracellularly.

Antibodies bind specifically to antigens forming antigen-antibody complexes. The specialized area of antibody attachment on an antigen is called an epitope. Depending on whether the antigen molecules are a toxin or part of a bacterial cell, the following reactions may occur:

— Toxin is neutralized, i.e. made harmless.
— Bacterial cell is destroyed following the activation and binding of complement, leading to lysis of the bacterial cell (cytolysis) or its phagocytosis and digestion within a phagocytic cell.

Complement consists of a group of enzymes which are normally present in the blood and tissue fluids. Over 18 distinct complement enzymes are involved in the destruction of microorganisms by cytolysis and phagocytosis. Ig M antibody is a powerful activator of complement. This is the type of antibody which is formed at the beginning of a humoral (antibody) response (explained in later text).

Complement is activated when antibody attaches to two adjacent antigen sites and a complement binding site is exposed on the antibody molecule (classical activating pathway). Complement can also be activated by Gram negative bacteria, *Entamoeba histolytica*, immature schistosomes, and enzymes such as fibrinolytic plasmin. The pathway by which complement is activated which does not involve antibody is referred to as the alternative pathway. Like the classical pathway it too ends in cytolysis.

The activity of complement in bacterial cell destruction is illustrated diagrammatically in 37:1 in Volume II of the Manual.

Antibodies

Antibodies are immunoglobulins (Ig) which react specifically with antigens. Immunoglobulins are composed of two types of polypeptide (amino acid) chains, i.e. heavy chains and light chains.

They are classified by their heavy chains because these are different for each class of immunoglobulin as follows:

Class of Ig	Heavy chains	
Ig G	gamma	(γ)
Ig M	mu	(μ)
Ig A	alpha	(α)
Ig D	delta	(δ)
Ig E	epsilon	(ε)

The light chains in each of the five immunoglobulin classes are of two types, i.e. kappa (κ) light chains and lambda (λ) light chains. In any one antibody molecule both light chains are either kappa or lambda. The part of the molecule to which an antigen can become attached is called the Fab (fragment for antigen binding) region.

Note: Ig G, Ig A (serum), Ig D and Ig E are monomeric (single molecule) antibodies consisting of a pair of heavy chains and a pair of light chains with two antigen binding sites per molecule. Secretory Ig A consists of two molecules. Ig M is a heavy pentameric (five molecule) immunoglobulin consisting of ten pairs of heavy chains and ten pairs of light chains with 5 to 10 antigen binding sites. The basic structures of monomeric and pentameric immunoglobulins are illustrated in 37:5 in Volume II of the Manual.

Ig G

Ig G is the main antibody which binds to foreign antigen at a later stage of a primary infection than Ig M and forms the rapid antibody response in repeated infections i.e. secondary response. Ig G crosses the placenta and therefore constitutes the main protective antibodies for an infant from birth to about 6 months. Killer lymphocytes and eosinophils can also attach to Ig G antibody bound to the cell surfaces of cancer cells, parasitic eggs or larvae, or virus-infected cells to bring about (with complement) their destruction.

Ig M

Ig M provides the early but short-lived antibody response in a primary infection, and therefore rises in Ig M levels indicate present or recent infection. It is the main immunoglobulin present on the surface of B lymphocytes before they become transformed. Ig M does not cross the placenta and therefore if found in a newborn baby it is indicative of active infection e.g. congenital syphilis, rubella, toxoplasmosis, or cytomegalovirus infection. Natural A and B isoagglutinins found in the blood are Ig M immunoglobulins. The 5-10 antigen attachment sites of Ig M molecules bring about strong complement binding (fixation) and rapid agglutination with phagocytosis, especially of Gram negative bacteria. Ig M is produced in large amounts in sleeping sickness (African trypanosomiasis). High levels of non-specific Ig M are occasionally found in malaria (see 15:2). Ig M neutralizes viruses.

Ig A

Ig A antibodies are found in secretions of the eye, nose, mouth, bronchi, and intestinal tract. They are locally active in neutralizing toxins and viruses, and assisting in phagocytosis. Ig A protects against respiratory tract infections, tapeworm infections, and gastrointestinal infections in breast-fed infants (breast milk contains high levels of Ig A and other important protective substances).

Ig D

Ig D is normally present in the body in small amounts. It is known to be active against food antigens and autoantigens of nuclear origin. It is also thought to be associated with the development of immunological tolerance, i.e. loss of capacity to react to a specific antigen when the antigen is met again. Raised levels of Ig D are found in acquired immune deficiency syndrome (AIDS), a serious immune disorder described in 11:4.

Ig E

Ig E, like Ig D, is also normally present in the body in very small amounts and is found in mucous membranes. Raised levels of Ig E are found in some intestinal helminth infections, schistosomiasis, filariasis, hydatid disease and trichinosis during migration stages. Macrophages are activated by antigen-Ig E antibody complexes. Ig E antibodies also bind to mast cells and basophils and are involved in drug allergies, asthma, and other immediate hypersensitivity reactions.

Note: A more detailed description of the characteristics and functions of Ig G, Ig M, Ig A, Ig D and Ig E can be found in Chapter 37 in Volume II of the Manual.

T lymphocytes and cell-mediated reactions

T lymphocytes like B lymphocytes also originate from lymphoid stem cells. Differentiation of the lymphoid stem cells which produce T lymphocytes takes place in the thymus early in life. Small T lymphocytes circulate between the blood and lymphoid tissues. Normally 60-85% of small lymphocytes in the blood are T cells.

T lymphocytes do not produce antibodies but they do possess specific protein molecules on their surfaces which act as receptors for corresponding antigens. Most T cells recognize antigens when presented on the cell membranes of macrophages. Following antigen recognition and attachment, a T cell becomes transformed, or sensitized, which results in its replication and the production of T memory cells.

Sensitized T lymphocytes secrete non-specific soluble substances called lymphokines which attract neutrophils and macrophages to those sites where they are needed. Lymphokines also promote phagocytosis, leading to the destruction of pathogen-containing cells. Lymphokines also stimulate the transformation of other T lymphocytes resulting in the release of more lymphokines.

T lymphocytes are therefore involved in immune responses in which cells directly destroy foreign antigens. This type of immunity is called cell-mediated immunity and is directed against intracellular pathogens such as *Mycobacterium tuberculosis*, *Mycobacterium leprae*, *Brucella* species, *Leishmania* species, *Toxoplasma gondii*, *Pneumocystis carinii*, *Cryptosporidium* species, *Trypanosoma cruzi*, viruses such as cytomegalovirus and herpesviruses, and fungi such as *Candida albicans*, *Cryptococcus neoformans*, *Aspergillus* species, and *Histoplasma capsulatum*.

T lymphocytes are also important in recognizing and destroying tumour cells and are essential in humoral (antibody) immune responses.

Those T lymphocytes that are directly involved in damaging and destroying cells are called T cytoxic (Tc) cells and T delayed (Td) cells. Sensitized Tc cells bring about cytolysis and Td cells secrete lymphokines and cause the tissue damage (delayed hypersensitivity) associated with some cell-mediated immune reactions, such as damage to nerves in tuberculoid leprosy, caseous necrosis in tuberculosis, reactions associated with insect stings and some drugs, and the rejection of transplanted tissue.

What are called T helper (Th) cells have a major role in regulating specific immune responses. They bring about the essential interactions between B and T lymphocytes and between different T cells.

Other T lymphocytes called T suppressor (Ts) cells are capable of inhibiting B cell activity and are involved in the overall regulation of specific immunity.

Natural killer cells

Natural killer (NK) cells are lymphocytes which have none of the surface characteristics (markers) of B or T lymphocytes.

NK cells are involved in natural non-specific immunity. They are capable of causing direct damage to tissue cells infected with viruses such as Epstein-Barr virus, coxsackie viruses and others. The development and cytotoxic effect of NK cells is influenced by interferon which is a substance secreted by virus-infected cells. NK lymphocytes are also able to attack tumour cells.

Macrophages

Macrophages are mononuclear (having single non-lobed nucleus) phagocytic cells that originate from bone marrow precursor cells (embryonic colony-forming stem cells). After differentiating and maturing in the bone marrow they are released into the blood where they circulate as monocytes for about 12 hours before entering the tissues and becoming tissue macrophages. Macrophages live for several months forming the body's mononuclear phagocytic immune response (formerly referred to as the reticuloendothelial system).

Macrophages are involved in both natural and specific immune responses. They are able to ingest and kill certain bacteria and remove from the blood and tissues unwanted debris and also damaged and antibody-coated cells. The phagocytic role of macrophages can often be demonstrated when examining blood films from patients with malaria, especially heavy *Plasmodium falciparum* infections, when monocytes can be seen containing black-brown particles of ingested malaria pigment (see colour Plate 41).

Large numbers of macrophages are found in the bone marrow, spleen, and Kupffer cells of the liver. They can also be found in lymph nodes, and lymphoid tissue of the intestinal tract, lungs and elsewhere.

In specific immunity, macrophages are able to kill pathogenic bacteria and parasites after having been activated by specific immune mechanisms involving T lymphocytes. Macrophages have cell membrane receptors for Ig G antibodies and complement (C_3). Stimulated T lymphocytes produce lymphokines which attract macrophages to where they are needed and increase their phagocytic action. Tissue macrophages are also involved in delayed hypersensitivity reactions.

Neutrophils

Polymorphonuclear (having a nucleus with several lobes) neutrophils, usually referred to simply as polymorphs or neutrophils, originate from embryonic colony-forming stem cells and like macrophages they too differentiate and mature in the bone marrow. They are released into the blood and circulate for about 10 hours before passing into the tissues. In an adult, neutrophils normally constitute up to about 70% of circulating white cells.

Neutrophils, like macrophages, are phagocytic cells but whereas macrophages are weakly mobile and are more associated with chronic inflammation, neutrophils are highly mobile and predominate in acute inflammation. The production of neutrophils increases in pyogenic infections but unlike macrophages, neutrophils are unable to replicate and die at the site of infection, forming pus cells.

Neutrophils (and also macrophages) kill bacteria in four stages referred to as chemotaxis, opsonization, ingestion, and killing. Chemotaxis is the movement of phagocytes to a site of infection by chemical substances (chemotoxins) produced following the activation of complement and other plasma proteins. In opsonization, activated complement factors and antibodies combine with bacterial surface antigens. Attachment of the antibody-coated bacterium to the membrane of the phagocytic cell brings about its ingestion. This is followed by intracellular killing in which antimicrobial substances present in the lysosome granule (organelle present in the cytoplasm of phagocytic cells) digest the engulfed bacterium.

Note: Phagocytosis is illustrated in 37:1 in Volume II of the Manual.

Eosinophils

Polymorphonuclear eosinophils are produced in the bone marrow. They are particularly important in parasitic helminth immune responses in which Ig G and Ig E antibodies are produced.

It is thought that lymphokines released from T lymphocytes stimulate the production of Ig E which binds to mast cells at the site of infection. This binding causes the release of substances which attract eosinophils, antibodies, and complement. Eosinophils attach to Ig G antibody-coated parasitic larvae and by enzymatic action, kill or damage the larvae. Antibody-coated schistosome ova are also killed by eosinophilic cytolysis.

Eosinophils are also involved in anaphylactic allergic reactions. Allergens (antigens which cause allergic responses) stimulate the production of Ig E antibodies which bind to mast cells. The allergens become attached to the bound Ig E, and cause the release of histamine and other toxic chemical substances which cause an allergic response. Eosinophils are attracted to the area and phagocytose the toxic substances. Large numbers of eosinophils are needed to neutralize toxins released from mast cells.

11:3 TISSUES OF THE IMMUNE SYSTEM

The organs and tissues involved in the immune system are shown in Fig. 11.1. They include:

- Bone marrow
- Thymus gland
- Lymph nodes and lymphatic vessels
- Spleen
- Lymphoid tissue of the tonsils and adenoids, intestine, lung, and elsewhere.

Bone marrow

Bone marrow is the tissue contained within the bones of the body. In an infant all the bones of the body contain active red coloured marrow full of developing cells. As life progresses, about half of the body's red bone marrow becomes replaced with yellow fatty inactive marrow. By adult life, red marrow is normally found only in the skull, vertebrae, ribs, sternum, pelvis, and ends of the long bones of limbs. When required, however, the yellow marrow in long bones is capable of reverting back to becoming red active marrow, e.g. in certain forms of anaemia and myeloproliferative diseases.

Red marrow

Red marrow consists of blood vessels, fat cells, reticulum cells, and developing blood and immune cells supported within a network of cancellous bony tissue. The production of blood cells in bone marrow is called medullary (bone marrow) haemopoiesis. When mature, haemopoietic cells enter the blood circulation through spaces in the walls of the small thin-walled blood vessels which pass through the marrow.

Development of haemopoietic cells

The different blood and immune cells are derived from a common cell called a pluripotential stem cell. This divides and differentiates to produce lymphoid stem cells and myeloid colony-forming units (CFU) from which the different haemopoietic cells originate. The cell lines which produce erythrocytes (red cells), thrombocytes (platelets), neutrophils, monocytes, basophils, eosinophils and lymphocytes are shown in Table 11.1. Neutrophils and monocytes originate from a common parent cell. The earliest committed cell in each cell series (precursor cell) is called a blast cell.

Lymphocytes after being processed in the bone marrow (B lymphocytes) or thymus gland (T lymphocytes), mature in the lymphoid tissues of lymph nodes and the spleen. Normally there are very few lymphoblasts found in the bone marrow.

A number of hormones and other factors influence which type of cells arise from the pluripotential stem cell. They are released in response to the body's normal needs and to inflammation, and other stimuli.

Thymus gland

The thymus gland lies in the thorax behind the sternum. It is lobed and at birth it is a relatively large gland which grows slowly until puberty after which it gradually reduces in size. By middle age it consists of only a few strands of tissue.

Differentiation of T lymphocytes

The thymus gland is particularly important in early life because it is the site where T lymphocyte precursor cells migrate to differentiate into the small T lymphocytes which are responsible for recognizing the body's own antigenic makeup and bringing about cell-mediated immunity against foreign (non-self) antigens.

The thymus is composed of a central medulla which contains reticular cells and a surrounding cortex which contains many dividing immature lymphocytes. The reticular cells are thought to regulate the replication of the lymphocytes in the cortex. Development and differentiation of T lymphocytes in the thymus is associated with acquiring Ly and other antigens. The different types of T lymphocytes produced by the thymus are T helper cells, T cytoxic cells, T suppressor cells, and T delayed hypersensitivity cells (see also 11:2).

The thymus also produces a number of hormonal factors which stimulate and influence immunological activity in lymphocytes and lymphoid tissues.

Lymph nodes and lymph vessels

Throughout the tissues, a network of lymphatic vessels (lymphatics) collect the excess tissue fluid not absorbed by blood capillaries. The tissue fluid originates from the blood plasma and is called lymph. Situated along the larger lymphatics are specialized areas of lymphoid tissue called lymph nodes. As the lymph passes through the lymph nodes, bacteria, cellular and other debris are filtered from it while immune cells and antibodies enter it. The lymph is then returned to the circulating blood through lymphatic vessels which drain into the lymphatic ducts which empty into veins in the neck.

The chemical composition of lymph may vary considerably from one lymphatic area to another. Also, the amount of lymph formed varies with different parts of the body at different times. In some tissues, lymph formation is almost continuous, such as in the intestinal tract, liver, and heart.

Structure of lymph nodes

Lymph enters a lymph node through one of several afferent lymphatics and leaves through an efferent lymphatic. A lymph node is made up of a mesh of reticular cells in which large numbers of lymphocytes are embedded in nodules called lymphoid follicles. These fill the cortex of a lymph node.

Dividing B lymphocytes form the germinal centres of the follicles while antibody producing plasma cells are found at the periphery. T lymphocytes occupy the paracortical areas of a lymph node and macrophages are found mainly in the medulla. Lymphocytes from the blood enter the lymph node through the blood vessels which supply the node.

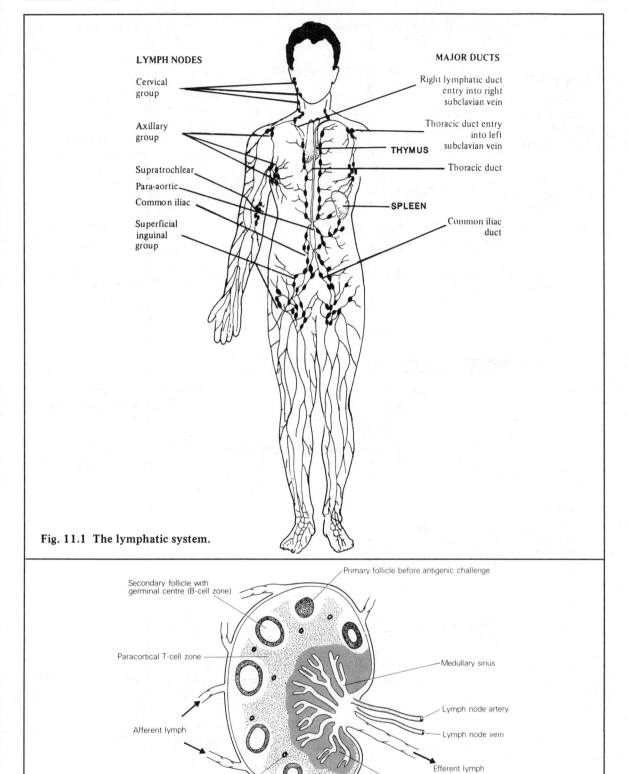

Fig. 11.1 The lymphatic system.

Fig. 11.2 Cross-section through a lymph node. *Reproduced from Integrated Clinical Science, Haematology, courtesy of William Heinemann Medical Books.*

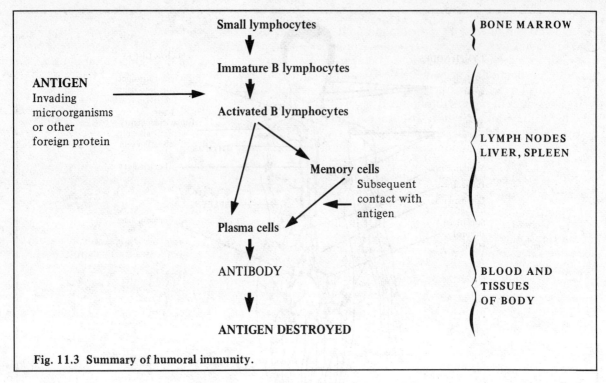

Fig. 11.3 Summary of humoral immunity.

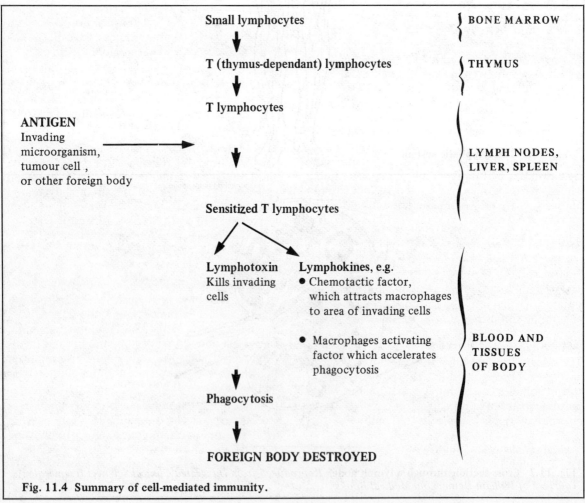

Fig. 11.4 Summary of cell-mediated immunity.

Role of lymph nodes

Foreign antigens filtered from the blood stimulate specific immune responses which result in lymphocyte transformation, multiplication, and specific antibody production. Antibodies and T lymphocyte cytotoxic cells leave the lymph node in the lymph and enter the circulating blood to be carried to where they are needed. By trapping and destroying microorganisms and debris and stimulating specific immune responses, lymph nodes are effective barriers against infection and prevent the spread of harmful substances in the body.

Lymphocytic memory cells are stored in lymph nodes. These cells are capable of developing rapidly into plasma cells to produce antibodies when the same foreign antigen which caused their original production is met again.

Enlargement of lymph nodes

The locations of the main groups of lymph nodes in the body are shown in Fig. 11.1. Inflammation of lymph nodes is called lymphadenitis. In African trypanosomiasis, especially gambiense infections, the cervical lymph nodes become greatly enlarged. In bubonic plague, the lymph glands draining the affected area become very inflamed, large, and tender (buboes). In throat infections, viral or bacterial, the lymph nodes in the neck often become swollen and painful. In tuberculosis, the lymph glands may become greatly enlarged especially in children.

Chyle

The lymphatic vessels which drain the villi of the intestine and discharge into the thoracic duct are called lacteals. During digestion, the lymph in the lacteals has a high fat content and appears milky white. It is known as chyle. In bancroftian filariasis, chyle may enter the urine following the rupture of a lymphatic vessel.

Spleen

The spleen is an ovoid shaped dark-red gland situated in the left upper abdomen below and behind the stomach.

Structure of spleen

The spleen is composed of splenic pulp enclosed in an elastic fibrous capsule. The pulp consists of splenic follicles containing lymphoid tissue (white pulp) surrounded by reticular fibres, blood vessels, macrophages, and blood cells (red pulp).

Role of spleen

The lymphoid tissue in the spleen performs a blood-filtering and immune role similar to that of lymph nodes. As the blood flows through the spleen, macrophages remove foreign bodies and microorganisms, especially capsulated bacteria such as pneumococci. B and T lymphocytes are activated and specific antibodies are produced.

The phagocytic cells in the spleen also remove from the blood:

— Red cells that have reached the end of their life-span.

— Red cell inclusions, e.g. Howell-Jolly bodies, Heinz bodies, and Pappenheimer bodies.

— Abnormal red cells, e.g. sickled cells, spherocytes, and target cells.

— Malaria-infected cells and malaria pigment.

— Antibody-coated blood cells.

The spleen is also a normal reservoir of platelets and to a lesser extent of red cells and neutrophils.

Enlargement of the spleen

Enlargement of the spleen is called splenomegaly. In tropical countries the main causes of splenomegaly are malaria, visceral leishmaniasis, intestinal schistosomiasis, sleeping sickness, brucellosis, cirrhosis of the liver, and haemoglobinopathies.

Enlargement is due to the proliferation of macrophages, lymphoid tissue and cells, the trapping and pooling of erythrocytes and other blood cells in splenic tissue and, or, the formation of infarcts.

Hyper-reactive malaria splenomegaly

This condition is sometimes found in immune adults living in malarious areas. The spleen becomes greatly enlarged due to an exaggerated immune response to malaria in which there is an overproduction of Ig M by sensitized B lymphocytes. The condition is further explained in 15:2.

Hypersplenism

In some cases of splenomegaly the spleen can become overactive and destroy red cells more rapidly than they can be produced (hypersplenism). This can lead to anaemia, leucopenia, and thrombocytopenia. In some forms of haemolytic anaemia, red cells are also removed and destroyed by the spleen more quickly than they can be formed.

Removal of the spleen (splenectomy) is sometimes undertaken as a treatment for severe hypersplenism or haemolytic anaemia. Following splenectomy, however, a person (especially a child) is more susceptible to pneumococcal septicaemia and other bacterial infections, and also to severe *P. falciparum* malaria.

11:4 TERMS USED TO DESCRIBE DISORDERS OF THE IMMUNE SYSTEM

Acquired immune deficiency syndrome (AIDS): A recently (1981) identified serious infectious disorder of the immune system in which cell-mediated immunity is defective. It is caused by T lymphocytes becoming infected with a lytic RNA retrovirus called human immunodeficiency virus (HIV).*

* HIV was formerly referred to as human T-cell lymphotropic virus type-3 (HTLV-III). It is identical with lymphadenopathy associated virus (LAV).

HIV is sexually transmitted by heterosexual and homosexual intercourse. It can also be transmitted by the transfusion of infected blood or blood products or by using needles or other objects contaminated with HIV infected blood when giving injections, or inoculations, or when performing ritual practices. An infected mother can transmit HIV to her infant as an intrauterine infection or at the time of birth. There is no evidence that HIV is spread through food, water, aerosols, or normal social contact.

Only a small percentage (5-20%) of those infected with HIV actually develop and die from AIDS or AIDS-related diseases. In some persons, infection may cause a fever-like illness whereas in others AIDS may develop several weeks or years after infection. The clinical features of AIDS include wasting with loss of weight, lymphadenopathy, enlarged liver and spleen, deficiency of T-helper lymphocytes (in most patients), low platelet count, raised Ig G, Ig A and Ig D, and often an accompanying fungal, protozoal, or viral infection.

AIDS patients often develop pneumonia caused by *Pneumocystis carinii* or thrush of the mouth caused by *Candida albicans*. Other AIDS-related opportunistic infections include cryptosporidial and *Isospora* enteritis, disseminated (widespread) cytomegalovirus infection, histoplasmosis, cryptococcal meningitis, *Strongyloides* infection, cerebral toxoplasmosis, and a disseminated infection with *Mycobacterium tuberculosis* or *Mycobacterium avium-intracellulare*. Some AIDS patients develop Kaposi's sarcoma or other cancers associated with defective cell-mediated immunity.

Severe disease of the central nervous system may occur with HIV infection when the virus infects brain cells.

The mortality rate from AIDS and AIDS-related diseases is high. In the absence of a vaccine and drugs to treat AIDS, the number of those infected with HIV is increasing and AIDS is spreading in many parts of the world including tropical Africa, parts of Asia, USA, Europe, and Japan. Tests to screen blood donors for antibody to HIV have been developed and are helping to detect the virus in blood and blood products.

Note: Further information and interim guidelines about HIV and AIDS, the risk of spread by heterosexual contact and HIV infection in pregnancy can be found in the 1986, Number 1 *IPPF (International Planned Parenthood Federation) Medical Bulletin*.[1] The epidemiology of AIDS in Africa has been reviewed by Chumeck.[2] A series of articles describing AIDS and AIDS-related diseaes can be found in *Postgraduate Doctor-Africa*

Anergy: Absence of cell-mediated immunity or lack of a response to a delayed hypersensitivity test after exposure to an antigen, e.g. negative lepromin test in lepromatous leprosy.

Autoimmune disease: Disorder of the immune system in which the body fails to differentiate between self and non-self antigens and damages or destroys its own tissues or tissue products. Although usual, the finding of autoantibodies is not diagnostic of autoimmume disease because such antibodies, especially antinuclear factor and rheumatoid factor, can be found in elderly persons or occur temporarily in response to drugs or infections. Rheumatoid factor is often found in sleeping sickness and visceral leishmaniasis. Many autoimmune diseases appear to be genetically linked, with some persons being more susceptible than others. Females are more commonly affected than males.

Examples of autoimmune diseases include:

● Systemic lupus erythematosus (SLE) in which antinuclear factor (ANF), anti-DNA autoantibodies, and immune DNA antigen-antibody immune complexes are formed which damage the skin, kidneys, joints, blood cells, clotting factors, and nerve cells. Common findings include a deficiency of lymphocytes, haemolytic anaemia, low platelet count, bleeding tendency, and neurological symptoms. The lupus erythematosus (LE) cell test is positive due to the presence of ANF.

● Rheumatoid arthritis in which rheumatoid factor (RF) is formed with immune complexes which cause severe and painful damage to the joints of the wrists, fingers, feet, ankles, hips and shoulders. Agglutination tests (e.g. latex test) for RF are positive.

● Insulin-dependent diabetes mellitus (IDDM) in which autoantibodies are formed against insulin secreting *beta*-islet cells which results in a deficiency of insulin to regulate blood glucose levels.

● Pernicious anaemia in which autoantibodies are formed against parietal cells and intrinsic factor, causing achlorhydria and a deficiency of intrinsic factor. Intrinsic factor is required for the absorption of vitamin B_{12} which is essential for the normal production of red cells.

- Autoimmune haemolytic anaemia in which autoantibodies are produced against antigens on red cells (often in association with other diseases) or against drug antigens attached to red cells. The antibodies coat the red cells leading to their removal and destruction usually by macrophages in the spleen.

Red cell autoantibodies that react at 35-37 °C are called warm autoimmune antibodies and are usually of the Ig G type. Blood films from persons with warm autoimmune haemolytic anaemia show spherocytic red cells and the direct Coomb's test is positive for Ig G and Ig G with complement. Warm autoantibodies occur in SLE, some forms of leukaemia and in autoimmune haemolytic anaemia due to drugs such as alpha-methyldopa.

Red cell autoantibodies that react at cooler temperatures are called cold autoimmune antibodies and are usually of the Ig M type. In cold autoimmune haemolytic anaemia, spherocytosis is less marked, and the direct Coomb's test is positive for complement. Cold Ig M autoantibodies usually show specificity for red cell antigens I or i. Cold autoantibodies (agglutinins) are often found in *Mycoplasma* pneumonia and infectious mononucleosis.

- Rheumatic heart disease (following infection with Group A *Streptococcus*) in which antiheart antibodies which damage the heart and its valves are produced because Group A streptococci carry an antigen which is similar to a human heart antigen. Other Group A streptococci (type 12) carry surface antigens similar to those in kidney glomeruli and therefore antibodies produced against these streptococci can damage glomeruli and lead to acute nephritis.

Note: Information about other autoimmune diseases can be found in the 2nd edition of *Immunology Simplified.*[4]

Hypersensitivity (allergy): Tissue damage which results from an antigen specific immune response. There are several types of hypersensitivity reaction:

- Type I, an immediate or anaphylactic (shock) type reaction as may occur in hay fever, some forms of asthma, or following insect bites, treatment with certain drugs, or hydatid cyst rupture.
- Type II, a cytotoxic type reaction as occurs for example when ABO incompatible blood is transfused.
- Type III, an immune-complex mediated type reaction as may occur in serum sickness, SLE, rheumatoid arthritis, or erythema nodosum.
- Type IV, a delayed hypersensitivity reaction, e.g. neuritis in leprosy, caseous necrosis in tuberculosis or granuloma formation in schistosomiasis.
- Type V, an anti-receptor type as in insulin-resistant diabetes, Graves' disease (excess of thyroid hormones in blood stream), or myasthenia gravis (fatigue and weakness of certain muscles).

Note: The different hypersensitivity reactions are fully described in the 2nd edition of *Immunology Simplified.*[4]

Immunodeficiency: Inherited, physiological, or acquired disorder in which there is a deficiency of one or more components of specific or non-specific immunity.

Examples of immunodeficiency disorders occurring in non-specific immunity include:

- Deficiency of complement factors, interferon, or lysozyme, as may occur in protein-calorie malnutrition or more rarely in inherited conditions.
- Defective phagocytosis as may occur in sickle cell disease, diabetes mellitus, protein calorie malnutrition, myeloid leukaemia, treatment with certain drugs, and in rare congenital disorders affecting neutrophils and monocytes. When phagocytosis is abnormal, infections occur more frequently especially with pneumococci and salmonellae.

Examples of immunodeficiency disorders occurring in specific immunity include:

- Acquired immune deficiency syndrome (AIDS) see previous text .
- Deficient cell-mediated immunity as occurs in malnutrition, measles, syphilis, miliary tuberculosis, some forms of leprosy, viral hepatitis, infectious mononucleosis, acute falciparum malaria, sleeping sickness, visceral leishmaniasis, chronic schistosomiasis and filariasis. Cell-mediated immunity is normally reduced in pregnancy and with aging.
- Deficiency of lymphocytes or defective lymphocytic responses due to cytotoxic drugs, corticosteroid therapy, or irradiation.
- Deficiency of immunoglobulins due to low protein levels, e.g. in the nephrotic syndrome or severe protein-calorie malnutrition.
- Deficiencies of immune responses due to diseases of the lymphoid tissues, e.g. Hodgkin's disease, multiple myeloma, leukaemias, Burkitt's lymphoma.

- Rare inherited disorders resulting in abnormalities and deficiencies of humoral and cell-mediated immunity e.g. agammaglobulinaemia in which gammaglobulin is not produced.

Immunosuppression: Generalized depression of the immune system due to malnutrition, drugs, irradiation, and diseases such as measles, whooping cough, infectious mononucleosis, acute malaria, visceral leishmaniasis, sleeping sickness, filariasis, and schistosomiasis.

References

1 International Planned Parenthood Federation. *IPPF Medical Bulletin*, 20: **1**, 1986. Copies of this two page Bulletin can be obtained from IPPF, 18-20 Lower Regent Street, London, SW1Y 4PW, UK.

2 Chumeck, N. AIDS in African Patients, *New England Journal of Medicine*, **310**, pp 492-495, 1985.

3 Farthing, C. (editor) AIDS Series. *Postgraduate Doctor-Africa*, beginning **8**, (8), pp 233-238 (12 part series), 1986.

4 Bowry, T. R. *Immunology Simplified*. Oxford University Press, 2nd edition, 1984, ELBS edition priced £1.95.

Recommended Reading

Bowry, T. R. *Immunology Simplified*. Oxford University Press, 2nd edition, 1984, ELBS edition priced £1.95.

Weir, D. M. *Immunology*. Churchill Livingstone, 5th edition, 1983, ELBS edition priced £2.25.

Chapel, H., Heaney, M. *Essentials of Clinical Immunology*. Blackwell Scientific, 1984, ELBS edition priced £3.

Govan, A. T., Macfarlane, P., Callander, R. *Pathology Illustrated*, Churchill Livingstone, 2nd edition, 1986. International Student edition priced £8.25. Highly recommended.

SECTION III

MEDICAL PARASITOLOGY

COLOUR PLATES

The parasites described in the following Chapters are illustrated in Colour Plates No. 1 to 56 between pages 288 and 289 in the Colour Section of the Manual.

Chart 12.1 Basic Classification of Parasites of Medical Importance

---

> **PROTOZOA**
>
> Single-celled Organisms

SARCOMASTIGOPHORA
Amoebae
Entamoeba histolytica
Naegleria species

Flagellates
Giardia lamblia
Trichomonas vaginalis

Haemoflagellates
Trypanosoma cruzi
Trypanosoma b. gambiense
Trypanosoma b. rhodesiense

Leishmania donovani
Leishmania braziliensis
Leishmania mexicana
Leishmania major
Leishmania tropica
Leishmania aethiopica

CILIOPHORA
Ciliates
Balantidium coli[a]

COCCIDIA
Sporozoa
Plasmodium falciparum
Plasmodium vivax
Plasmodium malariae
Plasmodium ovale

Isospora belli[a]
Cryptosporidium

Toxoplasma gondii[a]

> **HELMINTHS**
>
> Worms

> **PLATYHELMINTHES**
>
> Flatworms

> **NEMATHELMINTHES**
>
> Cylindrical Worms

TREMATODA
Flukes (digenetic)
Opisthorchis sinensis
Opisthorchis viverrini
Metagonimus yokogawai
Heterophyes heterophyes[a]
Fasciolopsis buski
Fasciola hepatica[a]
Paragonimus species

Schistosoma haematobium
Schistosoma mansoni
Schistosoma japonicum
Schistosoma mekongi[a]
Schistosoma intercalatum[a]

CESTODA
Tapeworms
Taenia solium
Taenia saginata
Echinococcus granulosus
Hymenolepis nana[b]
Diphyllobothrium latum

NEMATODA
Roundworms
Ascaris lumbricoides
Enterobius vermicularis
Strongyloides stercoralis
Trichuris trichiura
Ancylostoma duodenale
Necator americanus
Toxocara canis[a]

Wuchereria bancrofti
Brugia malayi
Brugia timori
Loa loa
Onchocerca volvulus
Dracunculus medinensis
Trichinella species

---

a   Parasite of low occurence.
b   Common parasite but of lesser medical importance.

12

Introduction to Parasitology

12:1 PARASITISM

Most plants and animals are able to live independently and are largely self-sufficient in obtaining and metabolizing the nutrients they require for their growth and reproduction. A small group of plants and animals, however, are not so independent and some of these have evolved a more or less intimate relationship with another organism of a different species so that both partners benefit from the relationship. This relationship in which neither partner is harmed is called commensalism. If, however, one partner benefits from the relationship and is unable to complete all its development and reproductive processes without the aid of the other partner, the relationship is then one of parasitism.

Parasitic relationships

In a parasitic relationship, the half of the partnership which benefits from the relationship is the parasite and that which provides the benefit is called the host. The degree of dependence of the parasite on the host varies considerably from one species of organism to another. For example, malaria parasites are unable to survive outside of a mosquito and a human body whereas some parasitic worms are capable of surviving for several generations independently of a host. The majority of parasitic species lie between these two extremes. The term free-living is used to describe the non-parasitic stages of active existence which are lived independently of a host. For example, hookworms have active free-living stages in the soil.

Other parasites have stages which can survive outside of the host for greater or shorter periods of time, but these stages are not strictly free-living in that they are in the form of eggs or cysts, e.g. the cysts of parasitic amoebae or the eggs of tapeworms and roundworms.

The eggs and cysts of parasites are resistant to adverse environmental conditions to a greater or lesser extent. They are usually passed in the host's excreta (most of the parasites which produce them are found in the intestine) and this is the normal way such infections are transmitted.

Endoparasites and ectoparasites

When a parasite lives within its host (for example, a malaria parasite), it is referred to as an endoparasite and is said to cause an infection. A parasite, however, which lives on the outer surface or in the superficial tissues of its host (e.g. a flea), is called an ectoparasite and is said to cause an infestation.

Most of the parasites which cause human disease are endoparasites. A basic classification of the medically important parasites is shown in Table 12.1. The characteristics of the different groups of parasites can be found in 12:4.

12:2 LIFE CYCLES OF PARASITES

All parasites pass through a series of developmental stages before a stage is reached when the organism reproduces and a new cycle of development begins. There may be few or several developmental stages, with at least one stage occurring in a host organism.

Within the developmental cycle (life cycle) there may be several phases of parasite multiplication or only one. According to species the phases of multiplication may be sexual or asexual. In some parasites sexual multiplication is followed almost immediately by asexual multiplication.

Direct and indirect life cycles

When a parasite requires only one species of host in which to complete its development it is said to have a direct life cycle, e.g. the life cycle of the parasite that causes amoebiasis in humans (*Entamoeba histolytica*) requires only a human host for its completion.

When two or more species of hosts are required, the life cycle is referred to as indirect, e.g. the filarial worms that parasitize humans require both a human host and an insect host in which to complete their development.

Parasites that have a direct life cycle and those that have an indirect life cycle are listed in Table 12.2

Definitive and intermediate hosts

When two or more species of hosts are required in the development of a parasite, i.e. an indirect life cycle, the terms definitive and intermediate are used to differentiate the hosts involved.

Definitive host
Depending on parasitic species, the definitive host is either:

— the host in which sexual reproduction takes place, e.g. a human is the definitive host for *Schistosoma haematobium* whereas an *Anopheles* mosquito is the definitive host for the malaria parasite.

The latter example in which an insect is a definitive host is rare (insects are usually intermediate hosts).

or,

— the host in which the mature or most highly developed form of the parasite occurs. When the mature or most highly developed form is not obvious, the definitive host is the mammalian host, e.g. a human is the definitive host for the trypanosomes that cause African trypanosomiasis.

Note: The life cycle of a parasite is often defined as the cycle of development of a parasite from definitive host and back to definitive host.

Intermediate host
This term is used to describe the species of host or hosts, other than the definitive host, that are essential to complete the indirect life cycle of a parasite, e.g. the tsetse fly is the intermediate host for the *Trypanosoma* species that cause African trypanosomiasis.

In the life cycles of parasitic worms, intermediate hosts harbour the larval forms. Snails serve as the intermediate hosts for all the flukes that parasitize humans (see Table 12.2).

In indirect parasitic life cycles, the term vector is usually applied only to blood-feeding arthropod intermediate hosts such as mosquitoes, tsetse flies, sandflies, and triatomine bugs.

The term mechanical vector is used to describe a vector which assists in the transfer of parasitic forms between hosts but is not essential in the life cycle of a parasite, i.e. no parasitic development occurs in such a vector. An example of a mechanical vector is a fly that transfers amoebic cysts from infected faeces to food that is eaten by humans. A non-arthropod mechanical vector is called a transport, or paratenic, host. In such a host a parasite remains viable but does not develop.

Reservoir host
A reservoir host is an animal in which a parasite usually resides or one in which a parasite which infects humans is able to be maintained in the absence of a human host.

A parasitic infection in which the normal host is an animal, but can produce disease in humans if they become infected accidentally, is called a zoonosis. Some of the most important parasitic diseases are zoonoses, e.g. leishmaniasis, South American trypanosomiasis, African trypanosomiasis, japonicum schistosomiasis, trichinellosis and echinococcosis. When a human becomes an accidental definitive or intermediate host of a parasite for which an animal is the normal host, the parasite may not be able to complete its normal life cycle (dead-end infection). Lack of adaptation of the parasite to a human host may also cause a serious infection in the person infected, e.g. echinococcosis.

Epidemiologically, reservoir hosts are important because they can maintain a nucleus of infection in an area which can be transmitted back to humans when human hosts become present again. For example, certain rodents are reservoir hosts for human cutaneous leishmaniasis in various parts of the world with infection being transmitted from rodent to rodent by sandflies and human infection occurring as and when the opportunity arises.

Identifying reservoir hosts of parasites that infect humans is therefore important in the control of parasitic diseases.

12:3 TRANSMISSION AND DISEASES CAUSED BY PARASITES

Routes of transmission
The infective stage of a parasite may be transmitted to a person in the following ways:

■ By ingesting the parasite in food, water, or from hands that have been contaminated with faeces that contain the infective form of the parasite. This method of transmission is often referred to as the faecal-oral (mouth) route. Examples of parasites transmitted in this way include:

Entamoeba histolytica
Giardia lamblia
Enterobius vermicularis
Trichuris trichiura

■ By ingesting the parasite in raw or under-cooked meat as occurs with:

Taenia saginata
Taenia solium
Trichinella spiralis

■ By ingesting the parasite in raw or under-cooked fish, crab, or water vegetation as occurs with:

Opisthorchis species
Metagonimus yokogawai
Diphyllobothrium latum
Paragonimus westermani
Fasciolopsis buski

Table 12.2 Life Cycles and Hosts of the Medically Important Parasites

Parasite	Host
DIRECT LIFE CYCLE	
Entamoeba histolytica	Human
Giardia lamblia	Human
Trichomonas vaginalis	Human
Balantidium coli	Pig, human
Ascaris lumbricoides	Human
Enterobius vermicularis	Human
Strongyloides stercoralis	Human
Trichuris trichiura	Human
Ancylostoma duodenale	Human
Necator americanus	Human
Trichinella spiralis	Pig, bushpig, rat, human

Parasite	Definitive Host	Intermediate Host
INDIRECT LIFE CYCLE		
Trypanosoma cruzi	Armadillo, oppossum, dog, cat, guinea pig, human	Triatomine bug
Trypanosoma b. rhodesiense	Game animals, human	Tsetse fly
Trypanosoma b. gambiense	Human, possibly pig	Tsetse fly
Leishmania donovani	Rodent, dog, human	Sandfly
Leishmania tropica	Dog, rodent, human	Sandfly
Leishmania braziliensis	Rodent, human	Sandfly
Plasmodium species	Mosquito	Human
Toxoplasma gondii	Cat, lynx	Herbivores, pig, bird, human
Wuchereria bancrofti	Human	Mosquito
Brugia malayi	Human, domestic and wild animals	Mosquito
Loa loa	Human	Horsefly
Onchocerca volvulus	Human	Blackfly
Dracunculus medinensis	Human, dog	Cyclops
Opisthorchis sinensis	Human, dog, pig, rat	1st Snail 2nd Fish
Fasciolopsis buski	Human, pig	Snail
Fasciola hepatica	Sheep, goat, cattle camel, pig, human	Snail
Paragonimus westermani	Human, tiger, cat, dog	1st Snail 2nd Crayfish, crab
Schistosoma haematobium	Human	Snail
Schistosoma mansoni	Human	Snail
Schistosoma japonicum	Cat, dog, rat, pig, buffalo, human	Snail
Taenia solium	Human	Pig
Taenia saginata	Human	Cattle
Echinococcus granulosus	Dog, wolf, fox, hyaena, jackal	Sheep, cattle, camel, human
Diphyllobothrium latum	Human, dog, cat, seal, bear, fox	1st Cyclops 2nd Fish

Note: The hosts mentioned are those that are epidemiologically important.

■ By ingesting the parasite in water containing infected Cyclops as occurs with:

  Dracunculus medinensis

■ By the parasite penetrating the skin when in contact with faecally polluted soil as occurs with:

  Hookworms
  Strongyloides stercoralis

■ By contact with water containing the parasite as occurs with:

  Schistosoma species

■ By the parasite entering through an insect bite as occurs with:

  Wuchereria bancrofti
  Brugia species
  Loa loa
  Onchocerca volvulus

■ By inoculation of the parasite into the blood by an insect as occurs with:

  Plasmodium species
  Trypanosoma b. gambiense
  Trypanosoma b. rhodesiense
  Leishmania species

■ By sexual contact as occurs with:

  Trichomonas vaginalis

■ By infected faeces from an insect being rubbed into the site of the insect bite as occurs with:

  Trypanosoma cruzi

Parasitic disease
Not all parasitic infections cause disease of clinical significance. Many factors influence whether an infection causes disease including:

Parasitic factors
— the strain of parasite.
— number of parasites (which may reflect the parasite's reproductive pattern and potential).
— size of parasite and site(s) occupied in the body.
— metabolic processes of the parasite, particularly the nature of any waste products.

Host factors
— age and level of natural immunity at the time of infection.
— immune responses to the infection.
— presence of co-existing disease or condition which reduces immune responses, e.g. pregnancy.
— whether there is undernutrition or malnutrition.
— life style and work of the person infected.

For example, a light infection with a small intestinal parasite which has little reproductive potential in a well nourished individual is likely to be of little or no consequence. An infection, however, with malaria parasites (which have a high reproductive potential) in a pregnant woman or non-immune malnourished infant could be serious or even life-threatening.

Further information concerning host responses to parasites and the local effects of parasitism can be found in the book of Knight called *Parasitic Disease in Man* (see Recommended Books).

Table 12.3 summarizes the main diseases caused by parasites, the tissues affected, the infective stages of the parasites, and methods of transmission.

Chart 12.3 Transmission and Diseases Caused by Medically Important Parasites

Parasite	Infective Stage	Transmission	Tissues Affected	Main Disease
PROTOZOA				
Entamoeba histolytia	Cyst	Ingestion	Large intestine, liver. Lungs,[a] brain,[a] skin[a]	Amoebic dysentery (10-20% of cases)
Giardia lamblia	Cyst	Ingestion	Small intestine	Giardiasis
Trichomonas vaginalis	Flagellate	Sexual	Vagina, urethra	Vaginitis
Balantidium coli	Cyst	Ingestion	Large intestine	Balantidiasis
Trypanosoma cruzi	Metacyclic trypomastigote	Contamination	Blood, macrophage system, heart muscle. Colon,[a] oesophagus,[a] brain,[a] etc	Chagas' disease

Parasite	Infective Stage	Transmission	Tissues Affected	Main Disease
Trypanosoma b. rhodesiense T. b. gambiense	Metacyclic trypomastigote	Bite of tsetse fly	Blood, macrophage system (especially lymph glands, bone marrow), c.s.f., CNS	African trypanosomiasis
Leishmania donovani	Promastigote	Bite of sandfly	Macrophage system (especially spleen, liver, bone marrow)	Visceral leishmaniasis
Leishmania braziliensis	Promastigote	Bite of sandfly	Skin, mucous membranes	Cutaneous, and mucocutaneous leishmaniasis
Leishmania tropica	Promastigote	Bite of sandfly	Skin	Cutaneous leishmaniasis
Plasmodium falciparum	Sporozoite	Bite of mosquito	RBCs, liver, spleen placenta. Brain,[a] kidney,[a] lung,[a] intestine[a]	Falciparum malaria
Other species of Plasmodium	Sporozoite	Bite of mosquito	RBCs, liver	Malaria
Isospora belli	Mature oocyst	Ingestion	Large intestine	Coccidiosis
Cryptosporidium	Mature oocyst	Ingestion	Large intestine	Enteritis[b]
Toxoplasma gondii	Oocyst	Ingestion	Muscle, endothelial cells, eye	Toxoplasmosis
	Toxoplasm	Congenital	CNS	Congenital toxoplasmosis

FLUKES

Opisthorchis sinensis	Metacercaria in fish	Ingestion	Liver, bile ducts	Opisthorchiasis
Fasciolopsis buski	Metacercaria on plant	Ingestion	Duodenal and jejunal wall	Fasciolopsiasis
Fasciola hepatica	Metacercaria on plant	Ingestion	Liver, bile ducts	Fascioliasis
Paragonimus species	Metacercaria in crab or crayfish	Ingestion	Lungs. Brain,[a] subcutaneous tissue[a]	Paragonimiasis
Metagonimus yokogawai	Metacercaria in fish	Ingestion	Small intestine, brain	Metagonimiasis
Schistosoma haematobium	Cercaria in water	Skin penetration	Adults in veins. Eggs in bladder, liver, brain[a]	Urinary schistosomiasis
Schistosoma mansoni S. japonicum	Cercaria in water	Skin penetration	Adults in veins. Eggs in intestine, liver, CNS[a]	Intestinal schistosomiasis

TAPEWORMS

Taenia solium	Cysticercus in pork	Ingestion	Adults in small intestine. Larvae in muscle, brain[a]	Taeniasis (adult) Cysticercosis (larvae)
Taenia saginata	Cysticercus in beef	Ingestion	Small intestine	Taeniasis
Echinococcus granulosus	Egg	Ingestion	Liver, lungs, brain, heart,[a] spleen,[a] kidney,[a] bone[a]	Hydatid cyst

Parasite	Infective Stage	Transmission	Tissues Affected	Main Disease
Hymenolepis nana	Egg	Ingestion	Small intestine	Hymenolepiasis
Diphyllobothrium latum	Plerocercoid in fish	Ingestion	Small intestine	Diphyllobothriasis

NEMATODES

Parasite	Infective Stage	Transmission	Tissues Affected	Main Disease
Ascaris lumbricoides	Embryonated eggs	Ingestion	Adults in small intestine. Migratory larvae in liver, lungs, trachea. Ectopic infections[a]	Ascariasis (Roundworm)
Enterobius vermicularis	Embryonated egg	Ingestion	Adults in caecum, rectum. Larvae in jejunal crypts	Enterobiasis (Threadworm)
Strongyloides stercoralis	Infective larva	Penetration	Adults in small intestine. Migratory larvae in lungs etc,	Strongyloidiasis
Trichuris trichiura	Embryonated egg	Ingestion	Adults in caecum. Larvae in crypts of small intestine	Trichuriasis (Whipworm)
Hookworms	Infective larva	Penetration	Adults attached to villi of small intestine. Migratory larvae in lungs, subcutaneous tissue[a]	Hookworm disease
Wuchereria bancrofti	Infective larva	Bite of mosquito	Adults in lymphatic system. Microfilariae in blood	Lymphatic (Bancroftian) filariasis
Brugia species	Infective larva	Bite of mosquito	Adults in lymphatic system. Microfilariae in blood	Lymphatic (Brugian) filariasis
Loa loa	Infective larva	Bite of horsefly	Adults in connective tissue Microfilariae in blood	Loiasis (Calabar swelling)
Onchocerca volvulus	Infective larva	Bite of blackfly	Adults in subcutaneous nodules. Microfilariae in skin, eyes[a]	Onchocerciasis (River blindness)
Dracunculus medinensis	Infective larva in Cyclops	Ingestion	Adults in connective tissue.	Dracunculiasis (Guinea worm)
Trichinella spiralis	Encysted larva in muscle	Ingestion	Larvae in muscle. Adults in small intestine	Trichinellosis

a   May also be affected in severe infections.
b   Commonly an opportunistic parasite, e.g. in persons with AIDS.

Acknowledge: The above Chart is reproduced from material kindly supplied by the Liverpool School of Tropical Medicine.

12:4 CLASSIFICATION AND CHARACTERISTICS OF PARASITES

A basic classification of the medically important single-celled parasites (protozoa), flukes (trematodes), tapeworms (cestodes) and cylindrical worms (nematodes) is shown in Chart 12.1 in 12:1. This subunit describes the basic characteristics of each of these groups of parasites.

Characteristics of protozoa

- Simple, single celled micro-organisms consisting of a nucleus and cytoplasm.
- Nucleus contains a karyosome and chromatin granules.
- Cytoplasm contains food vacuoles and other organelles.

The protozoa of medical importance belong to the following groups:

☐ Sarcodina   *Entamoeba histolytica*

☐ Mastigophora   *Giardia lamblia*
Trichomonas vaginalis
Trypanosoma species
Leishmania species

☐ Ciliophora   *Balantidium coli*

☐ Coccidia   *Isospora belli*
Cryptosporidium species
Toxoplasma gondii
Plasmodium species

Sarcodina

This subphylum includes the amoebae which have the following characteristics:

- Consist of a shapeless mass of moving cytoplasm which is divided into granular endoplasm and clear ectoplasm.
- Move by pushing out the ectoplasm to form pseudopodia (false feet) into which the endoplasm then flows.
- Reproduce by simply dividing into two (binary fission).
- Digested food substances are stored as glycogen and, or, chromatoid bodies.
- Form cysts by which they are transmitted.

Mastigophora

This subphylum includes the haemoflagellates (*Trypanosoma* and *Leishmania*), and flagellates of the gastrointestinal tract (*G. lamblia*) and urogenital tract (*T. vaginalis*). They have the following characteristics:

- Locomotion is mainly or wholly by a flagellum or flagella.
- Reproduce by simple binary fission.
- *Trypanosoma* and *Leishmania* species possess a kinetoplast. The flagellated forms have a single flagellum. They are transmitted by biting flies or bugs.
- *G. lamblia* is bilaterally symmetrical, having two nuclei, four pairs of flagella and two axonemes. It is transmitted by the ingestion of cysts.
- *T. vaginalis* has an undulating membrane bordered by a flagellum, four or five anterior flagella, and an axostyle. It is sexually transmitted.

Cilophora

This subphylum includes ciliates which have the following characteristics:

- Move by small hairs (cilia) which cover the organisms.
- Have two dissimilar nuclei (macronucleus and micronucleus).
- Reproduce by simple binary fission.
- Form cysts by which they are transmitted.

Coccidia

This subclass includes intestinal and tissue coccidian parasites and the malaria parasites which have the following characteristics:

- Reproduce asexually by a process called schizogony and sexually by a process called sporogony.
- Malaria parasites are transmitted by mosquitoes and the intestinal coccidia by the ingestion of oocysts.

Characteristics of tapeworms

- Body is tape-like and is made up of a head (scolex) and many proglottides (often called segments). Adults live in the intestinal tract with some species growing to great lengths.

  The head attaches the tapeworm to its host. It has suckers and in some species hooks also.

- Proglottides are formed from behind the head. Those that are newly formed are small and immature. Mature proglottides contain fully developed reproductive organs. The proglottides which contain eggs are known as gravid segments.

- Tapeworms are hermaphroditic with male and female reproductive organs being found in each mature proglottid. There are usually several testes, a bilobed ovary, and a uterus which may be coiled or as with *Taenia* species, consist of a central stem with side branches.

Where the male and female organs meet there is a common genital pore, which in some species, is situated ventrally in the mid line of each proglottid while in others it is situated on the side of the proglottid.

■ In most species, the eggs are released when a gravid segment becomes detached and ruptures.

■ There is no mouth or digestive system. A tapeworm obtains nutrients through its body surface. There is a simple excretory system.

The tapeworms of medical importance belong to the following two orders:

☐ Cyclophyllidea   *Taenia solium*
   Taenia saginata
   Echinococcus granulosus
   Hymenolepis nana

☐ Pseudophyllidea *Diphyllobothrium latum*

The characteristic features of these orders of tapeworms are as follows:

Cyclophyllidea
— Globular head with four suckers. The head of some species have hooks also.
— Common genital pore is laterally positioned on each segment.
— Uterine pore is absent. The vitelline glands are massed together below the ovary.
— Eggs are non-operculated. Each contains an embryo which has three pairs of embryonic hooklets. The embryo is released from the egg in the intermediate host.
— There is only one intermediate host.

Pseudophyllidea
— Elongated head with two slit-like sucking grooves.
— Common genital pore is positioned ventrally and in the mid-line of each segment.
— A uterine pore is present through which eggs are discharged. There are many vitelline glands and these are scattered, not massed together.
— Eggs are operculated. They develop and hatch in water, each producing a ciliated embryo.
— There are two intermediate hosts. The procercoid larva occurs in the first host and the plerocercoid larva in the second host.

Characteristics of flukes
The parasitic flukes, of medical importance belong to the subclass Digenea.

Digenetic flukes
These are trematodes for which two generations are required to complete their life cycle. There is an asexual generation in which multiplication occurs (in sporocyst or redia stage) and a sexual generation which produces eggs.

The following are the basic characteristics of parasitic flukes:

■ Unsegmented, mostly flat leaf-like worms (schistosomes are an exception).

■ Attach to their host by means of suckers. There is a sucker which surrounds the mouth (oral sucker) and another on the ventral surface (ventral sucker).

■ No body cavity.

■ Digestive system consists of a mouth and an oesophagus which divides to form two intestinal caeca. In some species the caeca are branched. There is no anus.

■ Excretory system is composed of excretory cells called flame cells, collecting tubules, and an excretory pore.

■ With the exception of schistosomes, trematodes are hermaphroditic (male and female reproductive organs in the same individual). Most trematode eggs are operculated (with lids). To develop, the eggs must reach water.

The hermaphroditic flukes of medical importance belong to the following superfamilies:

☐ Opisthorchioidea   *Opisthorchis sinensis*
   Opisthorchis viverrini
   Heterophyes heterophyes
   Metagonimus yokogawai

☐ Echinostomatoidea *Fasciolopsis buski*
   Fasciola hepatica

☐ Plagiorchioidea   *Paragonimus* species

The characteristic features of flukes belonging to these superfamilies are as follows:

Opisthorchioidea
— Adults live in the biliary ducts or small intestine.
— Testes are branched and arranged one in front of the other behind the ovary.
— Eggs are small and contain a miracidium when passed.
— First larval stage is found in a freshwater snail. The cercariae encyst in freshwater fish. Transmission is by the ingestion of metacercariae.

Echinostomatoidea
— Adults are large and live in the intestine or biliary ducts.
— Testes are large and branched.
— Eggs are large and contain an undeveloped ovum when passed.

— Cercariae encyst on water vegetation. Transmission is by ingesting metacercariae.

Plagiorchioidea
— Adults occur in the lungs and other tissues.
— Testes are arranged side by side behind the ovary.
— Eggs contain a large undeveloped ovum when passed.
— Cercariae encyst in crustacea. Transmission is by ingesting metacercariae.

Note: The characteristics of human schistosomes (non-hermaphroditic flukes) are described in 20:1.

Characteristics of roundworms
■ Non-segmented cylindrical worms that taper at both ends. The adults of some species are very long.
■ Possess a shiny cuticle (skin) which may be smooth, spined, or ridged.
■ Mouth is surrounded by lips or papillae. In some species the mouth opens into a buccal cavity which has cutting organs. The digestive system is a simple tube which ends in an anus.
■ Sexes are separate with the male worms being smaller than the females and usually curved ventrally.
■ In the male there is a testis at the distal end of a long tube which terminates in copulatory organs which may consist (according to species) of one or two projections called spicules, a copulatory bursa, caudal alae, or genital papillae.
■ Female worms possess (according to species) one or two tubular ovaries which lead to a uterus or uteri. The uterus or united uteri open to the exterior through the vulva which is situated anteriorly to the anus.
■ Females are either viviparous (produce larvae) or oviparous (lay eggs). The discharged eggs may hatch directly into infective larvae or may require special conditions in which to hatch and up to three developmental stages before becoming infective larvae. Each stage involves a shedding of the old cuticle, a process known as moulting.
■ Nematodes which infect humans live in the tissues or intestinal tract. Tissue nematodes are transmitted mainly by insect vectors. Most of the medically important intestinal nematodes are soil transmitted (i.e. spread by faecal pollution of the soil).

The intestinal nematodes of major medical importance belong to the following superfamilies:

☐ Ascaridoidea	*Ascaris lumbricoides*
☐ Oxyuroidea	*Enterobius vermicularis*
☐ Rhabditoidea	*Strongyloides stercoralis*
☐ Trichinelloidea	*Trichuris trichiura*
☐ Ancylostomatoidea	*Ancylostoma duodenale* *Necator americanus*

The characteristic features of each superfamily are as follows:

Ascaridoidea
— Large worms which live in the lumen of the gut.
— Mouth has three lips and the oesophagus is muscular and without a posterior bulb.
— Male has two spicules and the tail is curved ventrally.

Oxyuroidea
— Small thread-like worms that live in the colon and rectum.
— Oesophagus has a posterior bulb.
— Male has one or two copulatory spicules.

Rhabditoidea (Rhabdiasoidea)
— Very small worms that commonly live in the small intestine.
— Alternation of parasitic and free-living generations.

Trichinelloidea (Trichuroidea)
— Small worms with the anterior end narrower than the rest of the body.
— Oesophagus is a narrow non-muscular tube without a posterior bulb.
— One ovary in the female.

Ancylostomatoidea
— Small worms that live in the small intestine. Anterior end is hooked.
— Mouth of hookworms leads in to a well-developed buccal cavity, which depending on species, contains cutting plates or tooth-like plates. A hookworm sucks blood from its host.
— Bursa (expansion of cuticle at the end of the body) surrounds the cloaca of the male.
— Eggs are thin shelled and hatch larvae in the soil. Infection with hookworms is by infective larvae penetrating the skin.

The tissue nematodes of major medical importance belong to the following superfamilies:

☐ Filarioidea	*Wuchereria bancrofti* *Brugia malayi* *Brugia timori* *Loa loa* *Onchocerca volvulus*

Chart 12.5 Basic Differentiation of Tapeworms, Flukes and Nematodes

Features	Tapeworms (Cestodes)	Flukes (Trematodes)	Roundworms (Nematodes)
Shape	Tape-like	Leaf-like (except schistosomes) and unsegmented	Cylindrical and unsegmented
Anterior end	Suckers and often hooks on head. No mouth is present	Suckers on body but no hooks. A mouth is present	No suckers or hooks. A mouth is present
Digestive tract	Absent	Present, but no anus	Present with anus
Sexes	Hermaphrodite	Hermaphrodite except *Schistosoma* species	Separate male and female worms

☐ Dracunculoidea   *Dracunculus medinensis*
☐ Trichinelloidea   *Trichinella spiralis*

The characteristic features of these superfamilies are as follows:

Dracunculoidea
— Female worm is very long.
— Female is viviparous (producing larvae) with the larvae escaping from the ruptured uterus.
— Cyclops is the intermediate host.

Filarioidea
— Worms are long and slender. The tail of the male is coiled and bears papillae.
— Adults live in the lymphatic system, serous cavities, or connective tissues.
— Female is viviparous and the larvae which circulate in the blood or are found in the skin are called microfilariae.
— An insect is the intermediate host.

Note: The features of Trichinelloidea have been described previously under the intestinal nematodes.

12.5 QUALITY ASSURANCE IN PARASITOLOGY

Quality assurance is essential if consistently reliable results are to be obtained from parasitological investigations. Incorrect laboratory results can lead to misdiagnosis with incorrect or delayed treatment of patients. Unnecessary expense is incurred when tests are not performed well, drugs are wasted, or further investigations are performed to establish a diagnosis.

Quality assurance is the overall term used to describe the steps and procedures which need to be taken to ensure the reliability of results. It includes control of the collection and transport of specimens, and the control measures taken in the laboratory to ensure the reliable performance of tests and the correct reporting of results. As indicated in this subunit, the control of parasitological investigations requires very little expenditure. It mainly involves being aware of the areas which require control, the introduction of regular checks, and a responsible and careful way of work.

The following need to be controlled:

■ Collection and transport of specimens.
■ Use of equipment, especially a microscope.
■ Quality of reagents and stains.
■ Performance of techniques.
■ Detection and recognition of parasites.
■ Reporting and recording of results.

For all of these areas of control, adequate *written* instructions should be prepared and reviewed at regular intervals.

Collection and transport of parasitological specimens
Control of the following is important:

● Make sure specimen containers are leak-proof, clean, dry, and free from traces of disinfectant.

If an anticoagulated blood specimen is required, use a suitable anticoagulant, e.g. acid citrate dextrose (ACD) or sodium citrate for microfilariae (see 22:6) and EDTA for malaria parasites and trypanosomes. Mix the blood well but gently with the anticoagulant.

- Where applicable, collect specimens at the correct time, e.g. blood should be collected around midnight to detect nocturnally periodic microfilariae.

- Make sure the correct type of specimen is collected. Ensure that the container is labelled correctly with the date and the patient's name and number and where applicable, with the time of collection. A correctly completed request form must accompany the specimen.

  When received in the laboratory, check that the details on the form match those on the specimen.

- After collection, advise ward staff to protect specimens adequately, e.g. protect blood films from dust, flies, and ants. In high humidity climates, an incubator or fan may need to be used to dry thick blood films to prevent distortion of the parasites which can occur when films are left to dry slowly.

  Specimens need to be transported to the laboratory in a suitable container (which can be disinfected after use).

- Ensure all specimens arrive in the laboratory as soon after they are collected as is feasible.

  Some specimens need to be taken to the laboratory for examination *immediately*, e.g. a dysenteric faecal specimen or a rectal scrape for the detection of *E. histolytica* amoebae, cerebrospinal specimen for *T. b. gambiense* or *T. b. rhodesiense* trypomastigotes, or a discharge for *T. vaginalis* flagellates.

  In general, all other specimens for parasitological investigation should reach the laboratory within 1 hour of collection to avoid loss or distortion of parasites or the continued development of parasites to a stage which makes them more difficult to detect or identify e.g. if urine is left to stand for a prolonged time, *S. haematobium* eggs will hatch a miracidium. If EDTA blood is not examined within 2 hours of collection, malaria parasites (and also blood cells) will appear distorted and difficult to identify and trypanosomes will become immobile and lyze.

  When faecal specimens need to be sent to a referral laboratory for examination, a suitable fixative should be used to preserve the morphology of the parasites (see 13:9). The preservation of schistosome eggs in urine is also described in 13:9.

Use of equipment

Microscope

The most important piece of equipment which must be used correctly in parasitology work is a microscope. It is also an expensive instrument and therefore requires to be used with care.

The following are important points:

- Use an appropriate intensity of light. Less light is needed when using a low power objective than when using a high power objective. Less light is needed when using a monocular microscope than when using a binocular instrument. If needing to use daylight, direct the mirror at an outside white covered or painted board, *never* directly at the sun.

- Focus and centre the condenser (see 4:5).

- Obtain the best possible contrast by *adjusting the condenser iris*, especially when examining unstained preparations, e.g. wet faecal specimens, urine, cerebrospinal fluid, or discharges. Not closing the condenser iris sufficiently especially when using a 10× objective is one of the main ways in which unstained parasites are missed or identified incorrectly.

- When examining specimens, use the fine focusing knob to focus continuously. This is particularly important when examining unstained faecal and other suspensions and thick blood films.

- Always begin examining a specimen with a low power objective to detect parasites quickly or to scan a preparation to find areas of the correct thickness or staining to examine with a higher power objective. For example when examining blood films for malaria parasites, spread a small drop of oil over an area of the specimen and examine first with the 40× objective before using the 100× oil immersion objective (adding a further drop of oil if required). This will not only indicate the best area of the film to examine but will also help to detect larger parasites such as trypanosomes or microfilariae (examination with the 10× objective should also be made if filariasis is suspected), and give an indication of the type and number of white cells and red cell morphology.

- Use a calibrated eyepiece scale to measure parasitic cysts. The equipment needed to calibrate the scale for each objective and the technique of calibration are described in 4:11.

- Clean regularly the upper lens of the eyepiece, lower lens of the objectives, upper lens of the condenser, and mirror (if used). Follow the other instructions given by the manufacturer for maintaining the microscope in good condition. In high humidity climates, take adequate precautions to avoid the growth of fungi on the lenses.

Centrifuge

The force at which a specimen is centrifuged and the length of time of centrifugation are important when sedimenting parasites, e.g. when performing the formol ether concentration technique to sediment faecal parasites. If incorrectly centrifuged, the faecal debris may also be sedimented with the parasites.

Centrifuging at too great a force can destroy trypanosomes or cause the loss of sheath from pathogenic microfilaria species.

The centrifugal forces of a centrifuge will be given in the manufacturers' operations' manual.

Note: Guidelines regarding the correct and safe use of a centrifuge are given in 3:8.

Slides and coverglasses

Make sure slides and cover glasses are completely clean. After use, soak slides and cover glasses in separate containers (in a suitable disinfectant) to avoid damaging the fragile cover glasses.

Quality of reagents and stains

The following are the main stains and reagents which require checking:

Physiological saline

This is used mainly to make wet faecal preparations.

- Make up the reagent using distilled water, deionised water, or boiled filtered water and the correct amount of sodium chloride.
- Dispense the saline preferably from a small dropper bottle (which can be closed when not in use) to avoid contaminating the reagent.
- Check regularly for contamination (particularly for flagellates or ciliates) by examining a drop of the reagent on a slide using the 10× and 40× objective with condenser iris closed to give good contrast.

Dobell's iodine

This is used mainly to identify cysts in faecal preparations.

- Keep the reagent preferably in a dark brown dropper bottle or if this is not possible, cover the outside of the container with light opaque paper or tinfoil.
- Check the performance of the reagent by using it to stain the nuclei of *E. coli* cysts and the glycogen inclusions of *I. buetschlii* cysts.

Methanol (methyl alcohol)

Absolute methanol is required as a fixative for thin blood films and as a constituent of Giemsa and other alcohol-based Romanowsky stains.

- Use a good quality methanol. Technical grade methanol (lower priced) is suitable for making 70% v/v alcohol and acid alcohol, etc., but it contains traces of water and is therefore unsuitable as a fixative for blood films or for making Romanowsky stains.
- Avoid moisture from the atmosphere entering the methanol. Make sure the cap of the bottle is tight and transfer a small quantity from the stock bottle to another *dry* bottle for routine use.

Buffered reagents

Buffered water and buffered saline are used in parasitological techniques.

- Prepare the buffer correctly, weighing carefully the dry chemicals.
- Check that the pH of the buffer is correct.
- Store stock bottles of the buffer at 2-8 °C in tightly stoppered (preferably plastic) bottles. Check for contamination at regular intervals.

Giemsa stain

This is used mainly for staining malaria parasites, trypanosomes, leishmanial parasites and microfilariae.

- Use a reliable and if possible a ready-made standardized stain (e.g. BDH/Merck).
- Store the stain in a dark bottle and take precautions to avoid moisture entering the stain (see previous text).
- Check the quality of all new batches of Giemsa (especially if not using a ready-made stain) by using it to stain malaria parasites. If available, use a species that shows Schuffner's dots (*P. vivax* or *P. ovale*). Thick and thin blood films for control purposes can be prepared from fresh blood, dried, folded individually in paper, sealed in a plastic bag, and stored at −20 °C.

Note: If using stabilized Leishman stain, control this in the same way as described for Giemsa stain.

Field's stain

This is used for staining malaria parasites and is also useful (rapid *thin* film technique) for staining leishmanial parasites, trypanosomes, microfilariae, and *Giardia* flagellates.

- Prepare the staining solutions A and B using hot distilled water or heated boiled filtered water (at 70-100 °C). Filter the stains.
- Check the quality of the solutions by staining

thick films containing locally found species of malaria parasites (see under *Giemsa stain* for the preparation and storing of control films).

Note: Although Field's stains A and B are stable and the same staining solutions can be used many times (with regular filtering) for staining thick films (dip technique), to promote standardization and for safety reasons, it is better to change the stains frequently (see also 15:6).

Other reagents and stains

All other reagents and stains used to prepare parasitological specimens should be checked adequately for their performance and if applicable for contamination. They should be stored correctly.

Performance of a technique

Quality control of parasitological techniques includes:

- Preparing written instructions for all techniques and ensuring that these are followed by all members of staff.

- Standardizing as far as possible the amount of specimen used in films and suspensions, e.g. using a simple plastic bulb pipette and template for making thick blood films (see 15:6).

- Making faecal preparations of the correct density so that small parasites are not missed. Adequate mixing of the faeces in saline or iodine is also important.

- Standardizing the concentrations of working stains and staining times (may need to change for different batches of stain).

- Wiping the backs of slides after staining to remove particles of stain.

- Using correct speeds and times for centrifuging.

- Organizing the work of the laboratory so that parasitological specimens can be examined and reported with as little delay as possible, particularly blood films for the detection of malaria parasites and trypanosomes. All members of staff should be aware of the need to examine certain specimens immediately they are received (see text under *Collection and transport of specimens*).

Detection and recognition of parasites

This area of control is important. It should include:

- Adequate training of all members of staff and supervision of the work of newly qualified staff.

- Checking that specimens are being examined for a sufficient length of time, e.g. malaria thick films, especially in areas where *P. malariae*

occurs (parasitaemia is always low with this species).

Following the examination of a fresh faecal preparation with the 10× objective, a check should always be made with the 40× objective to avoid missing *G. lamblia* flagellates or other small parasites.

Skin snips for the detection of *O. volvulus* microfilariae should be left for sufficient time as explained in 22:7.

- Displaying charts and artwork which show the identifying features of parasites, e.g. microfilariae, malaria parasites, and faecal cysts, eggs, and flagellates.

- As mentioned under *Use of equipment*, making sure that the light, contrast, and magnification are correct when examining specimens microscopically and that the specimen is focused continuously.

- Preserving the less commonly seen faecal parasites as permanent microscopical preparations (formolised preparations sealed with nail varnish) or as suspensions of faeces preserved in Beyer's solution or formol saline (see 13:9).

Stained blood films showing malaria parasites, trypanosomes, and microfilariae can be mounted in DPX or a similar medium and kept for teaching purposes.

- Where there is doubt as to the identification of a parasite, further investigations should be carried out and if necessary a specimen should be sent to a Reference Laboratory for examination.

If cysts having the morphology of *E. histolytica* are seen, they should be measured to make sure they are not *E. hartmanni* (see 14:2).

A faecal specimen in which flagellates thought to be *G. lamblia* are found, should be stained by the rapid thin film Field's technique or other technique to confirm that the parasites are *G. lamblia* (see 14:4).

- Knowing which parasites are found only intermittently in specimens or in small numbers, e.g. trypanosomes, *G. lamblia* cysts, eggs of *Taenia* or *Schistosoma* species. Several specimens may need to be examined and, or, concentration techniques used.

- Participating in an external quality assessment scheme in which parasitological specimens are received from a Reference Laboratory and the laboratory staff examines them and reports back to the Reference Laboratory. This is one of the best ways of ensuring that parasites are being recognized correctly. Regional Laboratories should therefore consider operating such a scheme to assist peripheral laboratory workers.

External quality assessment scheme

Information about how to set up and run an external quality assessment scheme aimed at improving the reliability of parasitological results, can be obtained from Mr Anthony H. Moody, Chief MLSO, Laboratory, Hospital for Tropical Diseases, 4 St Pancras Way, London NW1 0PE, United Kingdom.

Reporting and recording of results

This area of quality assurance should include:

- Standardizing the reporting of microscopical preparations. An indication of the concentration of parasites should be given, e.g. for malaria parasites and for eggs in faeces.

- Writing reports clearly and neatly on forms which can be inserted in the patient's notes (see 1:6). Laboratory results should not be 'charted' by nursing staff.

- Ensuring that any abbreviations that are used are understood by those receiving the reports.

- Checking of reports by a senior member of staff before they are issued.

- Keeping a written record of the results of all parasitological investigations undertaken in the laboratory.

Recommended Reading

For the parasitology section, the following books are recommended for further information:

Bell, D. R. *Lecture Notes on Tropical Medicine*, 2nd Ed., Blackwell Scientific Publications, 1985 (£9.80).

Lucas, A. O., Gilles, H. M. *A Short Textbook of Preventive Medicine for the Tropics*, 2nd Ed, Hodder and Stoughton, 1984, (ELBS £3.95).

Knight, R. *Parasitic Disease in Man*, Churchill Livingston, Longman Group, 1982 (ELBS £4.50).

Parry, E. H. O. (Editor). *Principles of Medicine in Africa*, Oxford University Press, 2nd Ed, 1984 (ELBS £15.00).

Melvin, D. M., Brooke, M. M. *Laboratory Procedures for the Diagnosis of Intestinal Parasites*, 3rd Ed., US Dept of Health and Human Services, HHS Publication No (CDC) 82-8282, 1982, (US$ 13.00).

Crewe, W., Haddock, D. R. W. *Parasites and Human Disease*, Edward Arnold, 1985, (£22.50)

Peters, W., Gilles, H. M. *A Colour Atlas of Tropical Medicine and Parasitology*, Wolfe Medical, 2nd Ed, 1981, (ELBS £10.00).

WORLD HEALTH ORGANIZATION PUBLICATIONS

Technical Report Series

No 666 *Intestinal protozoan and helminth infections*, 1981.

No 680 *Malaria control and national health goals*, 1982.

No 701 *The leishmaniases*, 1984.

No 702 *Lymphatic filariasis*, 1984.

No 712 *Malaria control as part of primary health care*, 1984.

No 711 *Advances in malaria chemotherapy*, 1984.

No 728 *The control of schistosomiasis*, 1985.

No 735 *WHO Expert Committee on Malaria*, 1986.

No 739 *Epidemiology and control of African trypanosomiasis*, 1986.

Bench Aids for the Diagnosis of Malaria, Set 1, 1984, and Set 2, 1985, (Sw fr. 10 each set).

Special Programme for Research and Training in Tropical Diseases

Tropical Disease Research, Seventh Programme Report, 1 January 1983 - 31 December 1984, UNDP/World Bank/WHO, 1985 (free publication).

Venture for Health, UNDP/World Bank/WHO, 1984 (free publication).

Tropical Diseases Bulletin

This Journal gives abstracts of current papers and books concerning tropical medicine. It is published monthly, Further information can be obtained by writing to the Administrator, Bureau of Hygiene and Tropical Diseases, Keppel Street, London WC1E 7HT, United Kingdom.

13

Techniques used to Identify Parasites

13:1 SPECIMENS IN WHICH PARASITES ARE FOUND

The following are the main ways in which parasitic infections are diagnosed in the laboratory:

- By microscopical examination.
  The majority of intestinal, urinary, and blood parasites can be detected microscopically in unstained or stained preparations, either directly or following concentration.

- By cultural techniques.
  Only a minority of parasitic infections are diagnosed routinely by cultural techniques.

- By immunodiagnosis.
  With the development of reagents which are both more sensitive and specific, immunodiagnostic techniques are becoming increasingly used in diagnosis and in studies involving the epidemiology and control of parasitic diseases. Recent developments are discussed in 13:17.

Specimens in which parasites can be found and the form of the parasite which is normally found are listed in Table 13.1.

The examination of repeated specimens may be necessary to detect a parasite because an organism may be found in a specimen on one occasion and not on another, e.g. *Trypanosoma* species. Some intestinal parasites are excreted intermittently in faeces such the cysts of *E. histolytica* or *G. lamblia*, or the eggs of some helminths.

Table 13.1 Specimens in which Parasites are Found

Specimen	Parasite	Form
FAECES	*E. histolytica*	cyst, amoeba
	G. lamblia	cyst, flagellate
	T. hominis	flagellate
	B. coli	cyst, ciliate
	I. belli	oocyst
	Cryptosporidium	oocyst
	T. solium	egg, segment
	T. saginata	egg, segment
	H. nana	egg
	D. latum	egg[a]
	D. caninum	egg capsule[a]
	O. sinensis	egg
	O. felineus	egg
	H. heterophyes	egg
	M. yokogawai	egg
	F. hepatica	egg
	F. gigantica	egg
	F. buski	egg[b]
	Dicrocoelium	egg
	G. hominis	egg
	Schistosoma spp	egg
	A. lumbricoides	egg, worm
	E. vermicularis	worm[c]
	S. stercoralis	larva
	T. trichiura	egg
	A. duodenale	egg
	N. americanus	egg
	Trichostrongylus	egg
	Capillaria spp	egg
	Paragonimus spp	egg
BLOOD	*Plasmodium* spp	trophozoite, schizont[d], gametocyte
	Trypanosoma spp	trypoma-stigote
	W. bancrofti	microfilaria
	B. malayi	microfilaria
	L. loa	microfilaria
	Mansonella spp	microfilaria
URINE	*S. haematobium*	egg
	S. mansoni[e]	
	T. vaginalis	flagellate[e]
	W. bancrofti	microfilaria[c]
	O. volvulus	microfilaria[e]
SPUTUM	*Paragonimus* spp	egg[f]
CEREBROSPINAL FLUID	*Trypanosoma* spp	trypoma-stigote
	Naegleria	amoeba
BONE MARROW	*L. donovani*	amastigote
	T. gondii	toxoplasm
LYMPH GLAND ASPIRATE	*Trypanosoma* spp	trypoma-stigote
	L. donovani	amastigote
	T. gondii	toxoplasm
LIVER ASPIRATE	*E. histolytica*	amoeba
	L. donovani	amastigote
	T. gondii	toxoplasm
SPLEEN ASPIRATE	*L. donovani*	amastigote
	T. gondii	toxoplasm

SKIN	*Leishmania* spp	amastigote
	O. volvulus	microfilaria
	D. medinensis	larva in ulcer fluid
	E. vermicularis	egg on perianal skin
MUSCLE	*Trichinella*	larva
RECTAL SCRAPING	*E. histolytica*	amoeba
	Schistosoma spp	egg
DUODENAL ASPIRATE	*G. lamblia*	flagellate
	O. sinensis	egg
	F. hepatica	egg
	S. stercoralis	larva

Notes

a Sometimes segments are found in faeces.
b Occasionally flukes are found in faeces.
c Sometimes the egg is seen in faeces.
d Schizonts of *P. falciparum* are rarely seen in blood films.
e Not often found in urine.
f Occasionally flukes are found in sputum.

13:2 DIRECT EXAMINATION OF FAECAL SPECIMENS

Faeces, like other specimens received in the laboratory, must be handled with care to avoid acquiring infection. Faecal specimens may contain:

— the infective forms of parasites such as *S. stercoralis*, *G. lamblia*, *E. histolytica*, and *Cryptosporidium*.
— infectious bacteria such as shigellae or salmonellae.
— infectious viruses such as hepatitis viruses or rotaviruses.

Specimen: Faeces should be examined within a few hours of being passed. If amoebic dysentery is suspected, the specimen should be examined as soon as possible and kept in a warm environment (35-37 °C) until it is examined.

If needing to refer a specimen to a specialist laboratory, a suitable fixative should be used to preserve the parasites during transport (see 13:9).

Direct microscopical examination of faeces for parasites

1. Report the appearance of the specimen, mentioning:

— colour,
— consistency, i.e. whether it is formed, semiformed, unformed, or fluid,
— whether it contains blood, mucus, pus,
— whether it contains worms, e.g. *A. lumbricoides* (roundworm), *E. vermicularis* (threadworm) or tapeworm segments, e.g. *Taenia* species.

Blood and mucus in specimens
Blood and mucus may be found in faeces from patients with amoebic dysentery, intestinal schistosomiasis, invasive balantidiasis (rare infection), and in severe *T. trichiura* infections. Other conditions in which blood and mucus may be found include bacillary dysentery, *Campylobacter* enteritis, ulcerative colitis, intestinal tumour, and haemorrhoids.

Pus in specimens
This can be found when there is inflammation of the intestinal tract.

Pale coloured frothy specimens (containing fat)
Such specimens may be found in giardiasis and other conditions associated with malabsorption.

Note: Other appearances of faeces are described on p. 138 in Volume II of the Manual.

2. Place a drop of fresh physiological saline (Reagent No. 58) on one end of a slide and a drop of eosin stain (Reagent No. 33) on the other end. Using a wire loop or piece of stick, mix a small amount of specimen (about 2 mg, i.e. match stick head size) in the saline and a small amount in the eosin. Make smooth *thin* preparations.

Cover each preparation with a cover glass.

Note: When sampling, include material from the inside as well as from the surface of the faeces. If the specimen is mainly blood and mucus, do not mix it with saline but transfer a small amount to a slide and cover directly with a cover glass (press on the cover glass with a tissue to make a thin preparation).

Use of saline and eosin
In a saline preparation, motile parasites such as amoebae, flagellates, larvae, and ciliates can be detected and identified. Helminth eggs can be readily identified. Cysts can also be detected but they are much more easily seen against the pink-red background of the eosin preparation (must be thin). Amoebae (motile) are also easier to detect in an eosin preparation (see colour Plates 1, and 7a). The eosin does not stain the living amoebae or the cysts.

Note: Some workers prefer to use Dobell's iodine instead of eosin. Iodine should be used to confirm the identity of cysts (see later text) but it is not as good as eosin in the initial detection of cysts.

3. Examine systematically the entire saline preparation using the 10× objective with the condenser iris *closed sufficiently* to give good contrast.

Use the 40× objective to identify small parasites (always check several microscope fields with this objective before reporting a specimen as 'No parasites found').

If no cysts are seen in the saline preparation, examine the eosin preparation.

Use Dobell's iodine (Reagent No. 31) to confirm the identity of cysts. The iodine can be run under the cover glass of the saline preparation or a separate iodine preparation can be made using the method described in step 2.

Use of Dobell's iodine
Dobell's iodine stains the nuclei and glycogen inclusions of cysts. It does not stain chromatoid bodies.

Identification of cysts
In unstained preparations, cysts can be detected because they are refractile bodies, i.e. they shine brightly when focused. The identification of *E. histolytica* cysts and their differentiation from the nonpathogenic cysts which can be found in faeces are described in 14:2. The identification of *G. lamblia* cysts is described in 14:4.

Identification of flagellates
The flagellate of *G. lamblia* and its differentiation from the nonpathogenic flagellates which can be found in faeces are described in 14:4.

Identification of ciliates
B. coli is the only pathogenic ciliate which can be found in human faeces (it is a rare parasite). It is described in 14:6.

Identification of larvae
The identification of *Strongyloides* larvae in faeces is described in 21:4.

Identification of eggs
The common helminth eggs which can be found in faeces are shown in Plate 13.1. Below each illustration can be found the reference number of the text which lists the identifying features of the egg. The common helminth eggs are also shown in colour Plates 14-26.

4. Count the number of each type of parasite found in the entire preparation and report each as follows:

Scanty .... 1-3 per preparation
Few .... 4-10 per preparation
Moderate number ..... 11-20 per preparation
Many .... 21-40 per preparation
Very many .... over 40 per preparation

Report pus cells, red cells, fat globules and Charcot Leyden crystals (see Plate 13.2) as many, moderate number, or few per high power field (40× objective).

Note: Large numbers of pus cells can be found in bacillary dysentery, *Campylobacter* enteritis, and other conditions causing inflammation of the intestinal tract. They can be easily identified in a methylene blue preparation (see colour Plate 9). Large numbers of fat globules may be seen in malabsorption conditions. Charcot Leyden crystals may be found with intestinal coccidiosis, paragonimiasis and sometimes with amoebic dysentery, hookworm infection and other parasitic infections.

Normal structures found in faeces
Care must be taken not to report as parasites those structures which can be normally found in faeces such as muscle fibres, vegetable fibres, starch cells (stain blue-black with iodine), pollen grains, fatty acid crystals, soaps, spores, yeasts, and hairs (see Plate 13.2).

The yeast *Blastocystis hominis* can be confused with parasitic cysts but when stained with iodine it can be easily differentiated as shown on p. 181-183

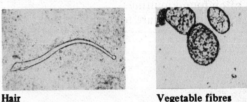

Hair   **Vegetable fibres**

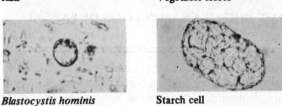

Blastocystis hominis   **Starch cell**

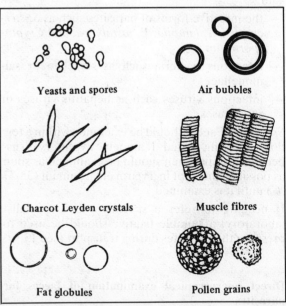

Yeasts and spores   **Air bubbles**

Charcot Leyden crystals   **Muscle fibres**

Fat globules   **Pollen grains**

Plate 13.2 Structures which may be found in faeces and can be confused with parasites.

μm

90

60

30

0

a b c d e f g h i j k l

μm

150

120

90

60

30

0

m n o p q r s t

a	*M. yokogawai*	f	*H. nana*	k	*D. latum*	p	*S. japonicum*
b	*H. heterophyes*	g	*E. vermicularis*	l	*H. diminuta*	q	*S. haematobium*
c	*O. felineus*	h	*T. trichiura*	m	*P. westermani*	r	*S. mansoni*
d	*C. sinensis*	i	*A. lumbricoides*	n	*Trichostrongylus*	s	*F. hepatica*
e	*Taenia*	j	Hookworm	o	*A. lumbricoides*, infertile	t	*F. buski*

Relative sizes of helminth eggs that can be found in faeces

PLATES OF HELMINTH EGGS

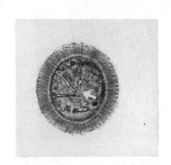

Taenia
See 18:2

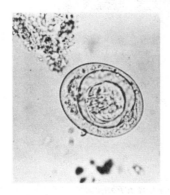

Hymenolepis nana
See 18:4

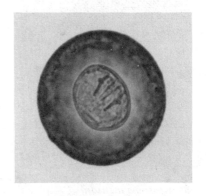

Hymenolepis diminuta
See 18:4

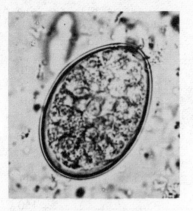

Diphyllobothrium latum
See 18:6

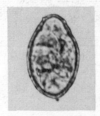

Opisthorchis sinensis
See 19:2

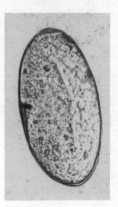

Fasciolopsis buski
See 19:3

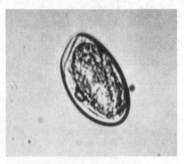

Paragonimus westermani
See 19:5
(More often found in sputum)

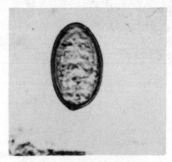

Metagonimus yokogawai
See 19:6

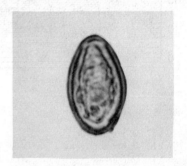

Heterophyes heterophyes
See 19:6

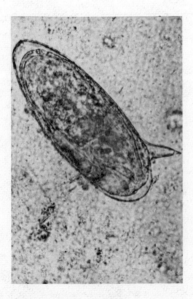

Schistosoma mansoni
See 20:3

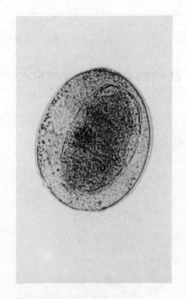

Schistosoma japonicum
See 20:4

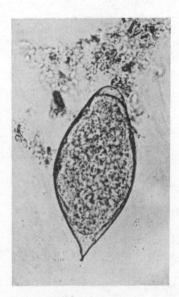

Schistosoma haematobium
See 20:2
(More often found in urine)

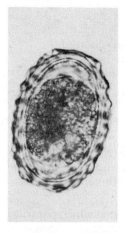

Fertilized *Ascaris*
lumbricoides. See 21:2

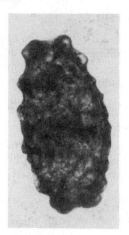

Unfertilized *Ascaris*
lumbricoides. See 21:2

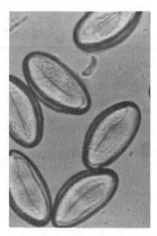

Enterobius vermicularis
See 21:3
(More often recovered from
perianal skin)

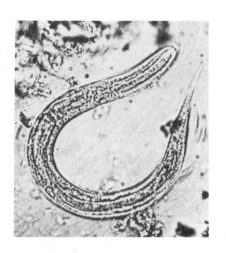

Strongyloides stercoralis
larva. See 21:4

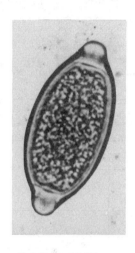

Trichuris trichiura
See 21:5

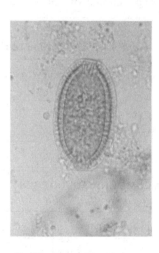

Capillaria
See 21:6

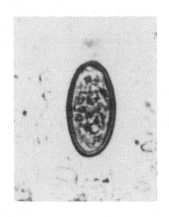

Dicrocoelium
See 19:6

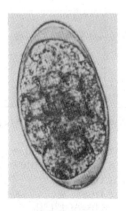

Trichostrongylus
See 21:8

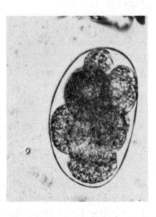

Hookworm
See 21:7

13:3 CONCENTRATION TECHNIQUES FOR FAECAL PARASITES

Concentration methods to detect parasites in faeces may be necessary for the following reasons:

- To detect parasites when they are not found in a direct examination but the symptoms of intestinal parasitic infection continue.
- To detect the eggs of parasites which are often few in number such as those of *Schistosoma* or *Taenia* species.
- To check whether treatment has been successful.
- To investigate the prevalence and incidence of parasitic infection as part of an epidemiological survey.

Choice of faecal concentration technique
The choice of concentration technique depends on:

- the species of parasite,
- the degree of concentration required,
- the number of specimens to be examined,
- the equipment and time available.

The following techniques are described in this Manual:

☐ Formol ether technique in which parasites are sedimentated by centrifugal force. Ether is used to dissolve faecal fat and to separate the faecal matter from the sedimented parasites (see 13:4).

☐ Formol detergent technique in which parasites are sedimentated by gravity using a solution of low specific gravity with detergent added to 'clear' the faecal matter (see 13:5).

☐ Sodium chloride floatation technique in which parasites are floated in saturated sodium chloride (see 13:6).

Table 13.2 Application of Faecal Concentration Techniques

Parasite	Formal Ether [a]	Saturated NaCl	Zinc Sulphate [b]
CYSTS *Giardia lamblia*	●[c]	—	●
Entamoeba histolytica	●	—	●
COMMONLY FOUND EGGS *Ascaris lumbricoides*	●	●[d]	—
Hookworm	●	●[e]	—
Trichuris trichiura	●	—	●[f]
Schistosoma species	●	—	—
Taenia species	●	—	—
Fasciola species	●	—	—
Opisthorchis species	●	—	●
LARVAE *Strongyloides stercoralis* [g]	●	—	—

Key: ● = Recommended   NaCl = Sodium chloride

a The formol detergent sedimentation technique is a suitable replacement when a centrifuge is not available.
b A 33% w/v solution with a specific gravity of 1.18 is used.
c The use of formol water instead of formol saline gives the best results.
d Fertile *Ascaris* eggs have a specific gravity of 1.130.
e Hookworm eggs have a specific gravity of 1.085.
f Fertile *T. trichiura* eggs have a specific gravity of 1.150.
g A simple water emergence technique in which the larve remain motile is also recommended (see 21:4).

☐ Zinc sulphate floatation technique in which parasites are floated in 33% w/v zinc sulphate (see 13:6).

The recommended technique for hospital laboratories is the formol ether technique. It is rapid and gives good concentration of parasitic cysts, eggs, and larvae, in fresh or preserved faeces. The formol detergent sedimentation technique is a suitable replacement for the formol ether technique if a centrifuge is not available and results are not required urgently (overnight sedimentation is required).

Floatation techniques are not recommended as routine concentration techniques because they concentrate only a small range of faecal parasites (see Table 13.2).

13:4 FORMOL ETHER CONCENTRATION TECHNIQUE

As shown in Table 13.2 in 13:3, the formol ether technique is recommended as the best overall technique for the concentration of parasites in faeces. A direct preparation of the faeces should also be examined (see 13:2) to detect motile protozoa such as *E. histolytica* amoebae and *G. lamblia* flagellates. The movement of these parasites will not be seen in a formol ether preparation because formalin kills living material. The formalin fixes the parasites and therefore their morphology is preserved.

In the Ridley modified method, faeces are emulsified in a formol water solution, the suspension is strained to remove large faecal particles, ether is added, and the mixed suspension is centrifuged. Cysts, eggs, and larvae (nonmotile) are fixed and sedimented and the faecal debris is separated in a layer between the ether and the formol water. Faecal fat is dissolved in the ether.

The formol ether technique is a suitable method for concentrating parasites in faeces that have been preserved in Beyer's solution, merthiolate iodine formaldehyde (MIF), and other faecal fixatives (see 13:9).

Required
— Formol water, 10% v/v *

    * Prepare by mixing 50ml of strong formaldehyde solution with 450ml of distilled or filtered water.

— Ether (diethyl)

    Use of ethyl acetate
    Diethyl ether is highly flammable and therefore its

replacement by a less flammable chemical such as ethyl acetate in the formol ether technique has been recommended by some workers. While faecal parasites are sedimented effectively when ethyl acetate is used, greater care needs to be taken when discarding the faecal debris layer to prevent remixing with the sediment. A further disadvantage in using ethyl acetate is the formation in some preparations of small bubbles under the cover glass, possibly formed by insoluble particles of ethyl acetate.[1] Compared with diethyl ether, ethyl acetate is more difficult to obtain and it also has an unpleasant smell.

— Sieve (strainer) with small holes, preferably 400-450 μm in size. The small plastic strainer available in most countries is suitable. It can be used many times and does not corrode like metal sieves.

Method
1. Using a rod or stick, emulsify an estimated 1 g of faeces in about 4 ml of 10% formol water contained in a screw-cap bottle or tube.

    Note: Include in the sample of faeces, parts from the surface and centre of the specimen.

2. Add a further 3-4 ml of 10% v/v formol water, cap the bottle, and mix by shaking for about 20 seconds.

3. Sieve the emulsified faeces, collecting the sieved suspension in a beaker.

4. Transfer the suspension to a conical (centrifuge) tube made of strong glass or polypropylene. Add an equal volume of ether, i.e. 3-4 ml.

    Caution: Ether is highly flammable, therefore use well away from an open flame, e.g. flame from the burner of a gas refrigerator, Bunsen burner, or spirit lamp. Ether vapour is anaesthetic, therefore make sure the laboratory is well-ventilated (see also 2:5).

5. Stopper the tube and mix for 1 minute. If using a Vortex mixer, leave the tube unstoppered and mix for about 15 seconds (it is best to use a boiling tube).

    Note: Do not use a rubber stopper in the tube because ether attacks rubber.

6. With a tissue or piece of cloth wrapped round the top of the tube, loosen the stopper (considerable pressure will have built up inside the tube). Centrifuge immediately at 750-1000 g (approx 3000 rpm) for 1 minute.

After centrifuging, the parasites will have sedimented to the bottom of the tube and the faecal debris will have collected in a layer between the ether and formol water as shown in Fig. 13.1.

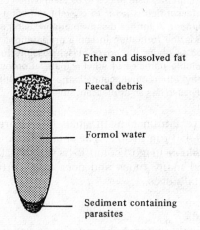

Fig. 13.1 Formol ether concentration technique for parasites, after centrifugation.

7. Using a stick or the stem of a plastic bulb pipette, loosen the layer of faecal debris from the side of the tube and rapidly *invert* the tube to discard the ether, faecal debris, and formol water. The sediment will remain.

8. Return the tube to its upright position and allow the fluid from the side of the tube to drain to the bottom of the tube.

9. Using a plastic bulb pipette or Pasteur pipette, mix the sediment. Transfer all the sediment to a slide, and cover with a cover glass.

10. Examine microscopically the entire preparation using the 10× objective with the condenser iris closed sufficiently to give good contrast. Use the 40× objective to identify the small cysts and eggs. If cysts are present, run a small drop of iodine under the cover glass to confirm their identity (see 14:2).

    Although the motility of *Strongyloides* larvae will not be seen, the nonmotile larvae can be easily recognized. A direct saline preparation, however, is required to detect *E. histolytica* amoebae and *G. lamblia* flagellates.

11. Count the number of each type of parasite in the entire preparation. This will give the approximate number of each parasite per gram of faeces.

Evergreen Faecal Parasite Concentrator (FPC) Kit
Evergreen Scientific have developed a formol ether acetate technique for concentrating faecal parasites (reagents are not supplied). The conical plastic tubes supplied in the

kit, however, are longer than those which can be accommodated in most swing-out rotor centrifuges. An angle rotor centrifuge is required (see 3:8).

13:5 FORMOL DETERGENT CONCENTRATION TECHNIQUE

The formol detergent technique for concentrating parasites in faeces is recommended when facilities are not available to perform a formol ether technique. The formol detergent technique is simple to perform, safe, and inexpensive. It is suitable for performing under field conditions and is recommended in preference to the Kato technique for the detection and quantification of schistosome eggs in faeces.[2]

In the formol detergent technique, a measured amount of faeces is mixed in a formol detergent solution of low specific gravity. After sieving the suspension, it is left undisturbed for the cysts, eggs, and larvae (nonmotile) to sediment under their own weight. This takes only 1 hour for heavy schistosome eggs and overnight for lighter eggs and cysts to sediment. While the parasites are sedimenting, the detergent 'clears' the faecal debris leaving only a fine precipitate through which cysts, eggs, and larvae can be seen and counted.

Required
— Formol detergent solution   Reagent No. 38
— Universal container with a conical base and measuring spoon (Sterilin type)
— Sieve (strainer) with small holes, preferably 400-450 μm in size. The small plastic strainer available in most countries is suitable.

Faecal formol detergent kit
A kit containing all the equipment (reusable) required to carry out the formol detergent concentration technique, is available to developing countries from Tropical Health Technology (see Appendix IV, Faecal formol detergent Schisto kit).

Method
1. Dispense about 10 ml of formol detergent solution into the Universal container.

2. Using the spoon attached to the cap of the Universal container, transfer a *level* spoonful of faeces to the container (approx. 335 mg when using a Sterilin spoon), and mix well in the formol detergent reagent to break up the faeces.

Tighten the cap and shake for about 30 seconds.

3. Sieve the emulsified faeces, collecting the sieved suspension in a beaker.

4. Return the sieved suspension to the conical based Universal container.

5. Stand the container upright in a rack for 1 hour (do not centrifuge).

6. Depending on whether schistosome eggs only or all faecal parasites are being concentrated, proceed as follows:

All faecal parasites
— Add a further 10 ml of formol detergent solution (judged by eye) and mix well for a minimum of 30 seconds.
— Leave to sediment overnight.

Schistosome eggs
— Using a plastic bulb pipette or a Pasteur pipette, remove and discard the supernatant fluid, taking care not to disturb the sediment which has formed in the base of the container.
— Add about 10 ml of the formol detergent solution, and mix well for a minimum of 30 seconds.
— Leave to sediment for a further 1 hour (do not centrifuge).

   Note: The schistosome eggs are fixed and will not overclear or become distorted.

7. Using a plastic bulb pipette or Pasteur pipette, remove and discard the supernatant fluid, leaving the fine sediment in the conical base of the container.

8. Transfer all the sediment to a slide and cover with a 40 × 22 mm cover glass or two smaller size cover glasses.

9. Examine microscopically the entire preparation, using the 10× objective with the condenser iris closed sufficiently to give good contrast.

   Use the 40× objective to identify the smaller parasites.

   Count the number of each type of parasite present and multiply by 3 to give the approximate number of each per gram of faeces.

13:6 FLOATATION CONCENTRATION TECHNIQUE

ZINC SULPHATE TECHNIQUE

As shown in Table 13.2 in 13:3, the zinc sulphate technique is recommended for concentrating the cysts of *G. lamblia* and *E. histolytica* and the eggs of *T. trichiura*. Other nematode eggs are concentrated less well while operculated trematode (fluke) eggs are not concentrated because they are ruptured in the zinc sulphate solution. The technique is not suitable for concentrating eggs or cysts in fatty faeces.

A zinc sulphate solution is used which has a specific gravity (relative density) of 1.180-1.200. Faeces are emulsified in the solution and the suspension is left undisturbed for the eggs and cysts to float to the surface where they are collected on a cover glass.

Required
— Zinc sulphate solution   Reagent No. 84
  33% w/v specific gravity
  1.180-1.200

  Use a hydrometer to check that the specific gravity (relative density) of the solution is correct. Adjust with distilled water or more chemical if required.

— Test tube (without a lip) of about 15 ml capacity which has a completely smooth rim.

Method
1. About one quarter fill the tube with the zinc sulphate solution.

2. Add an estimated 0.5 gram of faeces and using a rod or stick, emulsify the specimen in the solution.

3. Fill the tube with the zinc sulphate solution, and mix well.

4. Stand the tube in a completely vertical position in a rack.

5. Using a plastic bulb pipette or Pasteur pipette, add further solution to ensure that the tube is filled to the brim.

6. Carefully place a completely clean (grease-free) cover glass on top of the tube, avoiding trapping any air bubbles.

7. Leave undisturbed for 30-45 minutes to give time for the cysts and eggs to float.

Note: After 60 minutes, the eggs will begin to sink.

8. Carefully lift the cover glass from the tube by a straight pull upwards. Place the cover glass face downwards on a slide.

    The eggs and cysts will be found adhering to the cover glass.

9. Examine microscopically the entire preparation using the 10× objective with the condenser iris closed sufficiently to give good contrast. Use the 40× objective, and run a drop of iodine under the cover glass, to identify the cysts (see 14:2).

10. Count the number of eggs and multiply by 2 to give the approximate number per gram of faeces.

Note: Other floatation techniques are described in which the parasites are recovered from the surface of the fluid after centrifugation (for full details readers are referred to manuals of parasitology).[8]

SATURATED SODIUM CHLORIDE TECHNIQUE

The saturated sodium chloride technique is useful for concentrating hookworm eggs or *Ascaris* eggs, e.g. in field surveys.

The technique is the same as that described for the zinc sulphate floatation technique except that a saturated solution of sodium chloride (specific gravity of 1.200) is used. The eggs can be identified using the 10× objective.

13:7 CELLOPHANE THICK FAECAL SMEAR TECHNIQUE
(Kato)

In the original Kato technique, a cellophane rectangle soaked in glycerol and malachite green was placed on a sample of faeces and the preparation left until the glycerol had cleared sufficiently the faecal material to enable helminth eggs to be seen.[3]

Several modifications of the Kato technique have been developed and are widely used, particularly in schistosomiasis control work. In the modified techniques, the faeces is first passed through a plastic or wire screen to remove large faecal particles and a measured amount (usually 20-50 mg) of faeces is transferred to a slide and covered with a 30 × 22 mm piece of cellophane soaked in 50% v/v glycerol.[4] After clearing of the faeces, the eggs are counted to give a semiquantitative result. While the technique can be easily performed in the field, it is a messy technique and one in which the fingers can become easily contaminated.[2] An easier, safer, and more hygienic method for use in schistosomiasis work is the formol detergent 2 hour technique described in 13:5.

The Kato technique is not suitable for detecting cysts, larvae, or small fluke eggs. Thin-shelled eggs such as hookworm eggs may be easily missed or unrecognizable by being overcleared.

Note: Full details of the modified Kato technique can be found in the paper of Peters *et al.* [4]

13:8 COUNTING OF HELMINTH EGGS

The intensity of an intestinal helminth infection may sometimes be indicated by the concentration of its eggs in faeces. Parasite and host factors need to be considered.[5] Egg counts can be of value in epidemiological surveys.

The approximate number of eggs per gram of faeces can be calculated by using a formol ether technique (see 13:4) or a formol detergent technique (see 13:5). When a more accurate count is required the method of Stoll can be used.

Stoll's technique for counting helminth eggs

1. Weigh 3 g of faeces in a screw-cap container.

2. Add 42 ml of water to give a 1 in 15 dilution of the faeces. If the faeces is a formed specimen, use sodium hydroxide 0.1 mol/l (N/10) solution instead of water.

3. Using a rod, break up the faeces and mix it with the water.

4. Cap the container and shake hard to complete the mixing.

5. Using a graduated plastic bulb pipette, or a Pasteur pipette previously marked to measure the required volume, remove 0.15 ml of the suspension and transfer this to a slide.

6. Cover with a long cover glass if available or with two square cover glasses side by side.

7. Examine systematically the entire preparation, using the 10× objective with the condenser iris reduced to give good contrast. Include in the count any eggs lying outside the edges of the cover glass because these are also contained in the 0.15 ml sample.

8. Multiply the number of eggs counted by 100 to give the number of eggs per gram of faeces.

   Note: If the faeces is not a formed specimen, the following additional calculation is necessary to give the number of eggs per gram of faeces:

   Fluid specimen .... multiply by 5
   Unformed watery specimen .... multiply by 4
   Unformed soft specimen .... multiply by 3
   Semiformed specimen .... multiply by 2

9. Calculate the number of eggs per day, by multiplying the eggs per gram by the total weight of a 24 hour faecal specimen (the approximate weight of the daily faecal output of an inpatient is more easily estimated by the ward staff).

Note: For the interpretation of egg counts, readers are referred to the paper of Hall.[5]

13:9 PRESERVATION OF PARASITIES

Fixatives are required for preserving parasites in faeces when:
— specimens need to be sent to a reference laboratory for identification of a parasite or because microscopical examinations are not available locally.
— specimens are sent from a reference laboratory to peripheral laboratories as part of a parasitology quality assessment programme.
— individual laboratories wish to preserve faecal specimens for teaching purposes.
— specimens are collected in the field, e.g. during an epidemiological survey.

Several fixatives are available for the preservation of cysts and eggs in faeces. Special fixatives are required for preserving (with subsequent staining) the amoebae of *E. histolytica* and the flagellates of *G. lamblia*.

Preservation of cysts and eggs in faeces
If the specimen is to be examined for both cysts and eggs, a fixative which is free from iodine and other stains is preferable because stains are not required for the identification of parasitic eggs. Iodine preparations can be easily prepared from the preserved faeces for the identification of cysts.

A stain-free fixative which is recommended for preserving cysts and eggs in faeces is Beyer's solution.[6] It is a modified formalin solution containing copper chloride, glacial acetic acid, and formalin.

It maintains the morphology of cysts and eggs for long periods and allows the specimen to be examined as a direct preparation (sampling from sediment) or examined after concentration by the formol ether technique.

Fixation using Beyer's solution
1. Prepare a stock solution as described under Reagent No. 15. The stock solution is stable indefinitely at room temperature.
2. Before use, prepare a working solution by diluting the stock solution 1 in 10 (1 ml stock solution and 9 ml distilled or filtered water).
3. Emulsify approximately 1 g of faeces in 7-8 ml of Beyer's working solution. Use a leak-proof screw cap container.

Note: If the ingredients to prepare Beyer's solution are not available, 10% v/v formol saline can be used. This will also preserve cysts and eggs but not as well as Beyer's solution for long periods.

Preservation of amoebae and flagellates in faeces
Specimens containing fixed (non-motile) amoebae and flagellates require staining to identify the parasites. The choice of fixative depends on the staining technique to be used.

If specialist stains are to be used e.g. iron haematoxylin, a suitable fixative is SAF fixative (sodium acetate, acetic acid, formaldehyde).

Fixation using SAF solution
1. Prepare a solution of SAF as described under Reagent No. 62.
2. Emulsify approximately 1 g of faeces in about 10 ml of SAF solution. Use a leak-proof screw cap container.

Note: Another suitable fixative for preserving amoebae and flagellates in faeces is PVA (polyvinyl alcohol) solution. This fixative requires more ingredients, and is more toxic than SAF because it contains mercuric chloride. It is also difficult to prepare. Details of its preparation can be found in manuals of parasitology.[8]

MIF (merthiolate iodine formaldehyde) fixative
This fixative contains iodine and eosin and is therefore both a fixative and a stain. It stains cysts and *E. histolytica* amoebae can usually be recognized in wet preparations. It also stains eggs. Although widely used, it does not give the opportunity to use other stains and as mentioned previously the staining of eggs is not required.

Preservation of schistosome eggs in urine[7]
For teaching purposes and quality assessment

programmes, *S. haematobium* eggs can be preserved in urine by adding 1 ml of 1% v/v domestic bleach solution to every 10 ml of urine. The specimen can be examined after centrifugation (or 1 hour sedimentation by gravity) or by the Nuclepore filtration technique. The bleach also prevents the precipitation of phosphates.

Note: When preserved with bleach, the urine is unsuitable for chemical testing. It cannot therefore be tested for protein or blood.

Preservation of worms

Worms can be preserved in 10% v/v formol saline. Details of techniques used to clear and stain helminths can be found in the CDC Manual, *Laboratory Procedures for the Diagnosis of Intestinal Parasites*[8] and other textbooks of parasitology.

Preparation of permanent mounts of faecal sediments containing cysts and eggs

For the long term preservation of unstained cysts and eggs in mounted preparations, e.g. for teaching purposes, mixing of the specimen with glycerol (glycerine)-alcohol or glycerol and mounting in Permount is recommended.

Method using glycerol-alcohol[6]

1. Transfer a drop of faecal sediment (prepared after formol ether concentration) to a slide.
2. Mix with an equal volume of glycerol-alcohol (Reagent No. 42).
3. Cover with a cover glass.
4. Leave the preparation for several weeks to allow the alcohol and water to evaporate. The preparation can then be sealed using nail vanish.

Method using glycerol and Permount[9]

1. Prepare about 3 ml of faecal sediment containing the parasites (preserved in 10% formol saline or Beyer's solution).
2. Transfer the sediment to a conical tube. Add an equal volume of pure glycerol (glycerine). The glycerol will sink to the bottom of the tube. Leave the tube undisturbed for several days to give time for the parasites to sediment into the glycerol.
3. During the sedimentation period, run more glycerol down the side of the tube to ensure that the glycerol in the bottom of the tube is water-free.
4. After about 1 week, pipette off the supernatant fluid, taking care not to disturb the sediment in the bottom of the tube.

5. Mix the glycerol and sediment together and transfer a drop to a slide. Cover with a cover glass measuring 18 mm in diameter.
6. Apply a drop of *Permount* on top of the cover glass and cover with a square cover glass measuring 22 × 22 mm. Leave the preparation to dry (takes a few weeks to dry completely).

13:10 TRICHROME STAINING TECHNIQUE

The trichrome staining technique is recommended for staining *E. histolytica* amoebae in tissue (e.g. biopsies) and whenever a permanent stained faecal preparation is required to study nuclear detail of *E. histolytica* or other faecal protozoa. It is not recommended as a technique to replace the direct examination of wet faecal preparations because it is expensive, some helminth eggs become distorted and difficult to recognize, and the shrinkage of cysts makes it difficult to differentiate the cysts of *E. histolytica* from those of *E. hartmanni*. The chromatoid bars of *E. histolytica* cysts are more consistently stained using Burrow's stain or an acridine orange fluorescent technique (see 14:2) than by using a trichrome stain.

Caution: Smears to be stained by the trichrome technique require fixation in Schaudinn's fixative which contains the highly toxic chemical mercuric chloride.

Required
— Schaudinn's fixative   Reagent No. 65
— Ethanol iodine solution   Reagent No. 34
— Acidified ethanol solution   Reagent No. 6
— Trichrome stain   Reagent No. 82
— Ethanol, 70% v/v*
— Ethanol, 90% v/v*
— Ethanol, 95% v/v*
— Ethanol, absolute
— Xylene or toluene

*Prepare by diluting absolute ethanol. To make a 70% solution, mix 30 ml of distilled water with 70 ml of absolute ethanol.

To make a 90% solution, mix 10 ml of distilled water with 90 ml of absolute ethanol.

To make a 95% solution, mix 5 ml of distilled water with 95 ml of absolute ethanol.

Note: Keep all the alcohol solutions in screw cap airtight containers.

Method
1. Make a thin smear of the faeces on a slide. If the faeces is a formed specimen, emulsify it first

in physiological saline.

While the smear is still wet, fix it in Schaudinn's fixative for 5 minutes at 50 °C or 1 hour at room temperature (the smear must not be allowed to dry during staining).

2. Immerse the slide in a container of ethanol iodine solution for 2-5 minutes followed by 1 minute rinses in two containers of 70% v/v ethanol.

3. Stain in a container of trichrome stain for 10 minutes.

4. Rinse briefly in the acidified ethanol solution, followed by brief rinses in two containers of 95% v/v ethanol.

5. Immerse the slide in a container of absolute ethanol for 2-5 minutes.

6. Clear the smear by immersing the slide in a container of xylene or toluene for 3 minutes.

7. While still wet, mount the smear in Permount or another suitable mounting medium.

Results
Cytoplasm of amoeba .... Blue-green tinged and cysts   with purple
Nuclear chromatin .... Purple-red
Chromatoid bodies .... Purple-red
Ingested red cells .... Purple-red
Background material .... Pale green

13:11 ACRIDINE ORANGE TECHNIQUE FOR CHROMATOID BODIES IN CYSTS

The fluorochrome acridine orange can be used to demonstrate the blunt ended chromatoid bodies which can be found particularly in the younger cysts of *E. histolytica*. The presence of such chromatoid bodies can help to differentiate *E. histolytica* cysts from other protozoal cysts which can be found in faecal specimens (see 14:2).

The chromatoid bodies are composed of ribonucleic acid (RNA) and fluoresce yellow or yellow-orange (see colour Plate 2d). The method described enables a saline suspension of faeces to be used or a sediment from formol ether concentrated faeces.[10]

Required
Acridine orange stock solution   Reagent No. 8

Working acridine orange solution
Before use, prepare a working solution by mixing:
— 1 ml stock acridine orange solution
— 0.5 ml acetic acid (concentrated)
— 8.5 ml of phosphate buffered saline, pH 6.8-7.2

This provides a working solution of below pH 4 (the actual pH is not critical providing it is below pH 4.5).

Method
1. Add an equal volume of working acridine orange solution to a saline suspension of faeces or sediment from a formol ether concentration technique.

2. Mix and leave for 30 minutes (or longer) at room temperature.

3. Transfer a drop of the specimen to a slide and cover with a cover glass.

4. Examine the preparation by fluorescence microscopy using a dark field condenser, quartz halogen lamp, and a BG12 exciter filter with No. 44 and No. 53 barrier filters. The chromatoid bodies can be detected in the cysts when using the 40× objective.

No fading of the fluorescence occurs for several weeks.

Results
Chromatoid bodies ..... Yellow or yellow orange
Nuclei of cysts .... Green
Cytoplasm of cysts .... Pale green

13:12 BAERMANN'S METHOD FOR CONCENTRATING STRONGYLOIDES LARVAE IN FAECES

Required
— A small strainer
— Simple Baermann's apparatus (see Fig. 13.2)

Preparation of Baermann's apparatus
1. Attach a small piece of rubber or plastic tubing to the stem of a funnel, 6-8 cm in diameter.

2. Attach a short stem Pasteur pipette to the end of the tubing as shown in Fig. 13.2.

3. Close the tubing with a clip.

4. Support the apparatus in a stand.

5. Place a bottle containing a centrifuge tube beneath the tubing, to collect the fluid.

Method
1. Place about 5 g of fresh faeces in the bottom of the strainer.

2. Place the strainer in the funnel (see Fig. 13.2).

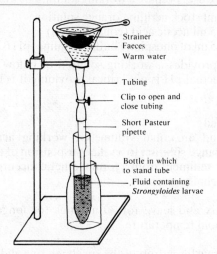

Fig. 13.2   Modified Baermann's apparatus for concentrating *Strongyloides* **larvae in faeces.**

3. Add warm water (about 40 °C) to cover the faeces in the strainer.

4. Leave undisturbed for 1½-2 hours to give time for the *Strongyloides* larvae to emerge from the faeces into the water.

5. Open the clip of the tubing and collect 7-10 ml of the fluid in the centrifuge tube.

6. Centrifuge the fluid at medium speed (about 1000 g) for 5 minutes to sediment the parasites.

7. Using a plastic bulb pipette or a Pasteur pipette, discard the supernatant fluid into a container of disinfectant.

8. Transfer the sediment to a slide and cover with a cover glass. Examine for motile larvae using the 10× objective with the condenser iris closed sufficiently to give good contrast.
Look for motile larvae.

Differentiation between the larvae of Strongyloides and hookworm
If the faecal specimen is more than 24 hours old, care must be taken to differentiate *Strongyloides* larvae from those of hookworm. This can be done as follows:

— Add a drop of Dobell's iodine (Reagent No. 31) to the preparation to kill the larvae.

— Using the 40× objective, examine the mouth-parts of the larvae.

The mouth-part of a *Strongyloides* larva is short, whereas that of a hookworm larva is relatively long (see Plate 21.4 in 21:4).

Note: *Strongyloides* larvae can also be detected in faeces using the simple water emergence technique described in 21:4.

13:13 FAECAL CULTURE TECHNIQUE TO DIFFERENTIATE HOOKWORM SPECIES

If required, the eggs of *Ancylostoma* and *Necator* hookworm can be identified by culturing faeces in distilled water and examining the filariform larvae ten days later.

Method
1. Spread a sample of the faeces on a strip of filter paper measuring 10 × 1.5 cm.

2. Place the inoculated strip in a large test tube containing about 7 ml of distilled water.

3. Seal the tube with cellophane and a rubber band and incubate at room temperature (20-25 °C) for 10 days.

4. After incubation, kill the larvae by submerging the tube to three-quarters of its length in a beaker of water heated to 50 °C for 15 minutes.
Caution: Following incubation, the larvae are directly infective.

5. Using forceps, remove the filter paper from the tube and discard it into a container of disinfectant.

6. Transfer the fluid from the culture tube into a conical (centrifuge) tube and centrifuge the fluid at medium speed (approx. 1000 g) for 2-3 minutes to sediment the larvae.

7. Examine the sediment for sheathed filariform larvae, using the 10× objective with the condenser iris closed sufficiently to give good contrast.
Identify the larvae as follows:

Ancylostoma duodenale filariform larvae
• The head and tail end bluntly.
• There is no gap between the oesophagus and the intestine.
• The oesophagus does not end in a thistle-funnel shape (see Fig. 13.3).

Necator americanus filariform larvae
• The head and tail are pointed.
• There is a gap between the oesophagus and the intestine.

- The oesophagus ends in a thistle-funnel shape (see Fig. 13.3).

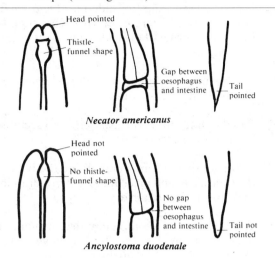

Necator americanus

Ancylostoma duodenale

Fig. 13.3 Differentiating characteristics between hookworm filariform larvae.
Courtesy of Churchill Livingstone Publishers.

Strongyloides filariform larvae
The filariform larvae of *S. stercoralis* may also be present in cultured faeces but they can be distinguished from hookworm larvae by being unsheathed and having a forked tail (not easily seen).

13:14 GIEMSA STAINING TECHNIQUE

Giemsa stain is an alcohol-based Romanowsky stain that requires dilution in buffered water (usually pH 7.1-7.2) or buffered physiological saline before use. Dilution in buffered saline often gives a cleaner background to the preparation.

A 3% v/v dilution of the stain with a staining time of 30 minutes is commonly used but the concentration of the stain can be increased to reduce the staining time, e.g. 10% v/v dilution with a staining time of 10 minutes.

During staining, care must be taken to prevent the fine particles of stain which form on the surface of the diluted stain from being deposited on a preparation. This can be avoided by placing the preparation face down in the stain and washing the stain from the dish at the end of the staining time. Alternatively, slides can be placed in a Coplin jar or in a staining rack in a staining trough (see 3:3), the diluted stain added and after staining the stain washed from the jar or trough.

Parasites which stain well with Giemsa include malaria parasites, trypanosomes, leishmanial parasites, and microfilariae (sheath of *L. loa* stains only with difficulty). Thick films must be thoroughly dry (preferably overnight) before being stained.

Required
— Giemsa stain   Reagent No. 41
— Buffered water, pH 7.1-7.2   Reagent No. 21
   or buffered saline, pH 7.1-7.2 (No. 20)

Method
1. Immediately before use, dilute the Giemsa stain as required:

   3% solution for 30 minute staining
   Measure 50 ml of buffered water (or saline) pH 7.1-7.2. Add 1.5 ml of Giemsa stain and mix gently. The stain can be measured using a graduated plastic bulb pipette or a small volume (2 ml) plastic syringe.

   10% solution for 10 minute staining
   Measure 45 ml of buffered water, pH 7.1-7.2 in a 50 ml cylinder. Add 5 ml of Giemsa stain (to 50 ml mark) and mix gently.

2. Place the slides face downwards in a shallow tray supported on two rods, in a Coplin jar, or in a staining rack for immersion in a staining trough. Thick blood films must be thoroughly dried and thin blood films must be fixed (methanol for 1 minute).

3. Pour the diluted stain into the shallow tray, Coplin jar, or staining trough. Stain as follows:

   30 minutes if using a 3% stain solution
   10 minutes if using a 10% stain solution

4. Wash the stain from the staining container using clean water (need not be distilled or buffered).

   Important: Flushing of the stain from the slides and staining container is necessary to avoid the films being covered with a fine deposit of stain.

5. Wipe the back of each slide clean and place it in a draining rack for the preparation to air-dry.

Results
Malaria parasites (see colour Plates 45-48)
Chromatin of parasite .... Dark red
Cytoplasm of parasite .... Blue
Schuffner's dots .... Red
Maurer's dots (clefts) .... Red-mauve

Trypanosomes (see colour Plate 52)
Nucleus .... Mauve-red
Kinetoplast .... Dark red
Cytoplasm .... Pale mauve
Flagellum .... Pale mauve

Leishmania parasites (see colour Plate 49)
Nucleus .... Mauve-red
Kinetoplast .... Dark mauve-red
Cytoplasm .... Pale mauve

Microfilariae (see colour Plates 32-38, 40)
Nuclei .... Dark purple
Sheath of *W. bancrofti* .... Pink
Sheath of *B. malayi* .... Dark pink
Sheath of *B. timori* .... Pale pink
Sheath of *L. loa* .... Pale grey or unstained

Blood cells
Red cells .... Grey to pale mauve-pink
Reticulocytes .... Grey-blue
Nuclei of neutrophils .... Dark purple
Granules of neutrophils .... Mauve-purple
Granules of eosinophils .... Red
Cytoplasm of mononuclear .... Blue or blue-grey
leucocytes

13:15 FIELD'S THICK FILM TECHNIQUE

Field's stain is a water-based Romanowsky stain. It is composed of two solutions called Field's stain A which contains eosin and phosphate salts and Field's stain B which contains methylene blue, azure I, and phosphate salts. It is pre-buffered to the correct pH and neither solution requires dilution.

Field's stain is stable and has the advantage that it is isotonic with malaria parasites and trypanosomes, penetrates rapidly unfixed parasites, and is particularly suitable for staining freshly made thick films. It is not suitable for staining microfilariae in thick films.

In the thick blood film staining technique the red cells are lyzed during the staining. The examination of thick films for malaria parasites is described in 15:6. It is particularly important to select a part of the preparation where the staining balance is correct.

Because thick blood films are not fixed, pathogens are not killed and therefore even after staining, preparations should be handled with care. A different technique is recommended when staining HIGH RISK blood specimens (see later text).

Required
— Container of Field's stain A   Reagent No. 35
— Container of Field's stain B   Reagent No. 36
— Two containers of clean water (need not be buffered or distilled but should be filtered water)

Note: By locating a thick film at one end of a slide, only a small amount of Field's stain A and B is required. While Field's staining solutions are stable stains, it is recommended that the stains should be changed frequently in a routine clinical laboratory to reduce the risk of infection and carry-over of parasites, and also to assist in the standardization of staining.

Method
1. Holding the slide with the *dried* thick film facing downwards, dip the slide into Field's stain A for 5 seconds. Drain off the excess stain by touching a corner of the slide against the side of the container.

2. Wash gently for about 5 seconds in clean water. Drain off the excess water.

3. Dip the slide into Field's stain B for 3 seconds. Drain off the excess stain.

4. Wash gently in clean water. Wipe the back of the slide clean and place it upright in a draining rack for the film to air-dry.

5. When the film is completely dry, examine it microscopically. Use the 40× objective to scan the smear *first* to find an area that is of the correct density and well stained to examine with the 100× objective (see 15:6).

Alternative thick film staining technique for HIGH RISK specimens
Thick blood films which may contain highly infectious pathogens, e.g. haemorrhagic fever viruses, hepatitis viruses, or AIDS virus, should not be stained by the dip technique (unless the solutions are discarded after use). A suitable alternative staining technique is as follows:

1. Holding the slide, apply a large drop of Field's stain A to cover the thick film.

2. Immediately wash off the stain with water. Apply the water to the side of the film or on the back of the slide to prevent loss of the blood. Drain off the excess water.

3. Apply a drop of Field's stain B. Immediately wash off the stain with water.

4. Stand the slide on a piece of absorbent paper to drain, supported against a suitable upright. When the film is dry, wipe the edge of the slide with a piece of absorbent paper soaked in 70% v/v alcohol. Discard this and the drainage piece of paper into hypochlorite disinfectant or bleach solution.

5. Before examining the dried film, mount a cover glass on top of it (immersion oil can be used as the mountant).

Note: Even after staining, a thick unfixed blood film containing parasites and pathogenic viruses remains infectious and must be handled with care.

Results
Malaria parasites (see colour Plates 41-44)
Chromatin of parasite .... Dark red
Cytoplasm of parasite .... Blue-mauve
Schuffner's dots .... Pale red
(often seen around *P. vivax* and *P. ovale* parasites)
Malaria pigment .... Yellow-brown
                                      or brown-black

Blood cells
Nuclei of small lymphocytes .... Dark purple
Nuclei of neutrophils .... Dark purple
Granules of eosinophils .... Red
Cytoplasm of mononuclear .... Blue-grey
leucocytes
Reticulum of reticulocytes .... Blue-grey
stippling in background

Trypanosomes (see colour Plates 54-55)
Nucleus .... Red-mauve
Kinetoplast .... Dark red
Cytoplasm .... Pale mauve
Flagellum .... Pale mauve

13:16 FIELD'S THIN FILM TECHNIQUE

The composition of Field's stain is described in 13:15. In the thin film technique, Field's stain B is diluted 1 in 5 before use.

The technique described in this subunit has been found useful in the rapid staining of malaria parasites in thin blood films, leishmanial parasites in films made from aspirates and skin ulcers, microfilariae in blood (when combined with Delafield's haematoxylin), and the flagellates of *G. lamblia* in faecal smears.[11]

Prior to staining, preparations require fixing in absolute methanol for 1-2 minutes.

Required
— Field's stain A   Reagent No. 35
— Field's stain B, diluted 1 in 5†   Reagent No. 36
— Buffered pH 7.1-7.2 water   Reagent No. 21

†Prepare by mixing 1 ml of Field's stain B with 4 ml of pH 7.2 buffered water. A syringe or graduated plastic bulb pipette can be used to measure the stain and buffered water.

Method
1. Place the slide on a staining rack and cover the methanol-fixed thin film with approximately 0.5 ml of diluted Field's stain B.

2. Add immediately an equal volume of Field's stain A and mix with the diluted Field's stain B. Leave to stain for 1 minute.

   Note: The stains can be easily applied and mixed on the slide by using 1 ml graduated plastic bulb pipettes. These inexpensive plastic pipettes can be used many times (see 2:4).

3. Wash off the stains with clean water.

4. Wipe the back of the slide clean and place it in

a draining rack for the film to air-dry.

Results
Malaria parasites (similar to colour Plates 45-48)
Chromatin of parasite .... Dark red
Cytoplasm of parasite .... Blue
Schuffner's dots .... Red
Maurer's dots (clefts) .... Red-mauve
Malaria pigment in white cells ..... Brown-black
Red cells .... Grey to pale mauve-pink
Reticulocytes .... Grey-blue
Nuclei of neutrophils .... Dark purple
Cytoplasm of mononuclear ... Blue or blue-grey
white cells
Granules of eosinophils .... Red

Trypanosomes (similar to colour Plate 52)
Nucleus .... Mauve-red
Kinetoplast .... Dark red
Cytoplasm .... Pale mauve
Flagellum .... Pale mauve

Leishmania parasites (similar to colour Plate 49)
Nucleus .... Mauve-red
Kinetoplast .... Dark mauve-red
Cytoplasm .... Pale mauve

Flagellates of G. lamblia (see colour Plate 7)
Nuclei .... Dark purple
Cytoplasm .... Pale mauve
Flagella .... Pale mauve

Note: The use of Field's stain with Delafield's haematoxylin for staining microfilariae is described in 22:6.

13:17 IMMUNODIAGNOSIS OF PARASITIC INFECTIONS

Immunodiagnosis is used to assist in the clinical diagnosis of parasitic infections and in the epidemiology and control of parasitic diseases.

Immunodiagnostic techniques are based on the detection of:

■ Antibody in a person's serum, produced in response to a particular parasitic infection. The antibody may persist for a long period in the serum after an infection has ended and therefore antibody tests are unable to distinguish between a past or present infection.

When used to assist in diagnosing parasitic diseases, antibody tests need to be interpreted with care (see later text). A wide range of parasitological antibody tests have been developed which have varying degrees of specificity and sensitivity. For only a few of these are reagents available commercially.

■ Antigen, which is excreted by parasites and can be found in serum, urine, cerebrospinal fluid, faeces, or other specimens.

Antigen tests provide evidence of present infection and are therefore of greater value than antibody tests in the clinical diagnosis of parasitic infections. The development of antigen tests is recent and very few tests are available commercially (see later text).

Immunodiagnosis of parasitic infections

Immunodiagnostic techniques are required when:

— parasites live in the tissues of internal organs and cannot therefore be easily removed for examination.

— parasites can be found in specimens only in certain stages of an infection, e.g. in the acute stage and not in the chronic stage.

— parasites are present only intermittently or in too few numbers to be easily detected in specimens.

— the techniques used to detect parasites are complex or time-consuming.

Those parasitic diseases for which immunodiagnosis is of particular value include:

● South American trypanosomiasis, chronic stage (see 16:3).
● African trypanosomiasis, when parasitaemia is low (see 16:2).
● Visceral leishmaniasis (see 17:2).
● Cutaneous and mucocutaneous leishmaniasis (see 17:4).
● Amoebic liver abscess (see 14:2).
● Toxoplasmosis (see 14:8).
● Hydatid disease (see 18:3).
● Filariasis, occult and chronic infections (see 22:2).
● Trichinellosis (see 22:9).
● Toxocariasis (see 21:8).
● Schistosomiasis, chronic stage (see 20:3).

Interpretation of antibody tests in parasitic infections

As already explained, the detection of antibodies in a person's serum does not indicate whether an active infection is present. In only a few parasitic infections can the demonstration of Ig M antibody help to indicate whether an infection is a recent one, e.g. toxoplasmosis. Testing for a rising antibody titre can be of value in indicating whether an infection is an active one and in some sensitive tests, changes in antibody titre can indicate

whether a patient is responding to treatment.

The results of antibody tests also require careful interpretation because false positive reactions may occur due to cross-reactions with other human and animal parasites. Different helminths share many antigens and therefore it is not always possible to provide a species diagnosis. False negative results may occur due to an excess of antigen removing the antibody.

Antibody (serological) tests

The range of antibody tests used in the serological investigation of parasitic infections include rapid slide agglutination tests, gel or cellulose acetate precipitin tests, indirect haemagglutination tests, complement fixation tests, indirect fluorescent antibody tests and enzyme-linked immunosorbent assays. The different types of antibody and the principles of antibody tests are described in Chapter 37 in Volume II of the Manual.

The choice of technique depends on a number of factors including the parasitic infection being investigated, the number of tests requested, the availability of reagents, sensitivity and specificity of the test system, and above all, the ability and facilities available in the laboratory.

The enzyme-linked immunosorbent assay (ELISA) has become a standard technique in the diagnosis and epidemiological studies of the important parasitic diseases.[12] It can be used for detecting antibody or antigen.

In the micro-ELISA for antibody detection, the antigen is coated on to the surface of wells in a microtitration plate. The patient's serum is then added and time allowed for an antigen-antibody reaction to occur. An enzyme-labelled specific antiglobulin is then added which attaches to the antigen-antibody complexes. Any unattached antiglobulin is washed away. An enzyme substrate is then added which is acted upon by the attached enzyme, producing a colour which can be measured colorimetrically or in some tests, interpreted visually. Commonly used enzymes are peroxidase or phosphatase. The intensity of the colour produced is proportional to the amount of attached enzyme and therefore to the amount of unknown antibody in the patient's serum.

In recent years ELISA have been used to assist in the diagnosis of malaria, amoebiasis, schistosomiasis, onchocerciasis, toxoplasmosis, echinococcosis, trypanosomiasis, leishmaniasis, and trichinellosis. The ELISA tends to be more sensitive and specific than other serological tests, provides a quantitative result using a single serum dilution, and has the added advantage that it can be automated in a central immunodiagnostic laboratory for epidemiological surveys.

Antigens used in serological tests

Most laboratories prepare their own antigens from parasites grown in cultures or developed in laboratory animals. Only a few antigens are available commercially and these may be very expensive and have only a short shelf-life.

Companies which supply parasitic reagents and test kits

These include Hoechst Behringwerke AG, Institut Pasteur, Fujizoki Pharmaceutical, Cordis Laboratories, Ismunit Immunologico Italiano, Dynatech Laboratories, Biotrol, and Wellcome Diagnostics (the addresses of these Companies can be found in Appendix II).

When purchasing a parasitic antibody test, always ask the manufacturer to supply a copy of the insert leaflet before ordering so that you can obtain information about the sensitivity and specificity of the antigen, the stability of the reagents, and suitability of the technique.

Laboratories wishing to set up tests routinely may have to rely on the different Schools of Tropical Medicine for their sources of antigen but as the importance of immunodiagnosis increases, both in clinical and epidemiological work, it is to be hoped that national and international antigen banks will be established from which inexpensive standardized reagents can be obtained.

Two new techniques which are developing rapidly and it is expected will provide specific antigens for use in serological tests are:

☐ Monoclonal techniques
☐ Recombinant techniques

Monoclonal antibodies

Monoclonal antibodies are made by fusing antibody producing lymphocytes (B lymphocytes) from an immunized mouse with a mouse myeloma cell line. Clones of the resultant hybridomas retain both the capacity to produce the particular antibody made by the lymphocyte and also the capacity for indefinite growth *in vitro*.

This allows the production *in vitro* of large quantities of a range of antibodies, each being usually against a narrow range of antigens. If the antigens which are useful in immunodiagnosis can be identified, the appropriate monoclonal can be used to extract and purify it, for example by affinity chromatography. Further information about the development of monoclonal antibodies in parasitic diseases can be found in the paper of Cohen.[13]

Recombinant DNA (DNA probes)

In simple terms this rapidly advancing technique involves, firstly, extracting and fragmenting the deoxyribonucleic acid (DNA) from one organism and hybridizing (incorporating) this with DNA fragments from another organism. The resulting hybrids are then reinserted into the latter which is known as a vector. This is usually a virus or a bacterial plasmid, nearly always from *Escherichia coli*, which is able to replicate itself very rapidly. If, for example the DNA coding for a certain antigenic protein in a parasite could be inserted into *E. coli*, large quantities of this protein could be produced. The technique is not fully developed but predictably it will be much more consistently effective in the future for the production of specific parasitic reagents.

Referral of blood samples for antibody tests

When a laboratory is unable to perform serological tests, venous blood can be collected from patients into dry leak-proof screw cap glass tubes or vials and sent (well-packaged) for testing to an immunodiagnostic laboratory. If the specimen is likely to take longer than 24 h to reach its destination, the serum must be separated from the red cells before the sample is dispatched and a cool box should be used to transport the serum. The specimen must be clearly labelled and show the date of collection. The accompanying request form should indicate whether the specimen is the 1st or 2nd specimen (the latter is usually collected 7-10 days later to look for a rising antibody titre).

Some immunodiagnostic centres may be able to accept capillary blood collected into plain or heparinised capillary tubes or on to absorbent paper. The latter method is often used in epidemiological surveys because it avoids the collection of venous blood. The dried blood samples remain stable for testing by ELISA and fluorescent antibody techniques for several weeks providing they are stored and transported under dry conditions. Several methods have been developed for the collection of capillary blood on absorbent paper and therefore the immunodiagnostic laboratory must be consulted as to the most suitable method to use.

Caution: Fresh or dried blood samples may contain highly infectious pathogens including hepatitis viruses, AIDS virus, viral haemorrhagic fever viruses, therefore always collect, handle, and transport blood specimens with care. Screw-cap airtight containers must be used and if whole blood or serum samples are being transported, sufficient packaging must surround the container to ensure that the blood or serum can be absorbed should a breakage occur. Packages should be labelled in red lettering URGENT, PATHOLOGICAL SPECIMEN. The regulations regarding the sending of pathological specimens through the post should be obtained from the Post Office and followed exactly.

Antigen tests

Monoclonal techniques are also being used to

develop highly reactive and specific antibody reagents, particularly for ELISA (sandwich assay).

Research laboratories have successfully used ELISA for the detection of amoebic antigen in faeces and in aspirates from liver abscesses.[14] ELISA tests based on secretory antigens have also been developed for the diagnosis of toxocariasis.

DNA probes have been researched for diagnosing malaria but they are not as yet as sensitive as microscopical diagnosis.

It is hoped that for the future, antigen tests will provide rapid, reliable, simple, and inexpensive tests for diagnosing reliably the major parasitic diseases and investigating immune responses.

10 Moody, A. H. A fluorescent technique for demonstrating the chromatoid bodies and nuclei in cysts of *Entamoeba histolytica* from faecal deposits. *Journal of Clinical Pathology*, **37**, (1), p 101-102, 1984.

11 Moody, A. H., Fleck, S. L. Versatile Field's stain. *Journal of Clinical Pathology*, **38**, 7, p 842-843, 1985.

12 Voller, A. ELISA - a widely applicable diagnostic tool. *Medicine Digest*, **10**, 6, p 5-10, 1984.

13 Cohen, S. Monoclonal antibodies in parasitic infectious diseases, *British Medical Journal*, **40**, 3, p 291-296, 1984.

14 Draper, C. C., Lillywhite, J. E. Immunodiagnosis of tropical parasitic infections, Ch 13 in *Recent Advances in Tropical Medicine*, ed. H. M. Gilles, Churchill Livingstone, London, 1984.

References

1 Erdman, D. D. Clinical comparison of ethyl acetate and diethyl ether in the formalin ether sedimentation technique. *Journal of Clinical Microbiology*, **14**, 5, p 483-485, 1981.

2 Moody, A. H. An introduction to selected diagnostic methods for parasites available as kits for smaller health units. *Laboratory in Health Care - Developing Country Proceedings of the 17th IAMLT Congress, 3-8 August 1986*. A limited number of copies are available from Tropical Health Technology, 14 Bevills Close, Doddington, March, Cambridgeshire, PE15 0TT, UK (free to developing countries, priced £5 to other countries).

3 Kato, K. and Miura, M. Comparative examinations, *Japanese Journal of Parasitology*, **3**, 35, 1954 (in Japanese).

4 Peters, P. A. *et al*. Quick Kato smear for field quantification of *Schistosoma mansoni* eggs. *American Journal of Tropical Medicine and Hygiene*, **58**, p 629-638, 1980.

5 Hall, A. Intestinal helminths of man: the interpretation of egg counts. *Parasitology*, **85**, (3), p 605-613, 1982.

6 Moody, A. H. The development of an internal quality control and external quality assurance in parasitology. *Laboratory in Health Care - Developing Country Proceedings of the 17th IAMLT Congress, 3-8 August, 1986*. For availability, see Reference 2.

7 Technique kindly supplied by Anthony H. Moody, Chief MLSO, Laboratory, Hospital for Tropical Diseases, London.

8 Melvin, D. M., Brooke, M. M. *Laboratory Procedure for the Diagnosis of Intestinal Parasites*, Health and Human Services Publication, No. CDC 82-8282, 1982.

9 Teschareon, S. Preparation of permanent slides of helminthic ova. *Journal of the Medical Association of Thailand*, **66**, 9, 1983.

Intestinal and Tissue Protozoa

14:1 CLASSIFICATION AND FEATURES OF INTESTINAL AND TISSUE PROTOZOA

The general characteristics of protozoa are described at the beginning of the Parasitology Section in 12:4.

Classification of intestinal and tissue protozoa of medical importance

Subphylum   SARCODINA
Species   *Entamoeba histolytica*
              Naegleria fowleri (low occurrence)

Subphylum   MASTIGOPHORA
Species   *Giardia lamblia*
              (Also known as *Giardia intestinalis*)
              Trichomonas vaginalis

Subphylum   CILIOPHORA
Species   *Balantidium coli*

Subclass   COCCIDIA
Species   *Isospora belli* (low occurrence)
              Cryptosporidium species
              Toxoplasma gondii

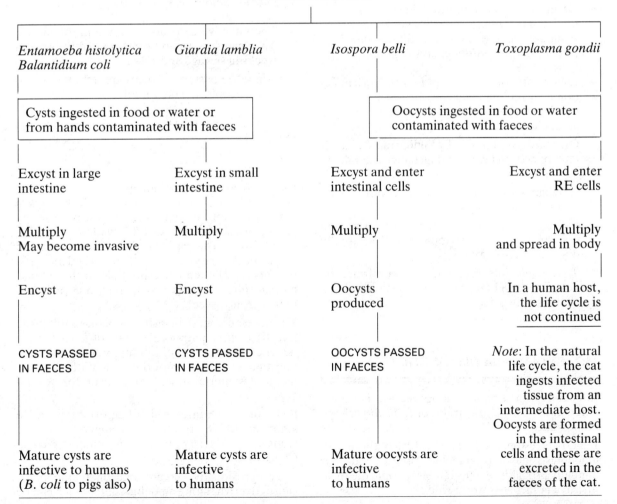

Intestinal and Tissue Protozoa of Medical Importance

SUMMARY LIFE CYCLES

Entamoeba histolytica *Balantidium coli*	*Giardia lamblia*	*Isospora belli*	*Toxoplasma gondii*
Cysts ingested in food or water or from hands contaminated with faeces		Oocysts ingested in food or water contaminated with faeces	
Excyst in large intestine	Excyst in small intestine	Excyst and enter intestinal cells	Excyst and enter RE cells
Multiply May become invasive	Multiply	Multiply	Multiply and spread in body
Encyst	Encyst	Oocysts produced	In a human host, the life cycle is not continued
CYSTS PASSED IN FAECES	CYSTS PASSED IN FAECES	OOCYSTS PASSED IN FAECES	*Note*: In the natural life cycle, the cat ingests infected tissue from an intermediate host. Oocysts are formed in the intestinal cells and these are excreted in the faeces of the cat.
Mature cysts are infective to humans (*B. coli* to pigs also)	Mature cysts are infective to humans	Mature oocysts are infective to humans	

Features of intestinal and tissue protozoa that infect humans

- E.histolytica, G. lamblia, and B. coli are motile organisms that multiply and encyst in the intestinal tract. They form cysts which are excreted in the faeces. Invasive strains of E. histolytica also multiply in the intestinal wall.

  I. belli multiplies intracellularly in the intestinal cells. It produces oocysts which are excreted in the faeces.

  T. gondii multiplies intracellularly in reticuloendothelial cells and in the cells of the brain and other organs of the body.

  T. vaginalis is motile and multiplies in the urogenital tract. Cyst forms are unknown.

- Infection is by ingesting cysts (E. histolytica, G. lamblia, B. coli) or oocysts (I. belli, Cryptosporidium, T. gondii) in food, water, or from hands contaminated with infected faeces. T. gondii can also be transmitted congenitally and by ingesting the parasites in under-cooked meat of intermediate hosts.

  T. vaginalis is transmitted sexually.

- Humans are the important hosts of E. histolytica, G. lamblia, I. belli and T. vaginalis. Animals are the natural definitive hosts of B. coli, Cryptosporidium and T. gondii.

- Laboratory confirmation of E. histolytica infection is by finding amoebae or cysts in faeces or by detecting antibodies in serum (invasive amoebiasis).

  Giardiasis is diagnosed by finding motile flagellates or cysts in faeces or flagellates in duodenal aspirates.

  A diagnosis of balantidiasis is confirmed by finding ciliates or cysts in faeces.

  Infection with I. belli is diagnosed by finding oocysts in faeces. Toxoplasmosis is usually diagnosed serologically.

  T. vaginalis infection is usually confirmed by detecting flagellates in vaginal or urethral discharges or in urine.

14:2 ENTAMOEBA HISTOLYTICA

Infection with Entamoeba histolytica is called amoebiasis. Only a few strains of E. histolytica are pathogenic.

It has been estimated that about 10% of those with amoebiasis develop amoebic disease and that annually probably 40 000-110 000 people die from invasive amoebiasis worldwide.[1]

Distribution

E. histolytica is endemic in many parts of tropical and subtropical Africa, Asia, Mexico, South America, and China. Distribution is related more to inadequate sanitation and poor personal hygiene than to climate.

Transmission and life cycle

E. histolytica is transmitted by the ingestion of infective cysts in food or water contaminated with sewage or from hands contaminated with faeces. Lack of personal hygiene among cyst carriers contributes to the spread of infection. Transmission may also occur by flies feeding on faeces containing cysts and subsequently contaminating food.

Life cycle

— Following ingestion, each cyst excysts in the large intestine to produce amoebae which multiply repeatedly.

— The amoebae form single-nucleated cysts which develop into infective cysts which have 4 nuclei. Once cysts are formed they do not become amoebae again in the same host.

— The infective cysts are excreted in the faeces. They can survive and remain infective several weeks in sewage and water.

  Amoebae passed in faeces are not infective to other people and die rapidly.

Note: The life cycle of E. histolytica is summarized in Fig. 14.1.

Clinical features and pathology

About 90% of persons infected with E. histolytica develop no clinical symptoms. Disease is caused by pathogenic strains of amoebae invading the wall of the intestine. They cause low abdominal pain and acute attacks of dysentery with blood and mucus in the faeces. The amoebae multiply in the submucosa, forming large flask-shaped ulcers which contain necrotic tissue.

The development of invasive amoebiasis following infection with a pathogenic strain of E. histolytica depends on the level of immunity, nutrition, and intestinal environment of the host. Without treatment, dysenteric attacks may recur for several years.

Some of the features which help to differentiate amoebic dysentery from bacillary dysentery (caused by Shigella species) are summarized in Chart 14.1.

Very occasionally, severe intestinal amoebiasis causes overwhelming amoebic colitis which can be

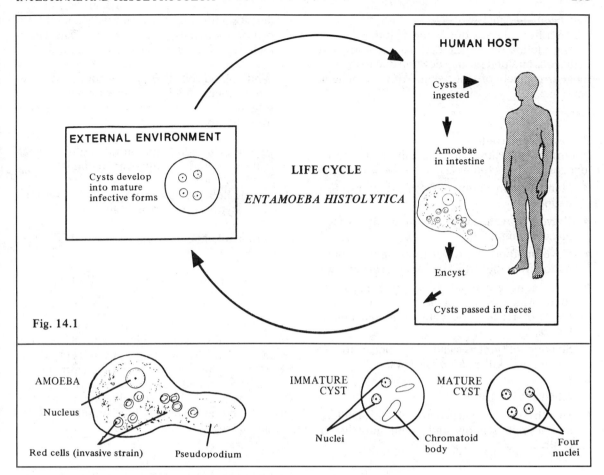

Fig. 14.1

EXTERNAL ENVIRONMENT

Cysts develop into mature infective forms

LIFE CYCLE

ENTAMOEBA HISTOLYTICA

HUMAN HOST

Cysts ingested

Amoebae in intestine

Encyst

Cysts passed in faeces

AMOEBA

Nucleus

Red cells (invasive strain)

Pseudopodium

IMMATURE CYST

Nuclei

Chromatoid body

MATURE CYST

Four nuclei

fatal. Other rare complications of invasive amoebiasis include appendicitis and inflammatory masses in the bowel referred to as amoebomas.

Chart 14.1 Differentiation of Amoebic and Bacillary Dysentery

Amoebic dysentery	*Bacillary dysentery*
• Gradual onset	• Acute onset
• No significant fever or vomiting	• Fever and usually vomiting
Faeces (fresh)	*Faeces (fresh)*
— Offensive odour	— Odourless
— Blood and mucus	— Often watery and bloody
— Acid pH	— Alkaline pH
— Few pus cells	— Many pus cells
— Motile amoebae containing red cells	— No motile amoebae containing red cells

Note: Pathogenic strains of *E. histolytica* are able to destroy polymorphonuclear cells and macrophages.

Liver abscess
Should an intestinal amoebic ulcer reach a blood vessel, amoebae may enter the blood stream and be carried to the liver and other parts of the body where they can form an abscess.

An aemobic liver abscess is a relatively rare complication of invasive amoebiasis. It is ten times more common in adults than in children with a higher frequency in men (3 to 1 ratio).[1] Most abscesses form in the right lobe of the liver. The clinical features include pain and tenderness in the region of the liver, wasting, and a fever associated with chills and night sweats. Patients with large or multiple abscesses may become jaundiced and anaemic.

The centre of the abscess contains a viscous red-brown or grey-yellow fluid consisting of digested liver tissue. It is referred to as pus but usually contains very few pus cells. Aspiration is an important part of treatment but neither aspiration nor surgery should be necessary to diagnose an amoebic liver abscess. Complications (such as generalised amoebiasis of the peritoneal cavity) may follow aspiration of a liver abscess and particularly after surgical investigation.

A serological test such as the cellulose acetate precipitin (CAP) test is helpful in diagnosing amoebic liver abscess. This test and the results of other laboratory tests in amoebic liver abscess are described under *Laboratory Diagnosis*.

Cutaneous amoebiasis
When a liver abscess drains through the skin following rupture or surgical drainage, a destructive cutaneous amoebiasis may develop due to the prolonged contact of the skin with pathogenic amoebae.

Prevention and control
Important measures to prevent and control amoebiasis are as follows:

- Hand washing after defaecation and before eating.

- Preventing water supplies from becoming faecally contaminated.

- Covering food and water to prevent contamination from flies which act as cyst carriers.

- Not eating green salads or other uncooked foods which may contain cysts, usually as a result of fertilization with untreated human faeces.

  Soaking of green salads in vinegar for 30 minutes will kill *E. histolytica* cysts.

- Boiling drinking water (*E. histolytica* cysts are killed at 55 °C).

- Health education, particularly of food handlers, and also in schools and community health centres.

LABORATORY DIAGNOSIS

Intestinal amoebiasis
Laboratory confirmation of intestinal amoebiasis is by:

▫ Examination of a fresh dysenteric faecal specimen or rectal scraping for motile *E. histolytica* amoebae.

  The finding of motile amoebae containing red cells is diagnostic of amoebic dysentery.

▫ Examination of formed or semiformed faeces for *E. histolytica* cysts.

  The finding of cysts indicates infection with either a pathogenic or nonpathogenic strain of *E. histolytica*.

Amoebic liver abscess
Laboratory tests which are helpful in diagnosing amoebic liver abscess include:

▫ Cellulose acetate precipitin (CAP) test to

detect significantly raised levels of anti-*E. histolytica* antibodies (see later text). The test is highly specific for invasive amoebiasis.

▫ White blood cell (WBC) total count and differential count. A leucocytosis with neutrophilia is found in about 80% of patients with amoebic liver abscess.

▫ Erythrocyte sedimentation rate (ESR), which is always raised, usually over 50 mm/h.

▫ Haemoglobin, which is frequently low (usually normocytic, normochromic anaemia).

▫ Serum alkaline phosphatase, which is often raised.

▫ Serum albumin, which is reduced in some patients.

Note: As already explained, the aspiration of pus from a liver abscess for diagnostic purposes is not recommended. If, however, pus is sent to the laboratory (aspirated as part of treatment), it should be examined for amoebae which can occasionally be found. The pus will contain very few pus cells and no bacteria will be found in a Gram stained smear.

Examination of faeces or rectal scraping for *E. histolytica* amoebae
Specimen: The specimen should be examined as soon as possible after it has been collected (within 15 minutes). It should be kept in a warm environment because amoeboid movement is reduced in cold surroundings.

The method of examination is as follows:

1. Using a warm slide, transfer a sample of mucus and blood to the slide, cover with a cover glass, and press gently with a piece of cloth or tissue to spread the specimen to make a thin preparation.

   Note: If possible avoid adding saline because unless this is isotonic and of the correct pH, it may kill the amoebae.

   Use of eosin
   Many workers recommend adding a drop of eosin solution (Reagent No. 33). The dye provides a pink-red background which may make it easier to detect the unstained moving amoebae as shown in colour Plate 1 (the dye does not penetrate the living amoebae).

2. Examine the preparation microscopically using the 10× objective with the condenser iris *closed sufficiently* to give good contrast. Look for very

small irregularly shaped clear objects (amoeboid movement will not be seen at this low magnification).

3. Use the 40× objective to identify an amoeba:

E. histolytica amoeba
— Look for characteristic active amoeboid movement. The amoeba will be seen to progress in one direction by pushing out projections of its cytoplasm (pseudopodia).

— Look for red cells inside the amoeba (see Plate 14.1 and colour Plate 1). The red cells will appear pale yellow-grey. The finding of ingested red cells identifies an amoeba as *E. histolytica* (pathogenic strain).

Occasionally, amoebae of nonpathogenic species may be found in faeces. In unstained preparations they can be differentiated from pathogenic *E. histolytica* by the absence of ingested red cells.

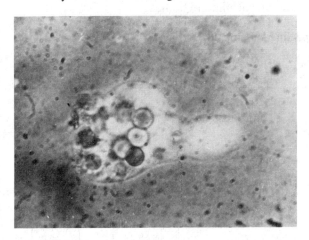

Plate 14.1 Amoeba of *Entamoeba histolytica* in faeces. Red cells can be seen in the amoeba, indicating that it is an invasive strain. *Courtesy of A. C. Rijpstra, Royal Tropical Institute, Amsterdam.*

Note: As will be seen by comparing colour Plate 1 with the hookworm egg shown, an *E. histolytica* amoeba is small (average size is 25 × 20 μm). The nucleus of the amoeba is difficult to see in fresh preparations.

Examination of fixed stained preparations for *E. histolytica* amoebae
When facilities are not available for the immediate examination of a faecal specimen for motile *E. histolytica* amoebae, a faecal specimen can be fixed and sent for examination to a parasitology Reference Laboratory. Suitable fixatives for preserving *E. histolytica* amoebae include polyvinyl alcohol (PVA) and sodium acetate formalin (SAF). The use of these fixatives is described in 13:9.

Examination of faeces for *E. histolytica* cysts
The cysts of *E. histolytica* may be found in formed and semiformed specimens.

Concentration
E. histolytica cysts can be concentrated by the formol ether technique, formol detergent sedimentation technique (overnight sedimentation), or by the zinc sulphate floatation technique. These techniques are described in Chapter 13.

Direct method of examining faeces for E. histolytica cysts
1. Place 1 drop of physiological saline or eosin solution (Reagent No. 33) on one end of a slide and 1 drop of Dobell's iodine (Reagent No. 31) at the other end.

   Use of eosin: The eosin provides a pink-red background against which the unstained cysts can be detected more easily (see colour Plate 2a).
   Use of iodine: The iodine stains the nuclei of the cysts.

2. Mix a small amount of faeces in the saline or eosin and a small amount of faeces in the iodine. Make smooth *thin* suspensions. Cover each preparation with a cover glass.

3. Examine the saline or eosin preparation microscopically using the 10× objective, with the condenser iris closed sufficiently to give good contrast.

   The cysts are round and small, measuring 10-15 μm in diameter. They can therefore just be seen with the 10× objective.

4. Identify the cysts using the 40× objective:

   E. histolytica cysts
   — Measure the cysts to see whether they are of the correct size for *E. histolytica*, i.e. 10-15 μm. The equipment required for measuring objects in microscopical preparations is described in 4:11.
   — Focus to see whether the cysts contain a blunt ended chromatoid body which is usually present in younger *E. histolytica* cysts (see Fig. 14.1 and colour Plate 2a). This structure will only be seen in the saline or eosin preparation, not in the iodine preparation. Some cysts contain several chromatoid bodies.

   Staining of chromatoid bodies: Several techniques are available. The simplest is to make a saline suspension of faeces in a small tube, add 2 or 3 drops of Burrow's stain (Reagent No. 22), and mix. Leave the suspension overnight or at least 6 hours for the chromatoid bars to stain. The chromatoid bars stain blue (see colour Plate 2c).

If facilities for fluorescence microscopy are available, acridine orange can be used to demonstrate chromatoid bars in *E. histolytica* cysts (see colour Plate 2d). The technique is simple, inexpensive, and takes about 30 minutes (see 13:11).

— Look for nuclei in the cysts and with focusing, count the number. The nuclei will be easier to count in the iodine preparation. No more than 4 nuclei will be seen in an *E. histolytica* cyst. Young cysts may contain only 1 or 2 nuclei (see colour Plate 2a and b, and Plate 14.2a).

Note: The detailed nuclear structure of *E. histolytica* cysts which is often described in textbooks of parasitology, is not easily seen unless the cysts are stained with special stains and examined with the 100× oil immersion objective. Such details are not required to identify *E. histolytica* cysts in routine work.

Differentiation of E. histolytica cysts from other cysts which can be found in faeces
The cysts of *E. histolytica* require differentiation from those of the following nonpathogenic species:

Entamoeba hartmanni
Entamoeba coli
Iodamoeba buetschlii
Endolimax nana

E. hartmanni cysts resemble morphologically those of *E. histolytica* but they can be differentiated by their smaller size. A cyst of *E. hartmanni* measures below 10 μm (average size 7-9 μm), whereas a cyst of *E. histolytica* measures 10-15 μm (see Plate 14.2b).

E. coli cysts are larger than *E. histolytica*, measuring 15-30 μm. They contain up to 8 nuclei (see Plate 14.2c). Occasionally needle-like chromatoid bodies are seen. The cysts show a greater variation in shape and size than those of *E. histolytica*.

I. buetschlii cysts are irregular in size and shape and are easily differentiated from *E. histolytica* in iodine preparations because they possess a glycogen inclusion which stains with iodine (see Plate 14.2d and colour Plate 6). They are often referred to as 'iodine cysts'. They contain a single nucleus and no chromatoid bodies.

Chart 14.2 Differentiation of Small Cysts in Faecal Specimens Using 40× Objective

Species	Size	Nuclei	Chromatoid body	Glycogen inclusion	Saline Eosin	Iodine
CYSTS OF AMOEBAE						
Entamoeba histolytica	10-15 μm	1-4	+ Blunt Immature cyst	Diffuse	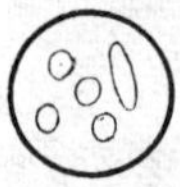	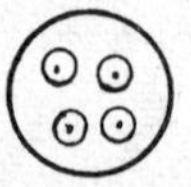
Entamoeba hartmanni	7-9 μm	1-4	+ Blunt Immature cyst	Diffuse	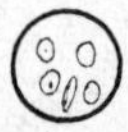	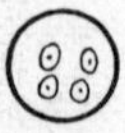
Entamoeba coli	15-30 μm	1-8	Rare Needle-like	Diffuse	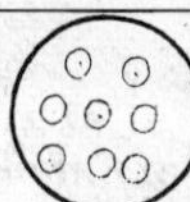	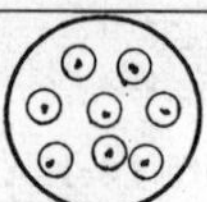
Iodamoeba buetschlii	9-15 μm	1	—	Compact mass	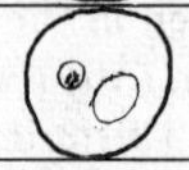	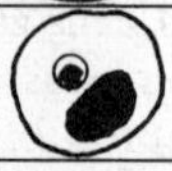
Endolimax nana	7-9 μm	4 Hole-like	—	—	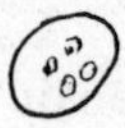	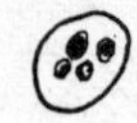

Species	Size	Nuclei	Contents of Cyst	Saline Eosin	Iodine
CYSTS OF FLAGELLATES					
Giardia lamblia	Oval 10×6μm average	4 Not obvious	Remains of axonemes and flagella	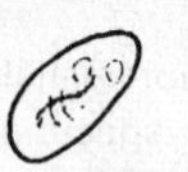	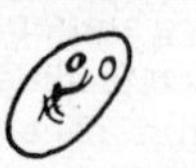
Chilomastix mesnili	Lemon-shaped 5-7 μm	1	Remains of flagella and cytostome	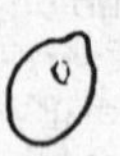	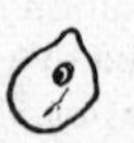

CYSTS OF AMOEBAE

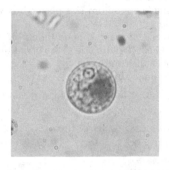 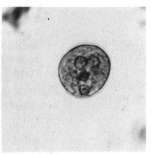 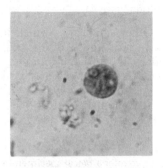

a Entamoeba histolytica. Left shows single nucleated cyst. *Right* **Four nucleated cyst.**

b Entamoeba hartmanni **with up to 4 nuclei.**

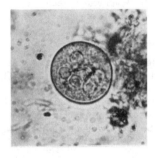 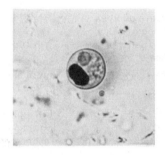 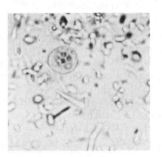

c Entamoeba coli **with up to 8 nuclei.**

d Iodamoeba buetschlii with large glycogen body.

e Endolimax nana **with 4 nuclei.**

CYSTS OF FLAGELLATES

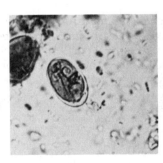 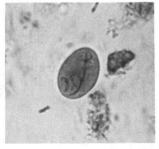 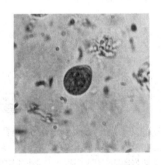

f **Cysts of** *Giardia lamblia* **showing nuclei, axonemes, and parabasal bodies.**

g Chilomastix mesnili, **lemon - shaped with 1 nucleus.**

Plate 14.2 Iodine preparations of cysts that can be found in faeces.

Acknowledgements Plate a (left), courtesy of V. Zaman, Plates a (right), b. c, d, f (left) and g, courtesy of A. C. Rijpstra and Royal Tropical Institute of Amsterdam, Plate e, courtesy of A. Moody, and Plate f (right), courtesy of W. Peters.

E. nana cysts are smaller than *E. histolytica* cysts, round to oval in shape, and possess four nuclei which look like punched out holes (see Plate 14.2e and colour Plate 4).

Note: Other small cysts which may be found in faeces include those of the flagellates *Giardia lamblia* (pathogen) and *Chilomastix mesnili* (non-pathogen). These cysts are easily differentiated from those of *E. histolytica* by their shape, size, and cyst contents as shown in Chart 14.2, Plate 14.2 and colour Plates 3 and 7.

Preservation of cysts in faeces
If needing to refer a faecal specimen for the identification of cysts to a parasitology reference laboratory, Beyer's solution (Reagent No. 15) is recommended as a fixative to preserve the cysts. Mix about 1 gram of faeces in about 8 ml of Beyer's working solution (see 13:9).

Beyer's solution is also an excellent preservative of other faecal parasites. It can be used in parasitology quality assessment programmes to send specimens to peripheral laboratories to assess whether *E. histolytica* cysts and other parasites are being identified correctly.

The following is a summary of the important microscopical features which identify the amoebae and cysts of *E. histolytica*.

Entamoeba histolytica

Amoeba
- Average size is about $25 \times 20\ \mu m$.
- Active amoeboid movement (directional) in fresh warm specimens.
- Contains ingested red cells (invasive strain).

Illustrations: See Plate 14.1 and colour Plate 1.

Cyst
- Round, measuring 10-15 μm.
- Contains 1, 2, or 4 nuclei.
- Chromatoid bar(s) can be seen in immature cysts.

Illustrations: See illustrations in Chart 14.2, Plate 14.2a and colour Plate 2.

Cellulose acetate precipitin (CAP) test to investigate invasive amoebiasis[2]
This is a simple inexpensive technique which is of value in confirming a diagnosis of amoebic liver abscess. It has a high specificity with positive results being obtained only if invasive amoebiasis is present. A positive result does not persist for more than a few months after cure.

The CAP test relies on the surface diffusion of specific globulins and soluble antigen to produce a line of precipitation where they meet which can be visualised by staining.

Required
— Plastic box containing foam sponge.

Preparation of the box
1. Take a shallow medium size plastic box with an airtight lid.
2. Take a piece of foam sponge (about 10-15 mm depth) and cut it to the size of the box. Cut a 5 cm square from the centre of it.
3. Place the sponge in the box.

— Piece of cellulose acetate paper, measuring 60 mm square.

— Template to make wells in the CAP to contain the antigen

Making a template
1. Take a piece of perspex or other thin rigid plastic.
2. Drill 5 bevelled holes, a central hole measuring 3 mm across the bevel, and four holes measuring 6 mm across the bevel and situated 1 cm apart and 1 cm from the central hole (see Fig. 14.2).

— Soluble amoebic antigen

Sources of amoebic antigen
Information can be obtained from Chief MLSO, Hospital for Tropical Diseases, 4 St Pancras Way, London NW1 0PE, UK. With the collaboration of the Hospital for Tropical Diseases, it is hoped that a CAP kit containing antigen will become available from Tropical Health Technology.

— Phosphate buffered saline   Reagent No. 56
(PBS), pH 7.0
— Nigrosin stain   Reagent No. 50

Method
1. Float the square of cellulose acetate paper onto PBS, pH 7.0 (contained in a shallow dish), and allow it to adsorb the buffer evenly. Immerse the paper in the buffer, remove, and blot to take up the excess buffer.

2. Using the template and a rod (e.g. wire loop holder), make 5 wells in the paper. Label one of the outer wells + (positive control) and another outer well − (negative control), and the other two wells with the patient's initials, as shown in Fig. 14.2.

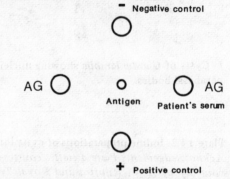

Fig. 14.2 Position of wells in CAP test.

14:2

3. Moisten the sponge with PBS, pH 7.0 and place the paper in the box over the hole in the sponge.

4. Using a fine capillary, place one drop (approx. 5 µl) of the patient's serum in each of the initialled wells, a positive serum in the positive well, and a negative serum in the negative well. Place one drop (approx. 3 µl) of amoebic antigen in the centre well.

5. Close the lid of the box and leave it at room temperature for 4 hours.

6. Remove the paper and wash it in physiological saline for 5 minutes.

7. Immerse the paper in nigrosin stain for 2 minutes. Rinse in water or 2% v/v acetic acid to clear the paper.

8. Holding the paper against a strong light, look for precipitin arcs. Check the positive and negative controls.

Results
A positive test is indicated by seeing a precipitin arc between the serum and the antigen as shown in Plate 14.3.

Report the test as 'CAP test Positive' or 'CAP test Negative'.

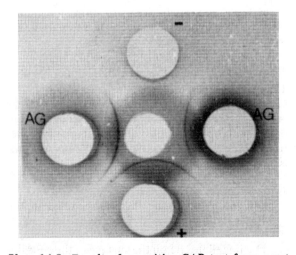

Plate 14.3 Result of a positive CAP test from a patient with amoebic liver abscess. Precipitin arcs (black curved lines) can be seen between the antigen well and patient's serum wells (left and right). There is no precipitin arc between the negative control serum well and the antigen well. A precipitin arc is shown with the positive control serum.

14:3 PATHOGENIC FREE-LIVING AMOEBAE

In recent years, about 150 cases of primary amoebic meningoencephalitis caused by free-living amoebae of the genus *Naegleria* have been reported worldwide in tropical and temperate regions.[4] The commonest pathogenic species is *Naegleria fowleri*.

Transmission
Naegleria attacks healthy persons, causing an acute and usually fatal meningoencephalitis. Although cysts are formed, it is the actively growing stages of *Naegleria* which infect the brain.

Most infections have been traced to bathing in stagnant freshwater lakes, pools contaminated with sewage or other decaying matter, and under-chlorinated swimming pools. *N. fowleri* is restricted to naturally warm water or to those which are thermally polluted. The organisms enter through the nose and are thought to invade the brain via the olfactory nerve.

The cysts of *Naegleria* (round in form) are killed by drying but can survive long periods if kept moist. *Naegleria* becomes an amoeboflagellate in water which helps it to spread, especially in fresh pools when it rains.

Clinical symptoms
Symptoms of acute meningitis generally follow within 5 days of exposure to contaminated freshwater containing *Naegleria*. The organisms enter through the nose and are thought to invade the brain via the olfactory nerve.

The cerebrospinal fluid (c.s.f.) is purulent with a raised protein concentration and cell count similar to that found in pyogenic bacterial meningitis. When the c.s.f. is examined microscopically (see below), the motile amoebae can usually be seen.

Unless diagnosed and treated at an early stage, irreversible brain damage occurs and the infection is fatal.

LABORATORY DIAGNOSIS

Look especially for *Naegleria* amoebae if the c.s.f. contains polymorphonuclear neutrophils but no bacteria can be detected in a Gram stained smear. The c.s.f. may also contain eosinophils and red cells. As in bacterial meningitis, the c.s.f. glucose will be reduced and protein raised.

Examination of a wet c.s.f. preparation for amoebae
1. Transfer a drop of uncentrifuged purulent c.s.f., or a drop of sediment from a centrifuged

specimen, to a slide and cover with a cover glass.

2. Examine the specimen, first using the 10× objective with the condenser iris *reduced sufficiently* to give good contrast.

Look for small, clear, motile elongated forms among the pus cells.

Use the 40× objective to identify the rapidly moving amoebae (even if the amoebae are not detected first with the 10× objective, *always* examine the preparation with the 40× objective).

Naegleria amoeba

- Elongate in form, measuring 10-22 × 7 μm.

- Rapidly motile (more than 2 body lengths per minute).

- When viewed with the 40× objective, vacuoles can usually be seen in the cytoplasm (the nucleus with its large nucleolus is not usually visible in an unstained preparation).

- Does not contain ingested red cells.

Note: *Naegleria* amoebae will remain motile for several hours at room temperature and up to 24 hours at 35-37 °C.

The amoebae can be stained with Giemsa stain, but they do not stain well by the Gram technique.

In distilled water, the amoebae develop flagella after 2-4 hours.

Illustration: See Plate 14.4

Important: If amoebae are seen in the c.s.f., immediately notify the medical officer attending the patient.

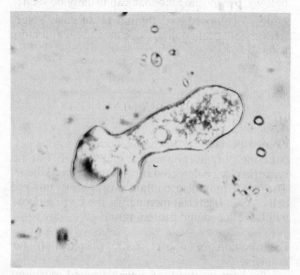

Plate 14.4 *Naegleria* amoeba.

Identification of Naegleria species
The amoebae can be identified as *Naegleria* by showing their utilization of *Escherichia coli* and ability to become amoeboflagellates in water. The technique is described on p. 165 in Volume II of the Manual.

Acanthamoeba species
Other free-living amoebae belonging to the genus *Acanthamoeba* have been reported as causing chronic granulomatous amoebic encephalitis, usually in immunocompromised persons. The brain is probably infected via the blood-stream, possibly from infected skin, eye, or lung.[4]

Acanthamoeba cysts as well as the amoebae are thought to be infective. Dry cysts can survive for several years in dust. They are angular in shape with a double wall. The amoebae are slow moving with spiky projections. Cerebrospinal fluid from patients with amoebic encephalitis usually contains only a few cells (polymorphs).

14:4 *GIARDIA LAMBLIA*

Infection with the intestinal flagellate *Giardia lamblia* is called giardiasis.

Giardia lamblia is also called *Giardia intestinalis*.

Distribution
G. lamblia has a worldwide distribution and is particularly common in the tropics and subtropics, in areas where water supplies and the environment become faecally contaminated.

In endemic areas, children are more frequently infected than adults, particularly those that are malnourished.

Transmission and life cycle
G. lamblia is transmitted by the ingestion of cysts in food or water contaminated with faeces containing cysts. Humans are the only reservoirs of infection. The cysts are infective directly they are passed in the faeces.

Life cycle
— Following ingestion, the cysts excyst in the upper small intestine to form flagellates.

— The flagellates lie on the surface of the cells lining the wall of the duodenum and jejunum. They become attached to the cells by a sucking disc and absorb nourishment through their body surface. They multiply rapidly. The flagellates of *G. lamblia* can also invade the bile duct.

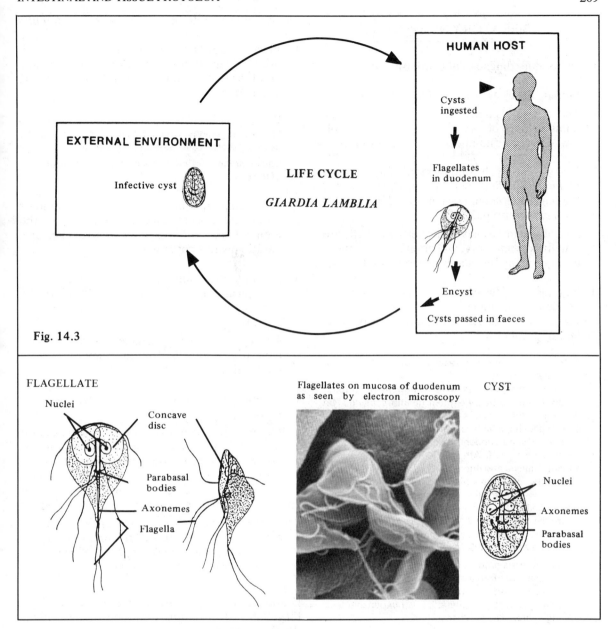

HUMAN HOST

Cysts ingested

Flagellates in duodenum

Encyst

Cysts passed in faeces

EXTERNAL ENVIRONMENT

Infective cyst

LIFE CYCLE

GIARDIA LAMBLIA

Fig. 14.3

FLAGELLATE

Nuclei

Concave disc

Parabasal bodies

Axonemes

Flagella

Flagellates on mucosa of duodenum as seen by electron microscopy

CYST

Nuclei

Axonemes

Parabasal bodies

— After becoming detached, the flagellates are carried down the intestinal tract during which they encyst.

— The infective cysts are excreted in the faeces.

Clinical features and pathology

Although many infections with *G. lamblia* are without symptoms, the parasites and their toxins can cause abdominal pain, severe diarrhoea, vomiting, lethargy, weight loss, and malabsorption with lactose intolerance. Faecal specimens are offensive, bulky, and pale coloured or watery.

People with gastrointestinal disorders or bacterial infections of the intestine appear to be more susceptible to *Giardia* infection. Both hypochlorhydria and pancreatic disease predispose to giardiasis.

Prevention and control

Giardiasis is prevented by improving sanitation and personal hygiene to prevent food, water, and hands from becoming contaminated with faeces containing cysts.

In water, the cysts of *G. lamblia* can remain infective for several weeks. The cysts are not killed in food or water stored at 4-6 °C. Like the cysts of *E. histolytica*, *Giardia* cysts are resistant to the concentrations of chlorine normally used for the treatment of domestic water supplies.

LABORATORY DIAGNOSIS

The laboratory diagnosis of giardiasis is by:

☐ Finding the cysts of *G. lamblia* in faeces.

The cysts are passed irregularly. Often large numbers may be present for a few days, followed by fewer numbers for a week or more.

☐ Less commonly, by finding motile flagellates of *G. lamblia* in diarrhoeic faeces. The identity of the flagellates should be confirmed by examining a stained preparation.

Faecal specimens have an offensive smell, are usually pale and fatty, and often contain mucus in which many flagellates may be found.

☐ Finding the flagellates of *G. lamblia* in duodenal aspirates. The aspirates are examined for flagellates in the same way as faecal specimens.

Enterotest capsule for recovery of *G. lamblia* in duodenal contents
The *Enterotest* consists of a strong nylon thread, coiled inside a small weighted gelatin capsule. The free end of the thread is attached to the cheek of the patient and the gelatin capsule is swallowed. The capsule reaches the duodenum and the gelatin dissolves around the thread. After 2 hours, the thread with attached mucus and duodenal fluid, is withdrawn and placed in a bottle containing about 15 ml of physiological saline. After shaking, the contents of the bottle are centrifuged and the sediment is examined for *G. lamblia* motile flagellates. A stained preparation should also be examined which will show the characteristic shape and 2 nuclei of *G. lamblia* flagellates.

The *Enterotest* is produced by the Health Development Corporation, California, USA and is available from Rocket of London Ltd, Imperial Way, Watford, WD2 4XX, UK and other suppliers. It is an expensive test, costing approx. £82 for 25 tests (1986).

Examination of faeces for *G. lamblia* cysts
Several specimens may need to be examined before the cysts are detected because, as mentioned previously, they are excreted irregularly. In some specimens very many cysts may be found while at other times only a few may be seen or none at all.

Concentration
G. lamblia cysts can be concentrated by the formol ether concentration technique, particularly when formol water is used instead of formol saline. The cysts can also be concentrated by the formol detergent sedimentation technique (overnight sedimentation) or by the zinc sulphate floatation technique. All these techniques are described in Chapter 13.

Direct method of examining faeces for G. lamblia cysts
1. Place 1 drop of physiological saline or eosin solution (Reagent No. 33) on one end of a slide and 1 drop of Dobell's iodine (Reagent No. 31) at the other end.

Use of eosin: The eosin provides a pink-red background against which the unstained cysts can be detected more easily (see colour Plate 7a).

Use of iodine: The iodine stains the internal structures of the cyst.

2. Mix a small amount of faeces in the saline or eosin and a small amount of faeces in the iodine. Make *thin* suspensions. Cover each preparation with a cover glass.

3. Examine the saline or eosin preparation microscopically, using the 10× objective with the condenser iris closed sufficiently to give good contrast.

The cysts are oval in shape and very small, measuring about $10 \times 6 \ \mu m$. They can just be seen with the 10x objective.

4. Identify the cysts using the 40× objective:
G. lamblia cysts
Examine the oval shaped cysts for parabasal rods, and the remains of axonemes, parabasal bodies, and flagella as shown in Plate 14.5 and colour Plate 7 (right). As will be seen from colour Plate 7c, the contents of the cyst will be more clearly seen in the iodine preparation.

The cysts contain 1-4 nuclei but these are not easily seen. The diagnostic features of *G. lamblia* cysts are their oval shape, small size, and contents (see also Chart 14.2 in 14:2).

Examination of faeces for *G. lamblia* flagellates
Flagellates of *G. lamblia* may be found in diarrhoeic faecal specimens.

1. Transfer a drop of faecal specimen (including a sample of mucus if present) to a slide and cover with a cover glass. Make a *thin* preparation.

2. Examine the preparation first with the 10× objective to locate a thin part to examine with the 40× objective for motile flagellates. Adjust the condenser iris to give maximum contrast.

Motile G. lamblia flagellates
The flagellates of *G. lamblia* measure 9-20 μm in length (usual size is 10-12 μm). They have a characteristic shape with a concavity at the front end. There are 8 flagella. The flagellates have a rotating and twisting movement. Some workers liken the movement to a falling leaf.

3. Confirm the identity of any flagellates seen, by preparing and examining a stained preparation of the faeces as follows:

— Make a thin smear of the faeces and allow it to air-dry.

— Fix the smear with absolute methanol (methyl alcohol) for about 1 minute.

— Stain the smear using Field's rapid staining technique for thin films as described in 13:16.

Field's modified *thin* film staining technique (see 13:16) is recommended because it takes just a few minutes, is easy to do, and shows well the two nuclei which differentiate the flagellates of *G. lamblia* from other flagellates which may be present in faecal specimens.

— When dry, examine the smear using the 40× and 100× objectives.

Note: Even when no flagellates are seen in a wet preparation, a stained preparation should always be examined if giardiasis is suspected. Occasionally the flagellates may be detected in a stained smear when they have been missed in a wet preparation.

Stained *G. lamblia* flagellates

The characteristic appearance of *G. lamblia* flagellates in a thin Field's stained preparation as seen with the 40× objective, is shown in colour Plate 7 (left).

Look for the 2 nuclei. Other flagellates which may be found in faeces have only 1 nucleus (see Chart 14.3). In a stained preparation, the flagella, axonemes, and parabasal bodies of *G. lamblia* flagellates will be seen.

Giardia lamblia

Flagellate
- Pear-shaped, usually measuring 10-12 × 6 μm.
- Upper end has a concavity with a sucking disc.
- There are 8 flagella.

Features which can be seen in stained preparations and are used to identify G. lamblia:
- 2 nuclei (other flagellates found in faeces have only 1 nucleus).
- Parabasal bodies.
- Axonemes.

Illustrations: See Plate 14.5, colour Plate 7 (left) and Chart 14.3.

Cyst
- Oval in shape.
- Small, measuring about 10 × 6 μm.
- Contains the remains of axonemes and parabasal bodies (stain with iodine).
- Thread-like remains of flagella may also be seen.
- 4 nuclei (difficult to see).

Illustrations: See Plate 14.5, colour Plate 7 a, b, c and Chart 14.2 in 14:2.

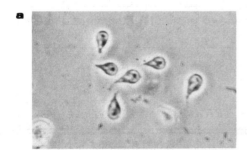
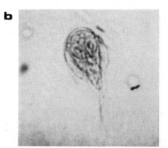
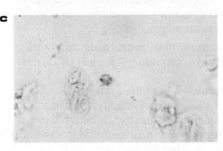
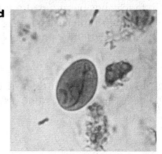

Plate 14.5 *a Giardia lamblia* **flagellates as seen with 40x objective.** *b* **Flagellate viewed with 100x objective.** *c Giardia lamblia* **cyst in saline preparation.** *d* **Cyst in iodine preparation.**
Plate a, courtesy of V. Zaman. Plate b, courtesy of A. C. Rijpstra, Plate d, courtesy of W. Peters.

Chart 14.3 Features which Differentiate Flagellates found in Faecal Specimens

Species	Size	Movement	Features	
Giardia lamblia	10-12 ×6 µm (usual)	Twists and rotates (likened to a falling leaf)	*Unstained* • Typical shape with 8 flagella. • Concavity at the anterior end. *Stained* • 2 nuclei • Axonemes • Parabasal bodies	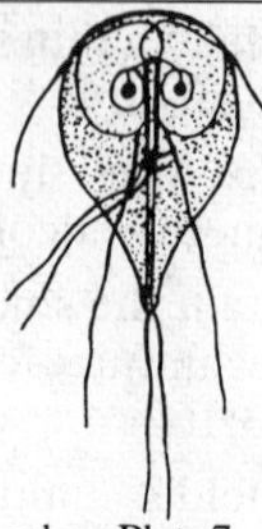 See also colour Plate 7
Chilomastix mesnili Nonpathogen	10-20 µm	Rotary	*Unstained* • Pointed tail. • 3 anterior flagella. • Spiral groove. *Stained* • 1 nucleus • Cytostome with fibril	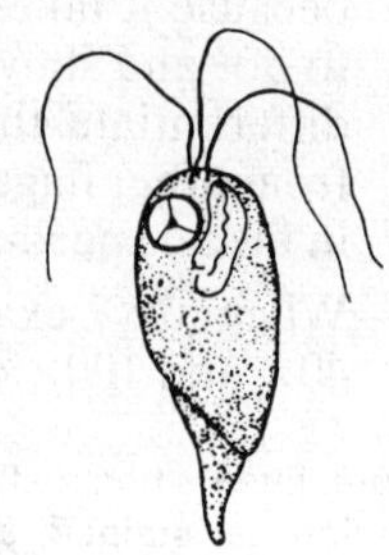
Trichomonas hominis Rarely pathogenic	7-15 µm	Jerky	*Unstained* • Oval to round. • 4 anterior flagella. • Axostyle extends beyond body. • Undulating membrane along length of body with free flagellum. *Stained* • 1 nucleus • Costa • Axostyle	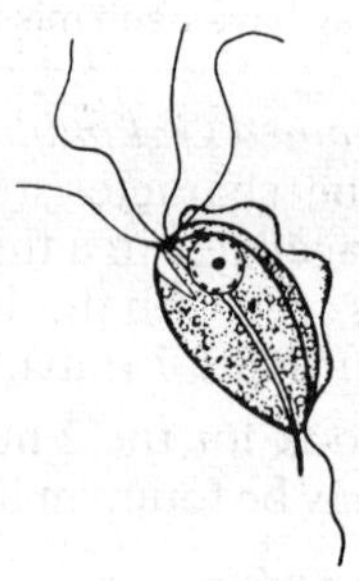

Note: Features which differentiate the cysts of G. lamblia and C. mesnili are summarized in Chart 14.2 in 14.2. T. hominis has no cyst stage.

Immunodiagnosis of giardiasis

A rapid visually read enzyme-linked immunosorbent assay (ELISA) for the detection of *Giardia* antigen in faeces has been developed by Green, *et al.*[5] Compared with microscopy, the sensitivity of the ELISA exceeded 98% and was 100% specific.

Because the test detects antigen, it detects active infection and is therefore of value both in diagnosis and epidemiology.

Reagents for the test are not yet available commercially. Further details of the test can be found in the paper of Green *et al.*[5]

14:5 *TRICHOMONAS VAGINALIS*

The flagellate *Trichomonas vaginalis* is a common cause of vaginitis in women. Infection is referred to as trichomoniasis.

T. vaginalis has a worldwide distribution. It is not especially common in tropical countries.

Transmission and life cycle

T. vaginalis is a sexually transmitted organism. The flagellates are the infective forms. They live and multiply in the urogenital tract of both women and men. There is no known cyst stage.

Clinical symptoms and pathology

In about 40% of infected women, *T. vaginalis*

causes acute inflammation of the vagina with a yellow-green purulent discharge, sometimes accompanied by urinary frequency.

In men, *T. vaginalis* infection is usually asymptomatic. Occasionally the organism causes urethritis with a non-purulent urethral discharge.

LABORATORY DIAGNOSIS

Laboratory confirmation of trichomoniasis is by:

☐ Finding *T. vaginalis* flagellates in unstained or stained preparations of vaginal or urethral discharges.

> **Vaginal discharge**: Differences in the appearances of vaginal discharges in *Trichomonas*, *Candida*, and *Gardnerella* infections and the microbiological investigations which are helpful in differentiating these infections, are described in 38:9 in Volume II of the Manual.

Note: *T. vaginalis* may also be found in the urine of men and women (see later text).

Examination of vaginal or urethral discharge for *T. vaginalis*

Wet preparations
1. Collect a small sample of discharge on a slide, add a drop of *fresh* physiological saline, and cover with a cover glass. Do not make the preparation too thick.

2. As soon as possible, examine the preparation microscopically using the 10× and 40× objectives with the condenser iris closed sufficiently to give good contrast.

   T. vaginalis flagellates
   Look for motile flagellates between the pus cells. *T. vaginalis* flagellates are round to oval in shape and a little larger than pus cells, measuring about 15-25 μm in length.

   Careful focusing is required to detect the flagellates. Movement is often slight (on-the-spot) and not progressional and may only be seen with the 40× objective.

   Note: If more than 10 minutes has passed since the collection of the specimen, motility can often be increased by incubating the preparation at 35-37 °C for a few minutes (in an airtight container with a damp piece of cotton wool).

Stained preparations
Make a smear of the discharge on a slide, air-dry, and fix with absolute methanol for about 1 minute.

If facilities for fluorescence microscopy are available, acridine orange can be used to demonstrate the flagellates as shown in colour Plate 12. *T. vaginalis* flagellates fluoresce orange among the green pus cells. A rapid acridine orange staining technique is described in 34:13 in Volume II.

If fluorescence facilities are not available, *T. vaginalis* can be stained using a Giemsa technique or the rapid Field's technique for thin films (described in 13:16).

In stained preparations, the morphological features of *T. vaginalis* can be seen, including the single nucleus, 3-5 anterior flagella, axostyle rod (extends beyond the body), and the undulating membrane with flagellum which extends along two thirds of the body. These structures, as seen with the 40× objective, are shown in Plate 14.7.

Trichomonas vaginalis
- Flagellate, measuring about 15-25 μm in diameter (little larger than surrounding pus cells).
- On-the-spot jerky motility in *fresh* specimens.
- Has an undulating membrane which extends along two thirds of the body.

In Giemsa or Field's (thin film) stained preparation:
- Single nucleus.
- Axostyle which extends beyond the body.
- 3-5 anterior flagella.
- Undulating membrane, bordered by a flagellum.

Illustration: See Plate 14.7.

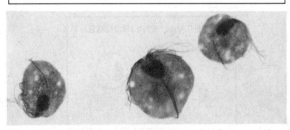

Plate 14.7 *Trichomonas vaginalis* **stained preparation.** *Courtesy of V. Zaman.*

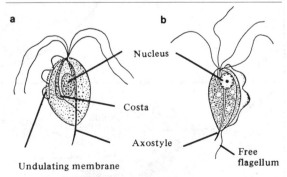

Fig. 14.4 *a Trichomonas vaginalis.*
b Trichomonas hominis.

Detection of *T. vaginalis* in urine

Motile *T. vaginalis* can sometimes be seen in the urine of men and women. *T. vaginalis* can be differentiated from *T. hominis* (which may be found in urine that has been contaminated with faeces) by its larger size and shorter undulating membrane and flagellum. The undulating membrane of *T. hominis* extends the full length of the body and is bordered by a flagellum which forms a free flagellum as shown in Fig. 14.4.

Note: *T. vaginalis* does not stain well in Gram stained smears. A Gram stained smear is useful in the investigation of acute vaginitis because yeast cells stain well by the Gram technique (Gram positive cells).

14:6 BALANTIDIUM COLI

Balantidium coli is a ciliate which is normally parasitic in pigs. Very occasionally it infects humans, causing balantidiasis. It is the only ciliate which can parasitize humans.

B. coli has a world-wide distribution, being more commonly found amongst those who keep pigs, especially in warmer climates.

Transmission and life cycle

B. coli is transmitted by the ingestion of cysts from hands, food, or drink contaminated with infective faeces.

Life cycle

— Following ingestion, the cysts excyst in the intestine, each cyst producing a single ciliate.

— The ciliates multiply in the colon by simple binary division often following conjugation during which nuclear particles are exchanged between individuals.

— Thick walled cysts are formed which are excreted in the faeces. The cysts are infective when passed.

Clinical features and pathology

Infection with *B. coli* can be without symptoms unless the ciliates invade the intestinal wall. Invasion can cause inflammation and ulceration, leading to dysentery with blood and mucus being passed in the faeces.

Intestinal perforation is a rare but serious complication of balantidiasis.

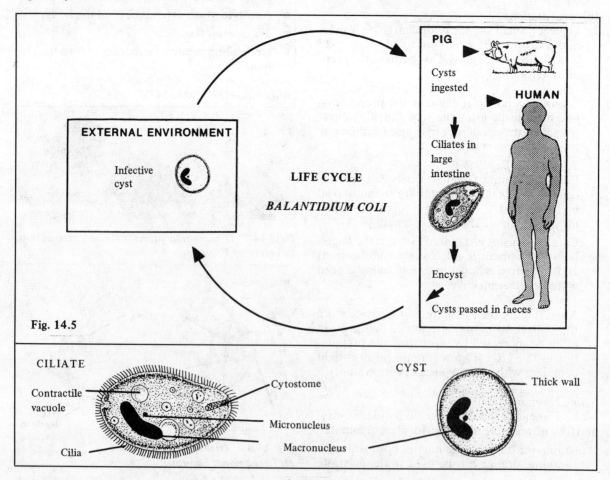

Fig. 14.5

LIFE CYCLE

BALANTIDIUM COLI

Prevention and control

Infection with *B. coli* can be avoided by not eating food which is likely to contain cysts and by improving personal hygiene especially among those who keep pigs. The cysts are rapidly killed by drying but in moist conditions they can remain infective for several weeks.

LABORATORY DIAGNOSIS

The laboratory diagnosis of balantidiasis is by:

☐ Finding *B. coli* ciliates in dysenteric faecal specimens.

☐ Finding *B. coli* cysts in formed or semiformed faeces.

Examination of faecal specimens for *B. coli* ciliates

1. Transfer a drop of fresh specimen to a slide and cover with a cover glass.

2. Examine the preparation microscopically using the 10× objective with the condenser iris closed sufficiently to give good contrast.

B. coli ciliates

Look for *large* oval shaped ciliates which have a rapid revolving motility. The ciliates are easily seen, measuring 50-200 × 40-70 μm. With focusing, the beating cilia can be seen especially in the region of the funnel-shaped cytostome (mouth), as shown in Plate 14.8 (upper).

In a stained preparation, a large bean-shaped nucleus (macronucleus) can be seen and also a small round nucleus (micronucleus) lying close to the macronucleus.

In dysenteric specimens the ciliates usually contain ingested red cells.

Note: *B. coli* ciliates degenerate rapidly in faeces and therefore specimens need to be examined while fresh.

Examination of faeces for *B. coli* cysts

1. Mix a small amount of faeces in physiological saline on one end of a slide and mix a small amount of faeces in Dobell's iodine (Reagent No. 31) on the other end of a slide. Cover each preparation with a cover glass.

2. Examine the preparations using the 10× objective with the condenser iris closed sufficiently to give good contrast.

B. coli cysts

The cysts are round or oval, *thick-walled*, and large, measuring 50-60 μm. In younger cysts, cilia are usually visible and also the macronucleus and micronucleus (seen in the iodine preparation.

An unstained cyst of *B. coli* is shown in Plate 14.8 (lower).

Balantidium coli

Ciliate
- Large, measuring 50-200 × 40-70 μm.
- Rapid revolving motility.
- Beating cilia can be seen, especially around the cytostome (mouth-end).

In stained preparations:
- Macronucleus and micronucleus can be seen.

Illustration: See Plate 14.8 (upper).

Cyst
- Large, measuring 50-60 μm.
- Thick-walled.
- Cilia may be seen in younger cysts.
- Macronucleus visible in stained preparations.

Illustration: See Plate 14.8 (lower).

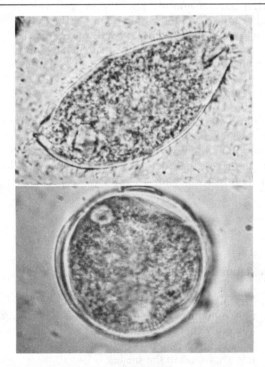

Plate 14.8 *Upper* **Ciliate of** *Balantidium coli* **(unstained) in faeces.** *Lower* **Cyst of** *B. coli*. **As seen with 40x objective.**

14:7   *ISOSPORA BELLI*
CRYPTOSPORIDIUM SPECIES

Isospora belli and *Cryptosporidium* are intestinal coccidian parasites.

ISOSPORA BELLI

Human infection with *Isospora belli* is uncommon but widely distributed. *I. belli* is thought to infect only humans.

Transmission and life cycle
Transmission of *I. belli* is by the ingestion of infective oocysts in water or food contaminated with faeces.

Life cycle
— Following ingestion, the parasites excyst and the sporozoites enter epithelial cells of the small intestine where they develop and multiply by schizogony.

— Oocysts are formed following sporogony and these are excreted in the faeces. The oocysts are immature when passed. Maturation to the infective stage takes place outside the body.

Clinical features and pathology
Human infection with *I. belli* is rarely serious and often asymptomatic. There may be abdominal pain and a mucous diarrhoea associated with malabsorption. Infection is self-limiting with any ulceration of the intestinal wall usually healing within a few weeks. There is often an eosinophilia.

Prevention and control
Infection with *I. belli* can be avoided by personal hygiene and adequate sanitation to prevent food and water becoming contaminated with faeces containing infective oocysts. After being excreted in the faeces, the oocysts take 4-5 days to develop to the infective stage.

LABORATORY DIAGNOSIS

The laboratory diagnosis of coccidiosis is by:

☐ Finding *I. belli* oocysts in the faeces. Usually only immature oocysts are found but occasionally more mature forms may be seen. In about 50% of infected persons, Charcot Leyden crystals are found in the faeces.

Examination of faeces for *I. belli* oocysts
If required, the oocysts can be concentrated by the formol ether technique or by the zinc sulphate floatation method (see Chapter 13).

The direct examination of faeces for oocysts is by mixing a small amount of faeces in saline on the end of a slide and a small amount of faeces in Dobell's iodine on the other end. The oocysts of *I. belli* can be detected with the 10× objective and identified using the 40× objective with the condenser iris adjusted to give maximum contrast.

I. belli oocysts
- Oval, measuring about 32 × 16 μm.
- Usually contain a central undivided mass of protoplasm (zygote) as shown in Plate 14.9, left.
- Occasionally, more mature oocysts may be seen as shown in Plate 14.9, right.

Illustrations: See Plate 14.9 and colour Plate 11.

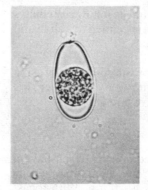 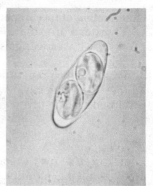

Plate 14.9 *Left* **Immature oocyst of *Isospora belli*.** *Right* **Mature oocyst of *I. belli*, as seen with 40x objective.**

CRYPTOSPORIDIUM

Cryptosporidium is associated with infection in persons with immunodeficiency such as those with acquired immune deficiency syndrome (AIDS, see 11:4), or other conditions which reduce normal immune responses, including treatment with immunosuppressive drugs.

Transmission and life cycle
Cryptosporidium species infect a wide range of animals and human infections may be zoonotic but person to person infection is also thought to occur. Infection is caused by ingesting oocysts from hands, food, or water contaminated with faeces containing infective oocysts.

The life cycle of *Cryptosporidium* is similar to that of other intestinal coccidia. The sporozoites bind to epithelial cells in the small intestine and multiply. Oocysts are produced which are excreted in the faeces.

Clinical features

In persons with abnormal immune responses e.g. AIDS patients (see 11:4), cryptosporidiosis can cause an acute and often fatal diarrhoeal disease and occasionally a respiratory infection.

Cryptosporidium can also cause gastroenteritis in persons with normal immune responses. Surveys carried out in several developing countries have indicated that *Cryptosporidium* is a significant cause of diarrhoea, especially in children below the age of 5 years. These reports have been reviewed in the paper of Baxby and Hart.[6] Infection is rare in breast fed infants.

Prevention and control

Human cryptosporidiosis is mainly prevented by personal hygiene and good sanitation. The oocysts of *Cryptosporidium* are resistant to many disinfectants but they can be killed in full-strength bleach, by formalin vapour, or in formalin solution.

LABORATORY DIAGNOSIS

The laboratory diagnosis of cryptosporidiosis is by:

☐ Finding the small oocysts of *Cryptosporidium* in stained faecal smears.

Faecal specimens from patients with acute cryptosporidiosis are watery and have an offensive odour. Pus cells are not found.

Examination of faeces for *Cryptosporidium* oocysts

Several staining techniques have been developed to detect *Cryptosporidium* oocysts in faecal smears and opinions differ as to the best technique. The techniques which are most frequently recommended are:

— A modified Ziehl-Neelsen technique.
— A safranin-methylene blue technique.

Concentration of the oocysts prior to staining is not necessary because many oocysts are usually excreted in acute infections.

Modified Ziehl-Neelsen staining technique[7]

1. Prepare a *thin* smear of a fresh faecal specimen.

   If the specimen is not a watery one, mix a sample of the faeces in fresh physiological saline and make a smear from this emulsified faeces.

2. Air-dry the smear. Fix the smear in absolute methanol for 3 minutes.

   Further fixation to ensure killing of the oocysts
   Further fixation is recommended using formalin vapour. Place the slide in an airtight container with a piece of cotton wool soaked in strong formalin solution. Leave for 20 minutes.

3. Stain the smear with cold carbol-fuchsin (Reagent No. 24) for 5-10 minutes. Wash off the stain with clean tap water.

4. Decolorize the smear using 3% hydrochloric acid in 95% ethanol until no more colour floods from the smear.

5. Rinse off the decolorizer with clean tap water.

6. Counterstain with 0.25% w/v malachite green for about 30 seconds.

7. Wash off the stain with clean water. Wipe the back of the slide clean and place it in a draining rack for the smear to dry.

8. Examine the smear microscopically for oocysts, using the 40× objective to identify the oocysts.

Cryptosporidium oocysts in a Ziehl-Neelsen stained smear
Look for small round to oval pink-red stained bodies, measuring about 5 μm in diameter, as shown in colour Plate 10. The oocysts may contain a single deeply stained dot. Some oocysts may stain palely.

Note: Yeasts and faecal debris often stain a dull red but these are easily distinguished from the oocysts. Some bacterial spores are also acid fast but these are too small to cause confusion. Very occasionally, the sporocysts of *Sarcocystis hominis* may be seen and although these are also acid fast, they are much larger than cryptosporidial oocysts.

Safranin-methylene blue staining technique[8]

1. Prepare a thin smear as described in the previous technique.

2. Air-dry the smear. Briefly pass the slide, smear uppermost, *once* through the flame of a spirit lamp or Bunsen burner.

3. Fix the smear in 3% v/v hydrochloric acid in absolute methanol for 3-5 minutes.

4. Wash with clean tap water.

5. Stain the smear with hot 1% w/v aqueous safranin solution for 1 minute.

   Heat the stain by holding a lighted spirited swab under the slide. Thorough heating is required but do not let the stain dry on the smear (add more stain if required).

6. Wash off the stain with clean tap water.

7. Counterstain with 1% w/v methylene blue for 30 seconds (other counterstains do not give as reliable results as methylene blue).

8. Wash with water. Wipe the back of the slide clean and place it in a draining rack for the smear to dry.

9. Examine the smear microscopically for oocysts, using the 40× objective (or if available 20× objective) to scan the smear and 100× objective to identify the oocysts.

Cryptosporidium oocysts in safranin-methylene blue stained smear

Look for small round to oval orange-pink bodies, measuring about 5 μm in diameter. The sporozoites within the oocyst stain slightly darker and are sometimes arranged around the periphery.

Yeasts, faecal debris, and cysts of other protozoa, stain blue. Bacterial spores stain red but they are generally smaller and do not have the same appearance as *Cryptosporidium* oocysts and the red staining sporocysts of *Sarcocystis hominis* are much larger.

Use of auramine phenol

If facilities for fluorescence microscopy are available, an auramine phenol staining technique can be used to demonstrate the oocysts of *Cryptosporidium*. This technique gives consistently good results.

14:8 *TOXOPLASMA GONDII*

Toxoplasma gondii is an animal coccidian parasite which causes toxoplasmosis, with congenital toxoplasmosis being the most serious form of human infection.

Distribution

T. gondii has a worldwide distribution. A wide range of animals serve as intermediate hosts of the parasites. The definitive hosts in which oocysts are formed are the cat and the lynx.

Transmission and life cycle

T. gondii is transmitted by the ingestion of oocysts in food, water, or from hands contaminated with faeces from an infected cat. Transmission can also occur by transplacental transmission or by ingesting the parasites in undercooked meat of an infected animal intermediate host.

Life cycle

In the natural life cycle of *T. gondii*, a cat or lynx ingests pseudocysts (containing the trophozoite forms of the parasite) in infected tissue from an intermediate animal host. After development in the intestinal cells of the cat, oocysts are produced which are excreted in the faeces of the cat. Oocyst excretion lasts up to 3 weeks. The natural life cycle is continued by an intermediate host ingesting infective oocysts.

Humans, with rodents, chickens, pigs, lambs and other animals, act as intermediate hosts of *T. gondii*. Following ingestion of infective oocysts, the parasites become intracellular and multiply in the lymph glands, liver, muscle, central nervous system, and other internal organs.

In the early acute stages of infection, the parasites (referred to as tachyzoites) invade phagocytic cells and mononuclear leucocytes. In the chronic stages of infection, the parasites (referred to as bradyzoites) multiply intracellularly in the tissues, forming cysts (pseudocysts).

Clinical features and pathology

Human toxoplasmosis may occur as an acquired infection or as a congenital infection in infants of infected mothers.

Although adult acquired infections are often asymptomatic, they can cause fever, a rash, enlargement of lymph glands with lymphocytosis, and occasionally inflammation of the eye (ocular toxoplasmosis), myocarditis, meningoencephalitis, and atypical pneumonia. In some infected persons the only clinical symptom is fever.

Serious and often fatal opportunistic *Toxoplasma* infections can occur in those with abnormal immune responses, e.g. patients with acquired immune deficiency syndrome (AIDS).

Congenital toxoplasmosis

Intra-uterine infection with *T. gondii* can cause severe and often fatal cerebral damage to a foetus. Infants who recover often show evidence of mental defects.

Infection occurring in early pregnancy may result in abortion or the still-birth of a foetus, while infection late in pregnancy may cause symptoms of infection to develop in the infant 2-3 months after birth.

Prevention and control

The risk of infection with *T. gondii* can be reduced by controlling the numbers of stray domestic cats and avoiding the contamination of hands, food, and water with cat faeces.

Transmission of trophozoites can be avoided by not eating raw or undercooked meat such as pork, mutton, beef, or game which may contain the parasites. Generally, meat that has been heated in all parts up to 65 °C and kept at that temperature for 4-5 minutes or longer, will not contain viable parasites. At 4 °C, *Toxoplasma* parasites in meat can survive for up to three weeks but they are killed if the meat is kept frozen at −15 °C for at least 3 days.

LABORATORY DIAGNOSIS

The laboratory diagnosis of toxoplasmosis is by:

☐ Serological tests, but the interpretation of results is often difficult because of the high prevalence of antibody in nearly all populations due to subclinical infections which are very common. A high antibody titre, particularly of Ig M, must be considered in relation to the clinical findings. It is important to test for a rising antibody titre.

☐ Occasionally in acute infections a diagnosis can be confirmed by identifying toxoplasms in Giemsa or Field's stained preparations of:

— lymph node aspirates
— bone marrow aspirates
— cerebrospinal fluid
— peritoneal or pleural fluids
— sputum

Animal inoculation in the diagnosis of toxoplasmosis
Animal inoculation is sometimes used in the diagnosis of toxoplasmosis. A specimen from the patient such as a bone marrow aspirate, cerebrospinal fluid, lymph node fluid, or peritoneal fluid is inoculated into white mice (known to be uninfected). If the inoculated specimen is infected with *Toxoplasma*, the parasites will produce a generalized infection in the mice 3-10 days after inoculation. The mice are tested for infection by examining wet preparations of peritoneal exudate, ventricular aspirates or biopsy from lymph nodes, liver, or spleen.

Other tests
☐ Total white blood cell count (WBC) and differential count. In acquired toxoplasmosis, a blood lymphocytosis is a common finding with many atypical mononuclear cells being seen in the blood film. The blood picture often resembles that seen in infectious mononucleosis (glandular fever).

☐ The results of cerebrospinal fluid tests (in meningoencephalitis) may include a raised protein level and presence of lymphocytes.

Serological diagnosis of toxoplasmosis
Tests used in the serological diagnosis of toxoplasmosis include the Sabin-Feldman dye test, an indirect fluorescent antibody test (IFAT), an indirect haemagglutination test (IHA), and a complement fixation test (CFT). More recently, enzyme linked immunosorbent assays (ELISA) have been developed and are claimed to be more specific than other tests, especially the IFAT.[9]

Sabin Feldman dye test
This test is sensitive but because it requires the use of live toxoplasms it is not as widely used as the other more recently developed tests which do not require the use of viable parasites.

IFAT
Antigens and reagents for the IFAT, together with instructions for use, are commercially available from several manufacturers and suppliers including Wellcome Diagnostics, Hoechst Company, and bioMérieux (for addresses see Appendix II).

In diagnosing congenital toxoplasmosis, it is necessary to test for Ig M antibodies in the serum of the infant. If such antibodies are present, they must have been formed by the infant in response to an active infection because Ig M antibodies cannot cross the placenta.

IHA
An IHA for the serological diagnosis of toxoplasmosis is available from Wellcome Diagnostics. The test, which is called *Tox-HA-Test*, is a valuable test because it indicates both the stage and degree of infection.

Microscopical examination of aspirates and fluids for toxoplasms
1. Make a smear of the specimen on a slide and air-dry.

   If the specimen is a fluid, centrifuge it first for 5-10 minutes at medium to high speed to obtain a sediment from which to make a smear.

2. Fix the smear with absolute methanol for 1-2 minutes.

3. Stain the smear using Giemsa staining technique (see 13:14) or Field's rapid *thin* film technique (see 13:16).

4. Examine the preparation microscopically using the 40× objective to detect the parasites and the 100× objective to identify the toxoplasms.

T. gondii toxoplasms

The parasites are crescent shaped and small, measuring about $3 \times 7\ \mu m$. One end is rounded and the other end is pointed as shown in Plate 14.10 and colour Plate 13. The cytoplasm stains blue and a dark red stained nucleus will be seen towards the rounded end of the toxoplasm.

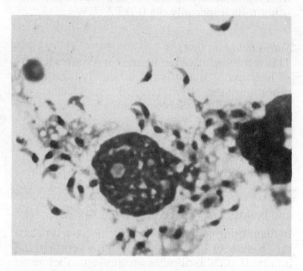

Plate 14.10 Stained *Toxoplasma gondii* as seen with the 100x oil immersion objective.
Courtesy of V. Zaman.

Toxoplasma in tissue sections

Toxoplasma may occasionally be found in a tissue section in which the organisms may appear round and resemble *Leishmania* amastigotes, but the infected tissue will have a characteristic histological appearance. A direct FAT is available to identify *Toxoplasma* parasites in tissue sections.

References

1 World Health Organization. *Informal Meeting on Strategies for Control of Amoebiasis*, WHO/PDP/845, WHO/CDD/PAR/84.2, 1984.

2 Stamm, W. P. and Phillips, E. A. A cellulose acetate membrane precipitin (CAP) test for amoebiasis. *Transactions of the Royal Society of Tropical Medicine and Hygiene*, **71**, 6, p. 490-492.

3 Moody, A. H. A. Fluorescent technique for demonstrating the chromatoid bodies and nuclei in cysts of *Entamoeba histolytica* from faecal deposits. *Journal of Clinical Pathology*, **37**, (1), p. 101-102, 1984.

4 Warhurst, D. C. Pathogenic free living amoebae, *Parasitology Today*, **1**, 1, p. 24-28, 1985.

5 Green, E. L., Miles, M. A., Warhurst, D. C. Immunodiagnostic detection of *Giardia* antigen in faeces by a rapid visual enzyme-linked immunosorbent assay. *Lancet*, **ii** (Sept. 28), p. 691-693, 1985.

6 Baxby, D. and Hart, C. A. Human cryptosporidiosis. *Postgraduate Doctor Africa*, **8**, (6), p. 176-181, 1986.

7 The modified Ziehl-Neelsen staining technique described has been kindly supplied by the laboratory of the Hospital for Tropical Diseases in London.

8 Baxby, D., Blundell, N., Hart, C. A. The development and performance of a simple, sensitive method for the detection of *Cryptosporidium* oocysts in faeces. *Journal of Hygiene*, **92**, p. 317-323, 1984.

9 Naot, Y., Remington, J. S. An ELISA for detection of Ig M antibodies to *T. gondii*. *Journal of Infectious Diseases*, **142**, p. 757-766, 1980.

Malaria Parasites

15:1 CLASSIFICATION AND BASIC FEATURES OF MALARIA PARASITES

Malaria parasites are protozoan parasites belonging to the subclass Coccidia. The general characteristics of protozoa are described at the beginning of the Parasitology section in 12:4.

Classification of malaria parasites of medical importance

Class	SPOROZOA
Subclass	Coccidia
Family	Plasmodiidae

Widespread species	*Plasmodium falciparum*
	Plasmodium vivax
Less widespread species	*Plasmodium malariae*
	Plasmodium ovale

Subdivision of *Plasmodium*

The genus *Plasmodium* is subdivided into the subgenus *Laverania* and the subgenus of the same name, i.e. *Plasmodium*.

P. falciparum belongs to the subgenus *Laverania* and *P. vivax*, *P. ovale* and *P. malariae* belong to the subgenus *Plasmodium*.

Features of malaria parasites infecting humans

- In their human host, malaria parasites have an asexual intracellular cycle of development called schizogony. The parasites live and multiply, first in the cells of the liver and then in the red cells.

  The forms of the parasite which rupture from the red cells infect new red cells. Some of these, instead of repeating red cell schizogony, develop into gametocytes which are the sexual forms of the parasite by which it is transmitted to the mosquito to continue its life cycle.

  In the mosquito, a sexual extracellular cycle of development occurs called sporogony. In this, male and female gametes are formed, fertilization occurs, and sporozoites are produced which are infective to humans.

- Transmission occurs when the sporozoites are injected by an infected female *Anopheles* mosquito when it takes a blood meal.

  For the *Plasmodium* species that infect humans, there are no natural animal reservoir hosts. Monkeys become infected with *Plasmodium malariae* but they are not thought to be important reservoirs of human infection.

- Laboratory confirmation of infection with malaria parasites is by finding the parasites in stained blood films. In malaria surveys and control work, immunodiagnosis is used.

- Malaria is the most important and widespread of parasitic diseases in tropical developing countries with falciparum malaria being responsible for more deaths than any other disease. As explained in 15:2, resistance of the parasite to drugs and of Anopheline mosquitoes to insecticides are serious problems in the control of falciparum malaria.

- Relapses due to hypnozoites (dormant forms which precede schizont development in the liver) occur in vivax malaria and less commonly in ovale malaria. Recrudescences of malaria (due to small numbers of erythrocytic parasites remaining in the blood after a previous attack) occur in falciparum malaria and over a long period in malariae infection.

15:2 *PLASMODIUM FALCIPARUM*

Malaria caused by *Plasmodium falciparum* is referred to as falciparum malaria, formerly known as subtertian (ST) or malignant tertian (MT) malaria. It is the most serious form of the disease and the most widespread, accounting for up to 80% of malaria cases worldwide.[1]

Varieties of *Plasmodium falciparum*

The species *Plasmodium falciparum* contains several 'varieties' which show differences in geographical distribution, vector susceptibility, human infection pattern, drug susceptibility, morphology and antigenic composition.[1]

Distribution

P. falciparum is found mainly in the hotter and more humid regions of the world. It is the main species found in tropical and subtropical Africa and parts of Central America and South America, Bangladesh, Pakistan, Afghanistan, Nepal, Sri Lanka, South East Asia, Indonesia, Philippines, Haiti, Solomon Islands, Papua New Guinea and many islands in Melanesia. It also occurs in parts of

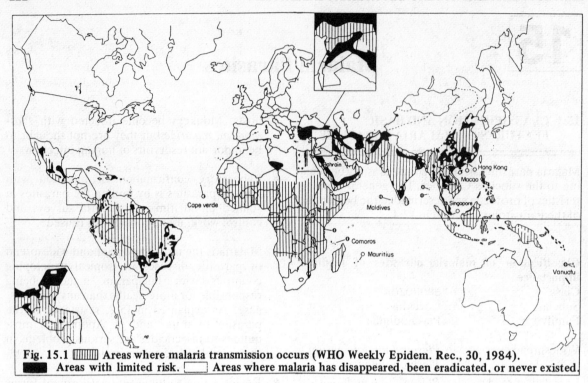

Fig. 15.1 ▦ **Areas where malaria transmission occurs (WHO Weekly Epidem. Rec., 30, 1984).**
■ **Areas with limited risk.** ☐ **Areas where malaria has disappeared, been eradicated, or never existed.**

India, the Middle East, eastern Mediterranean and countries of North Africa.

Areas of significant *P. falciparum* transmission are shown in Fig. 15.1.

Transmission and life cycle

The main factors which influence the epidemiology of falciparum malaria are the intensity of transmission and the immune response of the infected person.

Malaria transmission in an area may be:
- Stable
- Unstable

Stable malaria

In areas where malaria transmission is stable, transmission occurs for at least 6 months in a year and is intense. Children suffer repeated attacks from the age of a few months. Those who do not die, have a substantial immunity by the age of five or six years. When immunity is established, patients may still suffer attacks of malaria but these are comparatively mild and last for only a few days. Older people are little affected.

There is little variation in the incidence of malaria from year to year although there may be marked seasonal fluctuations, particularly in children.

Unstable malaria

In areas where malaria transmission is unstable, there are marked changes in transmission from one season to another and from one year to the next. The transmission season is short and infection of any one individual is comparatively infrequent so that immunity is unable to reach a high level.

When an outbreak of malaria occurs, usually following explosive breeding of mosquitoes, it does so in the form of an epidemic with people of all ages being susceptible and often severely at risk.

Terms used to describe the level of endemicity of malaria
The terms used are hypoendemicity (lowest level), mesoendemicity, hyperendemicity and holoendemicity (highest level). These terms define the increasing levels of prevalence of malaria as estimated by surveys of spleen and parasite rates in particular age groups.

Holoendemic and hyperendemic malaria are found in areas of stable transmission whereas mesoendemic and hypoendemic malaria are found in areas of unstable transmission.

P. falciparum is transmitted by many species of female Anopheline mosquitoes (see 23:3). The important species and their distribution are listed by Bruce-Chwatt in *Essential Malariology*.[2]

P. falciparum can also be transmitted by transfusion of infected donor blood or by injection through the use of needles and syringes contaminated with infected blood. Very occasionally, congenital transmission occurs, usually when a mother is non-immune.

Life cycle of P. falciparum
— Sporozoites contained in the saliva of an infected *Anopheles* mosquito are injected into

the blood of a human host when the vector takes a blood meal.

The sporozoites are elongate bodies measuring about 11 μm in length, with a central nucleus.

— After circulating in the bloodstream for not more than one hour, the sporozoites enter liver cells (hepatocytes) probably by way of the Kupffer cells.

— In liver cells, *P. falciparum* parasites grow, multiply and develop directly into schizonts (there is no hypnozoite stage). The schizonts in the liver are referred to as pre- erythrocytic (PE) schizonts.

PE schizonts of *P. falciparum* take 5½-7 days to develop. When mature each measures about 60 μm in diameter and contains up to 30 000 merozoites.

— When mature, the schizont and liver cell rupture and the merozoites enter the blood stream. To survive, the merozoites must enter red cells (erythrocytes) within a few minutes of being released from the schizont.

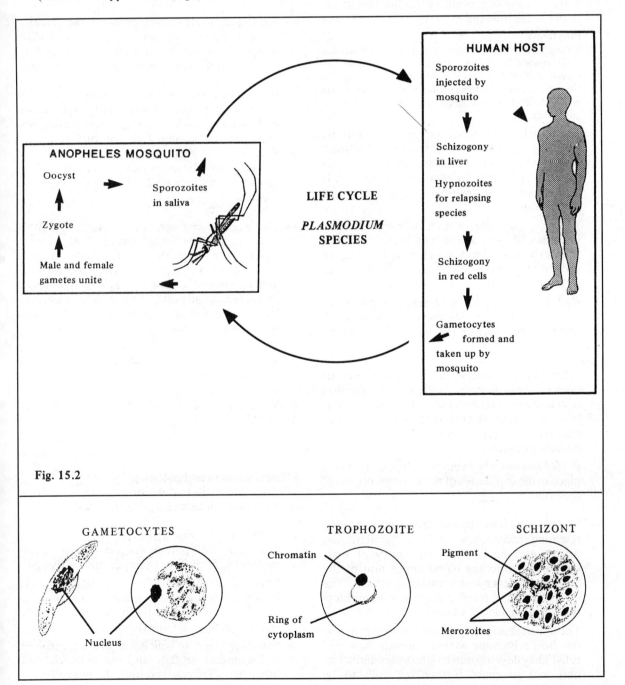

Fig. 15.2

— Most of the merozoites enter red cells in the sinusoids of the liver. A proportion are phagocytosed and destroyed.

How malaria parasites infect red cells

The merozoites become attached to red cells by special organelles which bind to specific glycophorin protein receptors on the red cell membrane. The membrane becomes indented and the parasite enters.

Entry of the parasites into red cells starts a cycle in the blood (erythrocytic cycle) which for *P. falciparum* takes 36-48 hours to complete.

— The merozoite develops into a trophozoite within a vacuole formed by the internal membrane of the host red cell.

Ring forms

Young trophozoites are concave disks which appear ring- shaped in stained preparations because the centre of the disk is very thin and does not stain. The ring of cytoplasm contains the organelles. The nucleus is clearly visible as a single or sometimes double chromatin dot.

The trophozoite feeds on haemoglobin by ingesting small amounts of red cell cytoplasm. Malaria pigment (haemozoin) forms as an end-product of haemoglobin breakdown. It accumulates as brown-black granules in the trophozoite.

As the trophozoite grows it becomes globular in form and the vacuole membrane enlarges. Maurer's clefts form which can be seen in stained preparations as irregular sized mauve-red staining 'dots'.

Red cells containing late stage trophozoites and schizonts of *P. falciparum* develop small knobs on their surface (visible by electron microscopy).

— When the trophozoite is fully developed, its nucleus begins to divide, followed by a division of cytoplasm. This process (schizogony) results in the formation of a schizont. A mature *P. falciparum* schizont contains 8-32 merozoites and malaria pigment.

P. falciparum erythrocytic schizogony takes place in the capillaries of the internal organs of the body.

— Mature schizonts rupture from the red cells, releasing merozoites, malaria pigment and toxins into the plasma. The entry of toxic metabolites into the blood circulation of the host causes fever and a 'malarial attack'. The incubation time for *P. falciparum* from infection to an attack is 9-14 days.

Those merozoites which are not destroyed by the host's immune system, invade new red cells. They develop into trophozoites and schizonts and so cause further red cells to be destroyed. In falciparum malaria, large numbers of red cells can become infected and many cells may contain more than one trophozoite.

— After several erythrocytic cycles, some of the merozoites enter red cells and instead of developing into schizonts they follow a sexual development and become gametocytes.

Gametocytes are thought to form in response to a developing immunity (raised antibody levels), lack of nutrients, or an accumulation of metabolites or parasitic debris. Their presence in the blood is not proof of active infection.

— For the life cycle to be continued, the gametocytes need to be ingested by a female *Anopheles* mosquito in a blood meal. If they are not taken up by a mosquito vector, they die.

— In the stomach of the mosquito, the male gametocyte rapidly divides into a number of male gametes each with a flagellum (exflagellation). These become free and highly motile. Following contact and entry into a female gamete, fertilization occurs. The male nucleus fuses with the female nucleus and a zygote is formed.

— The zygote develops into a motile ookinete which penetrates the stomach wall of the mosquito, forming an oocyst. Inside the oocyst, large numbers of sporozoites are formed. When mature the sporozoites leave the oocyst and spread to all parts of the mosquito, particularly to the salivary glands, ready to be transmitted when the insect next takes a blood meal.

Development of *P. falciparum* in the *Anopheles* mosquito (sporogony) takes 9-10 days at approx 28 °C.

Note: The life cycle of *P. falciparum* is summarized in Fig. 15.2 (see also p. 251).

Clinical features and pathology

The characteristic feature of malaria is fever. It usually occurs in three stages as follows:

— Cold stage, characterized by rigor and headache. The patient feels cold and shivers even though his or her temperature is rising.

— Fever stage, in which the temperature rises to its maximum and the headache is severe. Usually there are pains in the back and joints and often vomiting and diarrhoea.

— Sweating stage, in which the patient perspires, the temperature falls and the headache and other pains are relieved until the next rigor.

With falciparum malaria, attacks of fever may recur on alternate days or more commonly the fever tends to be continuous or irregular.

Pathogenicity of P. falciparum

P. falciparum is the most pathogenic of the human malaria species. Its pathogenicity is due mainly to:

☐ Erythrocytic schizogony taking place in the deep capillaries of organs such as the brain, heart, spleen, intestines, lungs, bone marrow and placenta.

☐ Changes on the surface of parasitized red cells (especially those containing mature forms of the parasite) which cause the cells to adhere to one another and to the cells lining the walls of capillaries. This leads to the sequestration (holding back) of infected red cells in the capillaries of internal organs, with subsequent congestion, hypoxia, blockage and sometimes rupture of small blood vessels. When in the capillaries of the internal organs, the parasites evade destruction by the spleen and continue their development, producing merozoites to invade new red cells.

☐ High levels of parasitaemia with the density of parasites often exceeding more than 250 000-300 000 /μl of blood. Up to 30-40% of the red cells may become parasitized in falciparum malaria. Such high levels of parasitaemia do not occur with other *Plasmodium* species.

Severe falciparum malaria

A falciparum infection should be considered as severe when more than 5% of the red cells become parasitized.[4]

Severe falciparum malaria is more likely to occur in a non-immune person (no previous exposure), person with lapsed immunity, pregnant woman (particularly primigravid), an immunosuppressed person, or following splenectomy.

The following complications are associated with severe falciparum malaria:

● Cerebral malaria: This is the commonest cause of death in falciparum malaria and is due to parasitized red cells and fibrin blocking capillaries and venules in the brain. Haemorrhaging from these small blood vessels may occur.

A recommended definition of cerebral malaria is 'the presence of unarousable coma, exclusion of other encephalopathies and confirmation of *P. falciparum* infection'.[3] This definition has been proposed to differentiate the serious condition of cerebral malaria from mental confusion, delirium, convulsions or other neurological symptoms associated with high fever, particularly in children.

Cerebral malaria usually occurs with heavy parasitaemia but it has been known to occur when the number of parasites are few. Children and non-immune adults are more commonly affected.

There is usually a neutrophilia and the cerebrospinal fluid (c.s.f.) may contain cells, a raised protein and low glucose. Raised c.s.f. lactate levels are also found in cerebral malaria.

● Anaemia: This can be severe and occur rapidly, particularly in young children.

Anaemia in falciparum malaria is due mainly to the mechanical destruction of parasitized red cells. Parasitized cells also lose their deformability and are rapidly phagocytosed and destroyed in the spleen. The production of red cells in the bone marrow is also reduced and there is a slow reticulocyte response. In a small number of patients, an immune destruction of red cells may occur.

Malaria attacks following treatment with iron
Iron is essential for the growth of *P. falciparum*. Rises in serum iron levels following treatment with iron, have been shown to increase the incidence of acute malaria attacks.

● Blackwater fever: This is a rare but acute condition in which there is a rapid and massive intravascular haemolysis of both parasitized and non-parasitized red cells, resulting in haemoglobinaemia, haemoglobinuria, and fall in haemoglobin. It is accompanied by high fever, vomiting, and jaundice and is often fatal due to renal failure. Following a haemolytic attack the parasites are difficult to find in the blood.

The urine appears dark red to brown-black (hence the name blackwater fever) due to the presence of free haemoglobin in the form of methaemoglobin and oxyhaemoglobin. The urine contains protein, hyaline and granular casts, and epithelial debris.

The exact cause of blackwater fever is not fully understood. It is thought that following repeated attacks of falciparum malaria, a person forms an autoimmune factor which results in a rapid haemolytic reaction if the person becomes infected with the same strain of *P. falciparum* that caused the autosensitivity. It occurs most frequently in non-immune persons who suffer repeated attacks of falciparum malaria and take antimalarials irregularly and inadequately to relieve their attacks. Excessive cold, abnormal physical activity, or alcohol abuse have also been reported as triggering a haemolytic attack.

Blackwater fever needs to be differentiated from haemoglobinuria caused by haemolysis due to heavy parasitaemia or glucose- 6-phosphate dehydrogenase (G6PD) deficiency. Haemolysis due to G6PD deficiency usually begins about 3 days after the deficient person ingests fava beans (or inhales fava bean pollen) or takes drugs such as phenacetin, sulphonamides, primaquine, pamaquine, pentaquine, nitrofurans, or para-aminosalicylic acid and ends when a new population of red cells is produced (only older red cells are normally affected).

● Diarrhoea and vomiting: These features are common in acute and severe falciparum malaria, especially in children and non-immune adults.

● Pulmonary oedema: This complication is rare but often fatal. It frequently accompanies renal failure and occurs when there is heavy parasitaemia especially during pregnancy or following childbirth.

● Hypoglycaemia: This finding is being increasingly reported in patients with severe malaria, especially children, pregnant women, and in those treated with quinine and quinidine.[4]

Falciparum malaria in pregnancy
Immunosuppression in pregnancy, particularly during the second half of pregnancy, can lead to heavy parasitic infection on the maternal side of the placenta with subsequent haemolysis, resulting in abortion, premature labour, and occasionally stillbirth and neonatal death. Placental infection is also associated with the birth of low weight infants.

It is also thought that heavy and prolonged infection of the placenta in late pregnancy can result in less Ig G crossing into the foetal circulation and therefore less protection against malaria in the first few months of life.

The protection normally afforded to sickle cell heterozygotes (HbAS) against severe falciparum is lost in pregnancy.

Immunity to malaria
As already explained under *Transmission*, the natural acquiring of immunity to malaria depends on repeated exposure to infection and is not easily developed in areas of unstable malaria transmission.

Even in areas of stable malaria transmission, the acquiring of immunity is slow. In the first few months of life, an infant (born of an immune mother) is normally protected by Ig G antibodies from its mother and by the high concentration of haemoglobin F in its red cells (Hb F is thought to discourage the growth of the erythrocytic forms of the parasite). Following repeated infection, an infant normally acquires a natural immunity to malaria by about the age of 5 years.

The antibodies produced in response to infection are directed mainly against merozoites, preventing the reinvasion of red cells, and also against erythrocytic schizonts resulting in a more rapid phagocytosis of parasitized cells or the intracellular death of parasites. Anti-sporozoite antibodies are also thought to be produced.

T lymphocytes are required for the development of effective immunity. Macrophages in the spleen, liver and bone marrow, phagocytose both parasitized and nonparasitized red cells, free parasites, and malaria pigment. T cells control macrophage activation and the intracellular destruction of parasites.

Acquired immunity is specific for a given species and strain of *Plasmodium* and is also stage-specific. When an immune person leaves a malaria endemic area, their acquired immunity is soon lost. Naturally acquired immunity can be suppressed in pregnancy (see previous text), in certain infections and serious illnesses, and when taking immunosuppressive drugs.

Acute falciparum malaria causes immunosuppression in the host. In young children, this leads to poor immune responses to vaccinations and inadequate immune responses to other parasitic infections, bacterial infections, and to viruses. Suppression of the normal immune response to Epstein-Barr virus (EBV), may lead to the development of Burkitt's lymphoma. It has been observed that the distribution of this form of cancer in Africa is particularly common in areas where falciparum malaria is endemic. In acute falciparum malaria, T cells are reduced and B cells increase.

Biological resistance against malaria
Some individuals living in malaria endemic areas of the world have a natural, or innate, resistance to malaria based on the inheritance of selected resistance genes expressed in red cells.

Genes which select against falciparum malaria include:

— Haemoglobin S gene
— Thalassaemia genes
— Glucose-6-phosphate dehydrogenase (G6PD) deficiency genes
— Ovalocytosis gene

With regard to some genes that confer resistance to falciparum malaria but themselves cause severe clinical effects and death such as HbS and the thalassaemia genes, there occurs a situation referred to as balanced polymorphism. In this, heterozygotes such as sickle cell trait individuals (HbAS) have a special protection against the serious effects of falciparum malaria compared with other members of the population who are not so protected and who are therefore more likely to die from falciparum malaria. These deaths thus balance those caused by the homozygous state of the gene (HbSS). In this situation falciparum malaria is actually responsible for maintaining the high frequency of HbS (or other gene causing severe disease) in a population. It is to be expected, therefore, that when falciparum malaria is brought under control that the frequency of the HbS gene and other severe genes selected by malaria will very slowly begin to decrease in populations.

Mechanisms by which resistance genes protect against malaria

Haemoglobin S
Protection is afforded only to heterozygous persons (Hb AS) against severe falciparum malaria. The protective mechanism is not fully understood. Cells containing HbAS sickle more quickly when they contain parasites than when they are nonparasitized, probably because the parasites lower the pH which leads to damage and sickling. The parasites in these cells are then thought to be rapidly phagocytosed. The parasites are therefore destroyed before they develop into schizonts. In homozygotes (HbSS), the phagocytic action of the spleen is frequently inadequate and the removal of parasitized cells will also need to compete with the removal of nonparasitized irreversibly sickled cells. Homozygous (HbSS) persons may die from severe falciparum malaria.

Thalassaemia genes
The protective mechanism of beta-thalassaemia trait is not yet fully understood. It has been suggested that parasites are able to invade thalassaemic cells but can be injured by the increased sensitivity of the cell membrane of such cells to peroxide damage.

G6PD deficient genes
The gene for G6PD is sex-linked and therefore only females can represent the heterozygous state for deficiency of the enzyme. Such individuals have a double population of red cells, one normal and one with G6PD deficient activity. Studies of females within the group who had malaria at the time, have shown that the G6PD positive cells contained more parasites than the G6PD negative cells. The reason for this is not yet understood. It seems that parasite development is normal in G6PD deficient males (hemizygotes) and therefore the protective mechanism in heterozygotes must in some way be associated with the fact that such females possess the double population of enzyme negative and positive red cells (genetic mosaicism) which interferes with the adaptation of the parasite to the G6PD deficient conditions in the cell.

Ovalocytosis
Ovalocytic (elliptical) red cells show a relative resistance to *P. falciparum*, probably due to their morphological abnormality but possibly also to the antigenic composition of their cell membrane. There is a high incidence of ovalocytosis in falciparum malaria endemic areas of Papua New Guinea.

Hyper-reactive malaria splenomegaly
Transient splenomegaly occurs with acute malaria in children and non-immune adults. In malaria endemic areas, a chronic form of splenomegaly can be found in children. These forms of splenomegaly (and splenomegaly which occurs in other tropical diseases), require differentiation from the condition referred to as tropical splenomegaly syndrome (TSS), or more recently called hyper-reactive malaria splenomegaly.[5]

Persons with hyper-reactive malaria splenomegaly are immune adults in malarious areas who have gross and chronic splenomegaly, with an overproduction of Ig M, high levels of malaria antibody and circulating immune complexes, and a moderately enlarged liver with hepatic sinusoidal lymphocytosis. The patient is usually anaemic (normocytic) and has a low white cell count and reduced platelet count.

The condition responds to prolonged treatment with antimalarial drugs. It is associated with vivax and quartan malaria as well as falciparum malaria and is thought to be due in part to inadequate T lymphocyte control.

Recrudescence of falciparum malaria
The occurrence of clinical falciparum malaria caused by parasites persisting in the circulation at a subclinical level following a previous attack, is referred to as a recrudescence.

A recrudescence is different to a malaria relapse, which can occur with vivax or ovale malaria (due to the delayed development of hypnozoites in the liver, see 15:3). There is no hypnozoite stage with *P. falciparum*.

A falciparum recrudescence can occur within a few weeks or months of a previous attack. If due to drug resistance, a recrudescence may occur within 2 weeks of the start of treatment. Most recrudescences die out within a year of the original attack.

A recrudescence may occur due to inadequate drug therapy, drug resistance, or when a person's natural acquired immunity is reduced, e.g. during pregnancy.

Prevention and control
In the 1986 Report of the *WHO Expert Committee on Malaria*, it is recommended that malaria control should be based on an epidemiological approach and that it should be planned and co-ordinated within primary health care with the active participation of the community.[6]

Control measures

Measures used to prevent and control malaria include:

- Avoiding mosquito bites by:
  - selecting healthy sites for houses on the tops of hills, exposed to prevailing wind, and away from known mosquito breeding sites whenever possible.
  - screening windows and doors with mosquito netting.
  - using effective mosquito bed nets during the biting hours of the local mosquito vector. The impregnation of nets with insecticides such as permethrin increases protection.
  - wearing protective clothing such as long trousers, long skirts, sarongs, and garments with long sleeves.
  - using mosquito repellents such as oil of citronella, dimethyl phthalate, mosquito repellent coils, or smoke from fires or from burning pyrethrum pellets.

- Using drugs to:
  - treat active infections, particularly in young children (early diagnosis and treatment are essential).
  - suppress infections until they die out.
  - prevent infections, especially in non-immune persons visiting or going to work in malarious areas or in persons with reduced immunity such as pregnant women.

- Preventing the breeding of mosquito larvae by:
  - altering the habitat to discourage breeding, e.g. preserving or planting vegetation where the vector needs sunshine or clearing vegetation where the vector needs shade.
  - flooding or flushing of breeding places.
  - draining to remove surface water and filling in ponds, pot-holes, drainage ditches, etc.
  - changing the salt content of the water.
  - regularly spraying breeding sites with oil or chemicals.

- Destroying adult mosquitoes by regular spraying of all houses with residual insecticides such as DDT (used twice yearly) or malathion (used every 3 months) as part of a control programme and providing there is no resistance of the mosquitoes to the insecticide.

- Health education in schools and villages, and training primary health care workers how to teach malaria control measures.

Important: Community measures aimed at the destruction of mosquito larvae and adults can only be applied intelligently when the breeding and feeding habits of the local vectors are known. A method which is effective in one area against one mosquito may fail or make the situation worse in another area which has a different mosquito vector.

It is necessary to use long term effective methods. The use of short term methods in an area of intense malaria transmission may have only a temporary effect and interfere with a valuable acquired immunity built up by people over the years at cost of life and suffering. Long-lasting control aimed at the eradication of malaria may be difficult to achieve.

Immunization against malaria

Because of the heavy loss of life, suffering and socioeconomic damage caused particularly by falciparum malaria, the World Health Organization within its *Tropical Disease Research Programme* and in collaboration with drug companies, has intensified its efforts in recent years to develop effective vaccines against malaria.

Three types of vaccines are being researched:

□ Anti-sporozoite vaccines, aimed at preventing disease. These types of vaccines are the most advanced and likely to become available first within the next few years.

□ Vaccines against the asexual forms of the parasite in the blood. Specific antigens have been characterized and cloned and clinical trials are due to begin in 1987.

□ Anti-gametocyte vaccines, with the purpose of controlling the transmission of malaria. When human blood containing anti-gametocyte antibodies is taken up by a mosquito vector, these antibodies will prevent the fertilization and development of the parasite in the vector. Such vaccines are therefore referred to as transmission-blocking vaccines and it is hoped that they will be effective, together with other control measures, in preventing malaria.

Most of the vaccine research and development work has been directed against *P. falciparum* because this is the most pathogenic species, but vaccines are also being researched against *P. vivax* and *P. malariae*.

Note: Further information about the transmission and control of malaria can be found in the:

- The 1982 World Health Organization report *Malaria Control and National Health Goals*, Technical Report Series No. 680.*
- The 1984 World Health Organization report *Malaria Control as Part of Primary Health Care*, Technical Report Series No. 712.*

- The 1986 World Health Organization report of the *Expert Committee on Malaria*, Technical Report Series No. 735.*

- The 1985 publication, *Essential Malariology* by L. J. Bruce-Chwatt.[2]

*Available from World Health Organization, 1211 Geneva, 27 Switzerland or other distributor of WHO publications.

LABORATORY DIAGNOSIS

With the spread of *P. falciparum* resistance to drugs and the increasing difficulty in controlling falciparum malaria in some areas, it is important to diagnose malaria accurately and to treat it correctly.

Where alternative more expensive drugs and those with greater side effects have to be used, the laboratory can help to ensure that such drugs are used only when necessary. The correct use of new drugs is essential to prevent resistance from developing.

Whenever possible, the laboratory diagnosis of malaria should form part of primary health care. The early diagnosis of a malaria attack is particularly important in young children (3 months-3 years) where severe untreated falciparum infections can be life-threatening and where chemoprophylaxis in areas of stable malaria transmission is undesirable because it delays the development of naturally acquired immunity. An early and accurate diagnosis of falciparum malaria in non-immune adults and pregnant women is also important (see previous text).

Laboratory investigations
The microscopical identification of parasites in blood is the most certain method of confirming infection with *P. falciparum*.

Currently available serological techniques are mainly of value in epidemiological work.

Microscopical laboratory techniques for investigating falciparum malaria include:

☐ Examination of stained thick blood films to detect the parasites and to examine white cells for malaria pigment.

☐ Examination of stained thin blood films to identify the species (when this cannot be done from the thick film) and to give an estimate of the percentage of red cells infected. Heavy parasitaemia in falciparum malaria is associated with severe disease which requires special treatment and follow-up.

Other methods of quantifying falciparum parasites can also be used (see later text).

☐ Examination of the buffy coat and red cells immediately below it after centrifuging blood in a small narrow bore tube. This can sometimes help to detect parasites when they are few in number, particularly late stage trophozoites and gametocytes (see 15:6). Malaria pigment is often more easily detected in this type of preparation because the white cells are concentrated.

Important: Whenever blood films are examined for malaria parasites, the opportunity should *always* be taken to look also for other parasites and any significant changes in the white cells (numbers, types, morphology), or red cells (clues for anaemia). Abnormalities which should be reported are listed in 15:6. In the presence of fever but absence of malaria parasites and pigment, an alternative diagnosis may be suggested such as a bacterial or viral infection, sickle cell disease, trypanosomiasis, or relapsing fever.

Future techniques
Future tests for diagnosing malaria and screening donor blood for parasites will probably involve the use of DNA probes or other techniques based on biotechnology and genetic engineering. While such techniques are capable of providing highly specific and rapid results, further research and development are needed to ensure adequate sensitivity, stability, and availability at affordable prices.

Other tests
☐ Measurement of haemoglobin. This should always be done when there is heavy parasitaemia, particularly in children below the age of 5 years when blood loss due to haemolysis, and anoxia, can be fatal. The haemoglobin should be tested at least daily.

☐ Blood urea or serum creatinine if renal damage is suspected.

☐ Testing of urine for free haemoglobin if blackwater fever is suspected. If haemoglobinuria is present, the patient should be screened for G6PD deficiency (see previous text for drugs which can cause acute haemolysis in G6PD deficient persons).

☐ Tests for liver function if liver cell damage is suspected. Measurement of serum bilirubin, albumin and aspartate aminotransferase can provide useful information.

☐ A platelet count and measurement of plasma fibrinogen, FDPs (fibrin/fibrinogen degradation products), activated partial thromboplastin time test (APTT) and prothrombin time (PT) if disseminated intravascular coagulation (DIC) or other abnormal bleeding is suspected.

Note: Although a transitory positive direct Coombs test can often be found in falciparum malaria (providing a Coomb's reagent capable of detecting Ig G and complement is used), the test is not usually required in the management of falciparum malaria.

Examination of blood

The blood must be collected and whenever possible the films reported before treatment is started. Malaria parasites are extremely difficult to find and recognise in blood films within a few hours of treatment (unless drug resistance is present).

Thick and thin blood films

The making of *both* thick and thin blood films is recommended. A thick and thin film can be prepared on the same slide. The technique of doing this and the staining of blood films are described in 15:6.

Microscopical examination of blood films for P. falciparum

In falciparum malaria, because parasitaemia is often heavy, it can be easily forgotten that small numbers of parasites can be present in light infections or if a blood film is taken when the parasites are mostly sequestered in the capillaries of internal organs. It must also be remembered that even when parasites are few in falciparum malaria, serious disease may be present.

It is therefore essential to examine carefully at least 100 high power microscope fields (thick film) before reporting 'No parasites found'. An undiagnosed serious falciparum infection can be fatal.

P. falciparum is also different from other *Plasmodium* species in that it is rare to find schizonts in blood films. Erythrocytic schizogony takes place in the internal organs and therefore only trophozoites (rings) and gametocytes are usually seen in blood films. If schizonts are seen (usually accompanied by heavy parasitaemia), this indicates a serious falciparum infection and the medical officer attending the patient should be notified as soon as possible.

In many areas where *P. falciparum* occurs, other *Plasmodium* species can be found and therefore it is possible to find mixed infections. Such mixed infections will only be reliably detected if the full number of microscope fields is examined even when falciparum parasites are seen in the first few fields examined.

The method of examining and reporting thick and thin blood films for malaria parasites is explained in 15:6. The following features (summarized also in Chart 15.1 in 15:6) can be used to identify *P. falciparum*.

Plasmodium falciparum
☐ Many parasites may be present.
☐ Usually only trophozoites and gametocytes are seen.

Host red cell
● Not enlarged.
● Cells containing late stage trophozoites often show irregular red-mauve staining Maurer's dots (clefts).
● May contain several parasites.
● Parasites may lie on red cell membrane (accolé forms).

Trophozoites (ring forms)
● Mainly small and delicate with thin ring (or part of ring) of blue cytoplasm and dark red staining chromatin dot.

In areas where there is drug resistance, the ring of cytoplasm of resistant strains may appear thick and distorted.

● May have double chromatin dot.
● In heavy infections, a few larger and more compact trophozoites may be seen with many small trophozoites.

Schizonts (dividing forms)
● Very rarely seen. Their presence in blood films (usually with many trophozoites) indicates a severe infection.
● If seen, they are often small and immature, containing only two or four merozoites and clumps of dark coloured pigment.

Gametocytes (sexual forms)
● Typically crescent (banana) shaped with rounded or pointed ends but oval forms may also be seen.

In the thicker parts of thick films, round shaped gametocytes can sometimes be seen due to the slow drying of the blood.

● Compared with the male gametocyte, the female gametocyte stains more deeply and bluer and has a more compact nucleus with less scattered pigment granules (these differences will be noticed but there is no need to differentiate the sexes in reports).

White cells
● In heavy and long-standing infections, brown-black malaria pigment can be seen in monocytes and sometimes also in neutrophils (always report it, especially if no parasites are found).
● Atypical mononuclear cells are often seen.

Illustrations: See colour Plates 41 and 45 and illustrations in Chart 15.1 in 15:6).

Estimating parasitic density in falciparum malaria
In falciparum malaria, because heavy parasitaemia indicates a severe infection for which the patient requires special treatment and care, a falciparum malaria blood film report should always include an estimation of the degree of parasitaemia.

Note: A low parasitaemia in falciparum malaria does not exclude a serious infection but most severe attacks are accompanied by heavy parasitaemia.

A quantitative report also enables a patient's response to treatment to be assessed where resistance to the drugs being used is suspected. Estimation of parasite numbers is required in epidemiological work.

Techniques to estimate parasite density
☐ Reporting the percentage of red cells infected. This provides the clinician with useful information in deciding treatment and in monitoring a patient's response. Field *et al* comment that when 10-20% of the cells are parasitized the prognosis is serious, with 20-30% it is grave, and over 30% it is exceptionally grave.[14]

The method of counting the percentage of parasitized red cells in thin blood films is described in 15:6.

☐ Reporting the number of parasites in 1 μl of blood. This way of reporting is preferred by some clinicians.

Absolute numbers of parasites (number/μl), can be estimated in thick films by counting the parasites against white cells and using a fixed white cell (WBC) count value or the patient's known WBC count (more accurate) to calculate the number of parasites per μl of blood.

☐ Reporting the parasitic density in plus signs (+ to ++++) with an accompanying interpretation of the grading scheme as described in 15:6. This is the simplest method and is recommended when it is not feasible to estimate parasitized cells or count the number of parasites per μl.

Note: Whichever method is used to estimate the degree of parasitaemia, to obtain a reliable result it is important to ensure that blood films are well made and stained correctly (see 15:6).

Laboratory indices of poor prognosis in falciparum malaria
The WHO Malaria Action Programme has suggested that the following laboratory indices should be considered as indicative of a poor prognosis in falciparum malaria:[4]

— Heavy parasitaemia with more than 5% of red cells parasitized (250 000 parasites/ μl).
— Presence of schizonts in peripheral blood films.
— Peripheral leucocytosis of more than 12 000/ μl.
— Low cerebrospinal fluid (c.s.f.) glucose and low c.s.f. lactate level (latter test requires the facilities of a specialist laboratory).
— Low antithrombin III levels (test requires the facilities of a specialist laboratory).
— Serum creatinine of more than 265 μmol/l.
— Blood urea nitrogen of more than 21.4 mmol/l.
— Packed cell volume of less than 20% or haemoglobin less than 7.1 g/dl (in previously non-anaemic person).
— Blood glucose of less than 2.2 mmol/l.
— Raised serum aminotransferases.

Blood transfusion in severe falciparum malaria
Blood transfusion may be necessary to correct severe anaemia or to replace deficient clotting factors (fresh blood is required). In blackwater fever, care must be taken because circulating haemolysins may haemolyze the transfused cells.

In patients with severe malaria, there may be difficulty in determining the blood group because of autoagglutination of the person's red cells. Testing of the patient's serum as well as red cells is necessary and autocontrols must be used.

Drug resistance of *Plasmodium falciparum*
Drug resistance has been defined by the World Health Organization as the ability of a parasite to multiply or to survive in the presence of concentrations of a drug that normally destroy parasites of the same species or prevent their multiplication. Such resistance may be relative (yielding to increased doses of the drug tolerated by the host) or complete (withstanding a maximum dose tolerated by the host).[7]

Drugs involved and distribution of drug resistance
Several new and effective antimalarial drugs were discovered between 1940 and 1960 but soon after each of these drugs was introduced, parasite resistance was reported and confirmed.

Of greatest concern has been the decrease in *P. falciparum* response to chloroquine (4-amino-quinoline compound) because this is the most widely used drug to treat malaria clinically.

Chloroquine resistance was first reported in Thailand and Colombia in the late 1950s. It has now spread to more than 40 countries in Asia, the Pacific region, South America, Central America, East and Central Africa and more recently resistance has been reported in West Africa. The countries involved are shown in Fig. 15.3.
The level and distribution of chloroquine resis-

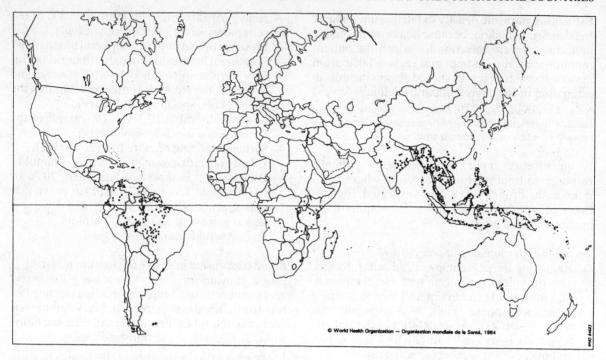

Fig. 15.3 Areas where chloroquine-resistant *Plasmodium falciparum* has been reported.
Reproduced from Weekly Epidemiological Record, 59, 1984 with the permission of the World Health Organization.

tance in the different countries varies. The greatest and most widespread resistance is in South East Asia and South America. The resistance is often noticed first in non-immune persons because higher doses of the drug are required for effective treatment.

Resistance to the suppressive drugs proguanil (*Paludrine*), and pyrimethamine (*Daraprim*) exists and is also spreading.

Resistant strains of *P. falciparum* to pyrimethamine/sulphadoxine (*Fansidar*) were reported from Southeast Asia in the early 1980s and more recently from some parts of Papua New Guinea, Brazil and Colombia. Sporadic reports of resistance to *Fansidar* have also come from East Africa. Serious toxic effects associated with *Fansidar* treatment have been reported from some places.

Reports of resistance to quinine and mefloquine are rare.

Reasons for resistance
Among the factors which are thought to have contributed to the emergence of chloroquine resistant strains of *P. falciparum*, the most important is the incorrect use of chloroquine particularly when inadequate amounts of the drug are taken by non-immune or semi-immune persons. When chloroquine is taken to relieve the symptoms of a malaria attack but not enough to kill all the parasites, the stronger parasites survive and multiply.

It is also thought that selective pressure favouring naturally occurring resistance mutations increases in areas of intense malaria transmission. Resistant strains may also develop in areas where small drug doses are used in prophylaxis.

WHO classification of drug resistance
Three levels of resistance (R) are defined by the World Health Organization:

RI — Following treatment, parasitaemia clears but a recrudescence occurs.

Patient's clinical response to treatment is satisfactory following a normal full course of chloroquine and there is clearance of parasitaemia (trophozoites) within 7 days, but within 3 weeks the illness recurs (recrudescence).

RII — Following treatment, there is a reduction but not a clearance of parasitaemia.

Patient improves when the chloroquine is given and the parasitaemia is reduced but not cleared during treatment. When the treatment ceases the patient's condition worsens.

RIII — Following treatment there is no reduction of parasitaemia.

Following treatment the patient does not improve clinically and the drug has no effect on the level of parasitaemia. In the absence of effective treatment, the parasitic density may continue to rise.

The above method of classifying resistance, based on counting trophozoites in blood films for up to 7 days after treatment and monitoring the patient for any subsequent recrudescence, is referred to as *in vivo* testing.

In vivo testing surveys

By studying suitable patients, *in vivo* testing can be used to establish whether chloroquine resistance is present in an area.[8] Reliable *in vivo* testing requires that the patient:

— is infected with only *P. falciparum* (mixed infections cannot be assessed satisfactorily) and the level of parasitaemia is at least 1000 trophozoites per μl of blood before starting treatment.

— has received no treatment for malaria within the previous 14 days (self or medically administered) and shows no aminoquinolines or sulphonamides in the urine when tested before starting treatment, see later text.

— is able to take and absorb the chloroquine administered as shown by a positive urine test for aminoquinoline 1 day after taking the drug.

Monitoring of patients in areas of suspected chloroquine resistance

In areas of suspected drug resistance (indicated by treatment failures), it is clinically important to check whether a patient with falciparum malaria is responding to treatment.

All patients with a falciparum parasitaemia (in a thick film) of more than 1 trophozoite in every high power microscope field ($+++$ or over), should be checked for a decrease and clearing of parasites following treatment. This is particularly important in children with high parasitaemia. Blood films should be taken and examined daily for a fall in parasitaemia by counting the parasites in thick films or the percentage of red cells infected with trophozoites. The haemoglobin should also be measured in young children with heavy infections.

Assistance should be sought from the World Health Organization (WHO) Malaria Action Programme in Geneva with regard to confirming drug resistance and determining its prevalence and degree using *in vitro* tests. Advice may also be obtained from WHO regarding malaria drug therapy and control measures.

WHO *in vitro* field testing kit to confirm and assess drug resistance

A field kit for *in vitro* drug sensitivity testing has been developed by WHO using a micro technique which requires only 100 μl of capillary blood.[9] Patients participating in the survey should not be severely ill. They should have parasite counts of more than 1000 trophozoites /μl (but not more than 80,000 μl) and should not have taken antimalarial drugs (negative urine tests) during previous 14 days.

The patient's blood is mixed in a culture medium and dispensed into wells of a culture plate which contain concentrations of chloroquine, amodiaquine, quinine, or mefloquine. One well contains no drugs and this acts as the control. After incubation at 37-38 °C for 24-30 hours in a carbon dioxide enriched atmosphere (candle jar), films are made and stained of the sedimented cells from each well. During incubation those trophozoites which are not inhibited by the drug, develop into schizonts.

The number of schizonts (containing 2 or more merozoites) per 200 parasites is counted in each film. The percentage of schizonts in each drug concentration is calculated by dividing the number counted by the number of schizonts per 200 parasites in the control well, multiplied by 100.

Resistance is indicated if schizonts develop in the presence of 5.7 pmol/well of chloroquine, 4 pmol/well of amodiaquine, 64 pmol/well of quinine, or 16 pmol/well of mefloquine.

Modifications of the micro *in vitro* test are being researched including extending the incubation period and developing a technique in which results can be read visually without a microscope (further details from WHO).

Note: Full details of *in vitro* sensitivity testing of *P. falciparum* to chloroquine, mefloquine, amodiaquine and quinine (for survey purposes), can be found in the WHO document, MAP/84.2, available from Malaria Action Programme, WHO Special Programme for Research and Training in Tropical Diseases, 1211 Geneva-27 Switzerland.

Further information: Details of malaria chemotherapy, control measures, and tests to establish and determine the prevalence and extent of drug resistance to *P. falciparum*, can be found in the 1984 WHO publication *Advances in Malaria Chemotherapy*.[15]

Information and guidelines on the use of drugs in the treatment and prevention of malaria can also be found in the 1985 publication *Essential Malariology* by L. J. Bruce-Chwatt.[2]

Papers published in 1985 concerning drug-resistant malaria and chemotherapy include those of Spencer[10] and Bisseru.[11]

Information about drug resistance and research into new malaria drugs, can be found in the 1985 WHO *Third Programme Review of the Scientific Working Group on the Chemotherapy of Malaria*.[12]

Testing urine for aminoquinolines and sulphonamides

Dill-Glazko test for chloroquine and amodiaquine[9]

In the presence of an organic base such as amodiaquine or chloroquine, the light yellow colour of ionized eosin in chloroform is changed into a violet-red ionized form of eosin. The test is performed as follows:

1. Using a small syringe or plastic bulb pipette,

transfer approximately 2 ml of urine into a small test tube.

2. Add 10 drops of Dill-Glazko eosin reagent (Reagent No. 29), stopper, and shake hard for about 15 seconds.

3. Examine for a violet-red colour in the lower chloroform layer. If seen, this indicates the presence of chloroquine or amodiaquine in the urine.

Note: The results of the test are fairly reliable for a period of 48 hours after an intake of chloroquine or amodiaquine.

False positive reactions may also occur if the urine contains quinine, pamaquine, primaquine, codeine, amphetamine, ephedrine, or pethidine.

Lignin test for sulphonamides[13]
This is a simple test in which sulphonamide compounds can be detected by a colour reaction using an acid solution. The test is performed as follows:

1. Dispense 1 or 2 drops of urine on to a piece of paper towel or print free area of newspaper.

   Note: Do not use filter paper or paper of bond quality.

2. Add a small drop of 25% v/v hydrochloric acid* to the centre of the moistened area.

   *Prepare by adding 2.5 ml of concentrated hydrochloric acid to 7.5 ml of water. Mix with care. *Caution*: Handle concentrated hydrochloric acid with great care. Do NOT mouth-pipette the acid.

3. Examine for the immediate appearance of an orange-yellow colour. If seen, this indicates the presence of a sulphonamide compound in the urine.

Note: The test usually becomes positive after the ingestion of sulphonamides and remains positive for 3 days. Some workers do not consider this simple test to be reliable. A more reliable test for sulphonamide detection in urine is that described in Volume II p 307-309 for the detection of dapsone (4:4 diaminodiphenylsulphone) in urine. Advice should also be sought from WHO.

Immunodiagnosis in malaria
Because antibody tests are unable to distinguish between active and past infections, they have only a limited value in the clinical diagnosis of malaria in countries where the disease occurs. Antibody tests are used mainly in epidemiological surveys to assist in the control of malaria.

Indirect fluorescent antibody test
The test which is most commonly used in epidemiological work is the indirect fluorescent antibody (IFA) test because it is the most easily standardized and has high sensitivity and specific-

ity. A thick blood film containing *P. falciparum* schizonts is used to provide the antigen. The schizonts are obtained by growing the parasites in continuous culture. *P. falciparum* antigen will react not only with anti-*P. falciparum* antibodies but also partially with antibodies formed against *P. vivax*, *P. ovale*, and *P. malariae*. For maximum sensitivity, however, antigens of these other *Plasmodium* species should be used.

The IFA becomes positive a few days after infection and antibodies can be detected for weeks, months, or even years afterwards depending on the amount of treatment given and whether the person has a previous history of malaria.

Other antibody tests
An indirect haemagglutination antibody (IHA) test has also been used in epidemiological work but compared with the IFA test, it lacks sensitivity and specificity.

Other tests used include enzyme linked immunosorbent assay (ELISA) and radioimmunoassay (RIA). These tests may become more important than the IFA test when monoclonal antibodies are used to produce specific purified antigens. Such tests enable large numbers of samples to be tested rapidly.

Future immunodiagnostic tests
Research continues within the WHO Malaria Action TDR Programme to produce inexpensive tests for the reliable detection of parasitic antigens, and the detection of parasite DNA or other components which could be used in the field to improve clinical diagnosis, to screen donor blood for parasites, and to assist in malarial epidemiology and control.

Note: An update on immunodiagnosis in malaria can be found in the 1985 World Health Organization document WHO/MAL/85.1018, available from the Malaria Action TDR Unit, WHO, 1211 Geneva-27, Switzerland).

15:3 *PLASMODIUM VIVAX*

Malaria caused by *Plasmodium vivax* is referred to as vivax malaria, formerly known as benign tertian (BT) malaria. It is a relapsing species and the main cause of malaria in temperate and subtropical regions.

Strains of *Plasmodium vivax*
The species *P. vivax* contains many strains which show differences in incubation time, relapsing pattern, morphology, number of parasites in red cells, and response to antimalarials. It has been suggested that *Plasmodium vivax multinucleatum* (reported from China and Papua New Guinea) and *Plasmodium vivax hibernans* (reported

from Russia) should be recognized as separate sub-species.

Distribution

P. vivax is capable of developing in mosquitoes at lower temperatures than *P. falciparum* and therefore has a wider distribution in temperate and subtropical areas. It is also found in some parts of the tropics.

P. vivax is the main *Plasmodium* species in South America (occurring as far south as northern Argentina), Mexico, the Middle East, northern Africa, India, Pakistan, Sri Lanka, Papua New Guinea and the Solomon Islands. It is also found in parts of South East Asia, Indonesia, Philippines, Madagascar, tropical and subtropical Africa, Korea, China, and the USSR.

P. vivax is rarely found in West Africa or other places where the red cells of the population lack the Duffy blood group antigens Fy^a and Fy^b (see later text).

Transmission and life cycle

P. vivax is transmitted in the same way as *P. falciparum* (see 15:2). Congenital transmission, although rare, occurs more frequently with *P. vivax* than *P. falciparum*.

Life cycle
— Following injection of sporozoites by the *Anopheles* mosquito, the parasites circulate in the blood stream for a short period before entering liver cells.

— In the liver cells, not all of the sporozoites develop directly into PE schizonts.

  Recent research has shown that the relapses which occur in vivax malaria are caused by some of the sporozoites developing into what are called hypnozoites. These are uninucleate forms, measuring 4-6 μm in diameter They remain dormant in the liver cells for a period of time after which they then become active and develop into PE schizonts. Not all the hypnozoites become activated at the same time. Their activation is strain determined.

  In some strains, the length of time before the primary attack can be as long as 6 to 12 months after infection due to the sporozoites developing first into hypnozoites. For most strains, however, the primary attack occurs 12-17 days after infection with subsequent relapses (activation of dormant hypnozoites) occurring at intervals up to 3 years or more after the first attack (in untreated persons).

  A PE schizont of *P. vivax* measures about 45 μm in diameter and contains about 10 000 merozoites.

— The mature PE schizont and liver cell rupture, releasing merozoites into the blood stream.

  The merozoites enter red cells (particularly young cells), become trophozoites and develop into schizonts within about 48 hours.

  With *P. vivax*, all stages of erythrocytic schizogony take place in the peripheral blood. Parasitized red cells become enlarged and irregular in shape and cells containing more mature parasites show stippling called Schuffner's dots. The parasites have an active amoeboid movement (as seen in wet preparations).

  A mature *P. vivax* erythrocytic schizont contains up to 24 or more merozoites and malaria pigment.

— Merozoites released from the schizonts invade new red cells and develop into schizonts which produce more merozoites.

  After a few erythrocytic cycles, some of the merozoites enter red cells and develop into gametocytes.

— The life cycle is continued by the *Anopheles* vector ingesting gametocytes in a blood meal.

  P. vivax sporogony in the mosquito is similar to that of *P. falciparum* (see 15:2). The cycle in the vector takes about 16 days at 20 °C (shorter at higher temperatures).

Clinical features and pathology

The incubation period for *P. vivax* varies according to the strain (see previous text). Parasite density in vivax malaria rarely exceeds 50 000 /μl or 2% of red cells infected. Infection is not usually severe and deaths from vivax malaria are less common than from falciparum malaria.

Erythrocytic schizogony becomes synchronised and therefore after a few days, a regular 48 h pattern of fever develops with cold, hot and sweating stages, often accompanied by nausea and vomiting. The temperature may rise to 40.6 °C (105 °F) or higher. All forms of the parasite (trophozoites, schizonts and gametocytes) can be found in blood films. The spleen enlarges and anaemia may develop, especially in children.

Relapses are a feature of vivax malaria. They may occur 8-10 weeks after a previous attack (short-term relapses) or about 30-40 weeks later (long-term relapses). As previously explained, the form and frequency of relapses depend on the infecting strain and occur due to the activation of hypnozoites in liver cells. During relapses, the parasites are often difficult to find in blood films.

Resistance to vivax malaria is naturally found in persons whose red cells lack the red cell Duffy antigens Fy^a and Fy^b. The glycophorin receptors which *P. vivax* needs to attach to and invade red cells are missing on Duffy negative (Fy^{a--}) red cells. The protection is absolute and afforded only to homozygotes.

P. vivax remains sensitive to chloroquine and to primaquine (kills hypnozoites). Reports of resistance to proguanil and pyrimethamine have been reported from many countries.

Prevention and control

The individual and community measures described for falciparum malaria in 15:2, apply to the prevention and control of vivax malaria. Knowledge of the breeding and feeding habits of local vectors is essential for effective control.

LABORATORY DIAGNOSIS

An accurate diagnosis of vivax malaria is required to ensure that the patient receives treatment both for the attack and against the relapsing forms of the parasite. The drug used to kill hypnozoites is primaquine.

Laboratory confirmation of *P. vivax* infection is by:

□ Examination of stained thick blood films to detect the parasites.

□ Examination of stained thin blood films to identify the species when this is not possible from a thick film and also to have the opportunity of examining the red cells for signs of anaemia and other abnormalities.

□ Examination of red cells just below the buffy coat layer after centrifuging blood in a narrow bore tube. *P. vivax* parasites are well concentrated by this technique (explained in 15:6).

Other tests
□ Measurement of haemoglobin if anaemia is suspected, especially in children.

□ G6PD screening test to detect G6PD enzyme deficiency. Primaquine can cause acute haemolysis in persons with G6PD deficiency.

Examination of blood

The blood must be collected and whenever possible the films reported before treatment is started. The preparation, staining and examination of blood films and buffy coat preparations for malaria parasites are described in 15:6.

The following features (summarized also in Chart 15.1 in 15:6) can be used to identify *P. vivax*.

Plasmodium vivax

□ Rarely more than 2% of red cells become infected. Young cells are preferentially parasitized.
□ Trophozoites, schizonts and gametocytes can be seen.

Host red cell
● Becomes enlarged and irregular in shape.
● Schuffner's dots are present (stain pH >7.1) in cells containing more mature parasites and can often be seen surrounding the parasites in thick films.
● May stain paler than non-parasitized cells.
● With some strains, red cells may become infected with several parasites.

Trophozoites
● Most are large and amoeboid. In thick films the cytoplasm appears fragmented.
● Fine pigment granules may be seen in cytoplasm.

Schizonts
● Large, round or irregular in form.
● All stages of developing schizonts can be seen, usually containing pigment granules.
● Mature schizonts contain 24 or more merozoites and a small amount of pigment.

Gametocytes
● Large, round or irregular in form. Small forms may also be seen.
● Contain scattered pigment granules.
● Compared with the male gametocyte, the female gametocyte stains more deeply and the nucleus appears more compact (these features will be noticed but there is no need to differentiate the sexes in reports).

Illustrations: See colour Plates 43 and 47 and the illustrations in Chart 15.1 in 15:6.

15:4 *PLASMODIUM MALARIAE*

Malaria caused by *Plasmodium malariae* is referred to as malariae malaria, formerly known as quartan malaria.

P. malariae has a much lower prevalence than *P. falciparum* or *P. vivax* and is able to persist in humans for many years.

Distribution
P. malariae is found in tropical and subtropical reg-

ions. In tropical Africa it accounts for up to 25% of *Plasmodium* infections. It is also present in many other countries where malaria occurs particularly in Guyana, India, Sri Lanka and Malaysia. In these countries it usually accounts for less than 10% of *Plasmodium* infections.

Transmission and life cycle

P. malariae is transmitted in the same way as *P. falciparum* (see 15:2). In tropical Africa, chimpanzees are naturally infected with *P. malariae* and may serve as reservoir hosts in some areas.

Life cycle

— Following injection of sporozoites by the *Anopheles* mosquito, the parasites circulate in the blood stream for a short period before entering liver cells.

— In the liver cells the sporozoites develop directly into PE schizonts. A mature *P. malariae* PE schizont measures about 55 μm in diameter and contains about 15 000 merozoites.

  Note: Although *P. malariae* can cause malaria attacks in an untreated person for several years following a primary attack, it has been shown that the parasite does not form hypnozoites. Subsequent attacks are thought to originate from small numbers of erythrocytic forms of the parasite remaining in the internal organs. Such recurring attacks are referred to as recrudescences, not relapses.

— When fully developed, the PE schizont and liver cell rupture, releasing the merozoites into the bloodstream.

  The merozoites invade red cells (usually older red cells), become trophozoites and develop into schizonts which produce merozoites. A considerable amount of pigment is produced. When mature, a *P. malariae* erythrocytic schizont contains up to 10-12 merozoites. Development is slow, with the erythrocytic cycle taking up to 72 hours to complete.

— After several erythrocytic cycles, gametocytes are formed. They are thought to develop in the internal organs, appearing in the blood only when they are mature.

— The life cycle is continued when the gametocytes are ingested by a mosquito vector in a blood meal.

  P. malariae sporogony in the mosquito is similar to that of *P. falciparum* (see 15:12). The cycle in the vector takes about 30-35 days at 20 °C (shorter at higher temperatures).

Clinical features and pathology

The incubation time for *P. malariae* varies according to the strain. The average is 18-40 days but longer times are associated with some strains.

Severe *P. malariae* infections are rarely seen. Only up to 1% of red cells become parasitized (less than 10 000 parasites /μl blood). The cycle of development in the red cells becomes well synchronized, with a malarial attack occurring regularly about every 72 hours. The spleen becomes enlarged in the early stages of the infection.

A serious complication of infection with *P. malariae* is nephrotic syndrome which may progress to renal failure. It occurs more frequently in children and is caused by damage to the kidneys following the depositing of antigen-antibody complexes on the glomerular basement membrane of the kidney. It produces oedema, marked proteinuria, and a low serum albumin level.

Recrudescences can occur over many years due to small numbers of erythrocytic forms of the parasite remaining viable in the host, possibly as a result of the parasites changing their surface antigens to remain free from host immune responses. Attacks up to 20-30 years after an original one have been reported.

Prevention and control

The individual and community measures described for falciparum malaria in 15:2, apply to the prevention and control of malariae malaria. Knowledge of the breeding and feeding habits of local vectors is essential for effective control.

LABORATORY DIAGNOSIS

Laboratory confirmation of *P. malariae* infection is by:

☐ Examination of stained thick blood films to detect the parasites. *Careful* examination of a thick smear is required to detect *P. malariae* infections because parasite numbers are normally very low (less than 1% of cells infected). In areas where *P. malariae* is found at least 200 high power microscope fields should be examined otherwise the parasites may be missed. Mixed infections are common in tropical Africa e.g. *P. malariae* with *P. falciparum*.

☐ Examination of stained thin blood films to confirm the species. A prolonged search is often required.

□ Examination of red cells just below the buffy coat layer after centrifuging blood in a narrow bore tube. This may help to detect the parasites.

Other tests
If nephrotic syndrome is suspected the following tests will provide useful information:

□ Estimation of urinary protein.
□ Measurement of serum albumin.
□ Measurement of serum sodium and potassium.
□ Measurement of blood urea or serum creatinine.

Examination of blood
The blood must be collected and whenever possible the films reported before treatment is started.

Note: The preparation, staining and examination of blood films and buffy coat preparations for malaria parasites are described in 15:6.

The following features (summarized also in Chart 15.1 in 15:6) can be used to identify *P. malariae*.

Plasmodium malariae

□ Rarely more than 1% of red cells become infected (a careful search is therefore required).
□ Trophozoites, schizonts and gametocytes can be seen.

Host red cell
● Not enlarged.
● No Schuffner's dots or Maurer's dots.
   Ziemann's stippling:
   This is rarely seen. Occasionally it may be seen as fine dark red stippling when staining is heavy.

Trophozoites
● Thick, compact and densely staining.
● Yellow-brown pigment is characteristically seen in late trophozoites.
● Band-forms containing pigment can sometimes be seen in thin films (trophozoite spreads across the cell).
● Bird's-eye form is occasionally seen in which a ring of cytoplasm surrounds a centrally placed chromatin dot.

Schizonts
● Small and compact with neatly arranged merozoites.
● Mature schizonts contain up to 12 merozoites.
● Yellow-brown pigment is characteristically seen.

Gametocytes
● Small, round or oval, and compact.
● Nucleus usually lies to one side.
● Yellow-brown pigment is easily seen.
● Compared with the male gametocyte, the female gametocyte is larger, stains more deeply and has a more compact nucleus (these features will be noticed but there is no need to differentiate the sexes in reports). Gametocytes are sometimes difficult to differentiate from late stage trophozoites.

Illustrations: See colour Plates 42 and 46 and the illustrations in Chart 15.1 in 15:6.

15:5 *PLASMODIUM OVALE*

Malaria caused by *Plasmodium ovale* is referred to as ovale malaria, formerly known as ovale tertian malaria. It is a relapsing species and has a restricted distribution and low prevalence.

Distribution
P. ovale is found mainly in West Africa where it accounts for up to 10% of malaria infections. It has also been reported from other parts of Africa, and from the Philippines, China and parts of the Far East, South East Asia and South America.

Transmission and life cycle
P. ovale is transmitted in a similar way to *P. falciparum* (see 15:2).

Life cycle
The life cycle of *P. ovale* resembles that of *P. vivax*, described in 15:3. There is a hypnozoite form and as in vivax malaria, activation of hypnozoites in the liver causes relapses.

Mature PE schizonts of *P. ovale* measure about 60 μm in diameter and contain about 15 000 merozoites.

All stages of erythrocytic schizogony take place in the peripheral blood. The erythrocytic cycle takes about 50 hours. No more than about 2% of red cells become infected (usually younger cells). About 20-30% of parasitized red cells become slightly enlarged and oval in shape with fimbriated (ragged) ends, especially those containing late stage trophozoites.

Infected red cells show dark red staining dots which are sometimes called James' dots rather than Schuffner's dots because they tend to appear brighter and larger than the Schuffner's dots that can be seen in vivax infected cells.`

Mature erythrocytic schizonts of *P. ovale* contain up to 10 merozoites. Gametocytes are formed after only a few erythrocytic cycles. Cells containing gametocytes do not become oval shaped.

Clinical features and pathology
The incubation period for *P. ovale* is 16-18 days but can be longer. Less than 2% of red cells usually become infected.

Clinically, ovale malaria resembles vivax malaria with attacks recurring every 48-50 hours. There are, however, fewer relapses with *P. ovale*.

Mixed infection is common particularly in West Africa with *P. ovale* often being found with *P. falciparum*.

Prevention and control
The individual and community measures described for falciparum malaria in 15:2, apply to the prevention and control of ovale malaria. Knowledge of the breeding and feeding habits of local vectors is essential for effective control.

LABORATORY DIAGNOSIS

The accurate diagnosis of ovale malaria is essential to ensure that the patient receives treatment both for the attack and against the relapsing forms of the parasite. Primaquine is used to destroy the hypnozoite forms.

Laboratory confirmation of *P. ovale* infection is by:

☐ Examination of stained thick blood films to detect the parasites.

☐ Examination of stained thin blood films to identify the species. This is particularly important in ovale malaria, when the form and stippling of the red cells greatly assist in identification.

☐ Examination of red cells just below the buffy coat layer after centrifuging blood in a narrow bore tube can sometimes help to detect the parasites.

Other tests
☐ Measurement of haemoglobin if anaemia is suspected, especially in a child.

☐ G6PD screening test to detect G6PD enzyme

deficiency. Primaquine can cause acute haemolysis in persons with G6PD deficiency.

Examination of blood
The blood must be collected and whenever possible the films reported before treatment is started.

Note: The preparation, staining and examination of blood films and buffy coat preparations for malaria parasites are described in 15:6.

The following features (summarized also in Chart 15.1 in 15:6) can be used to identify *P. ovale*.

Plasmodium ovale

☐ Rarely more than 2% of red cells become infected. Young cells are preferentially parasitized.
☐ Trophozoites, schizonts and gametocytes can be seen.

Host red cell
• About 20-30% of infected cells become oval or irregular in shape with fimbriated (ragged) ends, especially those containing late stage trophozoites and schizonts.
• Schuffner's (James') dots are present (stain pH >7.1) and can often be seen surrounding the parasite in thick films. The dots appear soon after the parasite infects the cell.

Trophozoites
• Small and compact (often resemble *P. malariae* trophozoites in thick films).
• Usually, very little pigment is seen.

Schizonts
• Small with little pigment.
• Mature schizonts contain up to 10 merozoites.

Gametocytes
• Small and usually round. They are often difficult to distinguish from late stage trophozoites.
• Nucleus often lies to one side.
• Compared with the male gametocyte, the female gametocyte is usually larger, stains more deeply and has a more compact nucleus (these features will be noticed but there is no need to differentiate the sexes in reports).

Illustrations: See colour Plates 44 and 48 and the illustrations in Chart 15.1 in 15:6.

15:6 EXAMINATION OF BLOOD FOR MALARIA PARASITES

With the spread of drug resistance, it is becoming increasingly important to confirm microscopically a diagnosis of malaria.

Role of the laboratory in malaria diagnosis and control

- Laboratory staff need to:
  - Standardize the preparation, staining, and reporting of blood films.
  - Introduce effective quality control in the preparation of blood films and laboratory diagnosis of malaria.
  - Report blood films rapidly.

  Standardization and adequate quality control of procedures will ensure that medical staff receive reliable information for treating patients and health authorities receive reliable data for evaluating malaria control measures. Rapid reporting will help to prevent the unnecessary use of drugs.

- District hospital laboratory staff should encourage, train, and supervise local community health workers in the laboratory techniques required to confirm a diagnosis of malaria.

  This will help to ensure that malaria is diagnosed correctly and at an early stage, particularly in pregnant women, young children and other non-immune or semi-immune persons living in rural areas.

- Senior laboratory staff in consultation with medical officers, nursing staff and community health workers, should decide and put into effect a *Safe Code of Practice* with regard to the:
  - Collection of blood.
  - Preparation, drying and handling of blood films.
  - Handling and disposal (in correct disinfectant) of prickers (lancets), needles, syringes, pipettes, slides and spreaders that are used in the collection of blood and preparation of blood films.
  - Identification and handling of known or suspect HIGH RISK specimens.

  By taking adequate safety precautions, accidental infection with malaria parasites will be avoided and also with other infectious pathogens which may be found in the blood, particularly haemorrhagic fever viruses, hepatitis viruses, human immunodeficiency virus (AIDS virus, formerly referred to as HTLV-III), and trypanosomes. All of these dangerous microorganisms can be transmitted by injection or passive entry of infected blood through small cuts, abrasions, insect bite wounds, or open ulcers on the skin.

Note: Further information regarding the safe handling and disposal of blood specimens and blood contaminated articles can be found in Chapter 33 in Volume II of the Manual.

Preparation of blood films for malaria parasites

As mentioned in subunits 15:2-15:5, blood for the examination of malaria parasites needs to be collected and whenever possible reported before treatment is started. If treatment needs to be started before the report is received, the laboratory should make the report available at the earliest opportunity.

Blood specimen

Blood films for malaria parasites can be prepared directly from capillary blood or from EDTA (sequestrene) anticoagulated capillary or venous blood providing the films are made within 1 hour of collecting the blood into EDTA. A thick film made from anticoagulated blood, however, needs to be handled with special care to avoid the blood being washed from the slide during staining. Whenever possible therefore, non-anticoagulated blood should be used.

Important: Specimens from patients with known or suspect hepatitis, viral haemorrhagic fever, or acquired immune deficiency syndrome (AIDS) should be marked 'HIGH RISK' in red writing and, or, a recognized warning symbol should be attached such as a red dot, star, or triangle.

A HIGH RISK specimen should be handled separately with special care. Blood slides should be kept in closed containers until they can be stained and examined and the specimen and equipment used to examine it must be disposed of safely, particularly prickers and needles.

It should be remembered that a thick film containing highly dangerous viruses and other pathogens remains infectious even after staining because there is no prior alcohol fixation stage as with thin films. A HIGH RISK thick blood film should not therefore be stained using a dip staining technique (see later text).

Need for thick and thin blood films

About twenty times more blood can be examined in a thick film than in a thin film in the same period of time. A thick film is therefore the most suitable for the rapid detection of malaria parasites. In areas where *P. malariae* exists, unless a thick film is examined, infection is likely to be missed because parasitaemia is normally low with this species.

More blood can be examined in a thick film because the film is not fixed and therefore the red cells are lyzed during staining. The parasites are not destroyed and after being stained they can be detected (with *careful* focusing) among the white cells, against a background of lightly stained haemoglobin and red cell stroma.

A thin blood film is required to confirm the *Plasmodium* species if this is not clear from the thick film. A thin film is fixed and therefore the parasites can be seen in the red cells. Depending on the species, parasitized red cells may become enlarged, oval in shape, and show stippling. These features, together with the parasitic forms present can greatly assist in confirming a mixed infection and in identifying *P. ovale* and *P. malariae* which are more difficult to differentiate in thick films (but best detected in thick films).

By counting the percentage of red cells infected before and after treatment, thin films are also of value in assessing whether a patient with severe falciparum infection is responding to treatment in areas where drug resistance is suspected.

Examination of a thin film also gives the opportunity to look for signs of anaemia and other abnormalities which may indicate an additional condition or, in the absence of malaria parasites, suggest an alternative diagnosis such as sickle cell disease, trypanosomiasis, relapsing fever, or leucocytosis indicating a bacterial or viral infection.

Making of thick and thin blood films
A thick and thin film can be made on the same slide which has the advantage that fewer slides are used and the thin film can be used for labelling the specimen when slides with frosted ends (for labelling) are not used. When slides are plentiful and frosted ended ones are available, thick and thin films are best made on separate slides.

To ensure good staining and standardization of reporting, the amount of blood used, particularly to make thick films, should be kept as constant as possible and the blood should be spread evenly over a given area of the slide. The simplest way of achieving these requirements is to use:

— A plastic bulb pipette or other suitable device to collect and dispense the blood. With reusable, inexpensive plastic bulb pipettes becoming more widely available, the collection of a drop of blood directly from the finger or heel, should be discontinued. It is impossible to control the amount of blood used to make blood films by such a direct collection technique.

— A template (pattern on which a slide can be placed), to indicate the sizes of the drops of blood to use and the area within which to spread the blood to make the thick film. The dimensions of the template shown in Fig. 15.4 for making thick and thin blood films on the same slide are also suitable for making the films on separate slides. The template can be used with slides having frosted or unfrosted ends.

The technique of making thick and thin blood films using a template is as follows:

1. Place a *completely clean* (grease-free) and scratch-free slide on the template (see Fig. 15.4).

2. Cleanse the lobe of the finger (or heel if an infant) using a swab moistened with 70% v/v alcohol or ether. Allow the area to dry.

3. Using a sterile lancet, prick the finger or heel. Squeeze gently to obtain a large drop of blood. Collect the blood in a small plastic bulb pipette or other suitable device (collecting the blood directly onto the slide should be avoided, see previous text).

4. Dispense the blood to fill the large circle of the thick film and the small circle of the thin film (only a *very small drop* of blood is required for a thin film).

5. Immediately spread the thin film using a *smooth* edged spreader (see Fig. 15.4 and Fig. 15.5).

   Using the plastic bulb pipette or other suitable device (do not use the glass spreader because this will encourage clotting and rouleaux formation of the red cells), spread the large drop of blood to cover evenly the area of the thick film as indicated by the template. When spreading, mix the blood *as little as possible*, to avoid the red cells forming marked rouleaux which may result in the blood being washed from the slide during staining.

   Spreading a thin film: It takes practice to make a good thin film. Laboratory staff should give practical training to ward staff on how to make an evenly spread thin film. A thin film which is too thick, has a ragged end, or appears lined horizontally or vertically, is extremely difficult to examine and report because the red cells and parasites will be distorted and the white cells will be concentrated in the end of the tail. It is essential to use a smooth edged spreader and a clean slide. The making of spreaders from glass slides (having ground glass polished edges) is shown in Fig. 15.5.

6. Using a black lead pencil, label the slide with the date and the patient's name and number. If

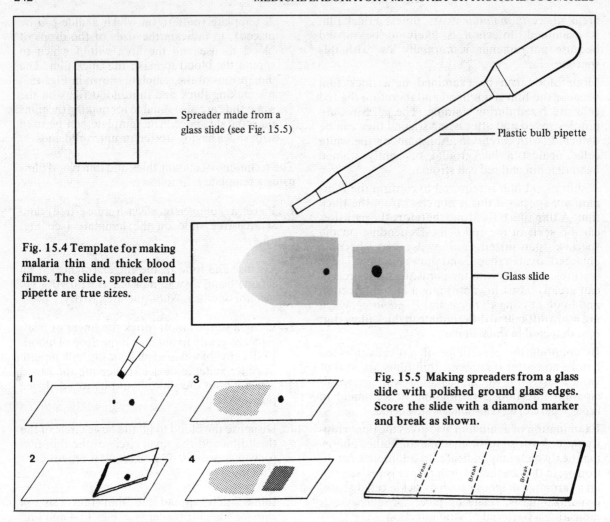

Spreader made from a glass slide (see Fig. 15.5)

Plastic bulb pipette

Glass slide

Fig. 15.4 Template for making malaria thin and thick blood films. The slide, spreader and pipette are true sizes.

1

2

3

4

Fig. 15.5 Making spreaders from a glass slide with polished ground glass edges. Score the slide with a diamond marker and break as shown.

Break   Break   Break

a slide having a frosted end is not used, write the information neatly on the dried thin film (along one side or along the top of the film).

7. Allow the blood films to air-dry with the slide in a horizontal position and placed in a safe place (where there is no risk of the blood coming into contact with any person or any object).

It is good practice to keep a separate box or deep tray for the drying of malaria blood films. The box should have a lid (but not made air-tight) to protect the films from flies, cockroaches, and dust. A cover made from mosquito netting is suitable. If the box or tray is placed in a warm sunny place, the thick film will dry rapidly (do not allow the blood to remain in the sun after it has dried).

In humid climates, it may be necessary to use an incubator to dry thick blood films.

Fixation of thin blood films

Absolute methanol (methyl alcohol) or ethanol (ethyl alcohol) is used to fix thin blood films. The

alcohol must be free from water otherwise it will not fix the cells properly. Always make sure the stock bottle of alcohol is kept tightly stoppered. For routine use, keep the alcohol in a dispensing bottle which can be closed when not in use (see 3:3).

The technique of fixing thin films is as follows:

1. Place the slide horizontally on a *level* bench or on a staining rack.

2. Apply two or three drops of absolute methanol or ethanol to cover the thin film, taking great care not to touch the thick film (if this is also on the same slide) with the alcohol.

3. Allow the film to fix for 1-2 minutes. Tip off the alcohol and allow the film to dry.

Note: Fixation of thin films in a container of methanol is not recommended if a thick film is on the same slide. Vapour from the alcohol will fix the thick film.

Staining of malaria parasites

Malaria parasites in thick and thin blood films are best stained at pH 7.1-7.2 using a Romanowsky stain (contains azure dyes and eosin). The stains most frequently used are:

- Giemsa stain
- Field's stain

(Stabilized Leishmann stain may also be used).

Giemsa stain

This is an alcohol-based Romanowsky stain that requires dilution in pH 7.1-7.2 buffered water before use. It gives the best staining of malaria parasites in thin films and also in thick films providing the thick films are left to dry overnight (or longer), the concentration of stain is low, and the staining time is sufficiently long. Less satisfactory results are obtained for thick films when the concentration of Giemsa stain is greatly increased to reduce the staining time. Care must be taken to ensure that water does not enter the stock solution of the stain. If this happens, the solution will not stain well.

Giemsa stain is commonly used in malaria survey work because many films can be stained at one time and differentiation of the different species in thin films is excellent providing a good quality standardized stain (e.g. BDH/Merck) is used. Giemsa staining technique is described in 13:14.

Field's stain

This water-based Romanowsky stain is composed of two solutions called Field's stain A and Field's stain B. It is buffered to the correct pH and neither solution requires dilution when staining thick films. When staining thin films, Field's stain B needs to be diluted. Compared with Giemsa working stain, Field's stain is more stable and has the advantage that it is isotonic with malaria parasites which prevents the parasites from becoming distorted in thick blood films.

Field's stain is commonly used in clinical malaria work because it gives the best staining of parasites in thick films when there is no time for prolonged drying of the films. Field's rapid staining technique for thin films is not as good as when Giemsa stain is used but it is adequate for most clinical purposes, particularly when reports are required urgently and when only a few films need to be stained. Standardized Field's stain is available (BDH/Merck). It can be purchased ready-made, but it can also be easily and more economically prepared in the laboratory from the bought powders (Field's stain A and Field's stain B).

Staining of thick and thin films on the same slide

When using Field's stain, the thin film should be fixed and stained first using *Field's rapid technique for thin films*, followed by staining of the thick film using *Field's rapid technique for thick films*. Each technique is extremely quick (see 13:15, 13:16).

When using Giemsa stain, it is possible to use a single staining technique for both films although some workers prefer to use separate stain concentrations and staining times for each type of film. For Giemsa staining of thick and thin blood films on the same slide, the World Health Organization recommends a regular technique in which the concentration of stain is 3% v/v and staining time is 30-45 minutes and a rapid technique in which a 10% solution is used and a staining time of 5-10 minutes. In both techniques the stain is diluted in pH 7.2 buffered water.

The malariologist P. G. Shute recommended substituting buffered physiological saline for buffered water, using a 6% concentration of Giemsa, and staining for 30 minutes. This gives a cleaner background to films and better preservation of the morphology of the parasites. It is also recommended for staining films that have been left unstained for a long period.

Reporting of stained thick and thin blood films for malaria parasites

Thick blood films

1. When completely dry, apply a drop of immersion oil to an area of the thick film which appears *mauve* coloured (usually around edges), indicating an area of good colour balance between the blue and red stains. Only in such an area will it be possible to see the correct staining of malaria parasites, i.e. chromatin stained dark red and cytoplasm stained blue.

   Note: If after staining the whole of the film appears yellow-brown (usually a sign that too much blood has been used), too blue or too pink, *do not* attempt to examine it. Restain it by dipping the slide into Field's stain A for 1 second, followed by a gentle wash in clean water, dip into Field's stain B for 1 second and a final gentle wash in clean water.

2. Spread the oil to cover an area of about 10 mm in diameter. This is to enable the 40× objective to be used *first* to examine the film, to select the best parts to examine with the 100× oil immersion objective. This preliminary scanning of a thick blood film should never be omitted (the more experienced you become the more you will value it).

   Preliminary scanning with the 40× objective will:

   — indicate quickly the best areas to examine with the 100× objective for malaria parasites,

— give an idea of white cell numbers and types,

— show the presence of malaria pigment in white cells,

— help to detect larger parasites such as trypanosomes and microfilariae,

— give a rapid indication of sickle cell disease in areas where this occurs (see later text).

3. Select an area that is well stained and of the correct thickness to examine for malaria parasites and move the 100× objective into place (if required add a further small drop of oil). The area selected should show a clear or pale coloured background and well balanced staining as judged by the nuclei of the neutrophils staining purple and the cytoplasm of the mononuclear cells staining blue.

4. Look for malaria parasites. The flow-chart shown on the opposite page can assist in the preliminary identification of parasites in thick films. If the species cannot be identified from the thick film, examine the thin film.

The features used to identify *Plasmodium* species in thick and thin blood films can be found in Chart 15.1.

5. Examine at least 100 high power (100× objective) microscope fields for parasites. In areas where *P. malariae* exists, examine approximately 200 fields (infections of this species rarely show more than 1% of red cells infected).

6. Report the species of *Plasmodium* and approximate numbers of parasites (trophozoites, schizonts, and gametocytes) found in the thick film as follows:

1-10   per 100 high power fields .... +
11-100   per 100 high power fields ...... ++
1-10   in every high power field .... +++
More than 10 in every high power field
                                    ++++

Note: With falciparum infections, because the gametocytes are easily recognized, it is possible to report separately the asexual and sexual forms (see *Example*).

Examples of reports
P. falciparum trophs +++, gametocytes +, with malaria pigment in white cells.

P. vivax parasites ++

Patients with P. falciparum infection of +++ or more
Patients with serious falciparum malaria as indicated by a +++ or more infection, require

further investigation. The percentage of red cells infected should be counted in the thin film and further blood films examined on a daily basis to ensure that the patient is responding to treatment (see later text). The patient's haemoglobin should also be measured and followed-up, particularly in a child.

Infection with more than one species of Plasmodium
Mixed infections are common and it is important for the laboratory to detect these to ensure that the patient receives a correct treatment and that health authorities receive reliable data as to the distribution of *Plasmodium* species in different localities. A mixed infection is more likely to be detected if the full number of high power fields is examined even when a falciparum infection is detected in the first few fields examined.

7. If no parasites are found after examining 100 fields (or if indicated 200 fields), report the film as:

Malaria thick film - NPF (meaning No Parasites Found)

Look for other clues in both the thick and thin blood films which may help to establish the reason for the patient's fever (see text below).

Abnormalities to be reported

☐ Malaria pigment in white cells (when found, make a further search for parasites).

☐ Increase in the total number of white cells (checked out by a total white cell count). It should be recalled that white cell counts are higher in infants than in adults (lymphocytes predominate).

☐ Sickle cell disease as shown by:
— In the thick film, a large amount of blue stippling in the background (indicating marked reticulocytosis) and nucleated red cells as shown by finding dark red nuclei (little larger than malaria chromatin dots). These features are shown in colour Plate 41 (right).

— In the thin film, a few sickled cells and nucleated red cells, marked anisocytosis (different sizes of red cells) and poikilocytosis (different shapes of red cells) and polychromasia (blue-mauve staining of red cells) indicating a reticulocytosis in response to marked haemolysis.

Confirm the condition by performing a sickle cell test and if possible haemoglobin electrophoresis.

☐ Features in the thin film indicating iron deficiency anaemia (hypochromic, microcytic red

**Flow-Chart to Assist in the Indentification of Malaria Parasites
Beginning with a Thick Blood Film**

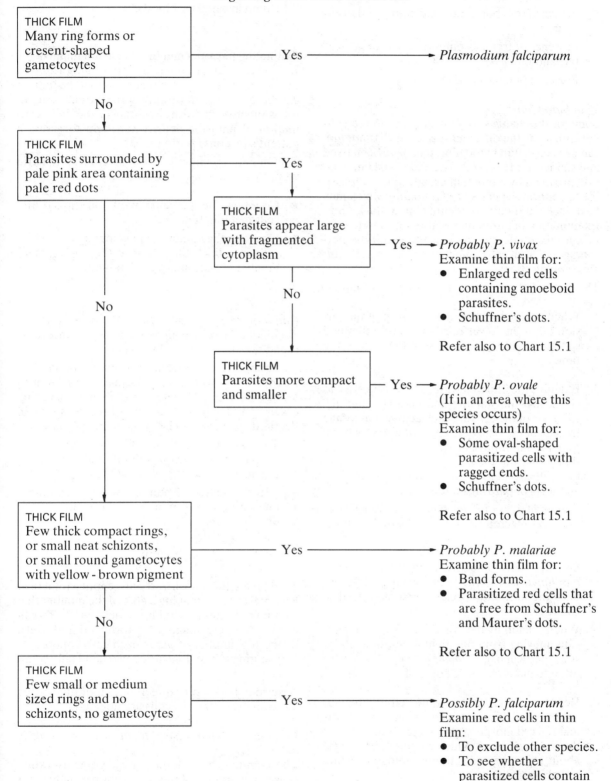

THICK FILM
Many ring forms or
cresent-shaped
gametocytes

— Yes ————————→ *Plasmodium falciparum*

No

THICK FILM
Parasites surrounded by
pale pink area containing
pale red dots

— Yes

THICK FILM
Parasites appear large
with fragmented
cytoplasm

— Yes —→ *Probably P. vivax*
Examine thin film for:
• Enlarged red cells
  containing amoeboid
  parasites.
• Schuffner's dots.

Refer also to Chart 15.1

No

No

THICK FILM
Parasites more compact
and smaller

— Yes —→ *Probably P. ovale*
(If in an area where this
species occurs)
Examine thin film for:
• Some oval-shaped
  parasitized cells with
  ragged ends.
• Schuffner's dots.

Refer also to Chart 15.1

THICK FILM
Few thick compact rings,
or small neat schizonts,
or small round gametocytes
with yellow - brown pigment

— Yes ————————→ *Probably P. malariae*
Examine thin film for:
• Band forms.
• Parasitized red cells that
  are free from Schuffner's
  and Maurer's dots.

Refer also to Chart 15.1

No

THICK FILM
Few small or medium
sized rings and no
schizonts, no gametocytes

— Yes ————————→ *Possibly P. falciparum*
Examine red cells in thin
film:
• To exclude other species.
• To see whether
  parasitized cells contain
  Maurer's dots.

Re-examine the thick film for parasite forms which could indicate a
different species. Remember the geographical distribution of the
four *Plasmodium* species. It also must be remembered that mixed
infections can occur. Refer also to Chart 15.1

cells), or macrocytic anaemia (macrocytic red cells and hypersegmented neutrophils).

□ Presence of borreliae, indicating relapsing fever.

□ Presence of trypanosomes (in areas of African trypanosomiasis).

□ Presence of microfilariae.

Thin blood films

Some of the changes which take place in red cells parasitized by the different species of *Plasmodium* can be seen in thin blood films that have been fixed and stained at pH 7.1-7.2. The additional information provided by a thin film usually makes it possible to confirm a species of *Plasmodium* which may have been difficult to identify in a thick film. Examination of a thin film is also required to confirm a mixed infection and also to count the percentage of red cells infected in serious *P. falciparum* infections.

The method of examining a thin film is as follows:

1. When completely dry, apply a drop of immersion oil to the lower third of the thin film and spread the oil to cover most of this part of the film.

2. Examine the film first with the 40× objective to check that the staining, morphology, and distribution of the cells are satisfactory. Late stage trophozoites, schizonts and gametocytes of all four *Plasmodium* species will be detected in a thin film using the 40× objective. This objective will also help to notice changes in the size and form of parasitized red cells.

   The small rings of *P. falciparum*, however, may only be detected when using the 100× objective.

3. Use the 100× objective to identify the *Plasmodium* species. The features which differentiate the different species are summarized in Chart 15.1.

   When examining the thin film, work systematically moving from one field to another. Parasites, particularly *P. malariae* and *P. ovale* are often found on the side edges of a thin film.

4. Report any increases in white cell numbers or an abnormal differential count, and also abnormal red cell morphology (see previous text). If the film is not well made or stained, be careful about reporting red cell morphology or white cell abnormalities.

   If the film has been made from EDTA anticoagulated *venous* blood, it should also be possible to comment on platelet numbers if the film has been well spread and stained. Do not,

however, attempt to report platelet numbers in films made from capilllary blood (platelets clump in capillary blood).

Estimating parasitaemia in falciparum malaria

In severe falciparum malaria it is important to know the degree of parasitaemia so that the patient can be given the most appropriate treatment. In areas of suspected drug resistance, the daily estimation of parasitic density can help to assess a patient's response to treatment.

Techniques commonly used in clinical malaria work for estimating parasite density are as follows:

■ Counting the percentage of parasitized red cells in a thin film.

■ Counting the number of parasites against white cells in a thick film, to give the approximate number of parasites per μl of blood.

Counting the percentage of parasitized red cells

Techniques used to count reticulocytes can also be used to count parasitized red cells.

One method is to insert in the eyepiece of the microscope a disc with a central square cut from it to reduce the size of the field. This will make counting easier by reducing the number of red cells seen in the field. The disc can be easily made as follows:

— Take a thin piece of card (light opaque) and cut from it a disc which will fit into the eyepiece of the microscope.

— Using a small sharp pair of scissors, cut a square measuring 6 × 6 mm from the centre of the disc.

— Insert the disc in the eyepiece. Rotate the eyepiece to straighten the square.

To estimate the parasitized cells, count a total of at least 500 red cells making a note of the number that contain parasites (excluding gametocytes). To calculate the percentage of parasitized red cells, divide the number of parasitized cells counted by 5. Counting is best done using two hand tally counters.

A serious falciparum infection is indicated when 5% or more of the red cells are infected.

Counting of malaria parasites against white cells in a thick film

The counting of malaria parasites against white cells is a method of obtaining an approximate parasite count. The accuracy of the method is dependent on knowing the actual white cell count and estimating the parasites against the white cells in an evenly spread and well stained thick blood film.

Note: In malaria surveys, it is common practice to use a white cell count of 8000/μl instead of performing an actual white cell count on every patient. In clinical work, the white cells should be counted.

Counting of the parasites is made easier if a grid is placed in the eyepiece.

A method of counting is as follows:

1. Select a part of the thick film where the white cells are evenly distributed and the parasites are well stained.

2. Using the oil immersion objective, systematically count 100 white blood cells (WBC), estimating at the same time the numbers of parasites (asexual) in each field covered. Counting is best done by using two hand tally counters.

   Repeat this in two other areas of the film and take an average of the three counts.

3. Count the number of parasites per μl of blood as follows:

Parasite count:

$$\frac{\text{WBC count} \times \text{Parasites counted against 100 WBC}}{100}$$

Example

Patient's WBC count = 4 000/μl

Parasites counted against 100 WBC = 680

Parasite count:

$$\frac{4000 \times 680}{100} = 27\,200/\mu\text{l}$$

Preparation and examination of buffy coat smears
Centrifuging of EDTA anticoagulated venous blood in a narrow bore tube gives excellent concentration of *P. vivax* parasitized red cells just below the white cells and platelets (buffy coat layer). Other species are less well concentrated but detection of the parasites in stained buffy coat preparations, especially late stage trophozoites and gametocytes, is often possible when no parasites are found in thick and thin blood films. In buffy coat preparations, the red cells are not destroyed and the parasites stain well and appear more clearly defined than in thick films. Phagocytosed malaria pigment is more easily detected because the white cells are also concentrated.

Method of preparing buffy coat preparations
While preparations can be made from centrifuging blood in capillary tubes and then breaking the tubes to obtain the buffy coat layer and red cells below it, this technique is dangerous and should be avoided.

A safer technique, but one that requires a longer period of centrifugation is as follows:

1. Using a small plastic bulb pipette or other suitable pipette, fill two small narrow bore plastic or glass test tubes with EDTA (sequestrene) anticoagulated venous blood. Tubes measuring 6 × 50 mm are suitable (each tube holds about 0.7 ml of blood).

Note: A narrow bore tube is best filled by inserting the tip of the pipette containing the blood to the bottom of the tube and withdrawing it as the tube fills.

Note: Clear reusable plastic test tubes measuring 6 × 50 mm and small plastic bulb pipettes suitable for filling 6 × 50 mm tubes (same as shown in Fig. 15.4) can be obtained from Tropical Health Technology Equipment Service (see Appendix IV).

2. Centrifuge the blood at medium to high speed for about 15 minutes.

   To judge the best time to use in the technique, individual laboratories should try centrifuging the blood at different times, e.g. 10, 15, 20, 25 minutes to evaluate the times which give the best concentration of locally found *Plasmodium* species.

3. Using a small plastic bulb pipette or other suitable pipette, remove and discard (into disinfectant) the supernatant plasma above the buffy coat layer.

4. Transfer the buffy coat layer and red cells immediately below it (to depth of about 1 mm) to one end of a slide and mix with the end of the pipette. Using a smooth edged spreader, make an evenly spread thin preparation. If the amount of specimen is more than is required for one film, transfer a drop to another slide and make a second preparation.

5. Allow the preparation(s) to air-dry. When dry, fix the films with absolute methanol or ethanol for 2 minutes.

6. Stain as described for a thin blood film (see previous text). Examine the preparation first with the 40× objective and then with the 100× objective. Use Chart 15.1 to identify the malaria parasites.

Note: Other parasites such as trypanosomes and microfilariae can also be concentrated by this technique. These parasites are concentrated in the plasma immediately above the buffy coat layer. In practice, when withdrawing the buffy coat layer and red cells below it, a small amount of supernatant plasma is always withdrawn and this will contain any trypanosomes or microfilariae which may be in the specimen.

Chart 15.1 Main Identification Features of Malaria Parasites in Stained Blood Films

Plasmodium falciparum

- ☐ Many parasites may be present.
- ☐ Usually only trophozoites and gametocytes are seen.

Host red cell
- Not enlarged.
- No Schuffner's dots but cells containing late stage trophozoites often show irregular red-mauve staining Maurer's dots (clefts).
- May contain several parasites.
- Parasites may lie on red cell membrane.

Trophozoites
- Mainly small and delicate rings (thin film) or small pieces of cytoplasm with chromatin dot (thick film).
  Ring of drug resistant strain may appear thick and distorted.
- May have double chromatin dot.
- In heavy infections, a few larger rings may be seen.

Schizonts
- Very rarely seen. Their presence in blood films (usually with many rings) indicates a severe infection which must be reported immediately.
- If seen, they are often small, containing only a few merozoites and a single clump of dark pigment.

Gametocytes
- Crescent (banana) shaped with rounded or pointed ends but oval forms may be seen.
- Pigment granules present, mainly around nucleus.

Distribution: Widespread in tropical Africa and other tropical countries. Also found in subtropics.

Recrudescences: Usually die out within 1 year of primary attack.

THIN FILM   THICK FILM

See Colour Plates 41 and 45

Plasmodium vivax

- ☐ Rarely more than 2% of red cells become infected.
- ☐ Trophozoites, schizonts, and gametocytes can be seen.

Host red cell
- Becomes enlarged and irregular in shape.
- Schuffner's dots are present and can also be seen surrounding the parasites in thick films.

Trophozoites
- Most are large and irregular in form (amoeboid). In thick films the cytoplasm appears fragmented.
- Fine pigment granules may be seen in cytoplasm.

Schizonts
- Large, round, or irregular in form.
- Mature schizonts contain 24 or more merozoites and small amount of pigment.

Gametocytes
- Large, round or irregular in form. Small forms may also be seen.
- Contain scattered pigment granules.

Distribution: Most widespread species in temperate regions and subtropics and is also found in tropics.

Relapses: Usually die out within 3-5 years after an attack.

THIN FILM   THICK FILM

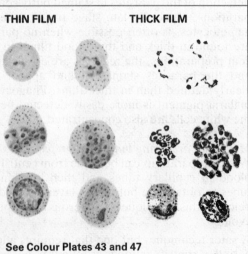

See Colour Plates 43 and 47

Plasmodium malariae
- ☐ Rarely more than 1% of red cells become infected (examine films carefully).

- ☐ Trophozoites, schizonts and gametocytes can be seen.

Host red cell
- Not enlarged
- No Schuffner's dots or Maurer's dots.

Trophozoites
- Thick, compact and densely staining.
- Band forms containing yellow-brown pigment can be seen in thin films.
- Bird's eye form occasionally seen (ring of cytoplasm surrounds a centrally placed chromatin dot).

Schizonts
- Small and compact with neatly arranged merozoites and abundant yellow-brown pigment.
- Mature schizont contains up to 12 merozoites and little cytoplasm.

Gametocytes
- Small, round or oval and compact. Difficult to distinguish from mature trophozoites.
- Nucleus usually lies to one side.
- Yellow-brown pigment is easily seen.

Distribution: Found in tropics and subtropics (has a low prevalence).

Recrudescences: Persist for many years after an attack.

THIN FILM   **THICK FILM**

See Colour Plates 42 and 46

Plasmodium ovale
- ☐ Rarely more than 2% of red cells become infected.

- ☐ Trophozoites, schizonts and gametocytes can be seen.

Host red cell
- About 20-30% of infected cells may become oval or irregular in shape with ragged ends.
- Schuffner's (James') dots are present and can also be seen surrounding the parasites in thick films.

Trophozoites
- Small and compact, similar to *P. malariae*.
- less pigment than *P. malariae*.

Schizonts
- Small and similar to *P. malariae* but with less pigment.
- Mature schizonts contain up to 10 merozoites.

Gametocytes
- Small and usually round. Difficult to distinguish from late stage trophozoites.
- Nucleus usually lies to one side.

Distribution: Found mainly in West Africa (has a low prevalence).

Relapses: Few

THIN FILM   **THICK FILM**

See Colour Plates 44 and 48

References

1 Walliker, D. Genetic variation in malaria parasites. *British Medical Bulletin*, **38**, 2, pp 123-128, 1982.

2 Bruce-Chwatt, L. J. *Essential Malariology*, William Heinemann Medical Books, 1985. ELBS edition, 1985, priced £7.50.

3 Warrell, D. A. *et al*. Dexamethasone proves deleterious in cerebral malaria. A double-blind trial in 100 comatose patients. *New England Journal of Medicine*, **306**, p 313-319, 1982.

4 World Health Organization Malaria Action Programme. Severe and complicated malaria. *Transactions of the Royal Society of Tropical Medicine and Hygiene*, **80**, (Supplement), p 1-50, 1986.

5 Bryceson, A. *et al*. Malaria and splenomegaly. *Transactions of the Royal Society of Tropical Medicine and Hygiene*, (letter), **77**, 6, p 879, 1983.

6 World Health Organization WHO Expert Committee on Malaria, *Technical Report Series*, No. 735, 1986.

7 World Health Organization *Terminology of Malaria and Malaria Eradication: Report of a Drafting Committee*. WHO, p 116, 1963.

8 World Health Organization *Practical Aspects of the in vivo Testing for Sensitivity of Human Plasmodium spp to Antimalarials*, WHO/MAL/82.988, Geneva.

9 World Health Organization. *Practical Aspects of the Use of the Standard WHO in vitro Macro and Microtest Systems for the Determination of the Sensitivity of Plasmodium falciparum to Chloroquine, Mefloquine, Amodiaquine and Quinine*, WHO/MAP.84.2, Geneva.

10 Spencer Harrison, C. Drug-resistant malaria changing patterns mean difficult decisions, *Transactions of the Royal Society of Tropical Medicine and Hygiene*, **79**, p 748-758, 1985.

11 Bisseru, R. Chloroquine resistance in Africa. *Postgraduate Doctor-Africa*, February, p 58-64, 1985.

12 World Health Organization. *Scientific Working Group on the Chemotherapy of Malaria - Third Programme Review*, TDR/CHEMAL/3rd Review/85.3.

13 Hepler, O. E. *Manual of Clinical Chemistry Methods*, 4th edition, p 21. C. C. Thomas, 1973.

14 Field, J. W., Sandosham, A., Jong, Y. L. *The Microscopical Diagnosis of Human Malaria*, Institute for Medical Research, Kuala Lumpur, 1963.

15 World Health Organization. Advances in malaria chemotherapy, *Technical Report Series*, No. 711, 1984.

16 Moody, A. H. and Fleck, S. L. Versatile Field's stain. *Journal of Clinical Pathology*, **38**, 7, p 842-843, 1985.

Recommended Artwork

The WHO Malaria Action Programme have produced an excellent set of colour plates to help in the microscopic diagnosis of malaria. The set has the code DSA/PROM/MAL/85.A and costs Swfr 10.00. It is available from World Health Organization, 1211 Geneva, 27-Switzerland.

Tropical Diseases Research Programme

MALARIA

Malaria is included in the *UNDP/World Bank/World Health Organization Special Programme for Research and Training in Tropical Diseases*.

Tropical Diseases Research (TDR) activities with regard to malaria as recorded in No. 5 of the 1985 *WHO Chronicle*, include:

● Development, testing and distribution of mefloquine, a new antimalarial drug, now registered for the treatment of multi-drug resistant *Plasmodium falciparum* malaria. Development was undertaken in collaboration with the Walter Reed Army Institute of Research (Washington).

● Research on the development of other antimalarial drugs, particularly those of the artemisinine (Qinghaosu) family. Artemisinine was originally extracted from the traditional Chinese herbal remedy Artemisia annua.

● Continuing research on malaria vaccines (see text under *Prevention and Control* in 15:2).

● Production of *Bench Aids for the Diagnosis of Malaria* see *Recommended Artwork*, at the end of the References.

Malaria Parasites

LIFE CYCLE SUMMARIES

Plasmodium falciparum	*Plasmodium malariae*	*Plasmodium vivax*	*Plasmodium ovale*
Sporozoites inoculated when *Anopheles* mosquito sucks blood		Sporozoites inoculated when *Anopheles* mosquito sucks blood	
Sporozoites enter liver cells		Sporozoites enter liver cells	
		Some sporozoites become hypnozoites (dormant forms)	
Develop into PE schizonts. Merozoites rupture from schizonts		Develop into PE schizonts. Merozoites rupture from schizonts	
RED CELLS INFECTED	RED CELLS INFECTED	RED CELLS INFECTED	RED CELLS INFECTED
Schizogony in blood in internal organs	Shizogony in peripheral blood	Schizogony in peripheral blood	Schizogony in peripheral blood
Gametocytes are formed and taken up by female *Anopheles* mosquito		Gametocytes are formed and taken up by female *Anopheles* mosquito	
Sporogony in mosquito. Sporozoites are formed		Sporogony in mosquito. Sporozoites are formed	

Trypanosomes

16:1 CLASSIFICATION AND FEATURES OF TRYPANOSOMES

Trypanosomes are protozoan parasites belonging to the subphylum Mastigophora and order Kinetoplastida, the general characteristics of which are described at the beginning of the Parasitology Section in 12:4.

Classification of trypanosomes of medical importance

Order	KINETOPLASTIDA
Genus	*Trypanosoma*

Subgenus	*Trypanozoon*
Species	*Trypanosoma (T.) brucei** complex
	* Usually the (T.) is omitted
Subspecies	*Trypanosoma brucei gambiense*
or variants	*Trypanosoma brucei rhodesiense*

Subgenus	*Schizotrypanum*
Species	*Trypanosoma (S.) cruzi**
	*Usually the (S.) is omitted

Note: Trypanosomes can also be classified by the type of development in their insect vectors and methods of transmission as follows:

The *T. brucei* complex belongs to the salivarian group of trypanosomes in which development takes place in the mid and fore gut of the vector and transmission is by inoculation when the vector bites.

T. cruzi belongs to the stercorarian group of trypanosomes in which development takes place in the hindgut of the vector and transmission is by faecal contamination after the vector bites.

General features of trypanosomes

- Trypanosomes are haemoflagellates i.e. actively motile flagellated parasites that live in the blood and lymph. The single flagellum arises from the kinetoplast which is situated posterior to the nucleus. The flagellum runs the length of the body along the undulating membrane and usually beyond it as an anterior free flagellum. The flagellated form of the parasite found in humans, in which the kinetoplast is positioned posterior to the nucleus, is called a trypomastigote, or simply a trypanosome.

T. cruzi in addition to its trypomastigote form also has a small non-flagellated form which lives in tissue cells. This intracellular form is called an amastigote.

- *T. b. gambiense* and *T. b. rhodesiense* trypomastigotes multiply in the blood and lymphatic system and possibly in epithelial cells. They are pleomorphic i.e. they vary in size and shape with some appearing short and stumpy, others long and slender, and some without a free flagellum.

The trypomastigotes of *T. cruzi* are monomorphic (one shape and size) and do not appear to multiply in the blood. The amastigotes multiply intracellularly.

- The vectors of *T. b. gambiense* and *T. b. rhodesiense* are tsetse flies. Most infections with *T. b. rhodesiense* are zoonotic with game animals being infected. Humans are the main hosts of *T. b. gambiense*. The vectors of *T. cruzi* are reduviid bugs with human infections being zoonotic. Many animals serve as hosts for *T. cruzi*.

In their insect hosts, the parasites develop into flagellated forms in which the kinetoplast is situated in front of and close to the nucleus with a short undulating membrane and free flagellum. These forms are called epimastigotes. They multiply and produce the infective, or metacyclic, trypomastigotes.

- Laboratory confirmation of infection with *T. b. rhodesiense* is mainly by finding trypanosomes in the blood and with *T. b. gambiense* by finding trypanosomes mainly in lymph node aspirates but also in blood. In the late stages of infection, trypomastigotes may also be found in cerebrospinal fluid, especially *T. b. rhodesiense*.

T. cruzi may be found in the blood in acute infections but most infections are diagnosed serologically, culturally, or by xenodiagnosis.

Trypanosomes of Medical Importance

LIFE CYCLE SUMMARIES

Trypanosoma b. rhodesiense *Trypanosoma b. gambiense*	*Trypanosoma cruzi*
Metacyclic trypomastigotes in saliva of tsetse fly are inoculated when vector sucks blood	Metacyclic trypomastigotes are deposited in faeces on the skin as triatomine bug feeds. Enter through the bite wound or are rubbed in
Trypomastigotes multiply at site of inoculation and then in the blood, lymph and tissue fluid	Trypomastigotes become amastigotes in reticulo-endothelial cells and multiply
TRYPOMASTIGOTES FOUND IN BLOOD AND LYMPH GLAND ASPIRATES AND IN LATER STAGES IN CSF	ENTER BLOOD AS TRYPOMASTIGOTES (found in blood in acute stage)
	Trypomastigotes are carried to muscle cells of heart, gut, etc. They become amastigotes and multiply
	Trypomastigotes enter blood
Tsetse fly ingests trypomastigotes in blood meal. In tsetse fly, trypomastigotes develop into epimastigotes and multiply	Triatomine bug ingests trypomastigotes in blood meal. In bug, trypomastigotes develop into epimastigotes and multiply
Metacyclic trypomastigotes form and migrate to the salivary glands. They are infective to humans and *T. b. rhodesiense* to many game animals. *T. b. gambiense* is infective to a few animals.	Metacyclic trypomastigotes form and are present in rectum of bug. They are infective to humans and many mammals.

16:2 *TRYPANOSOMA BRUCEI GAMBIENSE TRYPANOSOMA BRUCEI RHODESIENSE*

Trypanosoma brucei gambiense and *Trypanosoma brucei rhodesiense* cause African trypanosomiasis in humans. The disease is also known as sleeping sickness. The parasites are closely related and belong to the *Trypanosoma brucei* group, or complex.

Trypanosoma brucei complex

Trypanosoma brucei brucei (infective to animals but not humans) and the human pathogens *Trypanosoma brucei gambiense* and *Trypanosoma brucei rhodesiense* are morphologically indistinguishable.

Each trypanosomiasis endemic area seems to have associated with it several strains of biochemically and antigenically distinct trypanosomes. *T. b. gambiense* appears to be a homogeneous group whereas *T. b. rhodesiense* seems to be made up of many different strains. Enzyme studies support the view that *T. b. rhodesiense* is a set of variants of *T. b. brucei* rather than a subspecies of *T. brucei*.[1]

Distribution

African trypanosomiasis occurs in the tsetse fly areas of sub-Saharan Africa between 15 °N and 20 °S. Tsetse flies are found only in Africa.

It is estimated that about 50 million people in 34 countries are at risk of becoming infected and of these only 5 to 10 million have access to some form of protection or treatment.

T. b. gambiense is found in West Africa and western Central Africa, extending from Senegal across to Sudan and down to Angola. *T. b. rhodesiense* is found in East Africa, Central Africa, and Southern Africa, extending from Ethiopia down to Botswana (see Fig. 16.1).

Distribution of *T. b. gambiense* and *T. b. rhodesiense* overlaps in the region of the Great Lakes of East Africa. There are also extensive areas within the geographical boundaries where sleeping sickness is not found.

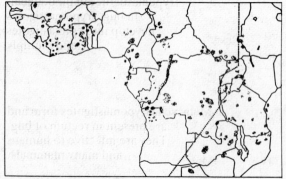

Fig. 16.1   Distribution of sleeping sickness foci in Africa. *Reproduced from WHO Technical Report Series, No. 739, 1986.*

Transmission and life cycle

African trypanosomiasis is transmitted by a small number of species of tsetse flies belonging to the genus *Glossina*. Both male and female tsetse flies suck blood and can therefore transmit the disease. The appearance, breeding and feeding habits of tsetse flies are described in 23:8.

T. b. gambiense is usually transmitted by lakeside and riverine tsetse flies, including *G. palpalis*, *G. fuscipes*, and *G. tachinoides*. *T. b. rhodesiense* transmission is associated with woodland and savannah tsetse flies, including *G. morsitans*, *G. pallidipes*, and *G. swynnertoni*. Both parasites, however, can be transmitted by either group of tsetse fly.

For *T. b. gambiense*, humans are the main reservoirs of infection. Semi-domestic animals may act as reservoir hosts.

Rhodesiense trypanosomiasis is a zoonosis with many game animals being naturally infected. Infection can persist for long periods in animals such as the reedbuck, warthog, hartebeest, hyaena, giraffe, and lion. Persons at greatest risk are therefore honey collectors, fishermen, hunters and members of trypanosomiasis control units, tourists, and other persons who enter tsetse fly infested game country in endemic areas. During epidemics, humans are the main sources of infection.

Trypanosomiasis can also be transmitted by blood transfusion (fresh blood) and therefore in areas in which the disease is endemic, blood donors should be checked for infection, especially the relatives of patients with trypanosomiasis. Tests used to screen fresh blood for infection are described at the end of this subunit.

Life cycle

— Metacyclic trypomastigotes are inoculated through the skin when an infected tsetse fly takes a blood meal. The parasites develop into long slender trypomastigotes which multiply at the site of inoculation and later in the blood, lymphatic system, and tissue fluid.

— The trypomastigotes are carried to the heart and various organs of the body and in the later stages of infection they invade the central nervous system.

— Trypomastigotes are ingested by a tsetse fly (male or female) when it sucks blood. In the midgut of the fly, the parasites develop and multiply.

— After 2-3 weeks, the trypomastigotes migrate to the salivary glands of the tsetse fly where

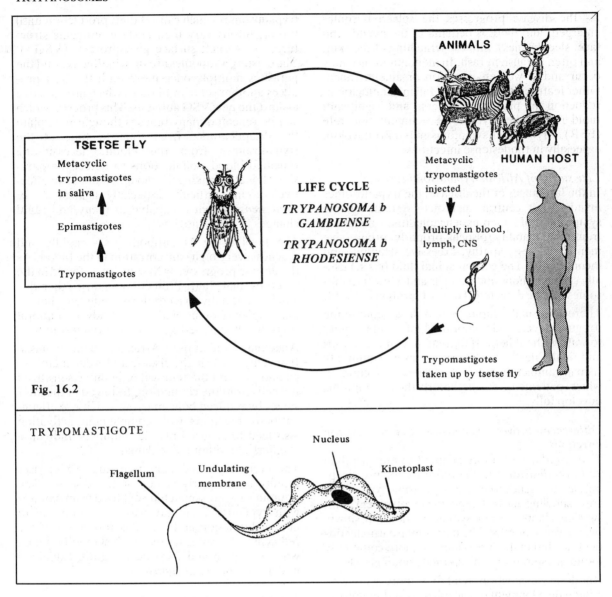

Fig. 16.2

they multiply further and become epimastigotes which in turn develop into metacyclic trypomastigotes.

Once infected a tsetse fly remains a vector of trypanosomiasis for the remainder of its life. The life-span of a tsetse fly is about 3 months. In an endemic area only a small proportion of tsetse flies actually become infected.

Clinical features and pathology
African trypanosomiasis is a wasting disease which is usually fatal unless treated. In rhodesiense trypanosomiasis and less commonly in gambiense infections, a painful swelling called a chancre develops and can be seen at the site of inoculation of the trypomastigotes. The chancre contains multiplying trypomastigotes. It disappears after about 10 days.

Early stages of African trypanosomiasis
In the early stages of the disease there is a high irregular fever with shivering, sweating, and an increased pulse rate. There is a persistent headache, and usually pains in the neck, shoulders, and calves, and occasionally a delayed intense pain to knocks and pressure known as Kerandel's sign.

The lymph glands near to the bite often become swollen. In gambiense infections the glands at the back of the neck are involved (Winterbottom's sign), while in rhodesiense infections it is usually the glands under the jaw, in the arm-pit, at the base of the elbow, or in the groin which are involved.

As the disease progresses the spleen becomes enlarged, and there is oedema of the eyelids and face, sleeplessness, aimless scratching of the skin, and often a transient rash. In men, impotence may occur and in women, abortion or amenorrhoea. Other features include a rapid fall in haemoglobin, reduction in platelet numbers, and significant rapid rise in the erythrocyte sedimentation rate (ESR). Myocardial symptoms may also develop, especially in rhodesiense infections.

Late stages of African trypanosomiasis
In the late stages of the disease, the trypanosomes invade the central nervous system, giving symptoms of meningoencephalitis, including trembling, inability to speak properly, progressive mental dullness, apathy, excessive sleeping, and incontinence. The cerebrospinal fluid (c.s.f.) usually contains mononuclear cells and a few trypanosomes may be detected. The c.s.f. protein is raised.

There is usually rapid weight loss, continuing irregular fever, oedema of the limbs and inability to walk without help. If untreated, coma develops and finally death. Such signs are more commonly seen in gambiense than in rhodesiense infections in which patients often die before these symptoms develop fully.

Differences between gambiense and rhodesiense infections
T. b. gambiense is more adapted to humans than *T. b. rhodesiense* and therefore gambiense sleeping sickness tends to be a more chronic type of disease showing early lymphatic involvement with swollen glands. Other symptoms develop slowly over several months. The parasites are usually difficult to find in the blood and are more commonly found in aspirates from enlarged lymph glands.

Rhodesiense infections tend to be more acute with a rapid development of encephalitis and symptoms leading to early death from toxaemia or heart failure.

Although *T. b. rhodesiense* trypanosomes are usually easier to find in the blood than *T. b. gambiense* trypanosomes, they can also be very few and difficult to detect in direct unconcentrated preparations.

Note: Occasionally infection with *T. b. gambiense* can be acute especially in epidemics and infection with *T. b. rhodesiense* may be chronic. 'Healthy' asymptomatic carriers of both *T. b. gambiense* and *T. b. rhodesiense* have been found in some areas.

Immunity in trypanosomiasis
The main immune response in African trypanosomiasis is a humoral one with stimulated B lymphocytes producing large amounts of Ig M followed in the later stages of infection by Ig G. The antibodies are effective in destroying the trypanosomes which caused their production until the organisms vary their surface antigenic structure, i.e. variant surface glycoproteins (VSG's). The existing antibodies are then ineffective and the parasites multiply once more until the host produces another set of antibodies which are effective against the new VSG antigens. This process, which can be repeated many times is thought to explain the disappearance from time to time of the trypanosomes from the blood, necessitating repeated blood examinations to detect the parasites. It is also making the development of an effective vaccine difficult, especially against *T. b. rhodesiense* which is capable of many and rapid changes in VSG antigens.

The level of Ig M antibody rises rapidly and reaches a very high concentration in the blood. As the disease progresses Ig M can also be found in the cerebrospinal fluid. Protection against other diseases, especially bacterial, is reduced due to immunodepression and the body's humoral responses being used against the trypanosomes.

Anaemia is a feature of African trypanosomiasis. It develops early in the disease and is due mainly to haemolysis and the removal of immune sensitized red cells from the circulation, followed in the later stages by reduced bone marrow activity. Antigen-antibody reactions with complement activation also lead to reduced platelet numbers and cause capillary and other tissue damage.

The erythrocyte sedimentation rate (ESR) rises rapidly in the early stages of the disease. The grouping and crossmatching of blood from patients with trypanosomiasis may cause difficulties due to autoagglutination and rouleaux formation of the red cells. The precautions which should be taken when grouping and crossmatching are explained under *Laboratory Diagnosis*.

Urine testing during treatment
The drugs used in the treatment of African trypanosomiasis may cause serious kidney damage. During treatment it is therefore recommended that a patient's urine be tested for protein, cells, and casts.

Prevention and control
Measures to prevent and control African trypanosomiasis include:

● Detecting and treating human infections at an early stage by:
— Using simple field diagnostic techniques.

  In survey work, capillary blood can be collected on filter paper and sent to a regional laboratory or trypanosomiasis control laboratory for serological testing (by an indirect fluorescent antibody technique or ELISA). Testing blood for rises in Ig M has not proved to be a reliable method of screening populations for infection.

— Informing communities of the risk of infection and importance of seeking early treatment if infection is suspected.

• Identifying animal reservoir hosts in endemic areas.

• In rhodesiense trypanosomiasis areas, restricting the movement of game animals to within fenced game reserves.

• Siting human settlements in tsetse fly infested areas only when there is adequate vector control.

• Reducing tsetse fly breeding by:

— Identifying and studying the breeding habits of local vectors.
— Selectively clearing the bush and wooded areas, especially around game reserves (rhodesiense trypanosomiasis areas), water-holes, bridges, and along river banks, combined with regular and careful spraying with insecticides.

• Using insecticide impregnated tsetse fly traps.

• Spraying of vehicles with insecticide as they enter and leave tsetse fly infested areas.

• Investigation of environmental change of land development which may allow the reintroduction of tsetse flies into a cleared area or encourage the flies to feed on humans.

• Use of biological methods aimed at the reduction of tsetse flies as part of a controlled eradication programme, e.g. introduction of sterilized male tsetse flies.

Further information on African trypanosomiasis
The biology and life cycle of pathogenic trypanosomes of the *Trypanosoma brucei* complex and information about the clinical features, treatment, and control of African trypanosomiasis can be found in a special 1985 issue of the British Medical Bulletin called *Trypanosomiasis*.[3]

A review of literature on *Trypanosoma brucei* trypanosomes published between July 1983 and December 1984 can be found in the Tropical Diseases Bulletin entitled *Trypanosomiasis, Salivaria*.[4]

Literature published by the World Health Organization on African trypanosomiasis can be obtained from the Trypanosomiasis Unit, Tropical Diseases Research Programme, WHO, 1211 Geneva-27, Switzerland.

LABORATORY DIAGNOSIS

Laboratory confirmation of African trypanosomiasis is by:

☐ Examination of blood for trypanosomes.

☐ Examination of aspirates from enlarged lymph glands for trypanosomes, especially when gambiense infection is suspected.

☐ Examination of cerebrospinal fluid (c.s.f.) for trypanosomes, cells, and raised protein when central nervous system (CNS) involvement is suspected.

Note: When trypanosomes are found in the blood or in lymph node aspirates, testing of the c.s.f. is necessary to determine whether the trypanosomes have invaded the CNS and further treatment is required.

☐ Testing serum for anti-trypanosomal antibodies, Serological tests are commercially available for the detection of antibodies against *T. b. gambiense*.

Other common laboratory findings in African trypanosomiasis
☐ Rapid fall in haemoglobin with reticulocytosis.
☐ Reduced platelet count.
☐ Significant and rapid rise in the erythrocyte sedimentation rate (ESR).
☐ High levels of Ig M in the serum and also in c.s.f. in the later stages of the disease.
☐ Occasionally, coagulation disorders with prolonged prothrombin and partial thromboplastin times, low fibrinogen levels, and increased fibrin degradation products (FDPs) when there is disseminated intravascular coagulation.
☐ Autoagglutination and rouleaux formation of patient's red cells.

Examination of blood for African trypanosomes
Repeated examinations and concentration techniques are often required to detect trypanosomes in the blood because their number varies at different stages of the infection. At times no parasites will be found (see *Immunity in trypanosomiasis*).

The following techniques are recommended:

— Thick stained blood film.
— Capillary tube centrifugation concentration technique, also referred to as the microhaematocrit centrifugation buffy coat technique.

— Test tube centrifugation concentration technique (especially in areas where *Mansonella* or other species of microfilariae may be present in the blood).

— Miniature anion exchange centrifugation (MAEC) technique.

Thick stained blood film

Although trypanosomes, when in sufficient numbers, can be detected by their motility in fresh unstained blood preparations, examination of a thick stained blood film is recommended because more blood can be examined in a shorter time.

The method of preparing and examining a thick blood smear for trypanosomes is as follows:

1. Collect a drop of capillary blood on a slide and spread it to cover evenly an area of 15-20 mm in diameter.

   Avoid making the smear too thick because it will not stain well and the trypanosomes will be difficult to detect. The thickness can be taken as correct if print from a page in this book can be seen but not read when the film is held just above the print. Alternatively, the template provided for making malaria thick blood films can be used (see 15:6).

   Note: Red cells from patients with trypanosomiasis will tend to form rouleaux. To avoid excessive rouleaux formation, mix the blood as little as possible when spreading it. Marked rouleaux will cause the preparation to be easily washed from the slide during staining. For the same reason it is also best to make thick films from non-anticoagulated blood.

2. Allow the smear to dry completely in a safe place and protected from flies, ants, and dust.

3. Stain the film using Field's rapid technique for thick blood films (see 13:15) or Giemsa staining technique (see 13:14). Allow the preparation to dry.

4. When dry, spread a drop of immersion oil on the film and examine it microscopically for trypanosomes using the 40× objective. Use the 100× objective to confirm that the organisms are trypanosomes (add a further drop of oil if required).

   Note: If no trypanosomes are seen, always check for other causes of a patient's fever such as malaria parasites or borreliae.

Morphologically the trypanosomes of *T. b. rhodesiense* and *T. b. gambiense* are indistinguishable from each other.

T. b. rhodesiense and T. b. gambiense trypanosomes

- Pleomorphic trypanosomes, i.e. showing a variety of forms, measuring 18-35 μm in length.

  Note: In the early stages of acute African trypanosomiasis, long slender trypanosomes (often seen dividing) can be found. In the later stages, intermediate and short trypanosomes appear, some having no free flagellum.

- Single flagellum arises from the kinetoplast and extends forwards along the outer margin of the undulating membrane and usually beyond it as a free anterior flagellum.

- Small dot-like parabasal body of the kinetoplast stains darkly.

- Nucleus stains dark-mauve and is usually centrally placed but posterior nuclear forms may also be seen.

- Cytoplasm stains palely and contains granules.

Illustrations: See Fig. 16.3, Plate 16.1, and colour Plates 52 and 54.

Acridine orange stained preparations

T. b. rhodesiense and *T. b. gambiense* can also be demonstrated in acridine orange (fluorochrome) stained preparations. The method is described in 34:13 in Volume II of the Manual. Trypanosomes contain RNA and therefore they fluoresce orange-red against a dark background. They can be rapidly detected using a 20× or 40× objective.

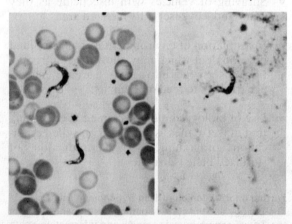

Plate 16.1 *Left* **Trypomastigotes in stained thin blood film.** *Right* **Trypomastigote in stained thick blood film.**

Capillary tube centrifugation concentration technique for trypanosomes

This technique is rapid and recommended where centrifuging facilities are available. If a haematocrit centrifuge is used, the packed cell volume can be measured at the same time to check whether the patient is anaemic. Anaemia is a common finding in African trypanosomiasis.

Note: The capillary tube technique is not suitable in areas where *Mansonella* or other species of microfilariae are likely to be present with trypanosomes in the blood. In such areas it is best to examine a stained preparation from a test tube concentration technique (see later text).

A method of performing the capillary tube centrifugation concentration technique is as follows:

1. Fill to about 10 mm from the top, two heparinized capillary tubes with capillary blood or two plain capillary tubes with fresh anticoagulated blood (EDTA or heparinized blood).

2. Seal the top end of each capillary tube by rotating it in a suitable sealant e.g. *Cristaseal, Sealease*, etc.

3. Centrifuge the capillaries in a haematocrit centrifuge for 5 minutes or if unavailable place the capillaries in a tube (preferably plastic) and centrifuge in a swing-out rotor centrifuge for 15 minutes.

   Caution: Handle the blood and capillary tubes with care. Infection can occur if viable organisms penetrate the skin or mucous membranes.

4. Wipe clean the area of each capillary where it will be viewed, i.e. where the red cell column joins the cellular layer (buffy coat) and plasma.

5. Mount the two capillaries on a slide, supported on two strips of plasticine or *Blutak* as shown in Fig. 16.4. Using a cloth or tissue, gently press to embed the capillaries in the plasticine.

6. Fill the space between the two capillaries with clean water and cover the preparation with a cover glass (see Fig. 16.4).

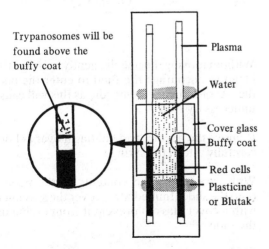

Trypanosomes will be found above the buffy coat

Plasma

Water

Cover glass

Buffy coat

Red cells

Plasticine or Blutak

Fig. 16.4 Examining centrifuged blood in capillaries for trypanosomes.

7. Examine immediately the plasma just above the buffy coat layer for motile trypanosomes. Use a 20× objective or if unavailable use a 10× objective, making sure the condenser iris is *closed sufficiently* to give good contrast, or preferably use dark-field microscopy. Use the 40× objective to confirm that the motility is due to trypanosomes.

The trypanosomes are very small but can be detected with *careful* focusing and providing the light is not too intense. The glass of the capillaries and cover glass must be completely clean.

Important: The preparation should be examined within a few minutes of the blood being centrifuged otherwise the trypanosomes will migrate into the supernatant plasma and be missed. Also, after centrifugation, the trypanosomes will gradually become less active and therefore more difficult to detect.

Note: If there are microfilariae present, their motility will make it impossible to see whether there are also trypanosomes. When this occurs it is best to examine a stained preparation from a test tube preparation as described in the following text. Breaking of capillaries to obtain a preparation for staining is not recommended for safety reasons.

Test tube centrifugation concentration technique
1. Collect venous blood into EDTA anticoagulant and mix well but do not shake. About 1.5 ml of blood is required.

   Important: The blood must be examined immediately (within 15 minutes) otherwise the trypanosomes will become inactive and difficult to detect.

2. Using a small plastic bulb pipette or other suitable pipette, fill two small narrow bore plastic or glass test tubes with EDTA (sequestrene) anticoagulated venous blood. Tubes measuring 6 × 50 mm are suitable (each tube holds about 0.7 ml of blood).

   Note: A narrow bore tube is best filled by inserting the tip of the pipette containing the blood to the bottom of the tube and withdrawing it as the tube fills.

   Availability of small tubes and plastic bulb pipettes
   Clear reusable plastic test tubes measuring 6 × 50 mm and plastic bulb pipettes suitable for filling 6 × 50 mm tubes are available from Tropical Health Technology, Equipment Service (see Appendix IV, Tubes, Plastic bulb pipettes).

3. Centrifuge the blood at medium to high speed for 15-20 minutes.

4. Using a small plastic bulb pipette, carefully

remove most of the supernatant plasma, leaving just 3 mm above the white cells and platelets (buffy coat). The trypanosomes will be concentrated in the plasma immediately above the buffy coat layer.

5. Transfer the remaining plasma with the buffy coat layer from each tube to a slide, mix gently and cover with a cover glass.

6. Examine immediately the entire preparation for motile trypanosomes, using the 40× objective with the condenser iris closed sufficiently to give good contrast.

Preparations containing microfilariae: If microfilariae are present, make a stained preparation. To do this, use forceps to remove the cover glass, allow the preparation to dry, fix it with two drops of absolute methanol (methyl alcohol) and stain using Field's thick blood film method (see 13:15)or Giemsa method (see 13:4). Examine the preparation for trypanosomes as described previously for a stained thick blood film.

Miniature anion exchange centrifugation (MAEC) technique to detect African trypanosomes
This technique is considered by most workers to be the most sensitive for detecting small numbers of *T. b. rhodesiense* or *T. b. gambiense* trypanosomes, but it is an expensive technique and therefore its use is recommended only when no parasites can be found by other methods.

The patient's heparinized blood is passed through a buffered anion (negatively charged) exchange column of diethyl-aminoethyl (DEAE)-52 cellulose. As the blood is eluted through the column, the strongly charged blood cells are adsorbed onto the cellulose while the less strongly charged trypanosomes are washed through the column with the buffered saline. The eluate is then collected, centrifuged, and the sediment is examined microscopically for motile trypanosomes. The technique *must be adequately controlled*. The cellulose column requires careful preparation and the pH of the buffer is critical to ensure adsorption of the cells and elution of the trypanosomes.

Full details of the technique, preparation and stability of reagents, and availability of MAEC kits for use in trypanosomiasis endemic areas can be obtained by writing to the Trypanosomiasis Unit, Tropical Diseases Research Programme, World Health Organization, 1211 Geneva-27, Switzerland.

Examination of lymph gland aspirates for African trypanosomes
In the early stages of African trypanosomiasis, especially in gambiense infections, trypanosomes can often be found in fluid aspirated from a swollen lymph gland. The fluid is collected and examined as follows:

1. Prepare a small syringe by rinsing it out with sterile isotonic saline. Pull back the plunger half way, ready for use.

   Note: Do not use sterile water to rinse the syringe because trypanosomes are rapidly destroyed in water.

2. Wearing sterile protective gloves, locate the swollen gland and holding it firmly, gently pull it towards the skin surface.

3. Cleanse the swollen area with a spirit swab.

4. Insert a sterile, size 18 gauge needle (without the syringe attached) into the centre of the gland (see Plate 16.2).

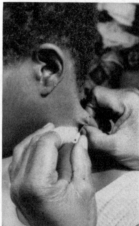

Plate 16.2 Collecting fluid from an enlarged lymph gland.
Courtesy of W. Peters.

Plate 16.3 Stained trypanosome and lymphocytes in lymph fluid.
Courtesy of W. Peters.

5. Without moving the needle, gently massage the gland to encourage the fluid to enter the needle. Avoid stirring the needle as this will cause unnecessary pain.

6. Remove the needle, and holding it over a slide, carefully attach the syringe.

7. With care, expel the contents of the needle onto the slide. Immediately cover the specimen with a cover glass to prevent it from drying on the slide.

8. Place a small sterile dressing over the needle wound.

9. With a minimum of delay, examine the entire preparation microscopically for motile trypanosomes using the 40× objective with the condenser iris *closed sufficiently* to give good contrast.

Note: If only a small amount of fluid is aspirated which is insufficient to examine as a wet preparation, allow the fluid to dry on the slide, fix it with two drops of absolute methanol (methyl alcohol), and stain by Field's rapid technique for thin films (see 13:16) or by Giemsa method (see 13:14). Examine the stained preparation as described previously.

The aspiration of fluid from an enlarged lymph gland is shown in Plate 16.2 and the appearance of a stained trypanosome in an aspirate is shown in Plate 16.3 and colour Plate 55.

Examination of chancre fluid for trypanosomes

When a chancre is present (more commonly seen in early *T. b. rhodesiense* infections than in *T. b. gambiense* infections), trypanosomes can often be detected in fluid aspirated from the swelling. The method of collecting and examining chancre fluid is as follows:

1. Cleanse the chancre with a spirit swab.

2. Wearing sterile protective gloves, puncture the chancre from the side with a small sterile needle. Blot away any blood.

3. Gently squeeze a small amount of serous fluid from the chancre and transfer it to a clean slide. Cover with a cover glass. Examine microscopically for motile trypanosomes as described previously for lymph node aspirates.

4. Place a sterile dressing over the needle wound.

Examination of cerebrospinal fluid for African trypanosomiasis

In the late stages of African trypanosomiasis, trypanosomes may be found in the cerebrospinal fluid (c.s.f.) together with Ig M-containing morula (Mott) cells, lymphocytes and other mononuclear cells. The protein content will also be increased.

Examination of the c.s.f. is required:

• To establish a diagnosis of trypanosomiasis when this is suspected clinically but the parasites cannot be found in blood (repeated examinations) or aspirates from swollen lymph glands.

• To determine whether the parasites have invaded the central nervous system (CNS). Further drug treatment is required if the CNS has become infected because Suramin, the drug commonly used to kill trypanosomes in the blood, does not destroy the parasites in the CNS.

Important: When trypanosomes have been found in the blood it is safer to collect a c.s.f. sample for testing after treatment has been started to kill the parasites in the blood. This will avoid the accidental introduction of trypanosomes into the CNS should the lumbar puncture be traumatic.

The c.s.f. must be examined *as soon as possible* after it has been collected. This is because the trypanosomes are unable to survive for more than 15-20 minutes in c.s.f. once it has been removed. The organisms become inactive, are rapidly lyzed and will not therefore be detected.

The method of examining c.s.f. is as follows:

1. Report the appearance of the fluid.

    A normal c.s.f. is clear and colourless. In meningoencephalitis due to trypanosomiasis, the c.s.f. usually appears clear to slightly cloudy depending on the number of cells present (large numbers of pus cells are not found as in bacterial meningitis).

2. Count the number of cells in the c.s.f. (see p. 162-163 in Volume II of the Manual).

    When trypanosomes have invaded the CNS, the c.s.f. will usually contain more than 5×10^6 cells/litre (5 cells/μl). The cells will be mostly lymphocytes and often morula cells will be found (see later text).

3. Centrifuge the c.s.f. at medium speed for 10-15 minutes to sediment the trypanosomes and cells.

4. Using a plastic bulb pipette or other suitable pipette, carefully transfer the supernatant fluid into another tube. This can be used for measuring the protein concentration.

5. Mix, and transfer the entire sediment to a clean slide. Cover with a cover glass. Examine immediately for motile trypanosomes using the 40× objective with the condenser iris *closed sufficiently* to give good contrast.

    Important: Usually only a few trypanosomes will be present and therefore a *careful* search of the entire preparation must be made. When searching, focus continuously and do not use too intense a light otherwise the trypanosomes will be missed.

6. If no trypanosomes are found but cells are present:

    — Using forceps, remove and discard the cover glass into a container of disinfectant, and allow the preparation to dry.

    — Fix the preparation with two drops of absolute methanol (methyl alcohol) and stain by

Field's rapid technique for thin blood films (see 13:16)or by Giemsa staining method (see 13:14).

— Spread a drop of immersion oil on the preparation and examine the area for trypanosomes and morula cells using the 40× objective.

Appearance of morula cells

Morula (Mott) cells are larger than small lymphocytes. The nucleus stains dark mauve, and the cytoplasm (may be scanty) stains blue. Characteristic vacuoles can be seen in the cytoplasm as shown in Plate 16.4 or colour Plate 53. When found in c.s.f., morula cells usually indicate trypanosome infection of the CNS.

7. Measure the total protein concentration of the c.s.f. (supernatant fluid) as described in 31:6.

When trypanosomes have invaded the CNS, the c.s.f. total protein will be raised. Very occasionally in the early stages of CNS involvement, trypanosomes can be found without a rise in c.s.f. protein but this is rare.

Ig M in c.s.f.

Ig M globulin, normally absent from c.s.f., can be detected in c.s.f. in the late stages of trypanosomiasis. Usually more than 100 μg IgM/ml of c.s.f. is found and as the disease progresses, amounts of IgM greater than 10% of the c.s.f. total protein may be found.

Ig M may also be detected in the c.s.f. of patients with viral meningitis, tuberculous meningitis and neurosyphilis but usually in amounts less than 10% of c.s.f. total protein. Tests to measure IgM in c.s.f. are expensive and not usually required when microscopy is possible to diagnose trypanosomiasis.

Summary of c.s.f. results in late stage trypanosomiasis with CNS involvement

Pressure .... Increased
Appearance .... Clear to slightly cloudy
Cell count .... Usually more than
5×10^6 cells/l
Total protein .... Raised
Pandy's test* .... Positive
Glucose (optional test) .... Reduced
Sediment .... May contain few trypanosomes
(fresh c.s.f.) and usually lymphocytes
and a few morula cells

*Pandy's test is of value only if unable to measure total protein

Serological diagnosis of African trypanosomiasis

Tests used in the serological diagnosis of trypanosomiasis to detect anti-trypanosomal antibodies, include an indirect fluorescent anti-

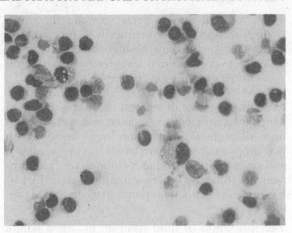

Plate 16.4 Morula cells (upper left and near centre) and lymphocytes in cerebrospinal fluid.
Courtesy of J. E. Williams.

body (IFA) test[5], an enzyme-linked immunosorbent assay (ELISA),[6][7] a capillary passive haemagglutination (HA) test,[8] and a capillary flocculation test.[9][10] Antigens for these tests are not commercially available, but details of their preparation can be found in the reference papers.

Serum for testing in the IFAT, ELISA, and capillary flocculation test can be collected on blotting or filter paper or into capillary tubes and sent to the nearest trypanosomiasis immunodiagnostic laboratory. Plasma is required for the HA test.

An antigen for a haemagglutination test to diagnose gambiense trypanosomiasis, is available from Hoechst Company.[11]

A card agglutination test (CATT) has recently been produced, to assist in the diagnosis and control of gambiense trypanosomiasis. It is available commercially from Smith Kline-RIT as Testryp CAAT.[12] The freeze dried reagents are stable for 1 year at 2-8 °C. After reconstitution, the reagents can be used for up to 2 weeks providing they are stored at 2-8 °C. Each vial of reagent is sufficient for 50 tests. Five vials are supplied with each kit. The CATT is claimed to have advantages in sensitivity and specificity as well as simplicity of use. It has yet to be fully evaluated.

Note: Because of the antigenic variations of trypanosomes it is becoming apparent that, for any serological test, it is necessary to use the local parasite for antigen to obtain maximum sensitivity.

Screening of blood donors for African trypanosomiasis

If donor blood can be stored for a few days at 2-8 °C, the risk of transmitting trypanosomes is removed because when stored at this temperature the parasites rapidly loose their infectivity. If the blood of donors from known trypanosomiasis endemic areas cannot be stored for a few days, such fresh blood should be screened for infection as follows:

☐ Testing for trypanosomes using the rapid capillary tube centrifugation technique (see previous text). If unable to perform this test, examine a stained thick blood film (taken at the time of donation).

☐ Measure the donor's haemoglobin (this test should always be performed before a person donates blood). Note whether the haemoglobin is lower than would be expected.

☐ Measure the erythrocyte sedimentation rate (ESR) or alternatively observe the time it takes for the red cells to settle in the unit of donated blood. A more rapid than normal sedimentation of the cells should alert laboratory staff as to the possibility of infected blood when taken from a donor living in a trypanosomiasis endemic area.

Blood grouping and crossmatching of blood from patients with trypanosomiasis
The grouping (typing) and crossmatching (compatibility testing) of blood from patients with African trypanosomiasis may cause difficulties due to autoagglutinins and rouleaux formation of red cells. When blood grouping, it is essential to test both the cells and serum of the patient and to check for autoagglutination. When crossmatching, autocontrols must be used and the use of antihuman globulin (Coombs crossmatch) is recommended.

16:3 *TRYPANOSOMA CRUZI*

Trypanosoma cruzi causes American trypanosomiasis, or Chagas' disease. The organism was first discovered in the vector by Carlos Chagas in 1907 and then shown to cause human disease.

T. cruzi is a complex group of organisms, the strains of which cannot be distinguished morphologically.

Trypanosoma cruzi complex
Enzyme electrophoresis of *T. cruzi* found in South America has shown the existence of three principal strain groups which differ in their infectivity to humans, their geographical distribution, transmission cycles, and may be linked to different forms of the chronic disease.

Distribution
Chagas' disease occurs only in the Americas, especially in tropical and subtropical Latin American countries. Its distribution is between latitudes 25 °N and 38 °S (see Fig. 16.5). It is thought that at least 65 million people live in areas where *T. cruzi* is found and are therefore at risk of infection, while 15 to 20 million people are probably infected.[18]

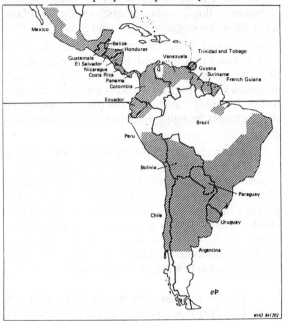

Fig. 16.5   Approximate distribution of Chagas' disease in Central America and South America. *Reproduced from WHO Chronicle, WHO 841202.*

Transmission and life cycle
T. cruzi is mainly transmitted through contact with the faeces of an infected blood-sucking bug of the family Reduviidae, subfamily Triatominae. The faeces containing infective trypomastigotes are deposited on the skin or mucous membranes as the bug feeds from its host. More than 80 species of triatomine bugs, both adults and nymphs, are capable of transmitting *T. cruzi* but the most important vectors are those that are well adapted to living in human dwellings. These include:

— *Triatoma infestans* in Argentina, Bolivia, Brazil, Chile, Paraguay, Peru and Uruguay.
— *Triatoma brasiliensis* in dry north-eastern Brazil.
— *Triatoma dimidiata* in Central America and the extreme north of South America.
— *Rhodnius prolixus* in Colombia, Ecuador, Venezuela, and parts of Central America.
— *Panstongylus megistus* in eastern Brazil.

Note: The epidemiologically important vectors of *T. cruzi* are illustrated and described in 23:12.

Adult triatomine bugs are winged and invade houses at night, often attracted by light. All bug stages can also be carried in to houses on roofing or with personal belongings. In houses colonized by bugs, several thousand may be found in the cracks of walls and in roofs, feeding from humans, domestic animals, and rodents. Chickens, although not infected with *T. cruzi*, often provide a source of blood for large numbers of triatomine bugs.

Important animal reservoirs of *T. cruzi* include opossums, dogs, cats, goats, sheep, rabbits, armadillos, mice, guinea pigs, and bats.

Besides those living in poorly constructed and overcrowded bug-infested dwellings in rural areas, those living in shanty towns are also at risk from infection when migrant workers and their families (often infected) travel from the countryside to the shanty towns bringing infected bugs in their luggage.

T. cruzi can also be transmitted by blood transfusion. It has been estimated that up to 20% of blood donors in non-endemic urban areas are infected with *T. cruzi* and therefore transmission of the parasite in blood is a serious problem.[18] Less commonly, transplacental transmission occurs with a foetus being infected from an asymptomatic mother. Such infected infants are often stillborn or born prematurely with a low birth weight.

Note: The precautions which need to be taken to avoid laboratory-acquired *T. cruzi* infections are described at the end of this subunit.

Life cycle
— In most infections, metacyclic (infective) trypomastigotes contained in the faeces of an infected bug, penetrate the skin through the bite wound or enter through the conjunctiva or membranes of the mouth or nose. The faeces are deposited as the bug feeds or soon after.

— The trypomastigotes invade the reticuloendothelial cells near the point of entry and multiply intracellularly as amastigotes.

    T. cruzi amastigotes: Each is round to oval in form, measures 2.5-6.5 μm in diameter and contains a nucleus, kinetoplast, and axoneme. Structurally the amastigotes of *T. cruzi* resemble those of *Leishmania* species.

— The amastigotes develop into trypomastigotes which are released into the blood when the cell ruptures. No multiplication of the parasite occurs in its trypomastigote stage in the blood.

— By way of the blood and lymphatic system, the trypomastigotes reach tissue cells, especially those of heart muscle, nerves, skeletal muscle, and smooth muscle of the gastrointestinal tract and elsewhere. The trypomastigotes become amastigotes and multiply, forming masses known as pseudocysts. One trypomastigote may give rise to 500 amastigotes within a single pseudocyst in as little as 5 days.

— Within the pseudocysts, a proportion of the amastigotes become elongated and develop first into epimastigotes and then into trypomastigotes which are released into the blood when the host cell ruptures. Some of these trypomastigotes continue to circulate while the majority infect further tissue cells.

— The life cycle is continued when a triatomine bug vector ingests circulating trypomastigotes in a blood meal. In the vector, the trypomastigotes transform and eventually develop into epimastigotes which multiply by binary fission in the gut of the bug.

— Within 10-15 days, metacyclic trypomastigotes (short, slender and highly motile) are formed and can be found in the hindgut of the bug, ready to be excreted when the vector defaecates as it takes a blood meal.

Clinical features and pathology
Geographically, there are differences in the clinical features and pathology associated with *T. cruzi* infection which may be due to variations in the strains of *T. cruzi* found in different areas, and to host factors.

Many people infected with *T. cruzi* remain asymptomatic and free from Chagas' disease, or experience only an acute infection without progressing to the chronic stage of the disease.

Multiplication of *T. cruzi* at the site of infection, together with a host cellular immune response, can produce an inflamed swelling known as a chagoma which usually persists for several weeks (see Plate 16.5). If the site of infection is the eye, usually the conjunctiva becomes inflamed and oedema forms. This is known as Romana's sign (see Plate 16.6).

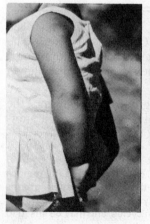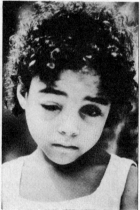

Plate 16.5 Cutaneous chagoma on forearm of a patient with Chagas' disease.
Courtesy of Dr M A Miles.

Plate 16.6 Romana's sign in acute Chagas' disease.
Courtesy of Dr M A Miles.

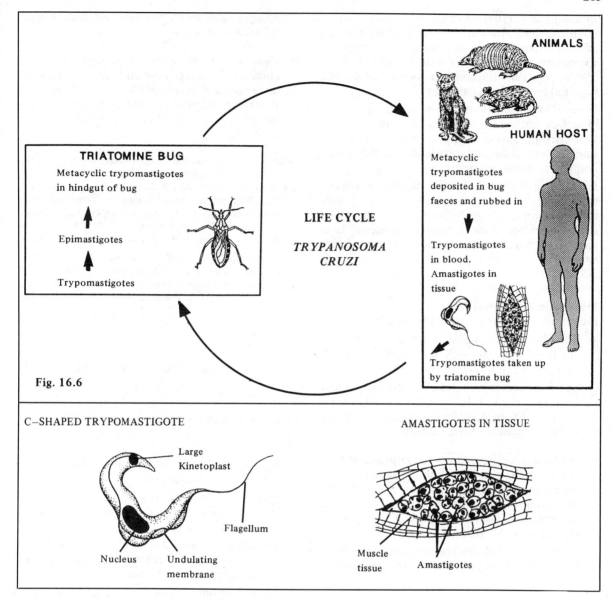

Fig. 16.6

LIFE CYCLE

TRYPANOSOMA CRUZI

TRIATOMINE BUG

Metacyclic trypomastigotes in hindgut of bug

↑

Epimastigotes

↑

Trypomastigotes

ANIMALS

HUMAN HOST

Metacyclic trypomastigotes deposited in bug faeces and rubbed in

↓

Trypomastigotes in blood. Amastigotes in tissue

Trypomastigotes taken up by triatomine bug

C–SHAPED TRYPOMASTIGOTE

Large Kinetoplast

Flagellum

Nucleus

Undulating membrane

AMASTIGOTES IN TISSUE

Muscle tissue

Amastigotes

Acute stage of infection

In this stage, trypomastigotes can be found circulating in the blood. They then multiply intracellularly as amastigotes and spread throughout the body. Symptoms may be minor and pass unnoticed or there may be fever, malaise, an increased pulse rate and enlargement of the lymph glands, liver, and to a lesser extent the spleen. Lymphocytosis is common and atypical mononuclear cells may be seen. Peripheral blood films often resemble those of glandular fever.

The acute form of the disease is most commonly seen in young children. Occasionally an acute attack can cause serious damage to the heart or result in other complications which may lead to death.

Early detection of *T. cruzi* infection, before there is nerve and muscle fibre damage, reduces the risk of chronic Chagas' disease developing.

Chronic stage of infection

If the person survives an acute attack, chronic Chagas' disease may develop with signs of cardiac muscle damage, including a weak and irregular heart beat, enlargement of the heart and oedema. Severe damage to heart muscle leads to heart failure. Approximately 10% of persons infected with *T. cruzi* develop chronic Chagas' cardiopathy. In some areas chronic Chagas' disease may be responsible for up to 10% of deaths among adult populations.[18]

Parasite infection of intestinal muscle may cause damage to nerves in the intestinal wall, causing loss of the muscular action necessary for the movement of food. The accumulation and slow movement of food leads to enlargement of the oesophagus (megaoesophagus) and colon (megacolon). These features are more commonly seen in central and eastern Brazil.

Immunity in T. cruzi infection

Soon after infection with *T. cruzi*, the humoral and cellular responses of the host reduce the number of trypomastigotes circulating in the blood and after a few weeks, xenodiagnosis or blood culture are required to detect the parasites.

T. cruzi organisms do not show marked variation in surface antigens like *T. b. rhodesiense* and *T. b. gambiense* but surface changes, related to the invasion of host cells and resistance to the host's immune response, do occur.

It is thought that autoimmunity may play an important part in the origin and development of myocarditis in chronic Chagas' disease[13] but the exact nature of anti-parasite immune responses to host tissues in Chagas' disease is not yet fully understood.[14]

Prevention and control

Preventive and control measures include:

- Spraying of bug-infested houses, furniture, sheds, latrines, etc, with insecticides every few months and checking for reinfestation.

   The insecticides used must be effective against local vectors and WHO test kits should be used to check for insecticide effectiveness and for the development of bug resistance.

- With community support, the improvement of rural housing and household hygiene to eliminate refuges for triatomine bugs, especially the plastering of all creviced wall surfaces with cement or if unavailable with a strong local clay-mud plaster that will not crack.

   In areas where *R. prolixus* is found, palm roofing should be replaced by corrugated metal sheets.

- Burning or spraying with insecticide, abandoned bug-infested houses and the spraying with insecticide of belongings transferred to new houses.

- Removal from houses of animal reservoirs which could harbour *T. cruzi*. Reservoir hosts include opossums, dogs, cats, goats, sheep, rabbits, armadillos, mice, and guinea pigs.

   Roosting chickens (from which bugs feed) should be removed from houses and encouraged to roost in trees. If a chicken house is essential, it should be a simple wooden frame structure, well-penetrated by daylight, and treated with insecticide at the same time as the house and associated out-buildings are sprayed.

- Selective destruction of infested mammal

refuges such as palm trees and hollow trees adjacent to houses.

- Periodic serological surveys (e.g. among school children) to detect new endemic foci in areas under control, combined with education about the transmission of *T. cruzi*, symptoms of early infection, and importance of treatment at an early stage.

Further information about Chagas' disease: A review of literature published between July 1983 - December 1984 entitled *Trypanosomiasis II Stercoraria* can be found in Tropical Diseases Bulletin.[14] Details of WHO published documents on American trypanosomiasis can be obtained by writing to the Trypanosomiasis Unit, TDR Programme, World Health Organization, 1211 Geneva-27, Switzerland.

A special 1985 issue of the British Medical Bulletin[3] entitled *Trypanosomiasis* contains information on the biology of *T. cruzi* and the epidemiology, pathology, immunology, diagnosis, chemotherapy, and control of Chagas' disease.

LABORATORY DIAGNOSIS

Laboratory confirmation of *T. cruzi* infection is by:

- Finding the trypanosomes of *T. cruzi* in blood in early acute infections.

- Detecting the parasites by xenodiagnosis in chronic and subacute infections when parasitaemia is low.

- Detecting the parasites by blood culture in the later stages of infection when facilities for xenodiagnosis are not available.

- Testing serum for anti-*T. cruzi* antibodies, to assist in the diagnosis of chronic Chagas' disease or congenital Chagas' disease, detection of infected donor blood, and the testing of populations as part of an epidemiological survey.

   When diagnosing congenital Chagas' disease, the tests used must distinguish between Ig M antibodies produced by an infected infant and maternal Ig G antibodies which have crossed the placenta and are present in the serum of the infant.

Other laboratory findings in T. cruzi infection

- In acute infections there is a raised ESR, and usually a marked lymphocytosis with atypical mononuclear cells (resembling glandular fever blood films) and often a positive Paul Bunnel test.

- In chronic infections, laboratory findings will

vary according to cardiac symptoms and other complications which may occur.

Examination of blood for *T. cruzi*

The detection of circulating trypanosomes in the early stages of *T. cruzi* infection is of great importance because at this stage effective treatment can be given which may prevent damage to heart muscle and other tissue cells and the development of chronic Chagas' disease in later life.

The trypanosomes of *T. cruzi* are fragile organisms. They tend to be easily lyzed in thick blood films (as the blood dries) and easily damaged when spreading blood to make thin films. The following techniques, which are based on detecting motile trypanosomes, are therefore recommended when examining blood for *T. cruzi* in acute infections:

— Careful microscopical examination of fresh blood for motile trypanosomes as a wet preparation.

— Capillary tube (microhaematocrit) centrifugation concentration technique. This is a rapid and sensitive technique.

— Test tube centrifugation concentration technique using venous blood.

Note: In areas where *Trypanosoma rangeli* (non-pathogenic species transmitted by *Rhodnius* bugs) is found with *T. cruzi*, i.e. mainly in Central America, Venezuela, Brazil, Columbia, all positive preparations should be checked to confirm that the motile trypanosomes seen are *T. cruzi* and not *T. rangeli* (see later text).

Miniature anion exchange centrifugation (MAEC) technique

This technique as used for detecting small numbers of *T. b. gambiense* and *T. b. rhodesiense* is not suitable for detecting *T. cruzi* in blood.

Examination of a wet blood preparation

1. Collect a small drop of capillary blood or fresh venous blood on a slide and cover with a cover glass. Do not make the preparation too thick otherwise the trypanosomes will be missed.

2. Immediately examine the entire preparation microscopically for motile trypanosomes. Use the 40× objective with the condenser iris closed sufficiently to give good contrast or preferably use dark-field or phase contrast microscopy.

   Up to 30 minutes may need to be spent examining the preparation to detect *T. cruzi* trypanosomes. The chances of detecting the parasites are increased if several preparations are examined or if a capillary tube centrifugation concentration technique is used (see later text).

Note: If motile trypanosomes are seen, and *T. rangeli* is known to occur in the area, identify the species by examining a stained thin blood film. To avoid damaging the parasites when spreading the blood, hold the spreader at an angle of 60-70° and use as little pressure as possible. Air-dry the film rapidly. Immediately fix the dried thin film with absolute methanol and stain using Field's thin blood film method (see 13:16) or Giemsa method (see 13:14). See later text for the features which differentiate *T. cruzi* from *T. rangeli*.

Capillary tube centrifugation concentration technique

This technique is as described for *T. b. gambiense* and *T. b. rhodesiense* in the previous subunit. Examination of four capillary tubes is recommended to increase the chances of detecting the parasites.

Note: If trypanosomes are seen and *T. rangeli* is known to occur in the area, identify the species by examining a stained preparation. For safety reasons, it is best not to break the capillary tubes to obtain a specimen for staining but to centrifuge anticoagulated venous blood in a narrow bore test tube and transfer the buffy coat and plasma *immediately above it* to a slide and make a preparation for staining. Spread the buffy coat and plasma on a slide (using minimum pressure) and air-dry rapidly. Fix the preparation with absolute methanol and stain using Field's rapid technique for thin films (see 13:16) or Giemsa staining technique (see 13:14). See later text for the features which differentiate *T. cruzi* from *T. rangeli*.

Test tube centrifugation concentration technique

The technique as described for *T. b. gambiense* and *T. b. rhodesiense* in the previous subunit can be used to detect *T. cruzi* in venous blood.

Alternatively, the Strout technique can be used in which 5-10 ml of freshly collected venous blood is allowed to clot and when the clot has retracted the supernatant serum is removed, centrifuged for 15 minutes, and the sediment examined as a wet preparation for motile trypanosomes.

Also recommended is the Hoff method in which about 1 ml of fresh EDTA anticoagulated blood is added to 3 ml of ammonium chloride solution (8.7 g/l aqueous solution) and the red cells left to lyze for 3 minutes. After centrifuging for 15 minutes, the sediment is examined as a wet preparation for motile trypanosomes.

Note: If motile trypanosomes are seen and *T. rangeli* is known to occur in the area, identify the species by examining a stained preparation.

Differentiation of T. cruzi and T. rangeli in stained preparations

Spread a drop of oil on the dried stained preparation and examine first with the 40× objective to detect the trypanosomes. Use the oil immersion objective to identify the species.

The following features can be used to differentiate *T. cruzi* and *T. rangeli* in Romanowsky stained blood films:

Trypanosoma cruzi trypanosomes

- Usually C-shaped, measuring 12-30 μm in length with a narrow membrane and free flagellum.
- Has a *large*, round to oval, dark-red staining kinetoplast at the posterior end.
- Nucleus is centrally placed and stains red-mauve.

Note: Occasionally slender forms of *T. cruzi* can be seen which have an elongated nucleus, subterminal kinetoplast, and shorter free flagellum.

Illustrations: See Fig. 16.6, Plate 16.7 and colour Plate 56.

Trypanosoma rangeli trypanosomes

Compared with *T. cruzi*, the trypanosomes of *T. rangeli* are longer and thinner, measuring 27-32 μm in length, have a long pointed posterior end and a much smaller kinetoplast which is situated a little way from the posterior end.

Illustration: See Plate 16.8.

Note: *T. rangeli* is transmitted by the bite of *R. prolixus* bugs. It is found in Brazil, Venezuela, Colombia, Panama, El Salvador and Guatemala.

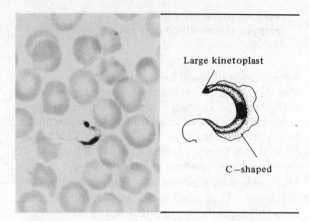

Plate 16.7 *Trypanosoma cruzi* in stained blood film as seen with 100x objective.

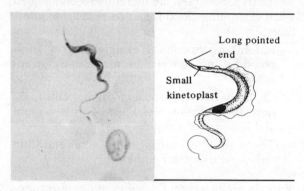

Plate 16.8 *Trypanosoma rangeli*. Compared with *T. cruzi* it is longer and thinner with a pointed end.

Artificial feeding technique

To avoid hypersensitive skin reactions in patients, especially when needing to use laboratory-reared *R. prolixus* bugs, an artificial feeding technique has been developed in which 5 ml of the patient's venous blood is injected into a bag (made of cow-gut membranes and containing heparin) inside a small pot containing the bugs. The bugs feed through the bag. The amount of blood ingested by the artificially fed bugs was shown to be directly comparable with that ingested during natural feeding.[15]

Method of examining bug faeces

1. Collect faeces from a bug into a drop of sterile isotonic saline on a slide. Cover with a cover glass.

   Note: Do not use unsterile saline because this may contain ciliates which could be confused with trypanosomal flagellates.

2. Examine the preparation microscopically for motile flagellates, using the 40× objective with condenser iris *closed sufficiently* to give good contrast, or preferably use phase contrast or dark-field microscopy.

Xenodiagnosis of T. cruzi

This method of diagnosis is of value to detect parasites during the chronic stage of infection when their number in the blood is usually very few.

Uninfected, *susceptible*, laboratory-reared triatomine bugs are starved for 2 weeks and then fed on the patient's blood. If trypanosomes are ingested they will multiply and develop into epimastigotes and trypomastigotes which can be found 25-30 days later in the faeces or rectum of the bug.

Note: The use of local bug vectors is important because there are differences in the susceptibility of vectors to infection by *T. cruzi*.

3. If flagellates are seen, identify the species in a Giemsa stained preparation. To avoid the faeces being washed from the slide during staining, mix a small drop of sterile human serum with the preparation before allowing it to dry. Fix the dried preparation with 2 drops of absolute methanol.

   Note: The parasites do not stain particularly well but staining can be improved by adding 1 drop of 10% v/v formol saline to every 10 ml of the diluted stain.

Differentiation between the epimastigotes of T. rangeli and T. cruzi

In mixed infections, the epimastigotes of *T. rangeli* can be differentiated from those of *T. cruzi*, mainly by their size. Compared with *T. cruzi*, the epimastigotes of *T. rangeli* are much longer and thinner, sometimes measuring more than 80 μm in length.

Note: Because the transmission of *T. rangeli* is by inoculation, the trypomastigotes and epimastigotes of this species are usually found in the salivary glands and not in the faeces of the bug (as is the case with *T. cruzi*).

Laboratory colonies of bugs bred for xenodiagnosis must be examined periodically for the presence of insect flagellates.

Blood culture to detect *T. cruzi*

A culture technique is used mainly to diagnose chronic Chagas' disease when the facilities for xenodiagnosis are not available. Culture methods are almost as sensitive as xenodiagnosis providing an aseptic procedure is used.

T. cruzi grows in many blood agar culture media. The preparation and use of a suitable medium is as follows:

Preparation of medium

1. Weigh the following ingredients and dissolve them by gentle heat in 100 ml of distilled water:

   Bacto blood agar base .... 1.4 g
   (Difco 00450)
   Bacto tryptose .... 0.5 g
   (Difco 0124-01)
   Purified agar .... 0.3 g
   (Oxoid 128)
   Sodium chloride .... 0.6 g

2. Mix and dispense 4 ml into clean culture tubes. Plug each tube with non-absorbent cotton wool. Wrap the rack of tubes in tinfoil and sterilize by autoclaving at 120 °C for 20 minutes.

3. When the medium has cooled to 45-50 °C, add aseptically to each tube, approximately 0.3 ml of sterile defibrinated rabbit blood, previously heat-inactivated at 56 °C for 30 minutes.

4. Allow the medium to set within the tubes in a sloped position.

5. Add aseptically to each tube, 0.5-1.0 ml of sterile physiological saline (0.9 g/litre) to which has been added 400 units benzylpenicillin and 400 units streptomycin sulphate per ml.

6. Incubate the tubes at 25-28 °C for 36 hours to test for sterility. If sterile, store the tubes of medium at 4-6 °C until required.

Use of medium

— Inoculate aseptically, 0.2 ml of the patient's blood and incubate at 25-28 °C. Inoculation of two tubes is recommended in case one tube should become contaminated.

— After 14-21 days, examine a few drops of the fluid for motile *T. cruzi* epimastigotes. Identify the species by examining a Giemsa stained preparation of the culture.

   Note: The appearance of *T. cruzi* epimastigotes from a blood agar culture is shown in Plate 16.9.

Field use: In surveys, blood samples can be inoculated aseptically, with the aid of a spirit lamp, through the rubber caps of re-used *Vacutainers*.

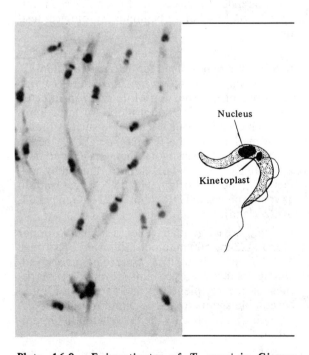

Plate 16.9   Epimastigotes of *T. cruzi* in Giemsa stained preparation of a culture. Note the position of the large kinetoplast and the nucleus.
Courtesy of Dr M. A. Miles.

Serological diagnosis of Chagas' disease

Serological tests are of value in diagnosing Chagas' disease in the chronic stage of infection when parasites cannot be found in the blood. Antibody testing is also important in mass surveys and to screen blood from blood donors in endemic areas.

Once infected with *T. cruzi*, a person remains infected for life and therefore antibodies persist throughout life.

Tests to detect anti-*T. cruzi* antibodies in serum include a complement fixation test (CFT), indirect fluorescent antibody test (IFAT), an indirect haemagglutination (IHAT), and an enzyme-linked immunosorbent assay (ELISA). These tests become positive about 1 month after infection and usually remain positive after treatment even if parasites cannot be found. The IFAT, IHAT, and ELISA are simpler than the CFT and can be performed on finger-prick blood collected onto filter paper. Filter paper blood samples should be stored frozen in a sealed bag containing a desiccant (e.g. silica gel) until they can be tested. Most antigens cross-react with *Leishmania* species and with *T. rangeli*.

Reagents for an IFAT, IHAT and ELISA are available commercially but not all the commercially available *T. cruzi* test kits are fully reliable. In most South American countries, there are immunodiagnostic centres to which blood samples can be sent or training given in *T. cruzi* serological techniques. District hospital laboratories are recommended to seek advice from a *T. cruzi* reference laboratory before beginning serological testing.

Screening of donor blood for *T. cruzi* infection

As mentioned under *Transmission*, there is a high incidence of transmission of *T. cruzi* in infected donor blood. Testing donor blood for infection is best achieved by using a technique such as the G-agglutination test. This test has been developed in Brazil. It uses epimastigote fragments coated onto graphite particles (details can be obtained by contacting the World Health Organization, Trypanosomiasis TDR Unit, 1211 Geneva-27, Switzerland).

In some areas, gentian violet is added to donor blood (125 mg/500 ml blood) followed by storage at 2-8 °C for 24 h to kill *T. cruzi*. The main disadvantage is that the dye stains (reversibly) the tissues of the recipient of the blood. New more acceptable agents to add to blood to kill *T. cruzi* are being researched by the World Health Organization.[16]

Avoiding *T. cruzi* infection in the laboratory[17]

Infection with *T. cruzi* can occur if viable parasites (even very few) penetrate the skin, conjunctiva, or mucous membranes. The following precautions are recommended to avoid laboratory-acquired infection with *T. cruzi*:

■ When working with live parasites and infected animals, wear good rubber gloves, a safety mask and eyeshields. Keep arms and legs covered. Wear shoes not open sandals.

■ When centrifuging, use tubes that can be closed.

■ Never mouth-pipette, eat, drink, chew gum, or smoke in the laboratory.

■ Protect all contaminated material from flies and before disposing of such material, immerse it overnight in 70% ethanol.

■ Use and dispose of contaminated needles, syringes, and lancets with great care.

■ Keep triatomine bugs in secure, unbreakable, double containers, and dissect bugs behind a small perspex screen or preferably use a microbiological safety cabinet (Class I or II).

■ Before any container of insects known or suspected of being infected is opened, chill the bugs by placing the container at 4 °C for at least 30 minutes. When working with the bugs, it is advisable to stand the container in crushed ice.

■ If personal contamination should occur, report the incident and obtain medical advice immediately.

If the skin has been punctured, wash the wound with running water and encourage bleeding. Apply a fresh solution of a germicide such as *Savlon*.

If the conjunctiva is contaminated, wash the eye well with clean water (do not apply a germicide because this could damage the eye), and immediately seek medical advice.

■ Laboratory and associated personnel working with live *T. cruzi* parasites should be tested two or three times a year for serum antibodies against *T. cruzi*.

References

1 Tait, A., Barry, J. D., *et al.* Enzyme variation in *T. brucei* ssp. II: Evidence for *T. b. rhodesiense* being a set of variants of *T. b. brucei*. *Parasitology*, **90**, pp 89-100, 1985.

2 Molyneux, D. H., Ashford, R. W. *The Biology of Trypanosoma and Leishmania*, Taylor and Francis, p. xii and p. 294, 1983.

3 Newton, B. A. (Editor) *Trypanosomiasis*, special issue, *British Medical Bulletin*, **41**, pp 103-199, 1985.

4 Taylor, A. E. R. (Editor) *Trypanosomiasis I Salivaria*, supplement in *Tropical Diseases Bulletin*, **83**, (2), R2-R15, 1986.

5 Wéry, M., Wéry-Paskoff, S., and Van Wettere, P. The diagnosis of human African trypanosomiasis by the use of a fluorescent antibody test. *Annales de la Société belge de Médecine tropicale*, **50**, pp 613-634, 1970.

6 Voller, A., Bidwell, D., and Bartlett, A. A serological study on human *Trypanosoma rhodesiense* infection using a microscale enzyme linked immunosorbent assay. *Zeitschrift fur Tropenmedizin und Parasitologie*, **26**, pp 247-251, 1975.

7 Voller, A., Draper, C. *et al*. Microplate enzyme linked immunosorbent assay for Chagas' disease. *Lancet*, **1**, p 426, 1975.

8 Boné, G. J., Charlier, J. L'haemagglutination indirecte en capillaire: une methode de diagnostic de la trypanosomiaise applicable sur le terrain. *Annales de la Société belge de Médecine tropicale*, **55**, pp 559-569, 1975.

9 Ross, J. P. J. The detection of circulating trypanosomal antibodies by capillary tube agglutination test. *Annals of Tropical Medicine and Parasitology*, **65**, pp 327-333, 1971.

10 Binz, G. An evaluation of the capillary and latex agglutination and heterophile antibody tests for the detection of *T. rhodesiense* infections, *Bulletin World Health Organization*, **47**, pp 773-778, 1972.

11 The Hoechst *Cellognost Trypanosomiasis Combipack* kit for IHA testing for antibodies to *T. b. gambiense* costs approx. £22.37 (1986) for 150 qualitative tests. The kit includes 5 ml IHA reagent, positive and negative control sera and 2 × 10 ml buffer solution pH 8. The reagents have a shelf-life of about 4 months before reconstitution and the IHA reagent after reconstitution can be used up to 4 weeks providing it is stored at 2-8 °C.

12 The Smith Kline *Testryp CAAT* test kit (No. 104155M) for 250 qualitative tests contains 5 vials of CAAT reagent (each vial is sufficient for 50 tests), 1 vial each of positive and negative control serum, and 1 vial of CAAT buffer. *Testryp CAAT* equipment (No. 104154L) for 250 qualitative tests consists of 250 heparinized capillary tubes, 1 capillary tube syringe, 25 plastic coated cards (10 tests each card), 1 syringe of 2.5 ml, 5 stirring rods, and 3 droppers. For the price of the kits, readers should contact Smith Kline (for address see Appendix II).

13 Hudson, L. Immunobiology of *T. cruzi* infection and Chagas' disease. *Transactions of the Royal Society of Tropical Medicine and Hygiene*, **75**, pp 493-498, 1981.

14 Taylor, A. E. R. (Editor). *Trypanosomias, II Stercoraria*, supplement in *Tropical Diseases Bulletin*, **83**, (3), R25-R60, 1986.

15 Cedillos, R. A. *et al*. *Boletin de la Oficina Sanitaria Panamericana*, **93**, pp 240-249, 1982.

16 WHO. Meeting on the development of trypanocidal compounds for the sterilization of blood. TDR/CHA/84.3, 1984. Copies can be obtained from TDR Unit, World Health Organization, 1211 Geneva-27, Switzerland.

17 Suggested guidelines for work with live *Trypanosoma cruzi* (formulated for research laboratories in UK), *Transactions of the Royal Society of Tropical Medicine and Hygiene*, **77**, pp 416-419, 1983.

18 Tropical disease research: TDR seventh programme report (1 January 1983 - 31 December 1984). WHO, 1985.

19 Cunningham, M. P., Bailey, N. M., Kimber, C. D. *Transactions of the Royal Society of Medicine and Hygiene*, **61**, p 688, 1967.

Recommended Reading

World Health Organization Epidemiology and control of African trypanosomiasis. Report of WHO Expert Committee. WHO, Geneva, 1986.

Tropical Diseases Research Programme
AFRICAN TRYPANOSOMIASIS CHAGAS' DISEASE

African trypanosomiasis and Chagas' disease are included in the *UNDP/World Bank/ World Health Organization Special Programme for Research and Training in Tropical Diseases*.

Tropical Diseases Research (TDR) activities with regard to African trypanosomiasis and Chagas' disease as recorded in No. 5 of the 1985 *WHO Chronicle* are as follows:

African trypanosomiasis:
- Research into new drugs such as DL-alpha-difluoromethylornithine (DFMO).

- Advances in vector control including an exchange of information among scientists working on traps enhanced by odour attractants and impregnated with insecticides. These are proving to be a remarkably successful practical means of reducing the tsetse fly population and controlling infection in some parts of West Africa.

Chagas's disease
- Continuing search for effective drugs to treat chronic Chagas' disease.

- Establishing more collaborating laboratories for the standardization of serodiagnoses of Chagas' disease. Such laboratories are now found in 11 countries of the Americas and the central laboratory in Sao Paulo, Brazil distributes reference sera to the collaborating laboratories.

- With a view to find a vaccine against Chagas' disease, TDR is supporting research on the standardization of animal models to provide information on the mechanisms of immune reactions and ultimately to help in the development and evaluation of vaccines.

17

Leishmanial Parasites

17:1 CLASSIFICATION AND FEATURES OF LEISHMANIAL PARASITES

Leishmanial parasites are protozoa belonging to the subphylum Mastigophora the general characteristics of which are described at the beginning of the Parasitology Section in 12:4.

Classification of leishmanial parasites of medical importance

Classification of *Leishmania* species is not yet complete. Recent advances in biotechnology make it possible to differentiate the species biochemically by their isoenzymes and other genetic characteristics. Accordingly, former classifications which were based on clinical, geographical, and epidemiological characteristics are now being reviewed.

The following is a generally accepted current classification of the *Leishmania* species and subspecies of medical importance:

Order	KINETOPLASTIDA
Species	*Leishmania donovani* complex
Subspecies	*L. d. donovani*
	L. d. infantum*
	East African *L. donovani*
	Sudanese *L. donovani*
	L. d. chagasi*
Species	*Leishmania braziliensis* complex
Subspecies	*L. b. braziliensis*
	L. b. guyanensis*
	L. b. panamensis*
	L. b. peruviana*
Species	*Leishmania mexicana* complex
Subspecies	*L. m. mexicana*
	L. m. amazonensis
	L. m. pifanoi
	L. m. venezuelensis
Species	*Leishmania major*
	Leishmania tropica
	Leishmania aethiopica

*Some workers consider these to be separate species

Features of leishmanial parasites
- In humans and other vertebrate hosts a small intracellular form of the parasite is found called an amastigote. It lives and multiplies in macrophages and other phagocytic cells in the internal organs (visceral leishmaniasis), in skin (cutaneous leishmaniasis), in organs and skin, or in mucocutaneous tissue and skin (mucocutaneous leishmaniasis).

In sandfly vectors and *in vitro* cultures at 25 °C, a flagellated highly motile form of the parasite is found called a promastigote. It multiplies in the gut of the sandfly, sometimes attached to the gut wall. A kinetoplast is found at the base of the single flagellum.

- Human infections with leishmanial parasites are with few exceptions zoonoses. The vectors are sandfly species that take up the parasites when feeding from the natural animal hosts of the parasites. Transmission to humans occurs when the infected sandflies feed from man. Less frequently man is an important reservoir of infection, e.g. in Indian visceral leishmaniasis.

There is considerable variation in human susceptibility, age at which infection occurs, and type of disease which results.

- Laboratory confirmation of visceral leishmaniasis is by finding intracellular or free amastigotes in aspirates from spleen, bone marrow, lymph glands, or occasionally by finding amastigotes in blood monocytes. Cutaneous leishmaniasis is diagnosed by finding amastigotes in material removed from skin ulcers. Mucocutaneous leishmaniasis is diagnosed by finding amastigotes in smears taken from infected mucocutaneous tissue.

17:2 *LEISHMANIA DONOVANI* COMPLEX CAUSING OLD AND NEW WORLD VISCERAL LEISHMANIASIS

Visceral leishmaniasis in the Old World is caused by:

- *Leishmania donovani* subspecies*
  * *L. d. donovani*
  * *L. d. infantum*
  * East African *L. donovani*
  * Sudanese *L. donovani*

In India and elsewhere, visceral leishmaniasis is known as kala-azar.

Leishmanial Parasites of Medical Importance

LIFE CYCLE SUMMARIES

Leishmania donovani complex	*Leishmania major* *Leishmania tropica* *Leishmania aethiopica* *Leishmania mexicana* complex *Leishmania braziliensis* complex
Promastigotes inoculated when a female sandfly sucks blood	Promastigotes inoculated when a female sandfly sucks blood
Promastigotes taken up by skin macrophages and become amastigotes. They multiply and spread throughout the body.	Promastigotes taken up by skin macrophages and become amastigotes. They multiply and spread to other skin macrophages.
AMASTIGOTES PARASITIZE MACROPHAGES OF MONONUCLEAR PHAGOCYTIC SYSTEM	AMASTIGOTES PARASITIZE MACROPHAGES IN SKIN and, or, MUCOCUTANEOUS TISSUE (see *Notes*)
Amastigotes taken up when sandfly takes a blood meal	Amastigotes taken up when sandfly takes a blood meal

Notes

☐ In post kala-azar dermal leishmaniasis, *L. donovani* is found in the skin.

☐ *L. b. braziliensis* and *L. aethiopica* parasitize mucocutaneous tissue.

Visceral leishmaniasis in the New World is caused by:

■ *Leishmania donovani chagasi*

Note: The term Old World refers to Africa, Asia, Europe. The term New World refers to the Americas which with respect to leishmanial parasites refers to South America and Central America.

Distribution

L. d. donovani is found in the Indian subcontinent and southwest Asia. Humans are the main reservoirs of infection. Young adults are more commonly infected and epidemics occur.

L. d. infantum is endemic in north Africa, Middle East, northeast China, and central Asia. Dogs and wild canids are reservoir hosts and young children are more often infected than adults.

L. d. chagasi is found in parts of Central and South America. Dogs and foxes are reservoir hosts and young children are commonly infected.

Other forms of *L. donovani* are found in East Africa and in the Sudan. In Sudan, rodents have been identified as reservoir hosts. The disease is more sporadic with herdsmen and migrant workers being commonly infected. In East Africa, humans are reservoirs of infection and the disease tends to be more sporadic with young males being more commonly infected.

Note: Further information of the known worldwide distribution of *L. donovani* and other *Leishmania* species can be found in the WHO 1984 Report on *The Leishmaniases*[1]

Table 17.1 Distribution, and Reservoir Hosts of Leishmania donovani complex

Species Subspecies	Distribution	Reservoir Hosts	Disease
OLD WORLD			
L. donovani donovani	Indian sub-continent, Southwest Asia	Humans	Epidemic visceral leishmaniasis (kala-azar) Post kala-azar dermal leishmaniasis
L. donovani infantum	North Africa, Middle East, Central Asia, North China	Dogs, foxes jackals	Infantile type visceral leishmaniasis
L. donovani (sensu latu) from East Africa	Kenya, Ethiopia, Somalia	Humans Possibly dogs	Visceral leishmaniasis‡
L. donovani (sensu latu) from Sudan	Sudan	Rodents and some wild carnivores	Visceral leishmaniasis‡
NEW WORLD			
L. donovani chagasi	Central and South America	Dogs and foxes	Infantile type visceral leishmaniasis

‡ Nodular or ulcerative lesions of the skin may occur

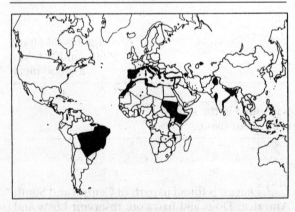

Fig. 17.1 Distribution of visceral leishmaniasis. Shading indicates endemic areas and dots show sporadic cases. *Reproduced from WHO Technical Report Series No. 701, 1984.*

Transmission and life cycle

The different forms of *L. donovani* have their own species of sandfly vectors and reservoir hosts.

Sandflies of the genus *Phlebotomus* transmit *L. donovani* except in Central and South America where the vector belongs to the genus *Lutzomyia*. The features and breeding habits of sandflies are described in 23:4.

Visceral leishmaniasis is a zoonosis except in the Indian subcontinent and some parts of East Africa. Important animal reservoir hosts of *L. donovani* are dogs, foxes, jackals and rodents as shown in Table 17.1.

A person becomes infected when promastigotes are inoculated at the time a female sandfly takes a blood meal.

L. donovani can also be transmitted congenitally, by sexual contact, and by blood transfusion. In endemic areas, blood donors should be screened serologically or if this is not possible at least by the formol gel screening test as described in this sub-unit.

Life cycle

— Following inoculation, the promastigotes are taken up by phagocytic cells and develop into amastigotes. The morphology of an amastigote is shown in Fig. 17.2.

— Amastigotes are spread in the blood and multiply in the macrophages of the spleen, liver, bone marrow, lymph glands, mucosa of the small intestine, and other tissues of the reticuloendothelial system (mononuclear phagocytic network).

— Intracellular and free amastigotes are ingested by a female sandfly vector when it sucks blood.

— After about 72 hours, the amastigotes become flagellated promastigotes in the midgut of the sandfly. The promastigote form is shown in Fig. 17.2.

— The promastigotes multiply and fill the lumen of the sandfly gut. After 4-18 days (depending on species) the promastigotes move forward to the head and mouth-parts of the sandfly ready to be inoculated when the vector next takes a blood meal. The salivary glands are not parasitized.

Note: The life cycle of *L. donovani* is shown in Fig. 17.2.

Clinical features and pathology

The incubation period for visceral leishmaniasis is usually from 6 weeks to 6 months but can be as little as 2 weeks or as long as 9 years. In the early stages of the disease there is a mild irregular fever which later becomes of daily occurrence, often accompanied by chills and sweating.

Other symptoms include cough, diarrhoea, dizziness, vomiting, bleeding gums, pains in the limbs and weight loss. Later there is enlargement of the spleen and liver, and lymphadenopathy which is more marked in infections with *L. d. infantum* and the Kenyan and Sudanese parasites than those caused by *L. d. donovani* in India.

Skin changes are common. The local Indian name of 'kala-azar' (meaning 'black sickness') is a reference to the greyish colour which the patient's skin becomes. In Kenyan and Sudanese visceral leishmaniasis, nodular or ulcerative lesions of the skin may occur.

Without treatment visceral leishmaniasis is usually fatal after periods varying from a few months to a number of years when the patient becomes thin, wasted, and exhausted.

The pathology of visceral leishmaniasis is due to blockage and destruction of the reticuloendothelial system with the most marked effects being seen in the spleen, liver, lymph glands, bone marrow, and intestines.

The spleen is grossly enlarged and its cells packed with amastigotes. The splenic pulp is greatly increased in amount and friability, and there may be many infarcts. The liver is usually enlarged and has a mottled brownish appearance. There is often fibrosis and cirrhosis of the liver in old untreated cases, and there are usually many parasites in the Kupffer cells.

The bone marrow appears a dark reddish colour with blood cell production becoming greatly depressed. The patient becomes anaemic, leucopenic, and thrombocytopenic and many amastigotes are found in the macrophages. The kidneys and lungs are not usually heavily parasitized but the villi of the jejunum and duodenum often become packed with infected macrophages.

Lymph glands are usually enlarged, particularly

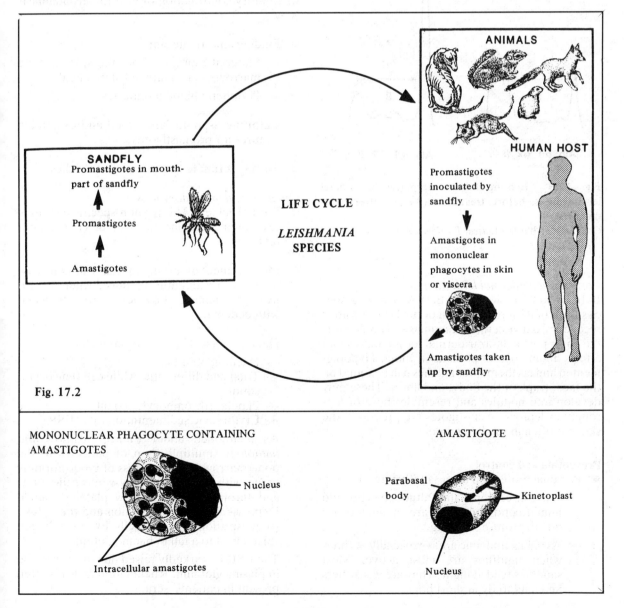

Fig. 17.2

those of the mesenteries. Amastigotes can frequently be seen in pharyngeal and nasal secretions and the parasites can sometimes be found in apparently normal skin.

In active visceral leishmaniasis there is a lack of a cell-mediated immune response to leishmanial antigens and therefore the parasites multiply rapidly. There is however a humoral response with large amounts of polyclonal non-specific immunoglobulin especially Ig G being produced and also specific anti-leishmanial antibody. Patients who have recovered from visceral leishmaniasis are immune from reinfection but relapses can occur.

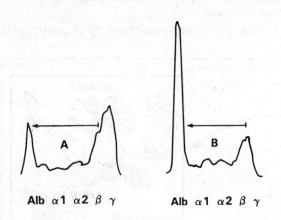

Fig. 17.3   Immunoglobulin response in visceral leishmaniasis, before treatment (A) and after treatment (B).
Courtesy of Wolfe Medical Publications.

Post kala-azar dermal leishmaniasis
In India and occasionally in East Africa, a cutaneous form of leishmaniasis can occur 1-2 years after recovery from visceral leishmaniasis. This is referred to as post kala-azar dermal leishmaniasis and affects about 20% of patients in India. Hypopigmented and erythematous patches can be found on the face, trunk of the body, and limbs. These may develop into nodules and resemble those of lepromatous leprosy. Amastigotes are present in the skin but often in small numbers.

Prevention and control
- Personal protection from sandfly bites by:
  - Using insect repellants, although in hot and humid conditions they are of limited use due to profuse sweating.
  - Avoiding endemic areas especially at times when sandflies are most active. Most sandflies feed at night. They are weak fliers and tend to fly in short hops.

Mosquito nets give little protection because sandflies will pass through all but the finest netting.

- Treating infected persons, especially in areas where humans are the only or important reservoirs of infection (see Table 17.1).

- Insecticide spraying of houses and farm buildings.

- Destruction of stray dogs in areas where dogs are reservoir hosts (see Table 17.1).

LABORATORY DIAGNOSIS

Laboratory confirmation of visceral leishmaniasis is by:

□ Finding amastigotes in:
  - Material aspirated from the spleen, bone marrow or an enlarged lymph gland.
  - Peripheral blood monocytes.

□ Culturing aspirates and blood and examining cultures for promastigotes.

□ Testing serum for leishmanial antibodies.

Other helpful laboratory tests
□ Formol gel test. This is a non-specific screening test for marked increases in Ig G (see later text).

□ Measurement of serum or plasma albumin (see 30:6). Serum albumin is reduced when there is liver cell damage. Low levels are associated with oedema.

□ Haematological investigations including:
  - Haemoglobin
  - Total and differential white cell (leucocyte) count
  - Platelet (thrombocyte) count
  - Erythrocyte sedimentation rate (ESR)

As mentioned under *Clinical features and pathology*, multiplication of parasites in the bone marrow leads to a loss of blood-forming tissue with leucopenia (low white cell count) and thrombocytopenia (low platelet count). Depressed red cell production and the uptake (sequestration) of red cells by an enlarged spleen lead to a fall in haemoglobin.

The ESR is markedly raised due to an increase in plasma globulin. Rheumatoid factor is often present in patients' sera.

Other haematological findings include a positive direct antiglobulin test and often auto agglutination of red cells. When slide and tube blood grouping, well washed red cells must be used. An indirect antihuman globulin technique should be included when crossmatching (compatibility testing).

Important: Before performing a splenic aspiration, measurement of the prothrombin time and a platelet count are recommended to detect abnormal clotting.

Leishmanin skin test (see 17:3)
This test is negative in active visceral leishmaniasis but may become positive in some patients within 1 year of recovery.

Examination of aspirates for amastigotes
The estimated percentage of patients in which amastigotes can be found in spleen, bone marrow, and lymph gland aspirates is as follows:

Aspirate	Positivity[1]
Spleen	98%
Bone marrow	54-86%
From enlarged lymph gland	64%

Splenic aspiration
Some workers regard the puncture of an enlarged spleen to be an unsafe procedure. Other workers consider the procedure to be safe when performed by an *experienced* person and the patient's platelet count is not less than 40×10^9 /l (40 000 /cu mm) and prothrombin time is normal.

Details of technique can be found in Annex 4 of the WHO publication, *The Leishmaniases*[1] and in the papers of Chulay and Bryceson[2] and Kager et al.[3]

Aspirated material is examined as follows:

1. Immediately after aspiration, make at least 2 thinly spread smears of the aspirate on *clean* slides.

   Only a small quantity of aspirate is required. Dilution with blood should be avoided.

   Note: Dispense any remaining aspirate into culture medium (see later text), or into a tube containing EDTA (sequestrene) anticoagulant and mix. If the aspirate is diluted with blood and the first two smears are negative, the EDTA sample should be centrifuged and examined as described for peripheral blood (see later text).

2. Air-dry the smears as rapidly as possible. Fix by covering each smear with a few drops of absolute methanol (methyl alcohol) or if more convenient, immerse the slides in a container of methanol. Fix for 3-5 minutes.

3. Stain the smears by the rapid modified Field's technique or by the Giemsa staining technique.

Rapid modified Field's technique
— Place the methanol-fixed smears on a staining rack and cover with approximately 1 ml of 1 in 5 diluted Field's stain B.

   To prepare a 1 in 5 dilution of Field's stain B, mix 2 ml of Field's stain B (Reagent No. 36) with 8 ml of pH 7.2 buffered water (Reagent No. 21).

— Immediately add an equal volume of Field's stain A (Reagent No. 35) and mix with the diluted Field's stain B. Leave to stain for 1 minute. Wash off the stains with clean water.

   The stains can be easily applied and mixed on the slides by using a 1 ml plastic bulb Pasteur pipette.

Note: The Giemsa staining technique is described in 13:14.

4. When dry, spread a drop of immersion oil on the smear and examine microscopically first using the 40× objective to scan the smear for large mononuclear phagocytic cells. Use the 100× oil immersion objective to identify the amastigotes (add a further drop of oil if necessary).

Amastigotes of Leishmania species

• Small, round to oval bodies measuring about 2-4 μm depending on species.

• Can be seen in groups inside mononuclear phagocytic cells or lying free between cells.

• Nucleus and rod-shaped kinetoplast in each amastigote stain dark reddish-mauve. Both structures must be seen.

• Cytoplasm stains palely and is often difficult to see especially when the amastigotes are in groups.

Illustrations: See Fig. 17.2, Plate 17.1 and colour Plate 49.

Note: Structurally the amastigotes of *Leishmania* species are similar. There are however variations in size between species.

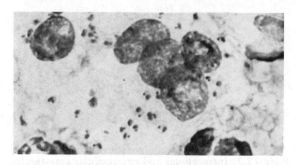

Plate 17.1 Amastigotes in stained smear of bone marrow as seen with 100x objective.

Reporting *L. donovani* amastigote numbers in splenic aspirate smears[1]

Parasite grading is useful because it provides an objective measure of the speed of response to treatment, distinguishes quickly between slow responders and non-responders, and provides useful information for research purposes. It also increases the frequency of parasite detection.

The following grading system is recommended (using 10× eyepiece and 100× oil immersion objective).[1]

Grade	Average parasite density
0	0 /1000 fields
1+	1-10 /1000 fields
2+	1-10 /100 fields
3+	1-10 /10 fields
4+	1-10 / field
5+	10-100 / field
6+	> 100 / field

Other findings in aspirates

Other parasites which may be found and should be reported in splenic and bone marrow aspirates include malaria parasites and trypanosomes.

If a smear contains pigment and eosinophils this may indicate *Schistosoma* infection. Eosinophils are absent or scanty in visceral leishmaniasis.

Smears that contain abnormal cells which could be malignant cells should be sent to a Cytology Laboratory for reporting.

Examination of peripheral blood for amastigotes

Occasionally amastigotes can be found in peripheral blood mononuclear leucocytes, especially in Indian and Kenyan visceral leishmaniasis. The white cells can be concentrated by centrifugation and the buffy coat (consisting of white cells) removed and stained as described in 16:2 (see *Test tube centrifugation concentration* technique). Examination of buffy coat preparations however, is not as sensitive a technique as examining a splenic or bone marrow aspirate.

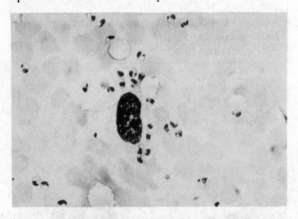

Plate 17.2 Intracellular and extracellular amastigotes in blood as seen with 40x objective.
Courtesy of J. E. Williams.

Culturing aspirates and blood for promastigotes

In the diagnosis of visceral leishmaniasis, culturing of aspirates is of value in detecting light infections. In Indian kala-azar, the culturing of blood may establish a diagnosis without the need for splenic aspiration. Culture is also of value in checking for infection during and after treatment. The form of leishmanial parasite found in cultures is the promastigote.

Aseptic technique

Aspirates or other tissue for culture must be collected aseptically to avoid introducing contaminating organisms. Bacterial contamination rapidly kills leishmanial parasites. Care must also be taken not to contaminate the culture with iodine or merthiolate which will also kill the parasites. If such antiseptics are used for sterilizing the skin they must be removed with 70% v/v ethanol. To allow for possible contamination, it is advisable to inoculate several bottles of culture medium at the same time.

Choice of culture medium

Both Novy-Nicolle-McNeal (NNN) medium and Schneider's enriched insect tissue culture medium are recommended for the *in vitro* culture of *Leishmania*.

Schneider's enriched medium has been shown to be more sensitive than NNN medium[4, 5] and has the additional advantage that it can be lyophilized and reconstituted with distilled water as required.

For those laboratories unable to obtain the ingredients required for Schneider's enriched medium, the use of NNN medium is also described.

SCHNEIDER'S ENRICHED MEDIUM

Required

Schneider's Drosophila Medium* .... 80 ml
Foetal calf serum* .... 20 ml
Antibiotic-antimycotic solution* .... 1.2 ml

*All the above ingredients are obtainable from Gibco Ltd. Schneider's Drosophila Medium is available as a liquid medium (100 ml, code 041-1720 H or 500 ml, code 041-1720 M).

Foetal calf serum is available in lyophilized form (20 ml, code 063-6145 D) or in liquid form (100 ml, code 011-6290 H). Foetal calf serum is also available from Institut Pasteur (50 ml, code 72 333).

The Antibiotic-Antimycotic solution contains penicillin, streptomycin, and *Fungizone*.[1] It is available in liquid form (20 ml, code 043-5240- D) or lyophilized (20 ml, code 061-5245 D).

For prices, storage and stability of the products, readers should write to Gibco Ltd and Institut Pasteur Company (for addresses, see Appendix II).

Preparation
1. Inactivate the foetal calf serum for 30 minutes at 56 °C. Allow to cool.
2. Aseptically add the 20 ml of inactivated foetal calf serum to 80 ml of Schneider's Medium and mix.
3. Add 1.2 ml of the antibiotic-antimycotic solution and mix.
4. Aseptically dispense the medium in 3 ml amounts in sterile 16 × 100 mm tubes, and stopper. If an inverted (tissue culture) microscope is available for viewing the cultures, dispense the medium in flat-bottomed tissue culture tubes.
5. Label and freeze at −20 °C. When stored at −20 °C, the medium can be kept for up to 1 year. It can be kept for up to 6 weeks at 4-6 °C.

If facilities are available, the medium can be lyophilized.

Use
— Allow 2 tubes of medium to thaw and reach room temperature.
— Aseptically inoculate each tube with approximately 0.1 ml of specimen.
— Incubate the cultures at 24 °C (± 2 °C) in the dark for up to 14 days. Room temperature is usually suitable. The cultures *must not* be incubated at the temperature used for culturing bacteria, i.e. 35-37 °C.
— Examine daily for promastigotes using an inverted microscope or if not available, use a sterile wire loop to transfer a drop of the culture to a slide for examination. Cover with a cover glass. Look for motile flagellated promastigotes using the 40× objective with the condenser iris closed sufficiently to give good contrast or preferably use dark-field or phase contrast microscopy.

Promastigotes in culture are shown in Plate 17.3 and colour Plate 50.

Note: Subculture negative cultures after 3-5 days into fresh medium. Examine daily for promastigotes for a further 10 days.

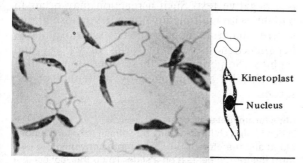

Plate 17.3 Promastigotes in culture.
Courtesy of A. Moody.

— Kinetoplast

— Nucleus

NNN MEDIUM
Required
Difco Blood Agar Base* .... 8 g
Glass-distilled water .... 200 ml
Defibrinated rabbit blood .... 0.6 ml in each 5 ml bottle of medium

*Difco Blood Agar Base is recommended because it has been shown to grow a wide range of *Leishmania* species including some of the more difficult to grow South American parasites. It is obtainable from Difco Company in powder form (114 g, code 0045-02-5). For the address of Difco, see Appendix II.

Preparation of defibrinated rabbit blood
Aseptically collect 20 ml of rabbit heart blood into a sterile flask containing about 100 glass beads of 4 mm diameter. Defibrinate the blood by rotating the flask for 5 minutes. To reduce the risk of contamination, add 200 IU of penicillin, 200 mg gentamicin, and 2 mg streptomycin per ml of defibrinated blood.

Preparation
1. Pour the 200 ml of water into a flask or bottle (one which will not crack in boiling water). Add the agar to the water and mix.
2. Stand the bottle or flask in a container of boiling water until the agar is completely dissolved.
3. Mix and dispense the medium in 5 ml amounts into screw-cap bottles of 20 ml capacity (McCartney type are suitable).
4. Sterilize by autoclaving (with caps loosened) at 121 °C for 15 minutes.
   After sterilizing, tighten the bottle tops.
5. Allow the agar to cool to 45-50 °C.
6. Aseptically add 0.6 ml of sterile defibrinated rabbit blood to each bottle of medium and mix *gently*.
7. Allow the medium to solidify with the bottles in a sloped position.
8. When the medium has set, stand the bottles in an upright position at room temperature for 24 hours to allow fluid of condensation to form. Store in the refrigerator at 4-6 °C until required.

Use
— Allow 2 tubes of medium to reach room temperature.
— Aseptically inoculate about 0.1 ml of specimen *into the fluid of condensation*.
— Incubate the cultures at 24 °C (± 2 °C) in the dark. Room temperature is usually suitable (but not 35-37 °C).
— Examine every 4 days for promastigotes using a sterile wire loop to transfer a drop of the culture to a slide for examination. Cover with a cover glass.

Look for motile flagellated promastigotes using the 40× objective with the condenser iris closed sufficiently to give good contrast or preferably use dark-field or phase contrast microscopy.

Promastigotes in culture are shown in Plate 17.3 and colour Plate 50.

Note: Subculture negative cultures after 8 days into fresh medium. Examine every 4 days for promastigotes for a further 20 days.

Serological diagnosis of visceral leishmaniasis

In active visceral leishmaniasis, specific antibody as well as non-specific polyclonal Ig G and Ig M are produced.

Several techniques have been developed to detect and measure specific anti-leishmanial antibodies in patients' sera. These include indirect fluorescent antibody test (IFAT), counterimmunoelectrophoresis (CIEP), and enzyme-linked immunosorbent assay (ELISA).

IFAT

This is a sensitive technique detecting antibody in about 93% of patients with visceral leishmaniasis. The test becomes positive in the early stages of the disease and negative within 6 months of cure. Positive reactions with low titres may occur with acute malaria and with sera from some patients with Chagas' disease, leprosy, tuberculosis and certain forms of cutaneous leishmaniasis especially the South American mucocutaneous form. The test uses *L. donovani* promastigotes or amastigotes as antigen. Details of technique can be found in the paper of Abdulla.[6] The technique requires a fluorescence microscope and training in fluorescent techniques.

CIEP

About 80% of patients with early visceral leishmaniasis are positive by CIEP and almost all patients with late infection. Details of the equipment, reagents and technique can be found in the papers of Rezai *et al*[7] and Aikat *et al*.[8]

ELISA

This test is reported as being both sensitive and specific but full evaluation of the technique is awaited. It can be carried out on serum or from eluates prepared from capillary blood collected onto absorbent paper. Reagents are stable and no special equipment is required. Compared with other techniques for the field diagnosis of visceral leishmaniasis, ELISA is less expensive and enables large numbers of samples to be examined at a single dilution that has previously been determined as giving acceptable sensitivity and specificity in a given area. Details of antigen preparation

and technique can be found in the papers of Hommel *et al*,[9] Ho *et al*,[10] and Diesfeld and Jahn.[11]

Note: Principles of IFAT, CIEP and ELISA techniqes are described and illustrated in Chapter 37 in Volume II of the Manual.

Formol gel (aldehyde) test

Because of its simplicity this non-specific test is still widely used to assist in the diagnosis of visceral leishmaniasis. It is based on the presence of large amounts of non-specific polyclonal globulin in the patient's serum. It is therefore a screening test which if positive requires further investigation. The test is positive in about 85% of patients with visceral leishmaniasis. It becomes positive about 3 months after infection and negative about 6 months after successful treatment.

Method
1. Collect about 5 ml of venous blood into a dry glass tube and leave to clot.
2. When the clot begins to retract (30-60 minutes after collection), centrifuge the blood to obtain clear serum. If a centrifuge is not available, leave the specimen to separate overnight.
3. Transfer about 1 ml of red cell free serum to a small tube. Add 2 drops of concentrated formalin solution (40% w/v), mix, and allow to stand for up to 20 minutes.

Results

Positive test: Serum whitens and gels like the white of a hard boiled egg usually within 5 minutes (see Colour Plate 51).

                A milky appearance without the serum solidifying may occur in early visceral leishmaniasis.

Negative test: Serum remains unchanged or gelling and whitening occur only after 20 minutes.

Note: If the serum solidifies without whitening this is a negative test. Such a reaction may occur in patients with multiple myeloma, trypanosomiasis, severe malaria, hepatosplenic schistosomiasis, hepatic cirrhosis, certain forms of leprosy and syphilis. Sometimes in these conditions gelling may also be accompanied by whitening of the serum.

Slide formol gel test

When testing children, it may be difficult to obtain venous blood and therefore it is usually more convenient to perform the formol gel test on a slide. To do this, collect in a small narrow bore tube sufficient capillary blood (avoiding haemolysis) to give a large drop of serum when clotted.

Allow to clot and when the clot has retracted, centrifuge the blood. Transfer a large drop of serum to a slide, add a *small* drop of concentrated formalin solution, and mix.

A positive test is indicated by a whitening and gelling of the serum usually within 5 minutes. Results are interpreted as described for the tube test.

17:3 *LEISHMANIA* CAUSING OLD WORLD CUTANEOUS LEISHMANIASIS

Cutaneous (skin) leishmaniasis of the Old World is caused by:

- *Leishmania tropica*
- *Leishmania major*
- *Leishmania aethiopica*

L. tropica was formerly referred to as *L. tropica minor*
L. major was formerly referred to as *L. tropica major*.

Old World cutaneous leishmaniasis is also referred to as oriental sore and local names are used to describe the disease in different parts of the world.

Distribution
L. tropica is found in the Middle East, Afghanistan, northwest India, eastern Mediterranean countries and North Africa. It is an urban disease with human beings thought to be the main reservoirs of infection.

L. major occurs in rural areas and has a wider distribution than *L. tropica*. It is found in the Middle East, Afghanistan, India, North Africa and subsaharan Africa from Senegal across to central Sudan. Infections are zoonotic with rodents, especially rats and gerbils, serving as reservoir hosts.

L. aethiopica is found only in the highlands of Ethiopia and Kenya. The disease is a zoonosis with rock and tree hyraxes serving as reservoir hosts.

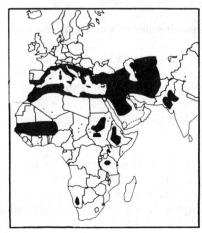

Fig. 17.4 Distribution of cutaneous and muco-cutaneous leishmaniasis in Old World.

A leishmanial parasite has also been reported as causing cutaneous leishmaniasis in the uplands of South West Africa and the Cape Province. Although isolated from hyraxes, the parasite is not the same as *L. aethiopica*.

Table 17.2 Distribution and Reservoir Hosts of *L. tropica, L. major,* and *L. aethiopica*

Species	Distribution	Reservoir Hosts	Disease
Leishmania tropica	Middle East, Afghanistan, India, eastern Mediterr-anean, North Africa	Humans	Urban cutaneous leishmaniasis Leishmaniasis recidivans
Leishmania major	Middle East, Afghanistan, India, North Africa, subsaharan Africa	Rodents, mainly rats and gerbils	Rural zoonotic cutaneous leishmaniasis
Leishmania aethiopica	Ethiopia, Kenya	Hyraxes	Cutaneous leishmaniasis Diffuse cutaneous leishmaniasis
Unidentified *Leishmania* species	South West Africa, Cape Province	Hyraxes	Cutaneous leishmaniasis

Transmission and life cycle
The vectors of *L. tropica*, *L. major* and *L. aethiopica* are *Phlebotomus* sandflies. The important reservoir hosts of the parasites are listed in Table 17.2.

Infection occurs when promastigotes are inoculated at the time a female sandfly takes a blood meal.

Life cycle
The life cycle of *Leishmania* species is summarized in Fig. 17.2. In cutaneous leishmaniasis, the parasites multiply in skin macrophages . In non-immune persons and when cell-mediated immunity is defective the parasites spread in cutaneous tissues.

Clinical features
L. tropica
The incubation period is usually 2-8 months. At the site of the bite a very small papule develops which may itch, but is painless. The skin above the papule soon flakes off and a moist crust forms over

a shallow ulcer. Usually the crust is dislodged leaving a crater-like sore with a raised margin. The sore enlarges by erosion of its edge until it is usually 25-70 mm in diameter and secondary papules may appear at its periphery. Infection with *L. tropica* is often referred to as a dry urban oriental sore.

If there is secondary bacterial infection with discharge of pus, an *L. tropica* ulcer may be confused with tropical ulcer. In general, however, the uncomplicated leishmanial ulcer is painless whereas tropical ulcer is extremely painful.

In some patients, multiple scattered lesions may be seen, due either to the repeated bites of infected sandflies or to the spread of parasites by way of the blood or lymphatics.

Oriental sore is usually self-healing after 1-2 years, leaving the patient firmly immune to re-infection with the same parasite. Rarely, however, there may develop multiple unhealing lesions, often on the face, which strongly resemble those of tuberculosis of the skin. The condition is referred to as leishmaniasis recidivans (LR) and is thought to be an allergic state in which cell-mediated immunity is over-developed. Parasites are scanty and difficult to find in smears but may sometimes be found after culturing infected tissue.

L. major
Infections with *L. major* are often referred to as wet oriental sore. The lesions develop and heal much more quickly than those of *L. tropica*. The early papule is often inflamed and resembles a boil of 5-10 mm in diameter which rapidly develops into a large uneven ulcer which is self-healing in as little as 3-6 months. Multiple lesions may occur in non-immune persons.

L. major infections protect against re-infection and against infection with *L. tropica*.

L. aethiopica
In the Ethiopian highlands, *L. aethiopica* is normally associated with a lesion similar to typical oriental sore, but may also give rise to diffuse cutaneous leishmaniasis (DCL) in patients who produce little or no cell-mediated immunity against the parasite. This is an incurable condition characterized by the formation of disfiguring nodules over the surface of the body. The nodules contain large numbers of amastigotes.

L. aethiopica can also cause mucocutaneous leishmaniasis.

Pathology
Following early massive monocyte and histiocyte invasion, the ulcer is then walled off or penetrated by macrophages, plasma cells, and lymphocytes, usually resulting in a reduction of parasite numbers (partial protection). This is followed by ulceration

of the dermis and healing with fibrosis and the formation of scar tissue except in those patients who develop diffuse cutaneous leishmaniasis or leishmaniasis recidivans.

Recovery from infection provides life-long immunity to re-infection with the same parasite but not necessarily to other *Leishmania* species or subspecies.

Prevention and control
Preventive and control measures are similar to those described for *L. donovani* infections in 17:2.

Measures to eliminate and control rodents should be taken in areas where these animals are sources of human infections. Whenever feasible, human dwellings should be sited away from the habitats of animal reservoir hosts where sandflies are known to breed, e.g. rodent burrows or rocks where hyraxes live.

LABORATORY DIAGNOSIS

Laboratory confirmation of cutaneous leishmaniasis is by:

☐ Detecting amastigotes in smears taken from infected ulcers or nodules.

In leishmaniasis recidivans, parasites are usually difficult to find in smears and culture is required.

☐ Culturing ulcer material and examining cultures for promastigotes.

Note: Because of the poor antibody response in cutaneous leishmaniasis, serological tests are of little value in diagnosis. There is, however, a cellular response which is the basis of the leishmanin skin test (see later text).

Collection and examination of smears for amastigotes
Material for examination should be taken from the *raised nodular or swollen edge* of an ulcer, not from its centre which usually contains only necrotic tissue.

Care should be taken to avoid contaminating the specimen with blood.

Note: Secondary bacterial contamination makes it difficult to find parasites and therefore if bacterial infection is present, examination for *Leishmania* amastigotes is best delayed until antimicrobial treatment has been completed.

Collection and staining of smears

1. Firmly squeeze the edge of the lesion between the finger and thumb to drain the area of blood (protective rubber gloves should be worn).

2. Using a sterile scalpel blade, make a small cut into the dermis and blot away any blood. Scrape the cut surface to obtain tissue juice and cells.

   Note: Some workers prefer to use a sterile dental probe or needle and syringe to obtain a specimen.

3. Spread the material on a clean slide using a circular motion and working outwards to avoid damaging parasites in those parts of the smear that have started to dry.

   The smear must be thinly spread and not left as a thick 'dab' smear. Parasites will be difficult to find in thick smears.

4. When dry, fix the smear by covering it with a few drops of absolute methanol (methyl alcohol). Fix for 2-3 minutes.

5. Stain the smear using the rapid modified Field's technique as described in 17:2 or Giemsa staining technique (see 13:14).

6. When the smear is dry, spread a drop of immersion oil on it and examine first with the 40× objective to detect macrophages which may contain amastigotes. Use the 100× oil immersion objective to identify the amastigotes (adding a further drop of oil if required).

   Note: The features which identify *Leishmania* amastigotes are described in 17:2.

Culture of ulcer material

Culture is of value when cutaneous leishmaniasis is suspected and parasites cannot be found in smears. In leishmaniasis recidivans, culture is usually required to detect parasites. Material for culture is best obtained by injecting and then aspirating a small quantity of sterile physiological saline in and then out of the hardened margin of the ulcer. A few drops of the final aspirate is used to inoculate the culture medium.

To allow for possible contamination, it is advisable to inoculate 2 or 3 bottles of medium.

Schneider's enriched culture medium is recommended.[5] If this is not available, NNN medium should be used. The preparation of both these media, and examination of cultures are described in 17:2. The form of the parasite found in cultures is the promastigote.

Note: *L. major* grows rapidly in culture.

Leishmanin test

The antigen used in the leishmanin test, or Montenegro reaction, is prepared from killed culture forms (promastigotes) of *L. braziliensis*, *L. mexicana*, or *L. tropica*, with a concentration of 10×10^6 parasites per ml.

The antigen is available from centres of leishmaniasis studies or from commercial manufacturers. In the test, 0.1 ml of well-shaken antigen is injected intradermally into the inner surface of the forearm. It is preferable to perform tests with an accompanying control solution. The diameter of induration is measured at 48 and 72 hours.

Positive reaction

The reaction is considered positive when the area of induration is 5 mm in diameter or more.

A positive reaction may be found in many persons from endemic areas who show no visible skin lesions but have been exposed to infection. A positive leishmanin test in children under 10 years of age from endemic areas, is highly suggestive of the disease.

In persons entering an endemic area for the first time, the development of skin lesions and positive leishmanin test indicate cutaneous leishmaniasis.

In South American mucocutaneous leishmaniasis, the leishmanin test is positive and the reaction may be sufficiently violent to cause necrosis in the centre of the area of induration.

Negative reaction

The leishmanin test is usually negative in *active* visceral leishmaniasis and diffuse cutaneous leishmaniasis. A negative reaction may also be found in some 15% of patients with uncomplicated cutaneous leishmaniasis.

There are no significant cross-reactions with other diseases.

17:4 *LEISHMANIA* CAUSING NEW WORLD CUTANEOUS AND MUCOCUTANEOUS LEISHMANIASIS

Cutaneous (skin) leishmaniasis in the New World is caused by:

■ *Leishmania braziliensis subspecies**
* L. b. guyanenis
* L. b. panamensis
* L. b. peruvaina

■ *Leishmania mexicana subspecies**
* L. m. mexicana
* L. m. amazonensis
* L. m. pifanoi
* L. m. venezuelensis

Mucocutaneous leishmaniasis in the New World is caused by:

■ *Leishmania b. braziliensis*

  Other as yet unidentified subspecies of *L. braziliensis* may also cause mucocutaneous leishmaniasis.

Note: Infections in humans have occurred with other leishmanial parasites of the *L. braziliensis* and *L. mexicana* complexes. Some of these isolates and their animal hosts have yet to be identified. There are thought to be many species of *Leishmania* in South and Central America each with their own vectors and mammalian hosts. Humans become infected when they intrude into areas of transmission and the sandfly vectors are both animal and human blood feeders.

Local names are used to describe the disease in different areas.

Distribution

Infections with parasites of the *L. braziliensis* and *L. mexicana* complexes are zoonoses and they occur therefore in and around the habitats of the parasites' natural animal hosts and sandfly vectors.

Leishmania braziliensis complex

Parasites of the *L. braziliensis* complex are much more widely distributed in the New World than those of the *L. mexicana* complex. Their distribution and reservoir hosts are summarized in Table 17.3.

Leishmania mexicana complex

L. m. mexicana is found in rain forests in Mexico (Yucatan), Guatemala and Belize. Rodents are the reservoir hosts. Woodcutters and gum (chicle) collectors are often infected. The vector bites in the early hours of the morning.

The distribution of the other subspecies of *L. mexicana* and known reservoir hosts are summarized in Table 17.3.

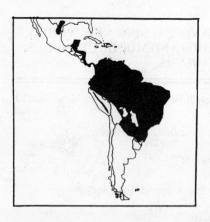

Fig. 17.5 Distribution of cutaneous and muco-cutaneous leishmaniasis in New World.

Figs. 17.4 and 17.5 reproduced from WHO Technical Report Series No. 701, 1984.

Note: Further information concerning the epidemiology and ecology of *L. mexicana*, *L. braziliensis*, and their subspecies and related species can be found in the paper of Lainson.[12]

Table 17.3 *Distribution, and Reservoir Hosts of L. braziliensis and L. mexicana Complexes*

Species Subspecies	Distribution	Reservoir Hosts	Disease
LEISHMANIA BRAZILIENSIS COMPLEX			
L. b. braziliensis	Amazon forest in Brazil	Possibly rodents	Mucocutaneous and cutaneous leishmaniasis
L. b. guyanensis	Guyanas, Brazil, Surinam	Sloths, anteaters	Cutaneous, often multiple sores
L. b. panamensis	Panama, Costa Rica, Colombia	Sloths	Cutaneous with single or few lesions
L. b. peruviana	Andes in Peru, Argentinian highlands	Dogs are naturally infected but there is probably a wild animal host	Self-healing cutaneous leishmaniasis
LEISHMANIA MEXICANA COMPLEX			
L. m. mexicana	Mexico, Belize Guatemala	Rodents	Self-healing body lesions. Destructive chronic ear lesions
L. m. amazonensis	Brazil, Venezuela, Trinidad	Rodents and other wild animals	Cutaneous single sore type. Sometimes diffuse cutaneous leishmaniasis
L. m. pifanoi	Venezuela	Possibly rodents	Diffuse cutaneous leishmaniasis. Single sore type also suspected
L. m. venezuelensis	Riverine forests in Venezuela	Unknown	Cutaneous leishmaniasis

*L. b. braziliensis or a closely related subspecies has also been found in Belize.

Transmission and life cycle

The vectors of *Leishmania* that cause cutaneous leishmaniasis in the New World are sandflies belonging to the genera *Lutzomyia* and *Psychodopygus*. Those that transmit *L. braziliensis* feed readily from man whereas those that transmit *L. mexicana* are less attracted to man. Reservoir hosts are listed in Table 17.3.

Note: Parasites of the *L. braziliensis* complex develop in both the posterior and anterior of the gut of their sandfly vectors, i.e. they have a peripylarian development. Other medically important *Leishmania* species develop only in the anterior part of the gut of their sandfly vectors, i.e. they have a suprapylarian development.

Infection occurs when promastigotes are inoculated at the time a female sandfly takes a blood meal.

Life cycle
The life cycle of *Leishmania* species is summarized in Fig. 17.2. In cutaneous leishmaniasis, the parasites multiply in skin macrophages (histiocytes). *L. b. braziliensis* parasitizes the skin and mucocutaneous tissues. When cell-mediated immunity in a human host fails, the parasites spread in the skin, causing diffuse cutaneous leishmaniasis.

Clinical features and pathology

Leishmania braziliensis complex
L. b. braziliensis causes the most severe and destructive form of cutaneous leishmaniasis in South America. Lesions are similar in development to those of oriental sore and the resulting ulcers may become very large and long-lasting. Early in the infection, parasites may migrate to tissues of the nasopharynx or the palate and sometimes after many years when the first lesion has healed there begins a slow continuous erosion of these tissues. Disfiguration is often extreme with complete destruction of the nasal septum, perforation of the palate, and damage to the tissues of the lips and larynx.

L. b. guyanensis in the Guyanas and north Brazil, may give rise to painless dry single ulcers or multiple lesions scattered all over the body. The disease is often referred to as 'forest yaws' ('pian bois'). There is no firm evidence that this parasite produces mucocutaneous leishmaniasis.

L. b. panamensis causes single or few skin ulcers which are not self-healing. Lymphatic involvement is common.

L. b. peruviana mainly infects children. The single or few lesions are painless and usually heal spontaneously after about 4 months. The infection is known locally as 'uta'.

Leishmania mexicana complex
L. m. mexicana causes chiclero's ulcer, or 'bay sore'. Lesions of the body caused by *L. m. mexicana*, like oriental sore, tend to be self-healing but those on the ear may last up to 30 years and entirely destroy the pinna of the ear.

Lesions of *L. m. amazonensis* resemble those of oriental sore but the parasite rarely infects man because he rarely goes into those areas of the forest where the vector is most abundant, and also because the vector is usually unattracted to humans. In the Amazon Region of Brazil up to 30% of cases registered as due to *L. m. amazonensis* have developed incurable diffuse cutaneous leishmanias.

L. m. pifanoi is known only from cases of diffuse cutaneous leishmaniasis but it is presumed that simple uncomplicated lesions of the skin must also exist.

L. m. venezuelensis lesions may be single or multiple and in some patients disseminated nodular lesions are formed.

Note: The pathology of cutaneous leishmaniasis is described in 17:3.

Prevention and control
Prevention of cutaneous and mucocutaneous leishmaniasis in South America and Central America is mainly by:

- Avoiding endemic areas especially during times when local sandfly vectors are most active.

- Using insect repellants although in hot and humid conditions such as the tropical rain forests of South America they are of limited use due to profuse sweating.

It would seem that the control of cutaneous and mucocutaneous leishmaniasis in the forests of Central and South America, both practically and economically, must depend on the development of chemoprophylactic drugs or vaccines.

LABORATORY DIAGNOSIS

Laboratory confirmation of infection with *Leishmania* of the *L. braziliensis* and *L. mexicana* complexes is by:

☐ Finding amastigotes in smears taken from infected lesions as described for Old World cutaneous leishmaniasis in 17:3.

In mucocutaneous leishmaniasis, the parasites are scanty and difficult to find in smears. Culture is recommended.

Note: *L. mexicana* amastigotes are larger than those of *L. braziliensis* and they have a more centrally placed kinetoplast.

☐ Culturing material from ulcers and examining cultures for promastigotes as explained in 17:2.

Note: *L. braziliensis* grows slowly in culture whereas *L. mexicana* grows rapidly. This can help to differentiate the two species. *L mexicana* promastigotes are larger than those of *L. braziliensis*.

Serology
In mucocutaneous leishmaniasis, antibodies can be found in the serum. In cutaneous leishmaniasis, antibody levels are usually low especially in *L. mexicana* infections.

Monoclonal antibodies have been developed to differentiate between *L. braziliensis* and *L. mexicana* in fluorescent antibody tests.[13]

Confirmation of species
Because there are differences in the prognosis and treatment of diseases caused by parasites of the *L. braziliensis* and *L. mexicana* complexes, it is important to know which organism is causing infection. Whenever possible, positive cultures should therefore be sent to Reference Laboratories for full identification.*

* Addresses of laboratories able to identify *Leishmania* isolates can be obtained from Chief of the Leishmaniasis Unit, Tropical Diseases Research Programme, World Health Organization, 1211 Geneva 27-Switzerland.

Leishmanin test
The leishmanin skin test is described in 17:3. It is usually positive in cutaneous and mucocutaneous leishmaniasis but negative in diffuse cutaneous leishmaniasis. Severe reactions may occur in patients with mucocutaneous leishmaniasis.

References
1. World Health Organization. *The Leishmaniases*. Technical Report Series, No 701, 1984. WHO, 1211 Geneva, 27-Switzerland.

2. Chulay, J. D. and Bryceson, A. D. M. Quantification of amastigotes of *Leishmania donovani* in smears of splenic aspirates from patients with visceral leishmaniasis. *American Journal of Tropical Medicine and Hygiene*, **32**, pp 475-479, 1983.

3 Kager, P. A. *et al*. Splenic aspiration: experience in Kenya. *Tropical and Geographical Medicine*, **33**, pp 125-131, 1983.

4 Lawrence, K. *et al*. Comparison of microscopy and culture in the detection of *Leishmania donovani* from splenic aspirates. *American Journal of Tropical Medicine and Hygiene*, **33**, (2), pp 296-299, 1983.

5 Shaw, J. J., Lainson, R. The *in vitro* cultivation of members of the *Leishmania braziliensis* complex. Correspondence Transactions of the *Royal Society of Tropical Medicine and Hygiene*, **75**, 1, 1981.

6 Abdullah, R. E. *Annals of Tropical Medicine and Parasitology*, **74**, pp 415-419, 1980.

7 Rezai, H. R., Farrell, J., Soulsby, E. L. *American Journal of Tropical Medicine and Hygiene*, **27**, p 1079, 1978.

8 Aikat, B. K., *et al*. *Indian Journal of Medical Respiration*, **70**, p 592, 1979.

9 Hommel, M., *et al*. *Annals of Tropical Medicine and Parasitology*, **72**, p 213, 1978.

10 Ho, M., *et al*. An enzyme-linked immunosorbent assay (ELISA) for field diagnosis of visceral leishmaniasis. *American Journal of Tropical Medicine and Hygiene*, **32** (5), pp 943-946, 1983.

11 Jahn, A., Diesfeld, H. J. Evaluation of a visually read ELISA for serodiagnosis and sero-epidemiological studies of kala-azar in the Baringo District, Kenya. Transactions of the *Royal Society of Tropical Medicine and Hygiene*, **77** (4), pp 451-454, 1983.

12 Lainson, R. The American leishmaniases: Some observations on their ecology and epidemiology. Transactions of the *Royal Society of Tropical Medicine and Hygiene*, **77** (5), pp 569-596, 1983.

13 Pratt, D. McM., David, J. R. Monoclonal antibodies that distinguish between New World species of *Leishmania*, *Nature UK*, 291 (June 18), pp 581-583, 1981.

Recommended Reading
Lainson, R. Chapter: Leishmaniasis. In: *Handbook Series in Zoonoses* (Ed. J. H. Steele), Section C: Parasitic Zoonoses, Volume I, CRC Press Inc., Boca Ratow, Florida, 1982.

Bell, D. R. *Lecture Notes in Tropical Medicine*, Blackwell Scientific Publications, 2nd Ed, 1985. Paperback priced £9.80.

Molyneux, D. H., Ashford, R. W. *The Biology of Trypanosoma and Leishmania, Parasites of Man and Domestic Animals*, Taylor and Francis, 1983.

Marinkell, le J. The control of leishmaniases. *Bulletin of the World Health Organization*, **55**, pp 807-818, 1980.

World Health Organization. *The Leishmaniases*, Technical Report Series, No 701, 1984, WHO, 1211 Geneva, 27-Switzerland.

Tropical Diseases Research Programme
LEISHMANIASIS
Leishmaniasis is included in the *UNDP/World Bank/ World Health Organization Special Programme for Research and Training in Tropical Diseases*.

Tropical Diseases Research (TDR) activities with regard to leishmaniases as recorded in No. 5 of the 1985 *WHO Chronicle* are as follows:

- Studies on nucleotide metabolism in *Leishmania* have led to the identification of allopurinol riboside as a potential therapeutic compound. This is being tested against cutaneous leishmaniasis in a limited clinical trial.
- Monoclonal antibodies and cloned kDNA probes specifically recognizing various *Leishmania* species have facilitated the identification and characterization of the parasite, and are being used to develop new diagnostic tests.
- It has been found that some types of T lymphocytes can aggravate leishmanial lesions in mice, a finding relevant to research on new approaches to vaccine development.
- Fourteen strains of *Leishmania* have been selected as reference strains to be used by all laboratories working on the identification and characterization of these parasites.

Acknowledgements
Colour Section

Acknowledgement and gratitude are expressed to all those who prepared and photographed the pathogens shown in the colour plates and to those who kindly supplied transparencies for reproduction.

Special thanks are due to:

Professor Wallace Peters of the London School of Hygiene and Tropical Medicine for supplying Plates 2b, 4, 5, 14—16, 19 left, 21, 22, 23a,c,d, 24, 26, 36, 37a, 39, 42 right, 43 right, 44 left, 45—48 most of right plates, and 54—56.

Mr Richard Suswillo of the London School of Tropical Medicine and Hygiene for supplying Plates 32a, 33a, 34a,b, 35a,b, 37b, 38a,b, 40a,b.

Mr Anthony Moody, Chief MLSO, Hospital for Tropical Diseases in London for supplying Plates 1b, 2a,c,d, 3, 7 left, 8, 10, 11, 17, 18, 23b, 25, 27 right, 28, 29, and 50.

Mr Martin Cannon and Director of the Huntingdon Research Centre in Huntingdon for kindly photographing and processing Plates 32b, 33b and 41 right.

Mrs. A. C. Rijpstra and Royal Tropical Institute, Amsterdam for supplying Plates 1a, 6, and 7a,c.

Dr Tito Alvarado, Program in Infectious Diseases, Texas University Medical School for supplying colour work for Plate 9.

Professor P. J. Fripp, School of Pathology, The South African Institute for Medical Research, for supplying Plate 12.

Dr John Baker for supplying Plates 13 and 53.

Plates 45—48 left are reproduced by courtesy of A. G. Bayer.

Plate 30 is reproduced by courtesy of the Center for Disease Control, Atlanta.

Plate 51 is reproduced from *A Colour Atlas of Tropical Medicine and Parasitology* with the permission of Wolfe Medical Publications Ltd.

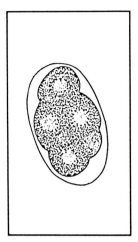

Hookworm egg for a comparison of size against amoebae and cysts shown on this page.

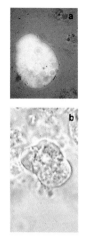

1 Amoebae of *E. histolytica*, average 25 × 20 µm. Note engulfed red cells. **a** Eosin, **b** Saline.

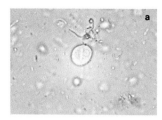
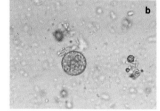
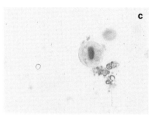
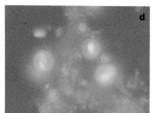

2 Cysts of *Entamoeba histolytica*, 10–15 µm, 1–4 nuclei. **a** Saline, showing chromatoid bar and nucleus. **b** Iodine, showing brown stained nuclei. **c** Burral's stain, showing blue chromatoid bar. **d** Acridine orange, showing yellow (RNA) chromatoid bars.

NONPATHOGENIC INTESTINAL CYSTS

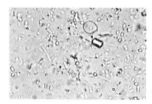

3 *Chilomastix mesnili* cysts, 5–7 µm, lemon-shaped. Saline preparation showing single nucleus.

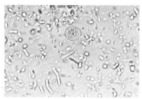

4 *Endolimax nana* cyst, 7–9 µm, round to oval. Iodine stained showing 4 hole-like nuclei.

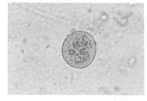

5 *Entamoeba coli* cyst, 15–30 µm. Iodine stained showing nuclei (up to 8 may be present).

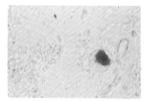

6 *Idoamoeba buetschlii* cyst, 9–15 µm. Iodine stained showing typical brown glycogen vacuole.

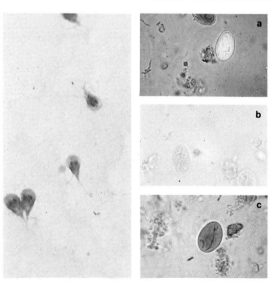

7 *Left:* Flagellates of *Giardia lamblia*, 9–20 µm in length. Stained by modified Field's technique. Motile in saline preparation. *Right:* Cysts of *G. lamblia*, oval, 8–12 µm in length. Rods and axonemes can be seen. **a** Eosin, **b** Saline, **c** Iodine.

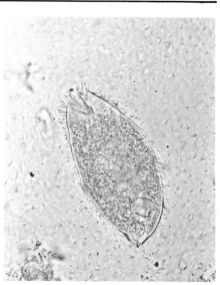

8 Ciliate of *Balantidium coli*, large, 50–200 × 40–70 µm. Has a rapid revolving motility in fresh saline preparation. Cytostome is visible (anterior), Cilia surround the organism.

As seen with 40× objective (except Plate 13)

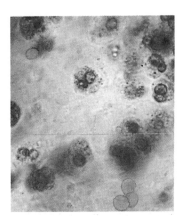

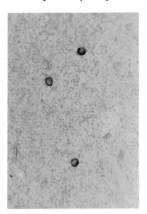

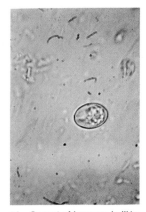

9 Pus cells and mononuclear white cells in methylene blue faecal preparation. Unstained red cells can be seen in bottom right.

10 Red stained oocysts of *Cryptosporidium* in Ziehl-Neelsen stained faecal preparation.

11 Oocyst of *Isospora belli* in faeces. It is immature when passed. Mature oocysts contain two sporoblasts.

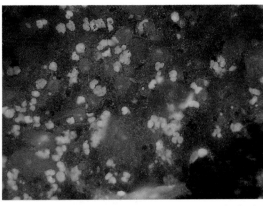

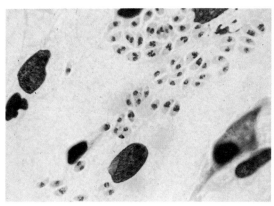

12 Red-brown flagellates of *Trichomonas vaginalis* in acridine orange fluorescent preparation of vaginal discharge. The green cells are pus cells.

13 Small spindle-shaped parasites of *Toxoplasma gondii* in Giemsa stained preparation as seen with 100× objective.

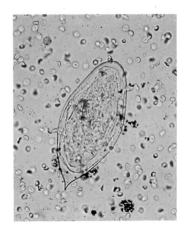

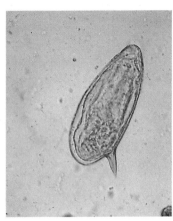

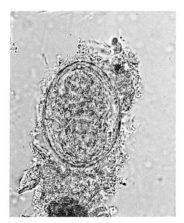

14 Egg of *Schistosoma haematobium* in urine. Note the terminal spine and presence of red cells. Proteinuria is usually found.

15 Egg of *Schistosoma mansoni* in faeces. The spine is lateral. Red cells and mucus are often present in faecal specimens.

16 Egg of *Schistosoma japonicum* in faeces. The knob-like spine is not visible. Note the debris covering the egg.

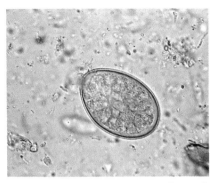

17 Egg of *Diphyllobothrium latum* in faeces. It contains yolk cells. The operculum can just be seen.

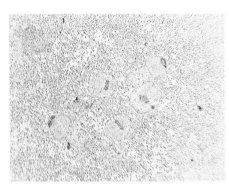

18 Protoscolices of *Echinococcus granulosus* in hydatid cyst fluid. With focusing the hooks of each scolex can be seen.

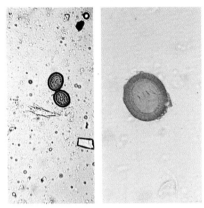

19 *Left:* Eggs of *Taenia* species in faeces, seen with 10× objective. *Right: Taenia* egg showing embryonic hooks, seen with 40× objective.

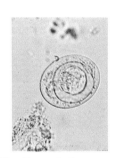

20 *Hymenolepis nana* egg in faeces. It is colourless and contains hooks and polar threads.

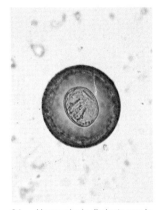

21 *Hymenolepis diminuta* egg in faeces. It is brown and contains hooks but no polar threads and is larger than *H. nana.*

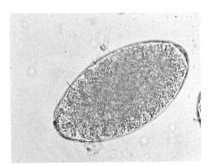

22 Egg of *Fasciola* species in faeces. The small operculum can be seen. *Fasciola* eggs resemble those of *Fasciolopsis buski.*

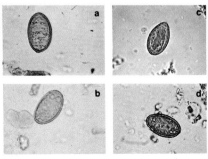

23 Small fluke eggs which are difficult to differentiate, **a** *Metagonimus,* **b** *Dicrocoelium,* **c** *Opisthorchis,* **d** *Heterophyes*

As seen with 40× objective (except Plate 29)

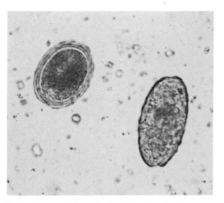

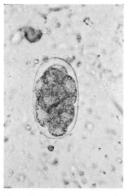

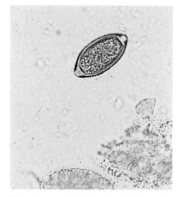

24 Eggs of *Ascaris lumbricoides* in faeces. *Left:* Fertilized egg. *Right:* Unfertilized egg.

25 Hookworm egg in faeces. It has a thin shell.

26 Egg of *Trichuris trichiura* in faeces.

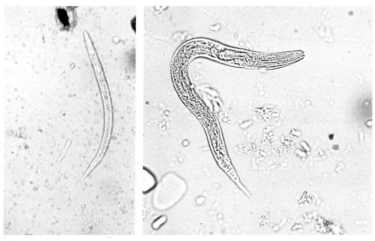

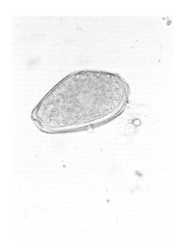

27 *Left:* Larva of *Strongyloides stercoralis* in faeces as seen with the 10× objective. *Right:* Larva of *S. stercoralis* as seen with the 40× objective. Larva is motile in saline.

28 Egg of *Paragonimus westermani* in sputum. The operculum can be seen.

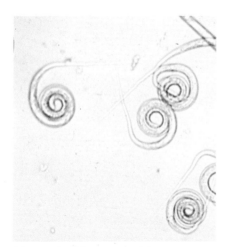

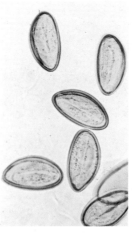

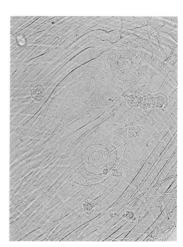

29 Larvae of *Dracunculus medinensis* expelled in water, as seen with 10× objective. They are motile.

30 Eggs of *Enterobius vermicularis* (pinworm) from perianal skin.

31 Coiled encysted larvae of *Trichinella spiralis* in striated muscle tissue.

FILARIAL WORMS

As seen with 10× and 40× objectives

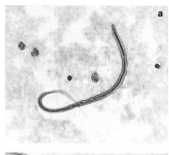
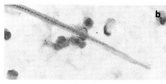

32 **a** *Wuchereria bancrofti* mf, sheathed, 10× obj, Giemsa. **b** Tail of *W. bancrofti* with no nuclei in tip, 40× obj, HE.

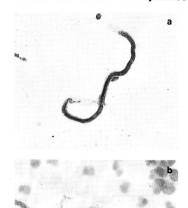

33 **a** *Loa loa* mf, sheathed, 10× obj, Giemsa. **b** Tail of *L. loa* with nuclei extending to tip, 40× obj, HE.

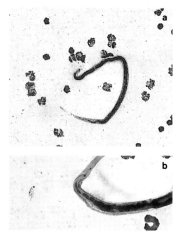

34 **a** *Brugia malayi* mf, sheathed, 10× obj, Giemsa. **b** Tail of *B. malayi* with two nuclei in tip, 40× obj, Giemsa.

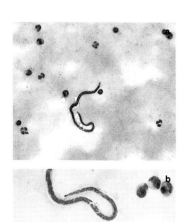

35 **a** *Mansonella perstans* mf, unsheathed, 10× obj, Giemsa. **b** Tail of *M. perstans* with a large nucleus in rounded tip, 40× obj.

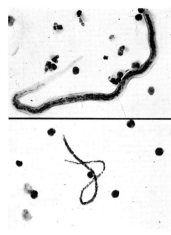

36 Comparison of size between *L. loa* (upper) and *M. perstans* (lower). Background cells are white cells. An eosinophilia accompanies filariasis.

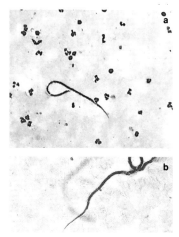

37 **a** *Mansonella ozzardi* mf, unsheathed, 10× obj, Giemsa. **b** Tail of *M. ozzardi*. It is long and pointed. No nuclei in tip, 40× obj.

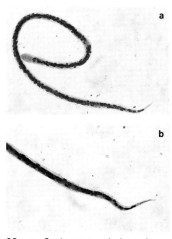

38 **a** *Onchocerca volvulus* mf, unsheathed, 10× obj, Giemsa. **b** Tail of *O. volvulus*. It is pointed. No nuclei in tip, 40× obj.

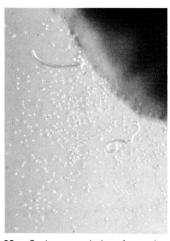

39 *Onchocerca volvulus* mf emerging from a skin snip. Saline preparation, 10× obj. The microfilariae are actively motile.

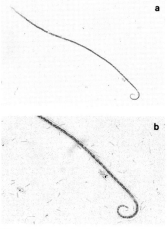

40 **a** *Mansonella streptocerca* mf, unsheathed, 10× obj, Giemsa. **b** Tail of *M. streptocerca*. It is hooked. Nuclei extend to tip, 40× obj.

Abbreviations: mf = microfilaria   obj = objective   HE = Haematoxylin and eosin stained

As seen with 100× objective, Fields stained

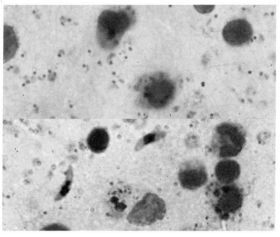
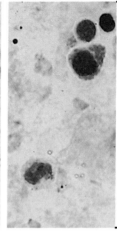

41 Plasmodium falciparum

Left: Many trophozoites and two gametocytes. Note the malaria pigment in the white cells. This is often seen in falciparum malaria, especially in heavy or long-standing infections.

Right: P. falciparum in patient with sickle cell disease. Note the nucleus from a nucleated red cell next to a small trophozoite (upper left). The malaria parasite consists of a red chromatin dot *and* blue cytoplasm. The blue stippling in the background is reticulum from reticulocytes. It is evidence of haemolysis.

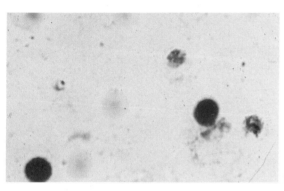
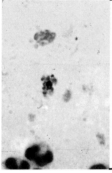

42 Plasmodium malariae

Left: Trophozoite (left) and early schizonts. Usually only a few trophozoites are found in *P. malariae* infections. Note the plentiful yellow-brown malaria pigment in the parasites.

Right: Gametocyte (upper) and late schizont (lower). Note their small size and presence of pigment.

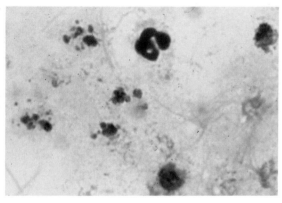
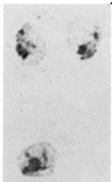

43 Plasmodium vivax

Left: Four trophozoites (left) and two gametocytes (lower and upper right corner). Note the large size and amoeboid fragmented appearance of the trophozoites.

Right: Trophozoites in thinner part of thick film. Note the outlines of the red cells, Schuffners dots surrounding the parasites, and malaria pigment.

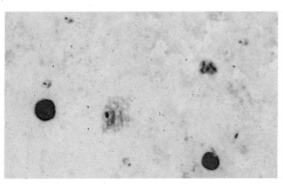
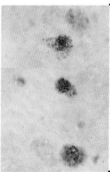

44 Plasmodium ovale

Left: Trophozoites and schizont (upper right). Note the late trophozoite (near centre) surrounded by James dots.

Right: Early schizont and gametocytes.

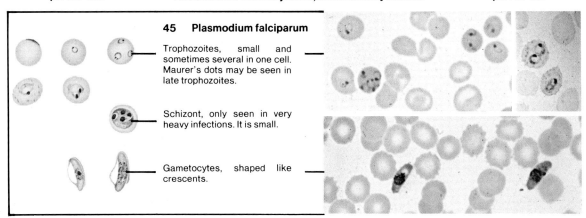

45   Plasmodium falciparum

Trophozoites, small and sometimes several in one cell. Maurer's dots may be seen in late trophozoites.

Schizont, only seen in very heavy infections. It is small.

Gametocytes, shaped like crescents.

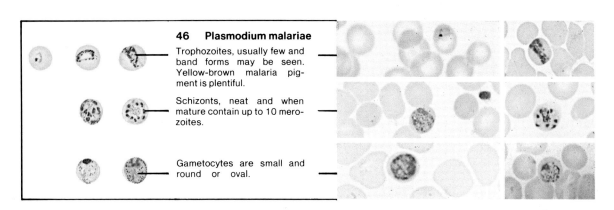

46   Plasmodium malariae

Trophozoites, usually few and band forms may be seen. Yellow-brown malaria pigment is plentiful.

Schizonts, neat and when mature contain up to 10 merozoites.

Gametocytes are small and round or oval.

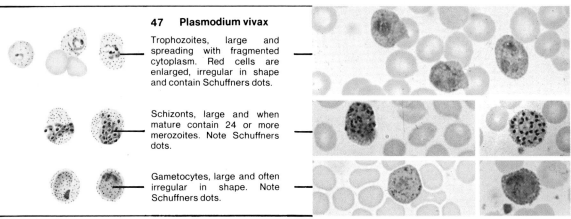

47   Plasmodium vivax

Trophozoites, large and spreading with fragmented cytoplasm. Red cells are enlarged, irregular in shape and contain Schuffners dots.

Schizonts, large and when mature contain 24 or more merozoites. Note Schuffners dots.

Gametocytes, large and often irregular in shape. Note Schuffners dots.

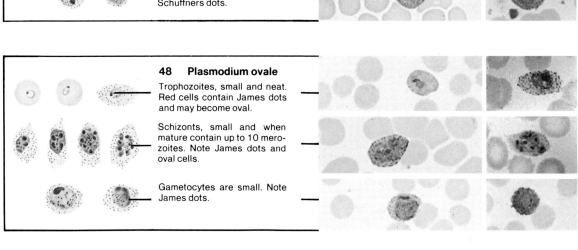

48   Plasmodium ovale

Trophozoites, small and neat. Red cells contain James dots and may become oval.

Schizonts, small and when mature contain up to 10 merozoites. Note James dots and oval cells.

Gametocytes are small. Note James dots.

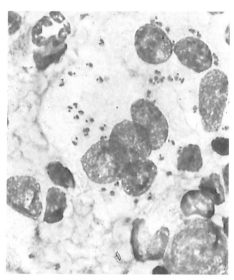

49 Amastigotes of *Leishmania donovani* in macrophage cells in Giemsa stained smear of spleen aspirate (structurally similar to amastigotes of other *Leishmania* species).

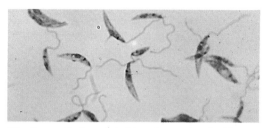

50 Promastigotes of *Leishmania* species in Giemsa stained culture smear.

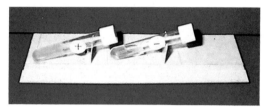

51 Formol gel test. *Left:* Positive test showing gelling and whitening of serum. *Right:* Negative test with no whitening or gelling of serum.

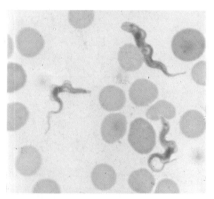

52 *Trypanosoma b. rhodesiense* in Giemsa stained thin blood film (morphologically indistinguishable from *T. b. gambiense*).

53 Giemsa stained Morula cell in smear of cerebrospinal fluid.

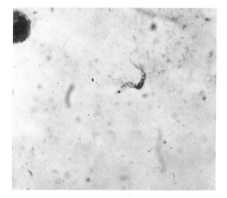

54 *Trypanosoma b. rhodesiense* in Field's stained thick blood film. The trypanosomes can also be stained by Giemsa.

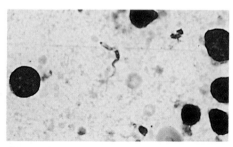

55 *Trypanosoma b. gambiense* in Field's stained smear of lymph gland aspirate.

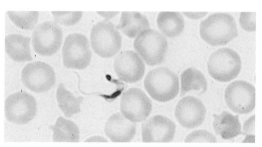

56 *Trypanosoma cruzi* in Leishman stained thin blood film in acute Chagas' disease.

18

Tapeworms

18:1 CLASSIFICATION AND FEATURES OF TAPEWORMS OF MEDICAL IMPORTANCE

The general characteristics of tapeworms (cestodes) are described at the beginning of the Parasitology Section in Chapter 12:4.

Classification of tapeworms of medical importance or common occurrence

Order   CYCLOPHYLLIDEA
Species *Taenia solium*
         Taenia saginata
         Echinococcus granulosus
         Hymenolepis nana

Order   PSEUDOPHYLLIDEA
Species *Diphyllobothrium latum*

Tapeworms of lesser medical importance or low occurrence

Order   CYCLOPHYLLIDEA
Species *Echinococcus multilocularis*
         Multiceps species
         Dipylidium caninum

Order   PSEUDOPHYLLIDEA
Species *Spirometra* species

Features of tapeworms that infect humans

- Adults of *T. saginata*, *T. solium*, *H. nana* and *D. latum* live in the small intestine. Humans are the only or main definitive hosts of *T. saginata*, *T. solium*, and *H. nana*. *D. latum* parasitizes fish-eating animals as well as humans.

    Note: Both adults and larvae of *H. nana* occur in man. Occasionally the larvae of *T. solium* are also found in man.

    Only the larval forms of *E. granulosus* and *Spirometra* species are found in humans.

- Transmission of *Taenia* species is by ingesting cysticercus larvae in undercooked beef (*T. saginata*) or pork (*T. solium*). *H. nana* is transmitted by ingesting embryonated eggs (from human faeces) or by internal autoinfection.

    D. latum is transmitted by ingesting plerocercoid larvae in raw or undercooked fish.

    Infection with *E. granulosus* is by ingesting embryonated eggs from dog faeces. *Spirometra* species are transmitted by ingesting procercoids in a crustacean host, ingesting plerocer-

coids in food, or by plerocercoids penetrating the skin when infected tissue is applied as a poultice.

- Laboratory confirmation of infection with *T. saginata* and *T. solium* is by finding gravid segments and eggs in faeces. The eggs of *T. saginata* are also found on perianal skin. *H. nana* and *D. latum* infections are diagnosed by finding eggs in faeces. Infection with *E. granulosus* is usually confirmed in the laboratory serologically or by examining the fluid from a removed cyst for protoscoleces.

Terms used to describe the eggs and larvae of tapeworms

Oncosphere (hexacanth embryo)
Embryo with six hooklets which is found in the egg of *Taenia* species and other Cyclophyllidea tapeworms. The oncosphere is surrounded by a wall called an embryophore. The remainder of the egg consists of yolk cells surrounded by an egg shell.

Cysticercus (plural: cysticerci)
Larval form (bladderworm) of *Taenia* tapeworms which is found in the intermediate host (pig or cow) and is infective to man. It consists of a small fluid-filled bladder containing a single invaginated (inward turning) scolex which when ingested and fully developed evaginates (turns outwards) in the small intestine and grows into a mature tapeworm.

Cysticercoid (plural: cysticercoids)
Solid larval form of *H. nana* containing a scolex which when fully developed emerges and attaches to the gut wall where it grows into a mature tapeworm. In nature it is found in the flea which serves as the intermediate host (also for *H. diminuta*). The larval form of *D. caninum* is also a cysticercoid. It is found in a cat or dog flea.

Hydatid cyst
This is the cystic larval form of *Echinococcus granulosus* which can develop in humans following the ingestion of embryonated eggs. In nature, it is found in sheep, cattle, pigs, goats and camels. It contains an inner germinal layer which usually produces many protoscoleces.

Coenurus (plural: coenuri)
This is the cystic larval stage of *Multiceps* species which is normally found in sheep or rodents. Very occasionally it is found in humans following the ingestion of eggs in dog faeces.

Coracidium (plural: coracidia)
Ciliated embryo with six hooklets which hatches from the egg of *Diphyllobothrium* species in water and is taken up by the first intermediate host.

Procercoid (plural: procercoids)
Immature larval stage of *D. latum* and other Pseudophyl-

lidea tapeworms which is found in the first intermediate host (crustacean).

Plerocercoid (plural: plerocercoids)
Elongated larval stage of *D. latum* and other Pseudophyllidea tapeworms which is found in the second intermediate host (fish). When fully developed it measures 6-20 mm and contains a scolex with sucking grooves. Pleroceroids of *D. latum* are infective to humans.

A plerocercoid larva is sometimes called a sparganum (plural spargana).

Tapeworms of Major Medical Importance or Common Occurrence in Humans
LIFE CYCLE SUMMARIES

Taenia saginata *Taenia solium*	*Diphyllobothrium latum*	*Hymenolepis nana*	*Echinococcus granulosus*
Cysticerci ingested in raw or insufficiently cooked beef (*T. saginata*) or pork (*T. solium*)	Plerocercoids ingested in raw or insufficiently cooked fish	Eggs ingested in food or from hands contaminated with human faeces	Eggs ingested in food or from hands contaminated with dog faeces
Tapeworm in small intestine	Tapeworm in small intestine	Tapeworm in small intestine	Eggs hatch embryos which are carried in blood and become lodged in liver, lung and elsewhere
EGGS AND SEGMENTS PASSED IN FAECES	EGGS PASSED IN FAECES	EGGS PASSED IN FAECES	HYDATID CYST IN TISSUE In humans only larval hydatid cyst stage found
Eggs ingested by cattle (*T. saginata*) or pigs (*T. solium*)	Eggs hatch in water and coracidia are ingested by a *Cyclops* and become procercoids		*Natural life cycle* Eggs ingested by sheep, goats, camels, cattle, or other intermediate host
			Embryos develop into hydatid cysts which contain protoscoleces
			Infective tissue eaten by dog or other definitive host
		Note: Internal auto-infection occurs. Eggs	Tapeworms in small intestine
Eggs hatch embryos which become infective cysticerci in muscle	Crustacean is ingested by a fish in which procercoids become infective plerocercoids	hatch embryos in small intestine which attach to intestinal villi and become tapeworms	EGGS PASSED IN ANIMAL FAECES

Note
T. saginata eggs are also found on perianal skin.

18:2 *TAENIA* SPECIES

Infection with *Taenia* tapeworms is called taeniasis. Humans are the definitive hosts of the following species:

- *Taenia saginata* (beef tapeworm)
- *Taenia solium* (pork tapeworm)

T. saginata and *T. solium* belong to the Taeniidae family of Cyclophyllidea tapeworms.

TAENIA SAGINATA

Distribution
T. saginata has a worldwide distribution with an estimated 61 million persons infected (1981 estimate).[1] It is found in countries where cattle are raised and beef is eaten. In Egypt and Morocco the camel is the main source of human infection.

Mass travel, the migration of workers, and inadequate disposal of sewage have contributed to an increase in the prevalence of infection with *T. saginata*.

Transmission and life cycle
T. saginata is transmitted by eating raw or insufficiently cooked beef or other animal meat which contains infective cysticercus larvae.*

* *Cysticercus bovis*
This name was used to describe the parasite in cattle before it was identified as the larval stage of *Taenia saginata*.

Life cycle
— Following digestion, the scolex (head) in the cysticercus is freed and becomes attached to the wall of the small intestine by its suckers. Segments (proglottides) are formed from the neck region and within 2-3 months the larva has grown into a long tapeworm with the gravid (egg-filled) segments being found at the tail end.

Mature *T. saginata* tapeworm: It measures 4-10 metres in length and consists of up to 2000 segments. The scolex is cubical in shape, measuring about 2 mm across, and has four suckers but no hooks (see Plate 18.1).

Gravid segments of *T. saginata* are described under *Laboratory Diagnosis*.

Usually only one tapeworm is present but multiple infections can occur.

— When fully developed the gravid segments become detached. The eggs are discharged only after the gravid segments have separated from the worm. Gravid segments containing eggs and eggs from ruptured segments are passed in the faeces.

T. saginata segments also migrate through the anus and release eggs on the perianal skin.

— For the life cycle to be continued the eggs must reach open ground where cattle feed. The segments are capable of movement and migrating to grazing sites. Each gravid segment contains about 80 000 eggs (mature and immature) which are released when the segment disintegrates. Mature eggs remain viable for many months.

— After ingestion by a cow or other suitable intermediate host, the embryos escape from the eggs, pass through the intestinal wall into a blood vessel and are carried in the blood circulation to muscles. In muscle tissue the embryos grow and develop into infective cystic larvae called cysticerci (singular cysticercus). The embryonic hooklets are lost after the embryo becomes embedded in the muscle tissue. The cysticerci can survive for several months after which they become calcified.

T. saginata cysticercus (*Cysticercus bovis*): It measures 5-10 × 3-5 mm and consists of a fluid filled sac, or bladder, containing a small invaginated (turned inwards) scolex which has suckers but no hooks.

Note: The life cycle of *T. saginata* is summarized in Fig. 18.1.

Clinical features and pathology
Clinically, infection with *T. saginata* rarely produces serious effects. There may be abdominal pain with intestinal disturbances and loss of appetite. Very occasionally migrating segments may cause appendicitis or cholangitis.

Prevention and control
- Avoiding eating raw or insufficiently cooked meat which may contain infective cysticerci. The cysticerci can be heat-killed at 56 °C or by deep-freezing meat for a minimum of three weeks.
- Inspecting meat and condemning any found to contain cysticerci.
- Providing health education and adequate latrines to ensure the containment of segments and destruction of eggs.
- Not using untreated human faeces to fertilize pastureland.
- Treating infected persons.

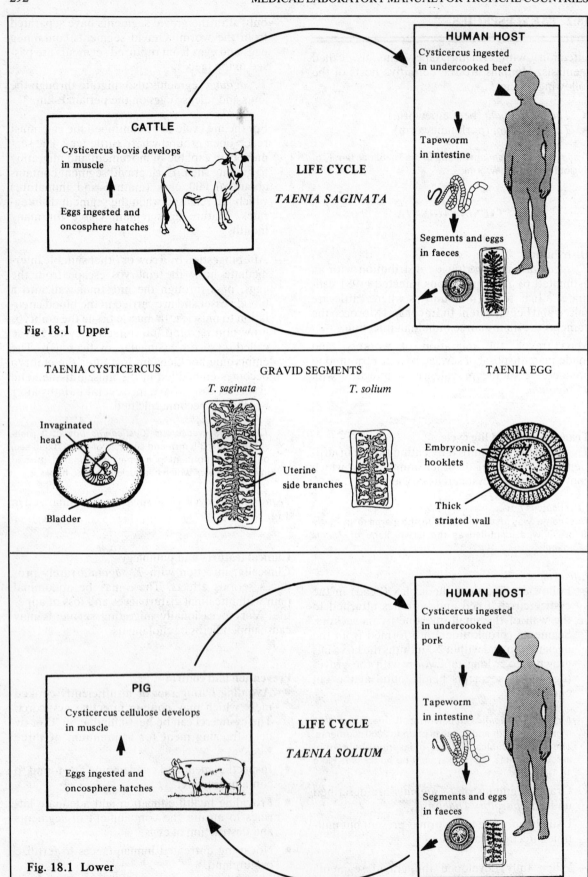

HUMAN HOST

Cysticercus ingested
in undercooked beef

Tapeworm
in intestine

Segments and eggs
in faeces

CATTLE

Cysticercus bovis develops
in muscle

Eggs ingested and
oncosphere hatches

LIFE CYCLE

TAENIA SAGINATA

Fig. 18.1 Upper

TAENIA CYSTICERCUS   GRAVID SEGMENTS   TAENIA EGG

T. saginata   *T. solium*

Invaginated
head

Uterine
side branches

Bladder

Embryonic
hooklets

Thick
striated wall

HUMAN HOST

Cysticercus ingested
in undercooked
pork

Tapeworm
in intestine

Segments and eggs
in faeces

PIG

Cysticercus cellulose develops
in muscle

Eggs ingested and
oncosphere hatches

LIFE CYCLE

TAENIA SOLIUM

Fig. 18.1 Lower

LABORATORY DIAGNOSIS

Laboratory confirmation of *T. saginata* infection is by:

☐ Identifying gravid segments recovered from clothing or passed in faeces. The segments are usually passed singly.

Following treatment the head and mature segments may be expelled and collected for identification.

☐ Detecting eggs in faeces. Morphologically the eggs of *T. saginata* and *T. solium* are indistinguishable.

Identifying *T. saginata* gravid segments
When freshly passed the segments are white and opaque. Viable (living) segments move by muscular contractions.

Caution: Because viable segments are actively motile, keep them in a closed container until they can be fixed and examined. Always use forceps to handle the segments.

Examination of a segment is as follows:

1. If recovered from faeces, wash the segment in clean water.

    If the segment is dry and shrivelled, soak it in water before examining it.

2. Press the segment between two slides and hold the slides together with an elastic band or adhesive tape at each end.

3. To kill the eggs, immerse the preparation for 10 minutes in a container of formol saline (Reagent No. 39) heated to 70 °C. Remove and wash in water.

    Caution: Formaldehyde has an irritating and harmful vapour, therefore when using formol saline make sure the room is well ventilated and cover the container of fixative with a tight fitting lid.

4. Firmly compressing the segment to give a thin preparation, hold it lengthways against the light and count the number of main branches arising from the central stem of the uterus (see Fig. 18.1). The branches are more easily counted with the help of a magnifying lens.

    The size of the segment and the number of uterine side branches can usually identify the segment as *T. saginata* or *T. solium*. Differentiation is also possible by examining a mature

segment or head of the tapeworm (expelled following treatment).

Gravid segment of Taenia saginata

• Appears white and opaque and measures about 20 mm long by 6 mm wide when freshly passed. It is therefore longer than a *T. solium* gravid segment.

• Uterus has a central stem which has more than 13 main side branches on each side. (*T. solium* has fewer than 13). The main side branches are subdivided into smaller branches.

Illustrations: See Fig. 18.1.

Note: If required, the uterine branches can be stained by injecting India ink through the opening (genital pore) on the side of the segment or by staining the segment with haematoxylin (Delafields or Harris').Staining is not usually necessary to identify fresh segments.

Identification of the scolex of *T. saginata*
The scolex (head) is very small, measuring only 2 mm across. It may be found among the smallest immature segments with the help of a magnifying lens. The scolex has 4 suckers but no hooks (see Plate 18.1). The absence of hooks distinguishes the scolex of *T. saginata* from that of *T. solium* which has hooks.

Caution: Use forceps to handle the small segments. If wishing to preserve the scolex and any of the segments for later examination, transfer them to a container of formol saline (Reagent No. 39) heated to 70 °C. This will kill the eggs and fix the segments. The scolex and segments can also be stored in formol saline solution (cold).

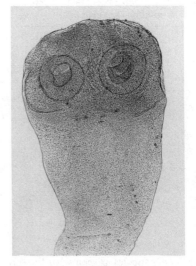
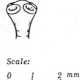

Scale:
0   1   2 mm

Plate 18.1 Head of *Taenia saginata*.
Courtesy of K. L. Frampton.

Detecting *Taenia* eggs in faeces or in a perianal preparation

Examination of faeces for Taenia eggs

A concentration technique and the examination of several specimens may be necessary to detect *Taenia* eggs in faeces because the eggs are not regularly discharged from the tapeworm in the intestine. The eggs are only released when gravid segments become detached and damaged.

The eggs can be concentrated by the formol ether technique described in 13:4. Floatation techniques are not suitable.

The following features identify a *Taenia* egg:

Egg of *Taenia saginata* or *Taenia solium*

- It is round or round to oval, measuring 33-43 μm in diameter.

- A thick, brown, radially striated wall (embryophore) surrounds the embryo.

- Hooklets are present in the embryo. Careful focusing is necessary to see the three pairs of hooklets.

   Hooklets
   These embryonic hooklets are present in the eggs of both *T. saginata* and *T. solium* (see previous text).

- Sometimes a clear membrane can be seen surrounding the egg but usually the egg shell and yolk cells are lost when the gravid segment becomes detached and disintegrates.

Illustrations: See Plate 18.2 and colour Plate 19.

Note: If required, the Ziehl-Neelsen staining technique (as used for AFB) can be used to differentiate *Taenia* eggs. The embryo of *T. saginata* is acid fast (i.e. stains red) whereas that of *T. solium* is not acid fast.

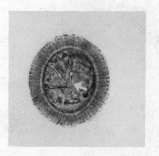

Plate 18.2 Egg of *Taenia* species as seen with the 40x objective. The white arrow shows the position of the hooklets. *Courtesy of K. L. Frampton.*

Collection and examination of a perianal specimen
The clear adhesive tape technique described in 21:3 for the recovery of *E. vermicularis* eggs from perianal skin can also be used to collect the eggs of *T. saginata* from skin around the anus.

TAENIA SOLIUM

Distribution
T. solium is not as widely distributed as *T. saginata* with an estimated 4 million persons being infected (1981 estimate),[1] mainly in Ethiopia, southern Africa, China, India, Central America, Chile, Brazil, and Papua New Guinea. It occurs where human faeces reach pigs and pork is eaten raw or insufficiently cooked.

Transmission and life cycle
T. solium is transmitted by eating raw or insufficiently cooked pork which contains infective cysticercus larvae*

*Cysticercus cellulosae
This name was used to describe the parasite in pigs before it was identified as the larval stage of *T. solium*.

Life cycle
The life cycle of *T. solium* is similar to that of *T. saginata*.

— Following digestion, the scolex in the cysticercus is freed and becomes attached to the intestinal wall by its hooks and suckers and grows into a long tapeworm. Within 2-3 months the tapeworm is mature and gravid segments are formed.

   Mature T. solium tapeworm: It measures 2-3 metres in length and consists of 800-1000 segments. The scolex is round, measuring about 1 mm in diameter, and has four suckers and a crown of hooks in two rows (see Plate 18.3).

Gravid segments of *T. solium* are described under *Laboratory Diagnosis*.

Usually only one tapeworm is present but multiple infections can occur and also infections with both *T. solium* and *T. saginata*.

— Gravid segments containing eggs and eggs from ruptured segments are passed out in the faeces. The eggs are not discharged from gravid segments attached to the tapeworm.

— The segments disintegrate and the eggs are released. Each gravid segment contains 30 000-50 000 eggs (mature and immature). Mature eggs can remain viable for several months.

— The life cycle is continued by the pig ingesting viable eggs. The embryos are released and are carried to the muscles of the pig where they develop into infective cysticerci. The embryonic hooklets are lost after the embryo becomes embedded in the muscle tissue. After several months the cysticerci die and become calcified.

> *T. solium cysticercus (Cysticercus cellulosae)*: It measures 5-18 × 5 mm and consists of a fluid filled bladder containing a small invaginated scolex which has a ring of hooks as well as suckers.

T. solium cysticerci in man
Occasionally in a human host, the gravid segments of *T. solium* are regurgitated and eggs reach the stomach. The embryos are freed and can be carried in the blood circulation to muscles, subcutaneous tissues, the brain, spinal cord, eyes and other parts of the body where they develop into cysticerci.

Human infection with *T. solium* larvae can also occur by ingesting viable eggs in infected food or from contaminated fingers.

Serious disease can result from infection with *T. solium* cysticerci (see *Clinical features and pathology*).

Note: The life cycle of *T. solium* is summarized in Fig. 18.1.

Clinical features and pathology
Infection with the tapeworm of *T. solium* rarely produces serious effects. There may be abdominal pain with intestinal disturbances and loss of appetite.

Infection with the larvae of *T. solium* (cysticercosis) can cause cystic nodules in subcutaneous tissues and muscles. Usually the larvae produce few serious clinical symptoms except when present in the brain where they can cause epilepsy and other central nervous system disorders. Dead and dying cysticerci may cause an inflammatory host response. When calcified the cysts can be detected by X-ray.

Prevention and control
- Avoiding eating raw or insufficiently cooked pork which may contain cysticerci ('measly' pork).
- Ensuring pigs do not have access to human faeces.
- Inspecting meat and condemning any found to contain cysticerci.
- Treating infected persons, and providing health education and adequate sanitary facilities.

The prevention of cysticercosis caused by internal autoinfection is by diagnosing *T. solium* infection and treating it effectively. Ingestion of eggs can be avoided by personal hygiene and by not eating food which may be contaminated with *T. solium* eggs such as raw vegetables grown on land fertilized with untreated human faeces.

LABORATORY DIAGNOSIS

Confirmation of taeniasis caused by *T. solium* tapeworm is by:

☐ Identifying gravid segments passed in faeces. The segments are often passed in chains.

  Following treatment, the head and mature segments may be expelled and collected for identification.

☐ Detecting eggs in faeces. Morphologically the eggs of *T. solium* and *T. saginata* are indistinguishable.

Note: Serum antibodies are formed in response to infection with *T. solium* cysticerci and serological tests have been developed to diagnose cysticercosis (especially cerebral disease). Most of these serological tests, however, are of low sensitivity and specificity and reagents are not commercially available. When available, hybridoma-derived reagents may provide tests with good specificity.[2]

Identifying *T. solium* gravid segments
The segments are examined in the same way as described for *T. saginata* (see previous text).
Caution: Use forceps to handle the segments. Viable segments are motile, therefore keep them in a closed container until they can be fixed and examined.

> **Gravid segment of *Taenia solium***
> - Appears grey-blue and translucent and measures about 13 mm long by 8 mm wide when freshly passed. It is therefore shorter than a gravid segment of *T. saginata*.
> - Uterus has a central stem which has up to 13 main side branches on each side (*T. saginata* has more than 13). The main side branches are subdivided into smaller branches.
>
> *Illustration*: See Fig. 18.1.
>
> *Note*: If required the uterine branches can be stained by injecting India ink through the opening (genital pore) on the side of the segment or by staining the segment with haematoxylin (Delafields or Harris').Staining is not usually necessary to identify fresh segments.

Identification of the scolex of *T. solium*
The scolex (head) is very small, measuring only 1 mm in diameter. It may be found among the smallest immature segments with the help of a magnifying lens. The scolex has 4 suckers and a crown of hooks (see Plate 18.3). The presence of hooks distinguishes the scolex of *T. solium* from that of *T. saginata* which has no hooks.

Caution: Use forceps to handle the segments. If wishing to preserve the scolex and any of the segments for later examination, transfer them to a container of formol saline (Reagent No. 39) heated to 70 °C. This will kill the eggs and fix the segments. The scolex and segments can also be stored in formol saline solution.

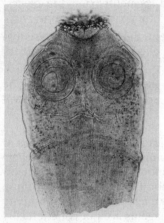

Scale:
0   1   2 mm

Plate 18.3 Head of *Taenia solium*.
Courtesy of K. L. Frampton.

Note: The examination of faeces for *Taenia* eggs is described under *Taenia saginata*. Morphologically the egg of *T. solium* is indistinguishable from that of *T. saginata*.

18:3 *ECHINOCOCCUS GRANULOSUS*

Development in man of the larval stage of the dog tapeworm *Echinococcus granulosus* causes echinococcosis. The disease is also called hydatid disease, or hydatidosis, because the larval stage is a hydatid cyst.

E. granulosus belongs to the Taeniidae family of Cyclophyllidea.

Distribution
Hydatid disease is known to occur in many parts of the world where sheep are in close association with dogs and humans or where dogs and wild carnivores are associated with livestock and wild herbivores. High infection rates occur in East Africa (especially the Turkana region in Kenya), North Africa, South Africa, India, the eastern Mediterranean, Middle East, and parts of South America and Australasia.

Transmission and life cycle
Hydatid disease is a zoonosis. Transmission is by ingesting *E. granulosus* eggs in food contaminated with dog faeces or from hands that have become contaminated when handling infected dogs.

Natural life cycle
Sheep, cattle, pigs, goats and camels serve as intermediate hosts of *E. granulosus*.

— When eggs are ingested by an intermediate host they are digested and the embryos are released in the duodenum. The embryos migrate through the intestinal wall into a blood vessel and are carried in the blood to the liver, lungs, and other organs of the host.

— The embryos develop into hydatid cysts which contain many protoscoleces.

— The natural life cycle is completed when infected tissue from a sheep (or other intermediate host) is eaten by the dog or occasionally by other animals that can serve as definitive hosts such as jackals, foxes and wolves.

— In the dog (or other definitive host), the scoleces evaginate, attach themselves to the wall of the small intestine and grow into mature tapeworms.

Mature E. granulosus tapeworm: It is small, measuring up to 9 mm long with usually only 3 or 4 segments. The scolex has 4 suckers and a crown of hooks in two rows.

— Eggs are produced which are released when the detached gravid segment (last segment) ruptures.

Morphologically, the eggs of *E. granulosus* are indistinguishable from those of *Taenia* species. The eggs of *E. granulosus* are able to survive for long periods. They are highly resistant.

Development in a human host
When man becomes an intermediate host of *E. granulosus*, the life cycle ends 'blindly'. There is no transfer of the parasite to a definitive host except in places where animal definitive hosts are able to feed on human remains.

Following ingestion of *E. granulosus* eggs, development of the parasite in a human host is as follows:

— The embryos are freed in the small intestine. They migrate through the intestinal wall into a blood vessel and circulate in the blood. Most of the embryos are filtered out in the liver and some in the lungs. A few may become lodged in other organs, bones and joints.

— The embryos become embedded in the tissues and after a few days they form sac-like structures. After several months or years they develop into hydatid cysts.

Hydatid cyst: It consists of an outer thick laminated cyst wall and an inner, thin, nucleated germinal layer. From the germinal layer, brood capsules are produced inside which small protoscoleces form (see Fig. 18.2). Occasionally

daughter cysts form within the main cyst when parts of the germinal layer become detached.

The brood capsules may break off and sink down through the fluid which fills the cyst. Free brood capsules and individual protoscoleces released from the capsules, form what is called hydatid sand.

There is a marked cellular response by the host to the presence of the hydatid cyst which leads eventually to it being surrounded by a fibrous wall. Older cysts may become calcified.

Note: The life cycle of *E. granulosus* is summarized in Fig. 18.2.

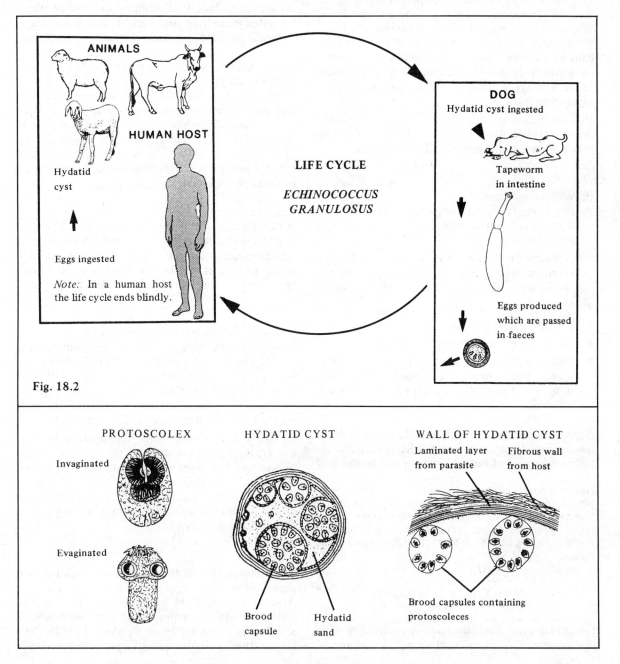

Fig. 18.2

Clinical features and pathology

Human infection with *E. granulosus* may produce serious symptoms depending on the site and size of the hydatid cyst. The cyst grows slowly but continuously and death can be caused by obstruction and pressure on vital organs or by rupture of the cyst with subsequent anaphylactic shock. Some cysts may grow for only a short time and then die and calcify.

Up to 60% of hydatid cysts are found in the right lobe of the liver (tests which may be helpful in distinguishing liver hydatid disease from liver carcinoma are listed under *Laboratory Diagnosis*).

Hydatid cysts may also occur in the lungs where they can cause pulmonary symptoms and the production of sputum containing blood and cyst fluid. When hydatid cysts develop in bone there is no fibrous wall formed and therefore the cyst spreads causing pain and leading to bone fractures. Other sites where hydatid cysts can form include the brain, kidneys, or spleen but these organs are only rarely infected.

Eosinophilia is not a constant feature of hydatid disease with only a minority of patients being reported as having generalized eosinophilia.

Prevention and control
- Practising personal hygiene, especially the washing of hands after handling dogs and before eating.
- Avoiding unnecessary handling of dogs that are in contact with sheep, and informing herdsmen and others at risk of the dangers of infection.
- Regular worming of dogs.
- Eliminating stray dogs.
- Not feeding dogs with uncooked meat or offal.
- Preventing dogs from entering places where sheep and other intermediate hosts are slaughtered and also inspecting carcasses for infection.

Note: Reasons for the high prevalence of hydatid disease in the Turkana district of Kenya are discussed in the paper of French, Nelson and Wood.[3]

Further information: More detailed information concerning the prevention and control of hydatid disease can be found in the 1981 FAO/UNDP/WHO *Guidelines for surveillance, prevention and control of echinococcosis/hydatidosis*, available from WHO, 1211 Geneva-27 Switzerland.

LABORATORY DIAGNOSIS

Hydatid disease is usually diagnosed clinically with the assistance of ultrasound scanning and other imaging techniques in places where these facilities are available.

Laboratory investigations include:

☐ Testing serum for antibodies produced in response to infection.

☐ Examining cyst fluid for brood capsules and protoscoleces following the surgical removal of a cyst.

Note: During surgery, care must be taken not to puncture a hydatid cyst because leakage of the fluid can cause anaphylaxis and massive reinfection from released protoscoleces.

Histological examination of the cyst wall should include PAS staining to show the laminated membrane and Ziehl-Neelsen staining to show the acid fast hooks of the protoscoleces.

Useful tests to differentiate liver hydatid disease from hepatoma

Serum glycoproteins, serum aminotransferases, and other liver function tests are usually normal with hydatid disease of the liver but abnormal with cancer of the liver. The erythrocyte sedimentation rate (ESR) is usually moderately raised with hydatid disease whereas with cancer of the liver it is markedly raised.

Casoni skin test

Although this intradermal test is still widely used to assist in the diagnosis of hydatid disease, it lacks standardization of the antigen, technique, and interpretation of results. The test is not sufficiently specific and false positive results occur frequently.

Serological diagnosis of hydatid disease

In general the sensitivity of serological tests is affected by the site and condition of a hydatid cyst. Sensitivity is higher with liver cysts than with lung cysts. Dead or calcified cysts may give negative results. False negative results may be obtained from patients with circulating immune complexes.

Serological tests used in the diagnosis of hydatid disease have been evaluated in the Turkana region of Kenya.[4] For most of the tests that have been developed, reagents are not generally available. Reagents for an indirect haemagglutination test are however commercially available from Behring Diagnostics, Hoechst Ltd.[5]

Examination of cyst fluid for brood capsules and protoscoleces

After centrifuging the cyst fluid or allowing it to settle by gravity, transfer a drop of the sediment to a slide and cover with a cover glass. Examine the preparation microscopically for protoscoleces using the 10× objective with the condenser iris *closed sufficiently* to give good contrast.

Protoscolex of Echinococcus

- It is colourless and round to oval in shape.
- With focusing the hooks of the invaginated scolex can be easily seen (use 40× objective).

Illustration: See Plate 18.3 and colour Plate 18.

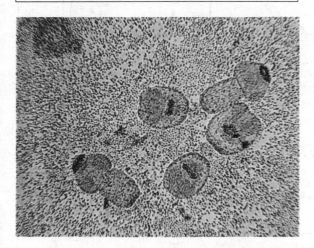

Plate 18.3 Hydatid sand from an hydatid cyst, showing protoscoleces of *Echinococcus granulosus* as seen with a 40x objective. *Courtesy of A. Moody.*

OTHER TAENIID TAPEWORMS WITH LARVAE THAT OCCASIONALLY INFECT HUMANS

Echinococcus multilocularis
Human infection with the hydatid cyst of this species causes multilocular or alveolar hydatid disease. Infections have been reported mainly from Canada, Alaska, USSR and Europe.

Definitive hosts are mainly foxes and wolves and the natural intermediate hosts are rodents and voles. Man becomes an intermediate host by accidentally ingesting eggs in food contaminated with faeces from a definitive host or from contaminated hands. In humans the hydatid cyst of *E. multilocularis* is invasive and spreads like a malignant tumour causing cavities and necrosis. It is not encapsulated like the hydatid cyst of *E. granulosus*. The liver is commonly infected. Surgical removal is rarely possible and the disease is usually fatal.

Multiceps species
The larval stage of these tapeworm species is a coenurus cyst and human infection with the larva is referred to as coenuriasis. Infection occurs following the ingestion of eggs in food or from hands contaminated with dog faeces.

Multiceps multiceps is found in North and South Africa and the coenurus infects the brain. There is no treatment and infection is usually fatal. *Multiceps brauni* is found in tropical Africa and causes a less serious disease because the coenurus does not infect the brain. The eyes and other parts of the body are infected.

The definitive hosts of *Multiceps* species are dogs and jackals. The intermediate hosts of *M. multiceps* are sheep and the intermediate hosts of *M. brauni* are rodents.

18:4 HYMENOLEPIS NANA

The dwarf tapeworm *Hymenolepis nana* is a common human parasite and is the smallest tapeworm known to infect humans.

H. nana belongs to the Hymenolepididae family of Cyclophyllidea tapeworms.

Distribution
H. nana is widely distributed in countries with warm climates including those of South America, Mediterranean region, Africa, and southeast Asia. Children are more commonly infected than adults.

Transmission and life cycle
Transmission is by ingesting eggs in food or drink or from contaminated hands. The eggs are infective when passed in the faeces. Internal autoinfection also occurs.

Life cycle
H. nana is unusual in that it has a direct life cycle with a human host serving as both definitive and intermediate host.

— Following the ingestion of eggs, the embryos are freed in the small intestine. They penetrate villi and within a few days develop into infective cysticercoid larvae.

— When fully mature, the cysticercoids rupture out of the villi into the lumen of the intestine. They become attached to other villi by their scoleces and grow rapidly into mature tapeworms. Eggs are produced after about 4 weeks.

Mature H. nana tapeworm: It is small, measuring only 10-44 mm in length. (See Fig.18.3). It consists of 100-200 short wide segments, a long neck and a scolex which has suckers and hooks.

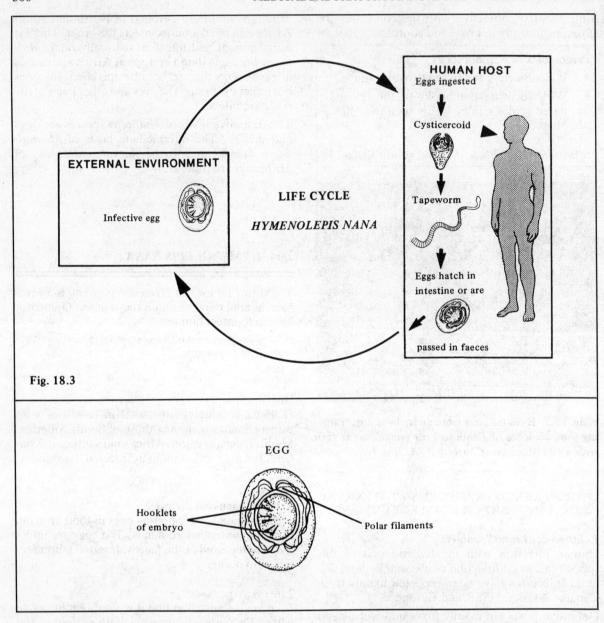

Fig. 18.3

— Gravid segments become detached and eggs are released in the intestine. Some of the eggs are passed in the faeces while others remain in the intestine. Those that remain hatch embryos which develop into cysticercoids.

The cysticercoids become attached to villi and grow into mature tapeworms.

Note: The life cycle of *H. nana* is summarized in Fig. 18.3.

Clinical features and pathology
Although many *H. nana* tapeworms can be found in the same host due to internal autoinfection, the life-span of the adult worms is only a few months.

Symptoms are rarely serious except in children when many tapeworms may cause abdominal pain and diarrhoea. Toxins released from the worms can cause allergic reactions.

Severe and sometimes disseminated infections can occur in malnourished or immunosuppressed persons.

Prevention and control
● Practising personal hygiene, especially the washing of hands before eating.

● Providing latrines and encouraging their use especially by children.

● Avoiding eating uncooked food which may be contaminated with human faeces.

LABORATORY DIAGNOSIS

Confirmation of *H. nana* infection is by:

☐ Finding the eggs of the parasite in faeces.

> *Caution*: *H. nana* eggs are infective directly they are passed.

Examination of faeces for *H. nana* eggs

The examination of faeces for helminth eggs in a direct physiological saline preparation is described in 13:2.

Concentration techniques and the examination of several specimens may be required to detect *H. nana* eggs. The eggs can be concentrated by the formol ether method or by the saturated sodium chloride floatation technique (see 13:6).

The following features identify the egg of *H. nana*:

Egg of Hymenolepis nana

- It is colourless, oval or round, measuring 30-45 μm in diameter.

- Hooklets are present in the embryo. Careful focusing is necessary to see the three pairs of hooklets.

- At each end of the egg thread-like structures called polar filaments are usually visible.

Illustrations: See Plate 18.5 and colour Plate 20, and Fig. 18.5.

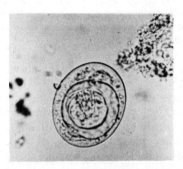

Plate 18.5   Egg of *Hymenolepis nana* showing polar filaments (threads) and hooklets.

Egg of Hymenolepis diminuta

H. diminuta is normally parasitic in the intestine of rodents. Very occasionally it infects man and eggs are passed in faeces which need to be distinguished from those of *H. nana*.

Compared with *H. nana*, the egg of *H. diminuta* is yellow-brown and larger, measuring 60-80 μm. It is without polar filaments. Like *H. nana* it contains

an embryo with 6 hooklets. The egg of *H. diminuta* is shown in Plate 18.6. and colour Plate 21.

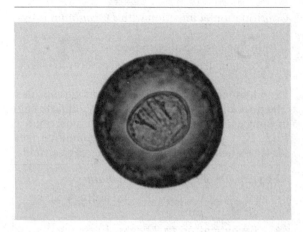

Plate 18.6   Egg of *Hymenolepis diminuta*. The hooklets can be seen.

18:5 *DIPYLIDIUM CANINUM*

Dipylidium caninum is a common parasite of dogs, foxes, jackals and cats. Very occasionally it infects humans.

D. caninum belongs to the Taeniidae family of Cyclophyllidea tapeworms.

Distribution

D. caninum has a worldwide distribution. Children are more commonly infected than adults.

Transmission and life cycle

Transmission of the parasite is by the accidental ingestion of an intermediate host of *D. caninum* such as a dog or cat flea which contains infective cysticercoid larvae.

— Following ingestion, the cysticercoids develop into mature tapeworms in the intestine. The eggs are passed in the faeces, often in egg capsules containing up to 20 eggs (see Plate 18.7).

  Mature D. caninum tapeworm: It measures 200-400 mm length. The scolex has 4 oval suckers and several rows of hooks which can be retracted.

— For the life cycle to be continued the eggs must be ingested by an intermediate host which is the larval stage of a cat or dog flea. Following ingestion, the larvae hatch from the eggs and develop into infective cysticercoids.

Clinical features

Infection with *D. caninum* rarely produces serious symptoms.

LABORATORY DIAGNOSIS

Confirmation of infection with *D. caninum* is by:

☐ Finding egg capsules in faeces.

☐ Occasionally finding gravid segments in faeces.

Examination of faeces for *D. caninum* egg capsules
The direct examination of faeces for helminth eggs in a physiological saline preparation is described in 13:2. If required a formol ether technique (see 13:4) can be used to concentrate the egg capsules.

Egg capsule of *Dipylidium caninum*

● A typical capsule measures about 60 × 100 μm.

● It contains up to 20 eggs. Each egg contains an embryo which has 3 pairs of hooklets and measures about 35 μm in diameter.

Illustration: See Plate 18.7.

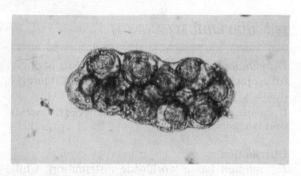

Plate 18.7   Egg capsule of *Dipylidium caninum* as seen with the 40x objective. *Courtesy of A. Moody.*

Examination of faeces for *D. caninum* gravid segments
The segments are elongate and resemble rice grains. They measure approximately 12 mm in length. A genital pore is present on each side of the segment. This is a characteristic feature of *Dipylidium* tapeworms.

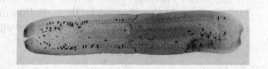

Plate 18.9   Gravid segment of *Dipylidium caninum*. A genital pore is present on each side of the segment.

18:6 *DIPHYLLOBOTHRIUM LATUM* AND SPARGANOSIS

Infection with *Diphyllobothrium latum* causes diphyllobothriasis.

D. latum and other *Diphyllobothrium* species are Pseudophyllidea tapeworms (see 18:1).

Distribution
D. latum is widely distributed in the lake areas of Europe, North America and the Far East. It is also found in parts of Asia, South America, and Central Africa.

Transmission and life cycle
Transmission is by ingesting the infective larva of *D. latum* which is known as a plerocercoid in raw or insufficiently cooked freshwater fish such as trout, perch or pike.

Life cycle
Unlike the other tapeworms described in this Chapter, the life cycle of *D. latum* requires two intermediate hosts, i.e. a crustacean and a fish. Definitive hosts include humans and fish-eating animals such as dogs, cats, foxes, bears and leopards. The life cycle beginning with the ingestion of a plerocercoid larva is as follows:

— The plerocercoid becomes attached to the wall of the small intestine and within 2-4 weeks develops into a mature tapeworm.

   Mature D. latum tapeworm: It is greyish white and long, measuring 3-10 metres with 3000-4000 segments. The elongated scolex has two slit-like suckers with grooves but no hooks. Mature segments are wider than they are long.

— Many eggs are produced which are discharged directly by the worm into the lumen of the intestine and passed in the faeces. Unlike the eggs of Cyclophyllidea tapeworms, the eggs of *D. latum* are operculated (with lids) and immature when passed. A mass of yolk cells surrounds an undeveloped ovum.

— For the life cycle to be continued the eggs must reach freshwater. Within 1-2 weeks the eggs mature and hatch, releasing spherical ciliated embryos called coracidia. Each coracidium has 3 pairs of embryonic hooklets.

— The coracidia are ingested by a crustacean of the genus *Cyclops* or *Diaptomus*. Within a few weeks, elongated larvae called procercoids develop inside the crustacean.

— The infected crustacean is ingested by a freshwater fish. In the second intermediate host, the procercoids are released and develop into infective plerocercoids which migrate to the muscles and connective tissue of the fish.

Plerocercoid larva: It is white and tape-like, measuring about 10 mm long by 2 mm wide (see Fig. 18.4). When full developed it contains a head with sucking grooves. A plerocercoid is also known as a sparganum.

— The life cycle is completed by a human or an animal definitive host eating fish containing the plerocercoids.

Note: The life cycle of *D. latum* is summarized in Fig. 18.4.

Clinical features and pathology

D. latum can live for many years in its human host. Diphyllobothriasis may cause gastrointestinal symptoms, weakness, weight loss, and other clinical features due to toxins released by the tapeworm.

Very occasionally a megaloblastic anaemia may develop due to the uptake of vitamin B_{12} by the tapeworm in competition with the host. This is more likely to occur when the tapeworm is situated in the upper part of the jejunum.

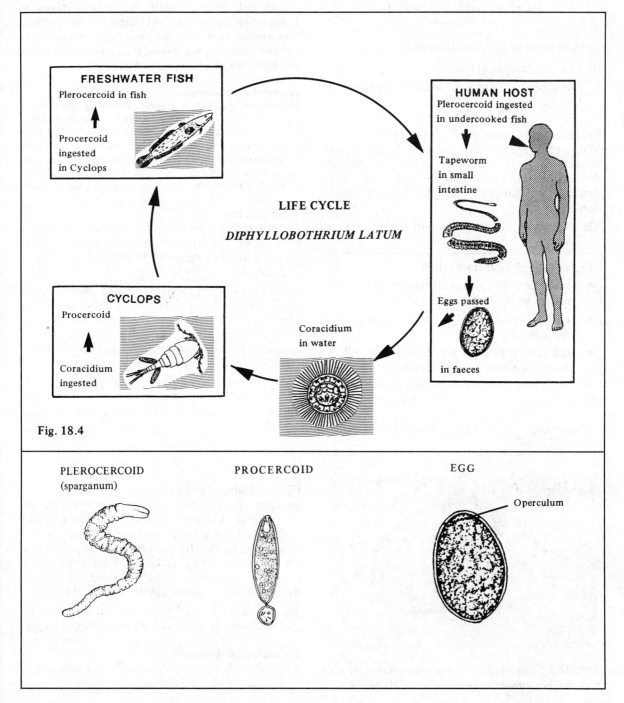

FRESHWATER FISH
Plerocercoid in fish

Procercoid ingested in Cyclops

HUMAN HOST
Plerocercoid ingested in undercooked fish

Tapeworm in small intestine

Eggs passed

in faeces

LIFE CYCLE

DIPHYLLOBOTHRIUM LATUM

CYCLOPS
Procercoid

Coracidium ingested

Coracidium in water

Fig. 18.4

PLEROCERCOID
(sparganum)

PROCERCOID

EGG

Operculum

Prevention and control

- Avoiding eating raw or insufficiently cooked freshwater fish which may contain plerocercoids. Viable plerocercoids may also be found in pickled or smoked fish.

- Killing the plerocercoids in fish by brine saturation or freezing at −10 °C for 24-48 hours.

- Preventing the eggs reaching water by providing adequate latrines combined with health education.

LABORATORY DIAGNOSIS

Confirmation of *D. latum* infection is by:

☐ Finding the eggs in faeces.

☐ Occasionally detecting mature segments in faeces.

Examination of faeces for *D. latum* eggs

Many eggs are usually present in the faeces because they are constantly discharged through the uterine pore and can therefore be easily detected in a direct physiological saline preparation (see 13:2).

The following features identify the egg of *D. latum*:

Egg of *Diphyllobothrium latum*

- It is pale yellow and oval in shape, measuring about 70 × 45 μm.

- Has an operculum (lid) which is usually difficult to see.

- Contains a mass of granulated yolk cells surrounding an undeveloped ovum.

- Sometimes a small projection is visible at the non-operculated end of the egg.

Illustrations: See Plate 18.8 and colour Plate 17).

Examination of a mature *D. latum* segment

Segments are not often found in the faeces because they tend to disintegrate in the intestines. When found, they often appear shrunken and empty.

Undamaged mature segments of *D. latum* are wider than they are longer, measuring 10-20 mm across by 3-7 mm long. The genital pore is found in the centre of the segment and not on the side as with Cyclophyllidea tapeworms.

SPARGANOSIS

Accidental infection with the larval stages of *Spirometra* tapeworms and other diphyllobothriid tapeworms that are not normally parasitic in humans causes sparganosis. It occurs mainly in the Far East, Southeast Asia and parts of Africa.

Spirometra tapeworms

Spirometra species are closely related to *Diphyllobothrium* species. Few details are known of the life cycles of most *Spirometra* tapeworms. Definitive hosts are known to include cats, dogs and possibly birds. First intermediate hosts are crustaceans and second intermediate hosts are frogs, birds and snakes. Plerocercoid larvae (spargana) are unable to develop into adult tapeworms in a human host.

Transmission

Infection is by ingesting a *Cyclops* infected with a procercoid. The larva migrates and develops into a plerocercoid (sparganum) in subcutaneous tissue and muscles.

Sparganosis of the eye is commonly caused by the application of infected frog tissue to eye sores. The plerocercoid migrates out of the tissue into the orbit of the eye. Infection with a plerocercoid may also occur by ingesting undercooked food prepared from secondary intermediate hosts.

The plerocercoids of some *Spirometra* species are able to multiply in a human host, usually in subcutaneous tissue where they encyst, forming large nodules.

Clinical features and pathology

Sparganosis may cause serious symptoms including painful inflamed swelling and occasionally widespread cystic lumps in muscles, lymph nodes, and subcutaneous tissue. Ocular sparganosis can cause serious damage to the eye. Occasionally serious symptoms can develop if spargana become sited in the nervous system or other vital organs.

Treatment is usually by the surgical removal of a plerocercoid or nodule containing a mass of larvae.

Prevention and control

- Boiling or filtering drinking water which may contain infected *Cyclops*.

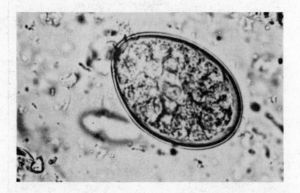

Plate 18.8   Egg of *Diphyllobothrium latum* as seen with the **40x objective**. *Courtesy of A. Moody.*

- Adequate cooking of animals capable of trans-mitting plerocercoids.

- Avoiding the application of frog tissue to eye sores and other parts of the body.

LABORATORY DIAGNOSIS

Sparganosis is usually diagnosed clinically or after removal of a larva or nodule. The larva is white and tape-like, measuring 10-35 mm long by 2-7 mm wide. The body is transversely wrinkled with a longitudinal groove.

A plerocercoid can be confused with the worm of *Dracunculus medinensis* (Guinea worm, see 22:8). Differentiation is made by recognizing the characteristic anterior end of a plerocercoid or by examining the larva histologically.

A species identification of a plerocercoid is only possible if the larva can be fed to an appropriate definitive host and the eggs subsequently identified. The eggs of *Spirometra* tapeworms are similar to but more pointed than those of *D. latum*.

World Health Organization. *Intestinal Protozoan and Helminth Infections*. WHO, Technical Report Series, No. 666,1981.

Knight, R. *Parasitic Disease in Man*, Churchill Livingstone, 1982. ELBS edition priced £4.50.

References
1 Peters,W., Gilles, H. M. *A Colour Atlas of Tropical Medicine and Parasitology*. Wolfe Medical Publications, 2nd Ed 1981, ELBS edition, 1985.

2 Craig, P. S. *et al. Australian Journal of Experimental Biology and Medical Sciences*, **58**, pp 339-350, 1980.

3 French, C. M., Nelson, G. S., and Wood, M. Hydatid disease in the Turkana district of Kenya, I. The background to the problem with hypotheses to account for the remarkably high prevalence of the disease in man. *Annals of Tropical Medicine and Parasitology*, **76**, pp 425-437, 1982.

4 Chemtai, A. K., Bowry, T. R., and Ahmad, Z. Evaluation of five immunodiagnostic techniques in echinococcosis patients. *Bulletin of the World Health Organization*, **59**, pp 767-772, 1982.

5 The Behring-Hoechst *Cellognost Echinococcosis Combipack* kit costs about £27.50 for 150 screening tests (1986). The kit contains 5 ml of Echinococcosis IHA Reagent, positive and negative controls and 2 × 10 ml Tris-buffer, pH 8.0. The reagents can be used in a tube test or in a microtitration plate test. For the address of Hoechst Ltd, see Appendix II.

Recommended Reading
Bell, D. R. *Lecture Notes on Tropical Medicine*. Blackwell Scientific Publications, 2nd edition 1985. Paperback priced £9.80.

Peters, W., Gilles, H. M. *A Colour Atlas of Tropical Medicine and Parasitology*, Wolfe Medical Publications, 2nd Ed, 1981. ELBS edition priced £9.00.

19 Hermaphroditic Flukes of the Liver, Intestinal Tract and Lungs

19:1 CLASSIFICATION AND FEATURES OF HERMAPHRODITIC FLUKES OF MEDICAL IMPORTANCE

The general characteristics of trematodes (flukes) are described at the beginning of the Parasitology Section in Chapter 12:4

Unlike the schistosomes described in Chapter 20, the flukes described in this Chapter are hermaphroditic, i.e. possessing male and female reproductive organs.

Classification of hermaphroditic flukes of medical importance or common occurrence

Superfamily	OPISTHORCHIOIDEA
Species	*Opisthorchis sinensis*†
	Opisthorchis viverrini

† Also known as *Clonorchis sinensis*

Superfamily	ECHINOSTOMATOIDEA
Species	*Fasciolopsis buski*
	Fasciola hepatica

Superfamily	PLAGIORCHIOIDEA
Species	*Paragonimus westermani*
	Paragonimus uterobilateralis
	Other *Paragonimus* species

Hermaphroditic flukes of lesser medical importance or low occurrence

Superfamily	OPISTHORCHIOIDEA
Species	*Heterophyes heterophyes*
	Metagonimus yokogawai

Superfamily	ECHINOSTOMATOIDEA
Species	*Fasciola gigantica*

Superfamily	PARAMPHISTOMATOIDEA
Species	*Gastrodiscoides hominis*

Superfamily	PLAGIORCHIOIDEA
Species	*Dicrocoelium dendriticum*

Features of hermaphroditic flukes that infect humans

- Adult flukes live (according to species) in the bile ducts, intestinal tract, or lungs.

- Animal reservoir hosts are important in the transmission of some species of medical importance.

- Transmission is by ingesting infective metacercariae. The metacercariae develop into flukes which produce operculated eggs. The eggs are excreted in the faeces of definitive hosts. The eggs of lung flukes can also be found in sputum. The eggs are operculated (with lids). Each egg hatches a miracidium.

  The first intermediate host is a snail. In this, the miracidium develops into a sporocyst which produces rediae. Some species produce more than one generation of rediae. From the rediae, cercariae are produced which are shed from the snail.

  The second intermediate host is (according to species) a freshwater fish, crab, crayfish or water plant. In or on these hosts the cercariae encyst and become metacercariae.

- Laboratory confirmation of fluke infections is by finding eggs in faeces or sputum(*Paragonimus*)

Note: The morphology of the medically important flukes is shown in the life cycle figures contained in the subsequent subunits of this Chapter.

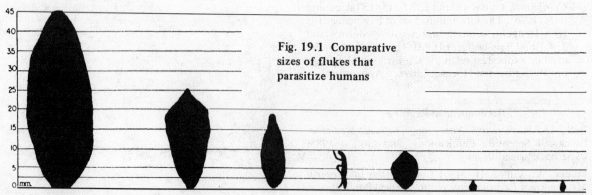

Fig. 19.1 Comparative sizes of flukes that parasitize humans

F. buski   *F. hepatica*   *O. sinensis*   *Schistosoma*   *P. westermani*   *H. heterophyes*   *M. yokogawai*

Hermaphroditic Flukes of Major Medical Importance
LIFE CYCLE SUMMARIES

Fasciolopsis buski *Fasciola hepatica*	*Opisthorchis sinensis* *Opisthorchis viverrini*	*Paragonimus westermani* Other *Paragonimus* species
Transmitted by ingesting metacercariae from uncooked water plants	Transmitted by ingesting metacercariae in undercooked freshwater fish	Transmitted by ingesting metacercariae in raw or undercooked crab or crayfish
Flukes in small intestine (*F. buski*) or biliary tract (*F. hepatica*)	Flukes in bile ducts	Flukes in lungs
EGGS PASSED IN FAECES	EGGS PASSED IN FAECES	EGGS PRESENT IN SPUTUM AND PASSED IN FAECES
	Eggs in water, ingested by snail	
Eggs hatch miracidia in water	Eggs hatch miracidia in snail	Eggs hatch miracidia in water
Miracidia penetrate snail		Miracidia penetrate snail
Sporocysts formed which produce rediae and finally cercariae	Sporocysts formed which produce rediae and finally cercariae	Sporocysts formed which produce rediae and finally cercariae
Cercariae leave snail, encyst on water plants and become infective metacercariae	Cercariae leave snail, encyst in or on fish and become infective metacercariae	Cercariae leave snail, encyst in crabs or crayfish and become infective metacercariae

19:2 *OPISTHORCHIS* SPECIES

OPISTHORCHIS SINENSIS

*Opisthorchis sinensis** is known as the Chinese or Oriental liver fluke.

* The name *Clonorchis sinensis* is also used and infection is referred to as clonorchiasis.

In 1981 it was estimated that a minimum of 28 million persons were infected with *O. sinensis*.

Distribution
O. sinensis is endemic in most of China and also in Japan, northern Vietnam, Taiwan and Korea. High infection rates are found especially in those parts of China where fish are cultured in ponds that are fertilized with human or animal faeces.

Transmission and life cycle

Infection is by eating raw, insufficiently cooked, smoked, or pickled fish which contains *O. sinensis* metacercariae.

Life cycle

— Following ingestion, the metacercariae excyst in the duodenum. Those young flukes that survive digestion, migrate to the bile ducts and occasionally to the pancreatic ducts where within about 4 weeks they develop into mature egg-producing flukes.

Mature O. sinensis flukes: They are small measuring about 10-25 × 2-5 mm, reddish-brown and almost transparent with a smooth outer surface. Morphological features are shown in Fig. 19.2.

— The eggs enter the small intestine in the bile and are excreted in the faeces. Each egg contains a fully developed miracidium.

For the life cycle to be continued, the eggs must reach fresh water which contains suitable snail hosts, e.g. of the genus *Bulimus*, *Parafossarulus*, or *Melanoides*.

— Following ingestion by the snail, the eggs hatch miracidia which develop into sporocysts which produce rediae and finally cercariae.

— The cercariae leave the snail and swim in the water for a few hours before encysting and becoming metacercariae under the scales and in the subcutaneous tissues of a suitable fish host. Many species of fish can serve as secondary intermediate hosts of *O. sinensis* especially those of the families Cyprinidae and Anabatidae.

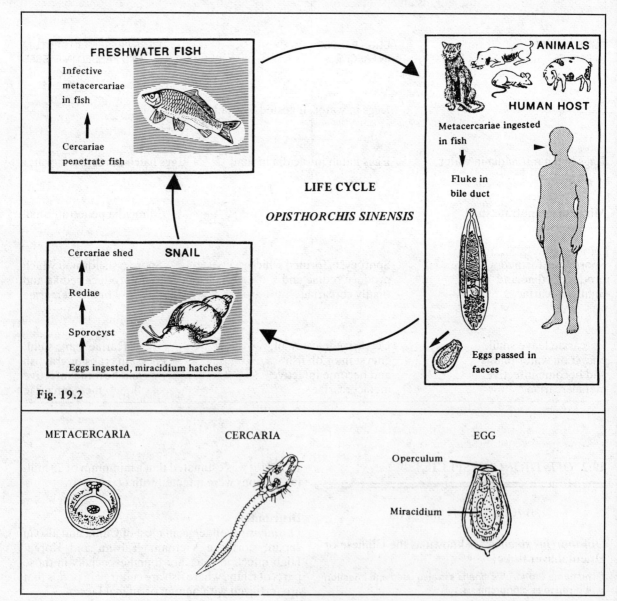

Fig. 19.2

The metacercariae are infective to humans and also to fish-eating animals such as dogs, cats, pigs and rats. In some areas, animal reservoir hosts are important in the human transmission of *O. sinensis*.

The life cycle of *O. sinensis* is shown in Fig. 19.2.

Clinical features and pathology

Symptoms of infection with *O. sinensis* are rarely serious. With heavy infections there can be damage to liver cells and bile ducts with jaundice, hepatitis, cirrhosis and biliary obstruction. The liver frequently becomes enlarged and in some cases cancer (adenocarcinoma) of the bile duct may develop. Other symptoms include epigastric pain and diarrhoea.

Chronic infection is associated with gall stones, recurrent attacks of cholangitis and pancreatitis.

Prevention and control

- Avoiding eating raw pickled, smoked, or insufficiently cooked fish which may contain metacercariae.

- Providing adequate latrines and health education to prevent contamination of fish ponds and other bodies of water that may contain snail hosts.

- Not using untreated faeces as fertilizer (night soil) in fish ponds.

- Using chemicals or other methods to eradicate snail hosts in areas where this is feasible.

LABORATORY DIAGNOSIS

Laboratory confirmation of *O. sinensis* infection is by:

- ☐ Finding eggs of the parasite in faeces.
- ☐ Detecting eggs in aspirates of duodenal fluid.

Other findings

An eosinophilic leucocytosis is common .

Anti-P_1 antibodies may be found in the sera of persons infected with *Opisthorchis* flukes who lack antigen P_1 on their red cells (i.e. P_2 positive). *Opisthorchis* flukes are known to contain P_1 substances that can stimulate the production of anti-P_1 antibodies.

Examination of faeces for *O. sinensis* eggs

The eggs can be few and because they are so small they can be easily missed. A concentration technique should therefore be used if infection is suspected and no eggs are found in a direct physiological saline preparation.

Direct saline preparation

Examination of a saline preparation for helminth eggs is described in 13:2. The 40× objective is required to identify *O. sinensis* eggs and the preparation must not be too thick otherwise the small eggs will be overlooked.

Concentration technique

O. sinensis eggs can be concentrated by the formol ether technique described in 13:4. Substitution of the formalin solution with a citric acid - Tween solution (Reagent No. 25) is recommended to increase recovery of *Opisthorchis* eggs.

The zinc sulphate floatation technique can also be used to concentrate *Opisthorchis* eggs but not the saturated sodium chloride floatation technique (see 13:6).

Egg of *Opisthorchis sinensis*

- It is yellow-brown and small measuring about 30 × 16 μm. It is shaped like an electric light bulb and contains a ciliated miracidium but this is difficult to see through the surface of the egg.

- Has a clearly seen operculum (lid).

- Often described as having 'shoulders' (rim on which the operculum rests).

- A small projection can sometimes be seen at the other end of the egg.

- When examined with the high power objective, an indistinct outer covering of the shell can be seen.

Illustrations: See Plate 19.1 and colour Plate 23.

Note: *Opisthorchis* eggs are not easily differentiated from those of other small trematodes such as *Heterophyes* and *Metagonimus* species. The clear operculum, 'shoulders', and outer shell covering of *Opisthorchis* eggs helps to identify them. The eggs of *Opisthorchis* show birefringence in polarized light.

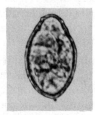

Plate 19.1 Egg of *Opisthorchis sinensis*.
Courtesy of K. L. Frampton.

Examination of duodenal fluid

A filtration technique can be used for the recovery of *O. sinensis* eggs from aspirates of duodenal fluid.[1] The equipment and filtration technique are similar to those described for filtering *S. haematobium* eggs except that a Nuclepore membrane of 8 μm pore size is required for filtering *O. sinensis* eggs. Staining the membrane with 1% w/v trypan blue in saline helps to show the eggs.

If unable to perform a filtration technique or the specimen is not suitable for filtration, transfer a drop of the aspirate (especially a piece of mucus) to a slide, cover with a cover glass and examine microscopically. Make sure the preparation is sufficiently thin otherwise the eggs will be missed. Use the 40× objective to identify the small eggs. If the aspirate is watery, centrifuge it first and examine a drop of the sediment.

Note: The *Enterotest* described in Chapter 14 for recovering *Giardia* parasites can also be used to obtain a sample of duodenal contents to examine for *Opisthorchis* eggs.

OPISTHORCHIS VIVERRINI

Opisthorchis viverrini is a similar fluke to *Opisthorchis sinensis*.

Distribution

O. viverrini can be found in the Mekong River Valley in Laos and Thailand. It is the commonest trematode infection in Thailand with an estimated 7 million people being infected in northeast Thailand (1982 estimate). Infection rates are as high as 90% in some villages with the heaviest infections being found in adults (40 y and over).

Transmission and life cycle

The transmission, hosts, and life cycle of *O. viverrini* are similar to those of *O. sinensis*. Fish-eating animals especially cats serve as reservoir hosts.

Clinical features and pathology

The mature flukes of *O. viverrini*, like those of *O. sinensis*, live in the bile duct and pancreatic ducts where they cause mechanical irritation and release toxic substances.

Commonest symptoms of infection are upper abdominal pain, gastrointestinal disturbances, oedema and weakness. Complications associated with severe infections include gallstones, obstructive jaundice, and cirrhosis. Recurrent attacks of cholangitis and pancreatitis can occur. Chronic infection can lead to cancer of the bile duct.

Prevention and control

The measures described for *O. sinensis* apply also to the prevention and control of *O. viverrini* infection.

LABORATORY DIAGNOSIS

The laboratory confirmation of *O. viverrini* infection is the same as that described for *O. sinensis* (see previous text). Eggs can be found in faeces and aspirates of duodenal fluid.

The egg of *O. viverrini* closely resembles that of *O. sinensis* except that it is smaller, measuring about 25 × 15 μm.

OPISTHORCHIS FELINEUS

O. felineus is normally parasitic in dogs and cats, but can infect humans. Infections have been reported from India, Japan, Europe and Siberia. The life cycle, clinical features, control, and laboratory diagnosis are similar to those described for *O. sinensis*.

The egg of *O. felineus* resembles that of *O. sinensis* except that is slightly narrower, measuring approximately 30 × 11 μm.

19:3 FASCIOLOPSIS BUSKI

Fasciolopsis buski is the largest fluke that infects humans. It is known as the giant intestinal fluke. The pig and buffalo are the normal definitive hosts of the parasite.

Distribution

Human infection with *F. buski* (fasciolopsiasis) is widespread in the Far East including southern and central China, Vietnam, Thailand, Laos and Taiwan. It also occurs in eastern India, Bangladesh and Indonesia.

It occurs particularly in areas where water plants are cultivated in ponds that are fertilized by pig or human faeces.

Infection rates are particularly high in school children.

Transmission and life cycle

Infection is commonly by peeling raw water chestnuts with the teeth or eating the fruits of water caltrop or other water vegetation on which *F. buski* metacercariae have encysted.

Life cycle
— Following ingestion, the metacercariae excyst in the duodenum, attach to the wall of the small intestine and within 3 months develop into mature egg-producing flukes. Many eggs are produced.

Mature F. buski flukes: They vary in size with the larger flukes measuring up to 70 × 20 mm by 3-7 mm thick. They are oval and covered with rows of small spines. Morphological features are shown in Fig. 19.3.

F. buski can be differentiated from *Fasciola hepatica* by its shape and intestinal caecae. *F. buski* has no anterior cone or 'shoulders' and its intestinal caecae have no lateral branches.

— Immature eggs are passed out in the faeces. Each egg contains an unsegmented ovum surrounded by many yolk cells.

For the life cycle to be continued, the eggs must reach fresh water. After a few weeks the eggs hatch miracidia which swim in the water in search of snails of the genus *Segmentina* or *Hippeutis*.

— After penetrating a snail host, the miracidia develop into sporocysts which produce two or more generations of rediae and finally cercariae. Development and reproduction in the snail takes about 2 months.

— The cercariae are shed from the snail and swim in the water until they find suitable water plants on which to encyst e.g. water chestnut or water caltrop. The encysted forms are called metacercariae and these are infective to humans and to the pig and buffalo.

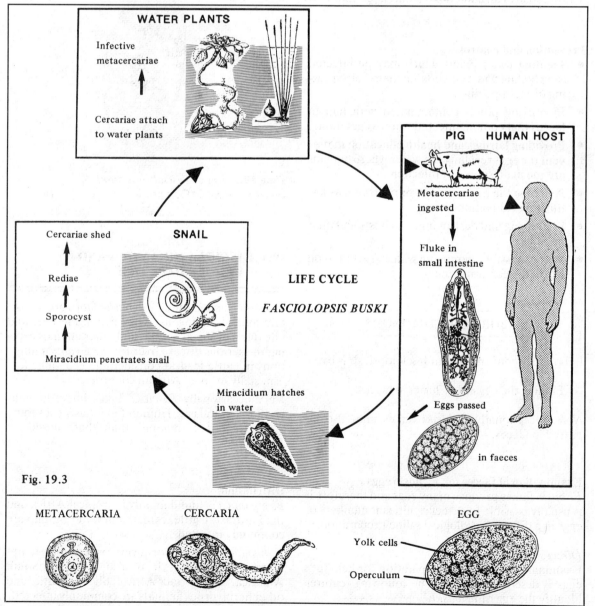

Fig. 19.3

The life cycle of *F. buski* is shown in Fig. 19.3.

Clinical features and pathology

Although infection with *F. buski* is often symptomless, the fluke can cause inflammation and ulceration of the intestinal wall with abdominal pain and diarrhoea. Large numbers of flukes can cause haemorrhage. Symptoms of malabsorption may develop with pale coloured and offensive faeces. In children, heavy infections may cause symptoms resembling protein calorie malnutrition with wasting.

Toxins produced by the flukes can cause oedema of the face and limbs, ascites and other allergic reactions. Plasma albumin levels may fall due to protein loss. There is usually a blood eosinophilia.

The life span of an adult fluke is only a few months.

Prevention and control

- Treating water plants which may be infected, using boiling water or cooking them before eating or teeth-peeling.
- Identifying ponds contaminated with human faeces that contain infected water vegetation.
- Providing latrines and health education to prevent the eggs reaching the water, where humans are the main source of infection.
- Avoiding the use of human or pig faeces as fertilizer in cultivation ponds.
- Identifying and destroying snail hosts and their habitats.
- Where possible, removing water vegetation on which the cercariae encyst.

LABORATORY DIAGNOSIS

Laboratory confirmation of fasciolopsiasis is by:

□ Finding the eggs of *F. buski* in faeces.

Note: Occasionally *F. buski* flukes may also be passed in faeces.

Examination of faeces for *F. buski* eggs

F. buski flukes produce many eggs and therefore it is usually possible to detect significant numbers of eggs in a direct physiological saline preparation.

Direct saline preparation

Examination of a saline preparation for helminth eggs is described in 13:2. The following features identify the egg of *F. buski*:

Egg of *Fasciolopsis buski*

- It is pale yellow-brown, large and oval, measuring about 140×85 µm.
- Contains an unsegmented ovum surrounded by many yolk cells.
- Has a small operculum which is usually difficult to see.

Illustrations: See Plate 19.2 and colour Plate 22.

Note: Morphologically the eggs of *F. buski* resemble those of *Fasciola hepatica*.

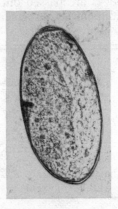

Plate 19.2 Egg of *Fasciolopsis buski*.
Courtesy of K. L. Frampton.

19:4 *FASCIOLA GIGANTICA* AND *FASCIOLA HEPATICA*

Fasciola gigantica and *Fasciola hepatica* are important animal pathogens. They live in the liver and bile ducts of sheep, cattle, and other animals causing the serious disease liver rot. *F. gigantica* infections in cattle lead to considerable economic loss especially in some African countries.

Very occasionally *Fasciola* flukes infect humans causing fascioliasis. Human fascioliasis caused by *F. hepatica* is commoner than that caused by *F. gigantica*.

Distribution

F. gigantica is found mainly in tropical Africa and the Far East. Cattle, camels and water buffalo are commonly infected.

F. hepatica is found worldwide, especially in temperate countries but it is also found in South America, Cuba, and Africa. Sheep, cattle and other herbivorous animals are commonly infected.

Transmission and life cycle

Fascioliasis is caused by eating wild watercress or other water vegetation on which metacercariae have encysted.

Life cycle

— Following ingestion, the metacercariae excyst in the duodenum and the young flukes migrate through the intestinal wall into the peritoneal cavity. They reach the bile ducts of the liver by penetrating through the liver capsule.

Mature Fasciola flukes: They are grey-brown and large. *F. gigantica* measures 25-75 × 12 mm. *F. hepatica* is smaller and more triangular in shape, measuring up to 30 × 12 mm. Both species have a characteristic cone-shaped anterior and branched intestinal caecae (unlike *F. buski*).

— About 3-4 months after infection, eggs are excreted in the faeces. To develop they must reach fresh water. After 9-15 days in water, the eggs hatch miracidia which enter snails of the genus *Lymnaea*. The species of snails infected by *F. gigantica* are aquatic whereas those infected by *F. hepatica* are amphibious.

— In the snail, the miracidia develop into sporocysts which produce generations of rediae and finally cercariae.

— After leaving the snail the cercariae encyst on water vegetation and grass.

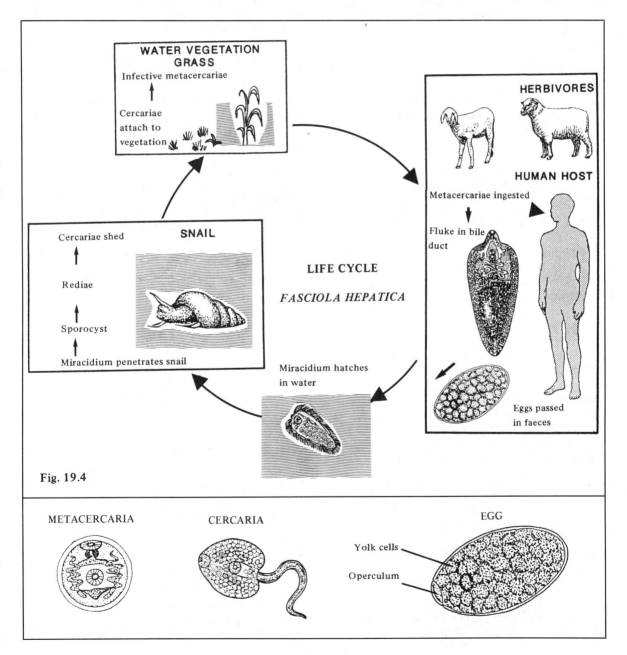

Fig. 19.4

Clinical features and pathology

Although light infections are usually asymptomatic, large numbers of flukes can cause serious liver damage especially during the migratory stage. With chronic infection there is thickening of the bile ducts due to a cellular immune response by the host. Very occasionally the flukes develop in other parts of the body.

Infection is usually accompanied by fever, pain, a marked blood eosinophilia, and urticaria. The liver becomes enlarged and blockage of the bile ducts can occur leading to obstructive jaundice.

Prevention and control

- Avoiding eating watercress or other uncooked water plants which may contain infective metacercariae.

- Reduce the infection rate in animals by fencing off grazing land known to be infected with metacercariae.

- Treating animals to reduce egg output.

- Identifying and destroying snail habitats where this is feasible.

LABORATORY DIAGNOSIS

Laboratory confirmation of fascioliasis is by:

☐ Finding the eggs of the parasite in faeces or aspirates of duodenal fluid.

☐ Testing serum for antibodies.

Examination of faeces for *Fasciola* eggs

In early and chronic infections, the eggs are usually difficult to find and therefore a concentration technique should be used if the eggs are not found in a direct saline preparation.

Direct saline preparation
Examination of a physiological saline preparation of faeces for helminth eggs is described in 13:2.

Egg of *Fasciola gigantica* and *Fasciola hepatica*

The egg of *Fasciola* species closely resembles the egg of *Fasciolopsis buski* except for the operculum which is less distinct. The egg of *F. gigantica* is larger than that of *F. hepatica*.

Illustration: The egg of *Fasciola* species is shown in colour Plate 22.

Note: If eggs are found in human faeces it must be confirmed that they are present due to a true *Fasciola* infection and not from eating animal liver containing *Fasciola* eggs. Repeated finding of the eggs in faeces establishes parasitic infection.

Concentration technique
Fasciola eggs can be concentrated by the formol ether concentration technique described in 13:4. Floatation techniques are unsuitable.

Examination of duodenal fluid

Aspirates of duodenal fluid can be examined for *Fasciola* eggs in the same way as described for *O. sinensis* in 19:2.

Serological diagnosis of fascioliasis

Reagents for the serological diagnosis of fascioliasis by immunoelectrophoresis (IEP) are commercially available from bioMérieux (for address, see Appendix II). Precipitating arcs can be seen from about the third week of infection. The sensitivity and specificity of IEP and other techniques used in the diagnosis of fascioliasis and follow-up testing of patients are discussed by Kagan in his 1980 review of immunological investigations of tropical diseases.[3]

Fasciola hepatica antigen
bioMérieux lyophilized antigen suitable for immunoelectrophoresis (IEP), is supplied in 2 × 20 mg vials which cost approx. £18 (1986). Each vial is reconstituted with 0.1 ml of distilled water. The reconstituted antigen is stable for 1 week at 2-8 °C and several months at −20 °C (divided in small amounts). Each test well is filled with 10 μl of antigen. Serum samples require concentration with *Lyphogel* before being tested. Further details can be obtained from bioMérieux.

Note: Details of a species specific indirect fluorescent antibody (IFA) test for diagnosing fascioliasis can be obtained from the Head of Laboratory, Hospital for Tropical Diseases, 4 St Pancras Way, London, NW1 0PE, UK.

19:5 *PARAGONIMUS* SPECIES

Paragonimus westermani is referred to as the Oriental lung fluke. It is the most well known species of lung fluke that infects humans but other species also cause paragonimiasis.[4, 5, 6, 7]

Distribution

P. westermani and its subspecies are widely distributed in the Far East, parts of Southeast Asia, Indonesia and some Pacific Islands.

Other less widely distributed species in the Far East include *P. miyazakii*, *P. pulmonalis*, *P. tuanshanensis*, *P.*

heterotremus, P. ohirai, P. iloktsuenensis, P. szech-uanensis and *P. heterotremus* is thought to be the main cause of human paragonimiasis in Thailand.

Paragonimus species are also found in Nepal. *P. compactus* and possibly other species are found in India.

In West Africa and Zaire, paragonimiasis is caused by *P. uterobilateralis* and *P. africanus.*

In South America (Peru and Ecuador) and Central America, *P. peruvianus* and possibly other species infect humans.

Transmission and life cycle

Infection is by ingesting the flesh or juice of raw, insufficiently cooked, or pickled crab or crayfish which contains *Paragonimus* metacercariae. In China, shrimps have also been found to be infected.

Infection can also occur by ingesting metacercariae from fingers contaminated during food preparation or less commonly by ingesting young flukes in undercooked meat from animals that have eaten infected crabs or crayfish.

In some areas, pigs are important carrier (paratenic) hosts of *P. westermani.*

Life cycle
— Following ingestion, the metacercariae excyst and the young flukes penetrate the intestinal wall. They migrate across the abdominal cavity, penetrate through the diaphragm into the thoracic cavity and into the lungs and bronchi. They reach the bronchioles where they become egg-producing flukes.

Occasionally the young flukes migrate to the liver, spleen, and other organs.

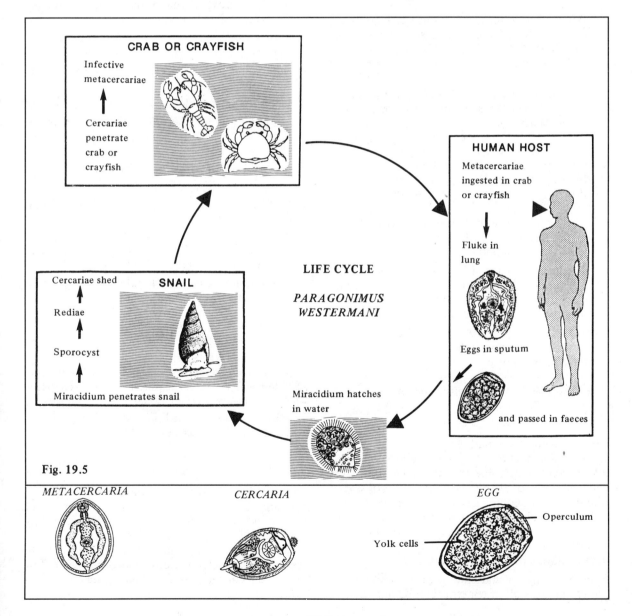

Fig. 19.5

— Following a host tissue response, the flukes becomes encapsulated in cysts.

Mature Paragonimus flukes: They are reddish-brown, small and oval, measuring about 12 × 6 mm by 5 mm thick (size varies according to species). They are covered with short spines.

Adults of *Paragonimus* species are identified by differences in the arrangement of spines on the surface of the body, differences in form of the ovary, and other features.

— About 3 months after infection, eggs containing an unsegmented ovum are produced. These pass into the sputum or are excreted in the faeces after being swallowed in sputum.

For the life cycle to be continued the eggs must reach water.

— After a few weeks, miracidia hatch from the eggs and swim in the water in search of suitable snail hosts. Snails of the genera *Semisulcospira* and *Thiara* serve as first intermediate hosts of *P. westermani*.

Snail hosts of other *Paragonimus* flukes include species of the genera *Brotia*, *Assiminea*, *Oncomelania*, *Tricula*, and *Potadoma*.

— After entering the snail, the miracidia develop into sporocysts which produce rediae and finally cercariae. Development and reproduction in the snail takes about 8 weeks.

— The cercariae are shed from the snail and swim in the water in search of crabs or crayfish in which to encyst and become metacercariae.

The metacercariae of *Paragonimus* species that infect humans are also infective to crustacean-eating animals. In some areas animal reservoir hosts are important in transmission.

The life-span of a *Paragonimus* fluke is usually 6-7 years but human infections of up to 20 years have been reported.

The life cycle of *Paragonimus* is shown in Fig. 19.5.

Clinical features and pathology
Light to moderate *Paragonimus* infections are usually asymptomatic. Heavy infections, however, can cause pulmonary disease. Symptoms of severe pulmonary paragonimiasis often resemble those of pulmonary tuberculosis with chest pain, cough, night sweats and haemoptysis (coughing up blood). In both conditions the erythrocyte sedimentation rate (ESR) is raised.

Sputum from patients with pulmonary paragonimiasis often contains blood, mucus, and rusty-brown particles in which masses of eggs can be found.

Occasionally *Paragonimus* flukes migrate to the liver and intestine causing enlargement of the liver, pain, and diarrhoea. Serious complications can arise when *Paragonimus* flukes migrate, or are carried in the blood circulation, to other parts of the body such as the central nervous system.

The flukes of some *Paragonimus* species, e.g. *P. szechuanensis*, migrate in subcutaneous tissue causing nodules and a marked eosinophilic leucocytosis.

Pulmonary symptoms associated with *P. miyazakii* infections include spontaneous pneumothorax and hydrothorax without haemoptysis.

Preventive and control measures
- Avoiding eating raw, undercooked, or pickled crabs or crayfish which may contain infective metacercariae.
- Not contaminating water with sputum or faeces.
- Detecting and treating infected persons in endemic areas.
- Identifying and destroying the snail hosts of local *Paragonimus* species where this is possible.

LABORATORY DIAGNOSIS

Laboratory confirmation of pulmonary paragonimiasis is by:

☐ Finding *Paragonimus* eggs in sputum or occasionally in aspirates of pleural fluid.

☐ Examining faeces for *Paragonimus* eggs that have been swallowed in sputum.

Other findings
With heavy infections there is a raised ESR and moderate blood eosinophilia.

Infections caused by *P. szechuanensis* and other *Paragonimus* species that migrate in subcutaneous tissue cannot be diagnosed by finding eggs in sputum or faeces.

In *Paragonimus* pericarditis many eosinophils can be found in aspirates of pleural fluid.

Examination of sputum for *Paragonimus* eggs
Sputum from patients with pulmonary paragonimiasis, often contains blood and stringy particles of rusty-brown gelatinous material in which masses of eggs can be found. Sputum from less heavily infected patients may contain very few eggs and a concentration technique may be necessary.

Examine the specimen as follows:

1. Report the appearance of the sputum, i.e. whether watery, mucoid, mucopurulent, or red and jelly-like, and whether it contains blood and rusty-brown particles.

2. If rusty-brown gelatinous particles are present, transfer a sample of this material to a slide and cover with a cover glass. Using a cloth or tissue, gently press on the cover glass to make a thin evenly spread preparation.

   If no rusty-brown particles are present or if no eggs are found when the particles are examined, carry out a concentration technique (preferably using sputum collected over 24 h):

   Concentration technique
   — Add an equal volume of 30 g/l (3% w/v) sodium hydroxide solution (Reagent No. 70) to the sputum, mix, and leave for 10 minutes to allow time for the sodium hydroxide to dissolve the mucus.

   — Mix well and centrifuge in a conical tube at slow to medium speed, i.e. not over 500 g (approx. 2000 rpm) for 5 minutes. Using a plastic bulb pipette, remove and discard the supernatant fluid and transfer a drop of the sediment to a slide. Cover with a cover glass.

3. Examine the unconcentrated sputum or sediment microscopically for eggs using the 10× objective with the condenser iris *closed sufficiently* to give good contrast. Use the 40× objective to identify the eggs.

Note: The eggs of *Paragonimus* species are identified from a knowledge of locally occurring species and by differences in egg size, shape and shell thickness.

FAR EAST

Egg of Paragonimus westermani

- It is yellow-brown or brown and usually asymmetrical in shape being slightly flattened on one side. It measures 70-100 × 50-65 μm.
- There is a flat operculum (lid).
- The thickness of the shell varies. It is thicker at the end opposite the operculum.
- Contains an unsegmented ovum and mass of yolk cells.

Illustrations: See Plate 19.3a and colour Plate 28.

Note: Details and illustrations of the eggs of other *Paragonimus* species that occur in the Far East can be found in the SEAMIC *Color Atlas of Helminth Eggs*.[2]

WEST AFRICA

Egg of Paragonimus uterobilateralis (Nigeria, Liberia, Guinea)

Similar to the egg of *P. westermani* but smaller, measuring 50-98 × 35-52 μm.[5] It is shown in Plate 19.3b.

Egg of Paragonimus africanus (Cameroon, Zaire)

This egg is larger than that of *P. uterobilateralis*, measuring 72-124 × 42-59 μm.[4] It is similar to *P. westermani* but thinner and is shown in Plate 19.3c.

SOUTH AND CENTRAL AMERICA

Egg of Paragonimus peruvianus

Similar to that of *P. westermani* except that it has a thin irregularly undulating shell. It measures 73-92 × 47-53 μm.[2]

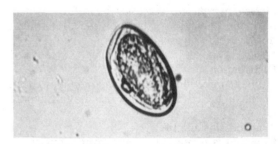

Plate 19.3a Egg of *Paragonimus westermani*.
Courtesy of V. Zaman.

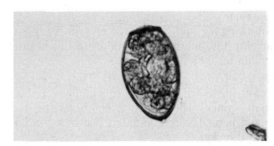

Plate 19.3b Egg of *Paragonimus uterobilateralis*.
Courtesy of J. Voelker.

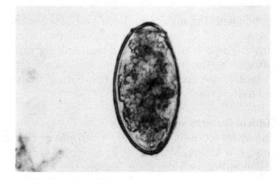

Plate 19.3c Egg of *Paragonimus africanus*.
Courtesy of J. Voelker.

Examination of pleural fluid for *Paragonimus* eggs

Aspirates of pleural fluid can be examined in the same way as described for sputum, except that there is no need to treat the fluid with sodium hydroxide before centrifuging.

Examination of faeces for *Paragonimus* eggs

A concentration technique should be used because only a few *Paragonimus* eggs are likely to be present in faeces. The formol ether concentration technique described in 13:4 is recommended. Floatation techniques are not suitable.

19:6 FLUKES OF LESSER MEDICAL IMPORTANCE

HETEROPHYES HETEROPHYES

Heterophyes heterophyes is a small fluke which is normally parasitic in the intestine of rats, cats, dogs, foxes, wolves and jackals.

Distribution

Human infection with *H. heterophyes* occurs mainly in the Far East and Nile delta in Egypt.

Transmission and life cycle

Infection is by eating raw or insufficient cooked fish which contains the metacercariae of *H. heterophyes*.

Life cycle

Following ingestion, the metacercariae excyst and develop into mature egg-producing flukes in the small intestine.

Mature H. heterophyes flukes: They are small, measuring less than 2 × 0.4 mm and covered with small spines. They have a characteristic large spined genital sucker situated just below a large ventral sucker.

Eggs contain a fully developed miracidium when passed in the faeces. In water, the eggs are ingested by snails of the genera *Pirenella* or *Cerithidia*.

In the snail, the miracidia hatch and develop into sporocysts which produce rediae and finally cercariae. The cercariae leave the snail and encyst on fish such as the mullet or minnow. The encysted metacercariae are infective to fish-eating animals and to humans.

Clinical features and pathology

Unless infection is heavy, *H. heterophyes* flukes cause few serious symptoms apart from intestinal inflammation and necrosis. Rarely the eggs may reach the heart and central nervous system where they can produce serious symptoms.

Prevention and control

H. heterophyes infection is prevented by not eating insufficiently cooked or pickled fish which may contain the metacercarial forms of the parasite.

LABORATORY DIAGNOSIS

Laboratory confirmation of infection with *H. heterophyes* is by finding the small eggs in faeces.

Egg of *Heterophyes heterophyes*

It resembles the egg of *Opisthorchis* and is very similar to the egg of *Metagonimus yokogawai*.

It differs from an *Opisthorchis* egg in being more oval with a less distinct operculum, lacking 'shoulders', and in being without an outer indistinct coat (see 19:2).

Illustrations: See Plate 19.4 and colour Plate 23.

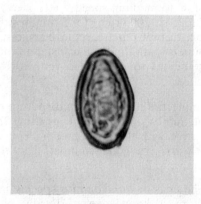

Plate 19.4 Egg of *Heterophyes heterophyes*.
Courtesy of K. L. Frampton.

METAGONIMUS YOKOGAWAI

Metagonimus yokogawai is the smallest fluke which parasitizes humans. It lives in the small intestine. Reservoir hosts include dogs, cats, pigs, and pelicans.

Distribution

M. yokogawai is found in the Far East and in the Mediterranean basin.

Transmission and life cycle

The transmission and life cycle of *M. yokogawai* are similar to that of *H. heterophyes*. Snail hosts of *M. yokogawai* belong to the genera *Semisulcospira* and *Thiara* and second intermediate hosts are cyprinid fish and sweetfish.

Mature M. yokogawai flukes: Unlike *H. heterophyes* flukes they have no genital sucker. The ventral sucker lies to one side of the body. The small fluke measures 1 × 0.5 mm and is covered with spines.

Clinical features and pathology

Most infections with *M. yokogawai* are asymptomatic. Heavy infections can cause inflammation of the intestinal wall with abdominal pain and watery diarrhoea.

Prevention and control

M. yokogawai infection is prevented by not eating insufficiently cooked or pickled fish which may contain the metacercarial forms of the parasite.

LABORATORY DIAGNOSIS

Laboratory confirmation of infection with *M. yokogawai* is by finding the small eggs in faeces. A concentration technique, such as the formol ether method may be necessary to detect the eggs (see 13:4).

Egg of *Metagonimus yokogawai*

It resembles the egg of *Opisthorchis* and is very similar to the egg of *H. heterophyes*.

It differs from an *Opisthorchis* egg in being more oval with a less distinct operculum, lacking shoulders, and in being without an outer indistinct coat (see 19:2).

Illustrations: See Plate 19.5 and colour Plate 23.

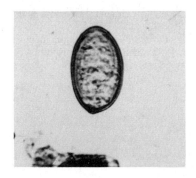

Plate 19.5 Egg of *Metagonimus yokogawai*.
Courtesy of W. Peters.

DICROCOELIUM DENDRITICUM

Dicrocoelium dendriticum is a small fluke which is normally parasitic in the biliary tract of sheep and cattle. It is found in China, North Africa, South America, and Europe.

Human infection is rare. Spurious infection (resulting from the ingesting of infected beef or sheep liver) is occasionally reported. A person becomes infected with a *Dicrocoelium* fluke by accidentally swallowing ants which contain metacercariae.

Following ingestion, the metacercariae develop into mature egg-producing flukes in the bile ducts and liver. Symptoms of infection are rarely serious.

Mature D. dendriticum flukes: They measure 5-15 mm long and are tapered at both ends.

LABORATORY DIAGNOSIS

Eggs of *D. dendriticum* can be found in faeces or in aspirates of duodenal fluid.

Egg of *Dicrocoelium dendriticum*

It is brown and resembles the eggs of *Heterophyes* and *Opisthorchis* species except that it is larger and asymmetrical, measuring about 42 × 25 μm.

Illustration: See Plate 19.6 and colour Plate 23.

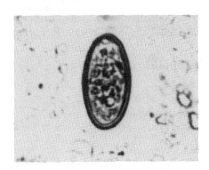

Plate 19.6 Egg of *Dicrocoelium dendriticum*.
Courtesy of A. Moody.

GASTRODISCOIDES HOMINIS

Gastrodiscoides hominis is an amphistome trematode (ventral sucker is situated at the posterior end of the fluke). The parasite is normally parasitic in the intestine of pig.

Distribution

Human infection with *G. hominis* is found mainly in India (Ganges river basin) and also in parts of Bangladesh, Vietnam, and the Philippines. High (up to 41%) infection rates have been reported from Assam.

Transmission and life cycle

Exact details of the transmission and life cycle of *G. hominis* are not known. It is thought to develop and reproduce in snails and encyst on water vegetation. Infection is probably by eating water plants or their fruits on which metacercariae have encysted.

Mature G. hominis flukes: They have a characteristic shape with the anterior end being cone-shaped and the lower half containing a large concavity. The ventral sucker is situated in the concavity. The flukes measure 5-10 mm long and 4-6 mm across the lower half.

The flukes live in the large intestine and eggs are passed in the faeces.

Clinical features and pathology

Large numbers of flukes can cause inflammation of the wall of the large intestine with mucous diarrhoea. Light infections are usually asymptomatic.

LABORATORY DIAGNOSIS

Laboratory confirmation of infection with *G. hominis* is by finding the eggs in faeces.

Egg of *Gastrodiscoides hominis*

- It is spindle shaped and large measuring about 150 × 60 μm.
- Has a small operculum.
- Contains an immature ovum and yolk cells.

Illustration: See Plate 19.7.

References

1   Feldmeier, H. and Horstmann, R. D. Filtration of duodenal fluid for the diagnosis of opisthorchiasis. *Annals of Tropical Medicine and Parasitology*, **75** (4), pp 463-465, 1981.

2   Suzuki, N. *Color Atlas of Helminth Eggs*. SEAMIC Publication No. 2, 1975. Available from SEAMIC, No. 6 Tokyo Kaiji Bldg., 7-2 Shimbashi 4-chome, Minato-ku, Tokyo, Japan.

3   Kagan, I. G. In: *Immunological Investigations of Tropical Diseases*, Ch 10, pp 148-156, 1980. Churchill Livingstone.

4   Yokoogawa, M. Newly introduced questions concerning *Paragonimus westermani*. *Journal of Formosan Medical Association*, **81**, pp 774-780, 1982.

5   Kum, P. N. and Nchinda, T. C. Pulmonary paragonimiasis in Cameroon. *Transactions of the Royal Society of Tropical Medicine and Hygiene*, **76**, pp 768-772, 1982.

6   Sachs, R. and Voelker, J. Human paragonimiasis caused by *Paragonimus uterobilateralis* in Liberia and Guinea, West Africa. *Tropenmedizin Parasitologie*, **33**, pp 15-16, 1982.

7   Zhong, H. L., He, L. Y., Xu, Z. B., and Cao, W. J. Recent progress in studies of paragonimus and paragonimiasis control in China. *Chinese Medical Journal*, **94**, pp 483-494, 1981.

Recommended Reading

Bell, D. R. *Lecture Notes on Tropical Medicine*. Blackwell Scientific Publications, 2nd edition 1985. Paperback priced £9.80.

Peters, W., Gilles, H. M. *A Colour Atlas of Tropical Medicine and Parasitology*, Wolfe Medical Publications, 2nd Ed, 1981. ELBS edition priced £9.00.

World Health Organization. *Intestinal Protozoan and Helminth Infections*. WHO, Technical Report Series, No. 666, 1981.

Knight, R. *Parasitic Disease in Man*, Churchill Livingstone, 1982. ELBS edition priced £4.50.

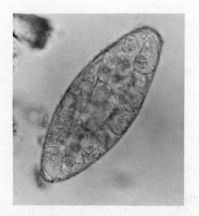

Plate 19.7 Egg of *Gastrodiscoides hominis*.
Courtesy of K. L. Frampton.

20 Schistosomes

20:1 CLASSIFICATION AND FEATURES OF SCHISTOSOMES

Schistosomes are trematodes (flukes) that live in the blood. The general characteristics of trematodes are described at the beginning of the Parasitology Section in Chapter 12:4.

Classification of schistosomes of medical importance

Superfamily	SCHISTOSOMATOIDEA
Widespread species	*Schistosoma haematobium*
	Schistosoma mansoni
	Schistosoma japonicum
Less widespread species	*Schistosoma intercalatum*
	Schistosoma mekongi

Animal schistosomes which occasionally infect humans

Schistosoma mattheei
Schistosoma bovis
Schistosoma rodhaini
Schistosoma margrebowiei

Features of human schistosomes

- They develop in the portal venous system and the adult flukes (depending on species) live in the veins of the intestine or bladder.

- Sexes are separate.

- Unlike most trematodes, schistosomes are not flattened and leaflike. They are long (up to 20 mm in length), worm-like and well adapted to life in the blood vessels of their hosts (see Plate 20.1).

  Most of the body of the male is folded inwards to form a groove (gynaecophoric canal) in which the female lives. The flukes have suckers which they use to attach themselves to the wall of blood vessels. They obtain food and oxygen from the blood in which they live.

- Humans are the only or most significant definitive hosts of *S. haematobium*, *S. mansoni* and *S. intercalatum*. *S. japonicum* parasitizes many animals as well as humans and dogs are important in the transmission of *S. mekongi*.

  Species of freshwater snails are required to complete the life cycle. No secondary intermediate host is required. Reproduction occurs in the sporocyst stage in the snail.

Unlike most other trematodes, there is no redia stage and there is no encysted metacercarial stage.

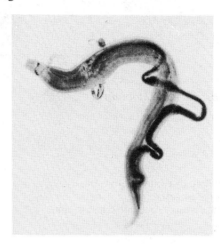

Plate 20.1 Male and female flukes of *Schistosoma mansoni*. The female is longer, thinner, darker and lies inside a groove in the body of the male. *Courtesy of Ciba-Geigy.*

- Transmission is by contact with water containing the infective forms of the parasite called cercariae. These develop in the snail and are able to penetrate unbroken skin. A schistosome cercaria has a forked tail and is shown in Plate 20.2.

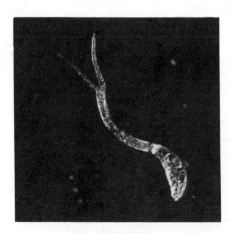

Plate 20.2 Cercaria of *Schistosoma* species, showing forked tail. *Courtesy of V. Zaman.*

• Laboratory diagnosis of schistosome infections is by finding eggs (depending on species) in urine, faeces, or occasionally in rectal scrapings. A schistosome egg is without an operculum but it has a spine, the position and form of which are used in species identification.

Note: The morphology of the schistosomes of major medical importance is shown in the life cycle figures contained in the subsequent subunits of this Chapter.

Schistosomes of Major Medical Importance

LIFE CYCLE SUMMARIES

Schistosoma haematobium

Schistosoma mansoni
Schistosoma japonica
Schistosoma mekongi
Schistosoma intercalatum

Transmitted by contact with water containing cercariae. After penetrating skin, the cercariae become schistosomules

Transmitted by contact with water containing cercariae. After penetrating skin, the cercariae become schistosomules

In blood, schistosomules pass through the heart and lungs

In blood, schistosomules pass through the heart and lungs

Adult flukes in portal veins

Adult flukes in portal veins

Migrate to veins of bladder Eggs are laid

Migrate to veins of intestine Eggs are laid

EGGS IN URINE

EGGS IN FAECES

Miracidia hatch in fresh water and infect snails

Miracidia hatch in fresh water and infect snails

Miracidia become sporocysts, multiply, and become infective cercariae which are shed from snail and swim in water

Miracidia become sporocysts, multiply, and become infective cercariae which are shed from snail and swim in water

Note: S. japonicum cercariae swim for only a short time in the water after which they become attached to vegetation or other objects in the water.

20:2 *SCHISTOSOMA HAEMATOBIUM*

Schistosoma haematobium causes urinary schistosomiasis. The species contains several strains.

Note: The term bilharziasis is also used to describe human schistosomiasis.

It is estimated that at least 180 million persons are at risk of infection with *S. haematobium* and that about 90 million persons are infected.[1,2]

Distribution

S. haematobium is endemic in 52 African and eastern Mediterranean countries. It is found in much of tropical and subtropical Africa and also occurs in Iran, Iraq, Saudi Arabia, Yemen, Syria, in Maharashtra State in India and in several Indian Ocean islands including Malagasy Republic, Mauritius, Pemba, Zanzibar, and some smaller islands off the East African coast.

The development of irrigation channels and dams for hydroelectric power and flood control have altered the distribution and greatly increased the prevalence of *S. haematobium* infections in several countries, e.g. Aswan Lower Dam in the United Arab Republic (Egypt), Akosombo Dam in Ghana, and the Sennar Dam in Sudan.

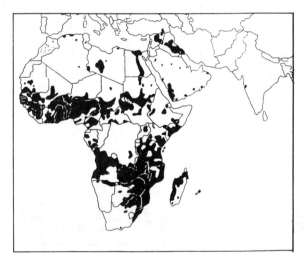

Fig. 20.1 Distribution of *Schistosoma haematobium*. *Reproduced from WHO Technical Report series No. 728, 1985.*

Transmission and life cycle

Urinary schistosomiasis is caused by persons passing urine containing *S. haematobium* eggs into water which is used by others for bathing, washing clothes, agricultural purposes, fishing, or recreation. The parasite is not infective or able to multiply immediately after it is passed in the water. It requires an aquatic snail in which to reproduce and develop to its infective free-swimming cercarial stage.

The snail hosts of *S. haematobium* belong to the genus *Bulinus*. The snails are found among vegetation in stagnant or slow moving fresh water irrigation channels, large natural and man-made lakes, and smaller collections of water.

In most endemic areas a high proportion of children and teenagers become infected.

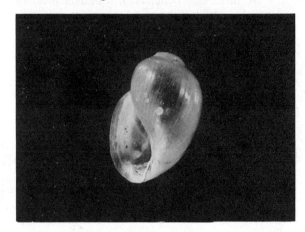

Plate 20.3 Shell of a *Bulinus* snail. *Courtesy of K. L. Frampton.*

Life cycle

— A person becomes infected by contact with water containing infective cercariae. The cercariae become attached to the skin and are able to penetrate unbroken skin.

  Note: If ingested, cercariae can penetrate mucous membranes.

— During penetration, the cercariae shed their tails and develop into schistosomules which migrate through subcutaneous tissue into blood vessels.

  In the blood the young flukes are carried through the right side of the heart to the lungs. From the lungs most of the schistosomules pass through the left side of the heart, enter the abdominal aorta, and from there reach the portal (liver) circulation.

— In the blood vessels of the liver, the young flukes reach maturity.

  Mature S. haematobium flukes: The body surface of the male is covered with small tubercles (rounded knobs). The male fluke is short and cylindrical, measuring 10-15 × 0.8-1.0 mm. There are 4 or 5 testes. The female is longer and thinner, measuring 20-26 × 0.25 mm and appears darker than the male due to the presence of blood pigment in the gut. The ovary is situated posteriorly and the long uterus contains 10-100 eggs at a time.

— Following mating, the paired flukes migrate to the veins surrounding the bladder (vesical plexus). Occasionally, mature flukes can be found in the veins of the rectum and portal system.

— The female lays eggs in the venules (small veins) of the bladder. The estimated egg output of *S. haematobium* is 20-200 eggs per day. Many of the eggs penetrate through the mucosa into the lumen of the bladder and are passed in the urine. Eggs can be found in the urine from about 6-8 weeks after infection. Each egg contains a fully developed miracidium.

About 20% of eggs remain in the wall of the bladder and become calcified. *S. haematobium* eggs can be found also in the ureters, rectal mucosa and reproductive organs, especially in heavy infections.

— In fresh water and in the presence of light and a warm temperature, the miracidia hatch rapidly. They are ciliated and swim in the water in search of a suitable species of *Bulinus* snail. Penetration of the snail host must occur within 32 hours of the miracidia hatching. After this time the miracidia die.

Bulinus snails: They are ovoid with a short spire and measure 9-18 mm in length, depending on species (see Plate 20.3). They are aquatic and hermaphroditic (male and female).

S. haematobium in Africa south of the Saraha is transmitted by snails of the *Bulinus africanus* group, in the Mediterranean area and South-West Asia by the *B. tropicus/truncatus* complex and in Arabia and Mauritius by the *B. forskali* group.

In India the snail host of *S. haematobium* is *Ferrissia tenuis*.

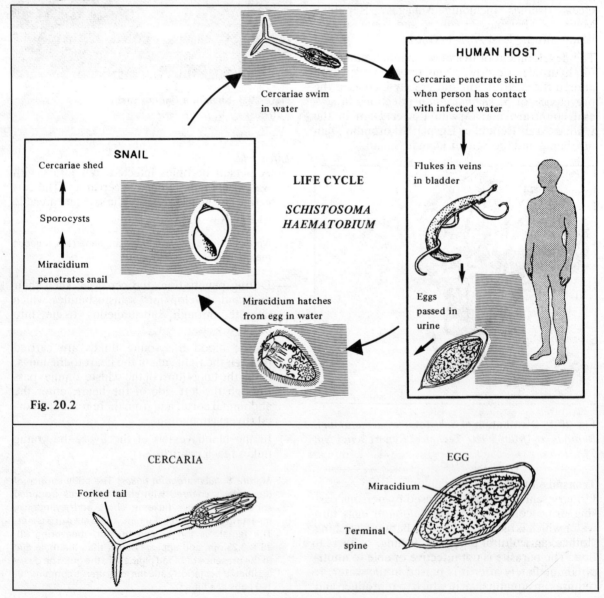

Fig. 20.2

— In the snail, the miracidia develop into sporocysts which reproduce to give further sporocysts and finally cercariae. Development in the snail takes two to several weeks depending on species and particularly on temperature. A single snail sheds many hundred cercariae. They are shed during daylight hours with sunlight encouraging shedding.

— The cercariae leave the snail and are able to survive and swim in the water for up to about 48 h. For the life cycle to be continued, the cercariae must enter a human host.

Schistosome cercariae:They measure 200-400 μm in length (just visible to the naked eye) and have a forked tail (see Plate 20.2).

Note: The life cycle of *S. haematobium* is shown in Fig. 20.2.

Clinical features and pathology

Within 24 hours of infection an intense irritation and skin rash, referred to as 'swimmer's itch', may occur at the site of cercarial penetration.

Note: A severe dermatitis can be caused by cercariae of bird and other animal schistosomes (not normally parasitic in man) accidentally penetrating human skin.

Within a few days after penetration, the young flukes become coated with host red cell antigens and histocompatibility antigens. In this way the schistosomes are not recognized as being foreign and live free from host attack to develop and produce eggs for long periods. It is the eggs not the adult flukes which are responsible for the clinical features and damage to the bladder and ureters which occurs in *S. haematobium* infections.

Haematuria and proteinuria

Haematuria (blood in urine) caused by eggs penetrating through the wall of the bladder is a characteristic feature of urinary schistosomiasis. Several studies in *S. haematobium* endemic areas have shown that up to 80% of infected children have haematuria and of those infected with more than 50 eggs/10 ml of urine, 98-100% have haematuria. Proteinuria (protein in urine) is also found and in most endemic areas proteinuria and haematuria are related to the intensity of infection, especially in children. Serious urinary disease and complications are related to heavy infection but significant disease can also occur in light infections.

S. haematobium eggs in tissues

Eggs trapped in the wall of the bladder and surrounding tissues cause inflammatory reactions with the formulation of granulomata. The granulomata contain eggs, toxic products, eosinophils, epithelioid cells, and lymphocytes.

The urine often contains eosinophils derived from the inflammatory reactions around eggs in the bladder wall. There is also a blood eosinophilia.

Many of the eggs die and become calcified eventually producing what are known as 'sandy patches' in the bladder. In heavy infections, eggs can be carried to other parts of the body. Following prolonged untreated infection and a marked cellular immune response, the ureters may become obstructed and the bladder wall thickened, leading to abnormal bladder function with painful and frequent urination, urinary infection, and eventually kidney damage. Severe and chronic urinary schistosomiasis is associated with squamous cell bladder cancer.[3]

In some areas, *S. haematobium* infection has been linked to an increase in *Salmonella typhi* and *Salmonella paratyphi* carriers following acute infection with these salmonellae.

In Egypt, up to 25% of persons with chronic urinary schistosomiasis are reported as having calculi (stones) in the bladder and urinary tract. A further complication associated with urinary schistosomiasis is the nephrotic syndrome.

Prevention and control

In the prevention and control of urinary schistosomiasis a combination of some or all of the following methods is nearly always necessary:

- Avoiding contact with water known to contain cercariae by:
  — Providing safe water supplies in villages to reduce as much as possible contact with infested water.
  — Constructing footbridges across infested rivers and streams.
  — Providing safe recreational bathing sites, especially for children.

- Preventing water becoming contaminated with eggs by:
  — Health education and providing sanitation facilities.
  — Treating infected persons.

- Minimising the risk of infection from new water conservation and irrigation schemes and hydroelectric developments by:
  — Not employing infected workers.
  — Siting settlements away from canals, drains, and irrigation channels and providing latrines and sufficient safe water for domestic use.
  — Lining canals with cement and keeping them free from silt and vegetation in which snails can breed.

— Varying the water levels in the system.

— Using molluscicides (chemicals to kill snails) at regular intervals.

- Destroying snail intermediate hosts by:

— Using molluscicides without harming important animal and plant life. Molluscicides, however, are becoming increasingly expensive. They are most cost-effective when treating small bodies of water and when transmission is seasonal and the affected area is limited. Careful selection of a molluscicide is essential. Niclosamide (e.g. *Bayluscide*, *Mollutox*) is the most frequently used chemical.

— Introducing fish or other predators which will feed on the snails, or introducing other species of snails which will compete with the unwanted snails in a given habitat. So far this method of control has not been shown to be very effective.

— Removing vegetation from locally used water places, draining swamps, flooding, and other measures to eradicate snail habitats. Some snails, however, can resist drying or become preserved in mud between rainy seasons.

- Treating water supplies by:

— Using a chlorine disinfectant.

— Storing water for 48 hours after which time any cercariae in the water will be dead.

— Positioning horizontal sand or other filter systems at water inputs to prevent cercariae entering.

Filtering systems
Low cost, effective, simple to operate and maintain filtration systems suitable for use in remote areas in developing countries are available from SWS Filtration Ltd (for address, see Appendix II).

Note: Further information about the control of schistosomiasis can be found in the 1985 World Health Organization report *The Control of Schistosomiasis*, Technical Report Series No. 728, available from WHO, 1211 Geneva 27 Switzerland.

The findings of a 1982 *Symposium on Schistosomiasis Control* in Brazil, Egypt and the People's Republic of China have also been published.[4]

LABORATORY DIAGNOSIS

Laboratory confirmation of *S. haematobium* infection is by:

□ Finding the eggs or occasionally the hatched miracidia of *S. haematobium* in urine. Miracidia can be found if the urine is dilute or has been left to stand for a few hours before being examined.

Examination of a 24 h urine may sometimes be necessary to detect the eggs when they are few in number.

Occasionally *S. haematobium* eggs can be found in faeces.

□ Detecting eggs in a rectal biopsy or bladder mucosal biopsy when an infection is light or a patient has been partially treated.

Other findings
— Haematuria is a common finding particularly among children (see previous text).

— Proteinuria is frequently present (see previous text).

— Cells, especially eosinophils can often be found in the urine. Eosinophils can be easily differentiated from pus cells by adding a small drop of weak eosin solution (1 in 10 dilution of Field's stain B) to a urine sediment. The granules of eosinophils stain bright red whereas the granules of pus cells remain unstained or stain a pale pink. There is usually also a blood eosinophilia.

— Bacteriuria may accompany urinary schistosomiasis.

Examination of urine for *S. haematobium* eggs
Specimen
Collect at least 10 ml of urine into a clean dry container. Instruct the patient to include in the specimen the last few drops of urine passed. These drops often contain the highest number of eggs. Specimens collected around midday may also contain more eggs than those collected at other times.

In moderate to heavy infections, the urine will usually contain blood and appear red or red-brown and cloudy.

Testing of the urine should take place as soon as possible after collection before the miracidia have time to hatch from the eggs. To avoid hatching, the specimen should be kept in the dark (e.g. inside a box) until it is examined.

24 h urine specimen
In light infections or when it is necessary to make an accurate egg count, collect urine over a 24 h period. The procedure for collecting a 24 h urine is explained in 26:5.

Note the appearance of each sample of urine passed over the 24 hours. If blood is not visibly present, test the sample for protein and traces of blood using reagent strip tests. After testing for protein and blood, add 2 drops (approx 0.1 ml) of 10% v/v formol saline or 1% v/v domestic bleach to each sample (50-100 ml of urine) to preserve the eggs. At the end of the 24 hour period deliver the samples to the laboratory for testing.

Recommended techniques for detecting and counting *S. haematobium* eggs in urine are as follows:

- Filtration quantitative technique
- Sedimentation quantitative technique

Note: A quantitative technique should be used because this will give an indication of the intensity of infection. Quantitative results are also of value in planning the prevention and control of urinary schistosomiasis.

Filtration technique for S. haematobium eggs
This technique is recommended because it has been shown to be the simplest and the most sensitive, rapid, and reproducible for detecting and quantifying *S. haematobium* eggs in urine.[5, 6, 7]

Note: Since publication of the 1st edition of this Manual in 1981, inexpensive filtration kits have become available (see later text).

Required
— 10 ml Luer syringe
— Syringe filter holder (Swinnex type), 13 mm diameter. This is suitable for holding filters of 12 mm or 13 mm diameter.
— Nuclepore polycarbonate membrane filter of 13 mm diameter and 12-14 μm pore size. This is a clear filter which can be disinfected in domestic bleach and reused several times providing it is handled with care using blunt-ended forceps.

If a polycarbonate membrane filter is not available, a *Nytrel* woven filter of 12 mm diameter and 20 μm pore size can be used. When using a *Nytrel* filter the eggs are viewed against the fibres of which the filter is made and therefore they are not seen as distinctly as on a polycarbonate filter but the eggs can be stained with 50% Lugol's iodine. The reuse of *Nytrel* filters is not recommended.[26]

Sources of schistosomiasis urine filtration kits
Low priced kits are available to developing countries from the non-profit organizations PATH and Tropical Health Technology (for addresses, see Appendix II). PATH kits contain filter holders, polycarbonate membranes and blunt-ended forceps. Tropical Health Technology kits contain filter holders, polycarbonate membranes, blunt-ended forceps, reusable autoclavable 10 ml Luer syringes, (see Appendix IV, Schisto urinary filtration kit).

Method
1. Collect a specimen of urine as described previously. Report the appearance of the urine, i.e.

colour, whether clear or cloudy, and whether blood is present.

2. If the urine does not appear to contain blood, test it for protein (see 28:3) and if possible also for red cells (see 28:6).

3. Using blunt-ended (untoothed) forceps, carefully place a polycarbonate or *Nytrel* filter on the filter support of the filter holder. Re-assemble the filter holder and attach it to the end of a 10 ml Luer syringe (see Plate 20.4).

4. Remove the plunger from the syringe.

5. Fill the syringe to the 10 ml mark with well-mixed urine, and replace the plunger. Hold the syringe over a beaker or other suitabler container.

Note: This method of filling the syringe is preferred to drawing up the urine into the syringe because it does not require tubing and the air which passes through the membrane after the urine, helps to stick the eggs to the filter.

6. Pass the urine through the filter as shown in Plate 20.4.

Clogging of filters
If a membrane filter clogs, remove the filter holder and attach it to another syringe containing 3% v/v acetic acid. Pass the acid through the filter. This may help to clear it. If, however, the blockage does not clear, use another membrane to filter the remaining sample of urine. Both filters must be examined to give the number of eggs in the 10 ml of urine.

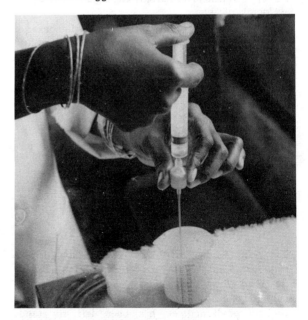

Plate 20.4 Filtering urine for schistosome eggs.
Courtesy of K. E. Mott/World Health Organization.

7. Remove the filter holder and unscrew it. Using blunt-ended forceps, carefully remove the filter and transfer it to a slide. Place the filter face upwards (eggs on surface) on the slide, add a drop of physiological saline, and cover with a cover glass.

8. Using the 10× objective with the condenser iris *closed sufficiently* to give good contrast, examine systematically the entire filter for *S. haematobium* eggs.

Count the number of eggs and report their number per 10 ml of urine.

Note: If more than 50 eggs are present there is no need to continue counting (50 eggs or more/ 10 ml of urine is considered a heavy infection). Report the count as 'More than 50 eggs/10 ml'.

Reuse of filters

Immediately after use, carefully remove the filter and soak it for 4-5 hours or overnight in a disinfectant such as domestic bleach diluted 1 in 5 with water (do not use a disinfectant containing phenol). Recover the filter by straining the disinfectant through a small plastic strainer. Wash the filter by agitating the strainer (with filter inside) in warm water containing detergent followed by several rinses in clean water. After the final wash, dry the *underside* of the strainer. Remove the filter from inside the strainer and transfer it to a slide, add a drop of water, and cover with a cover glass. Check microscopically that the filter is clear of eggs and does not appear damaged. If suitable for reuse, dry the filter and return it to its storage box.

Caution: If using polycarbonate membranes also for filtering microfilariae, soak and wash separately the two different filters and store them in separate boxes labelled clearly, '12 μm filters for schistosome eggs', and '5 μm filters for microfilariae'.

Note: the filter holder and syringe should also be soaked in disinfectant before being washed and reused.

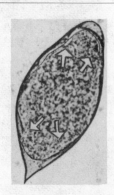
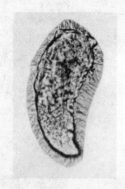

Plate 20.5 Egg of *S. haematobium*. White arrows show the position of the flame cells..
Courtesy of Wellcome Museum of Medical Science.

Plate 20.6 Ciliated, and rapidly motile miracidium hatched from an *S. haematobium* egg, in urine that has been left to stand. *Courtesy of Ciba-Geigy.*

Egg of *Schistosoma haematobium*

- It is pale yellow-brown, large and oval in shape, measuring about 145 × 55 μm.

- Has a characteristic small spine at one end (terminal spine).

- Contains a fully developed miracidium. If the urine is very dilute or has been left to stand the ciliated miracidium may hatch from the egg and be seen swimming in the urine (see Plate 20.6).

- Shell is not acid fast (Ziehl-Neelsen staining). The egg shell of other terminally spined *Schistosoma* species is acid fast.

- A viable egg (in fresh unpreserved urine) shows what is called flame cell movement i.e. flickering of the excretory flame cells (see Plate 20.5).

  A non-viable egg is dark-coloured and shows no structural detail or flame cell movement. It may be surrounded by fibrous cells.

- A calcified egg is usually smaller and appears black and often distorted with a less distinct terminal spine.

Illustrations: See Plate 20.5, Plate 20.6, and colour Plate 14.

Note: *S. haematobium* eggs are sometimes found in faecal specimens. In West and Central Africa they require differentiation from *S. intercalatum* eggs which can also be found in faeces and have a terminal spine (see Plate 20.11 in 20:3).

Occasionally the eggs of *S. mansoni* can be found in urine (see Plate 20.9 in 20:3).

Viable and non-viable schistosome eggs

In assessing the severity of infection or in judging whether treatment has been successful, it is often important to know whether Schistosome eggs are viable or non-viable.

Although it is often possible to see flame cell movement in viable eggs (see previous text), a more reliable way of differentiating viable from non-viable schistosome eggs is to examine a preparation stained with 1% w/v trypan blue in physiological saline.[8] A drop of stain is added and the preparation is left for 30 minutes at room temperature (in a damp chamber to prevent drying out). Non-viable eggs take up the stain and appear blue whereas viable eggs remain unstained and can be seen clearly against the pale blue stained filter.

Alternatively, another simple but less reliable method to test for viability in fresh unpreserved urine, is to add two or three drops of water to the preparation and leave it on a warm and well-lit part of the bench to encourage hatching of the miracidia. After several minutes and gentle pressure on the filter, examine the preparation for hatched miracidia or any movement of the miracidia in the eggs. Movement indicates that the eggs are viable.

Urine sedimentation technique for S. haematobium eggs

The following sedimentation technique is recommended if the equipment to perform a filtration technique is not available. The eggs are sedimented by centrifugation or if a centrifuge is not available by gravity.

Method

1. Collect a specimen of urine, report its appearance, and test for protein and red cells as described previously.

2. Mix the urine well and transfer 10 ml to a conical tube. If the urine contains blood, add two drops of saponin reagent (Reagent No. 63) to lyze the red cells. Centrifuge at slow to medium speed, i.e. not over 500 g (approx. 1500-2000 rpm) for 5 minutes to sediment the eggs. Do not exceed 500 g because this may cause hatching of the miracidia.

   If a centrifuge is not available leave the tube in a cool *dark* place for 1 hour to give time for the eggs to sediment by gravity.

3. Using a Pasteur pipette, remove and discard all the supernatant fluid. Transfer the entire sediment to a slide and cover with a cover glass.

4. Examine the preparation microscopically for *S. haematobium* eggs and count the eggs as described in step 8 of the previous method.

   Report the number of eggs/10 ml of urine.

Examination of a 24 h urine

Collect and preserve the 24 h specimen as described previously.

After measuring the volume, allow the eggs to sediment by leaving the urine in a narrow covered cylinder overnight. Remove and discard all but the last 15 ml (approx.) of specimen and continue as described in steps 2 and 3 of the previous method. Examine the entire sediment and count the number of eggs.

Report the volume of 24 h urine in ml and number of eggs/24 h urine.

Detection of schistosome cercariae in infested water

Details of a field filtration technique (using a 50-90 μm porosity *Nytrel* filter) to locate schistosomiasis transmission sites by recovering cercariae from water, can be found in the paper of Prentice.[11]

Caution: When sampling water which may contain cercariae, great care must be taken, including the wearing of gloves and other protective clothing.

Once collected, the cercariae can be killed and preserved by stirring in 5 ml of concentrated formalin solution to each litre of water. Stirring is required to prevent the cercariae sticking to the sides of the sampling container.

Examination of biopsies for S. haematobium eggs

The laboratory examination of rectal and bladder mucosal biopsies for schistosome eggs is described in 20:3. *S. haematobium* eggs found in biopsies are often non-viable and appear black (calcified).

20:3 SCHISTOSOMA MANSONI AND SCHISTOSOMA INTERCALATUM

SCHISTOSOMA MANSONI

Schistosoma mansoni causes intestinal schistosomiasis. There are several different strains of *S. mansoni*. In 1981 the minimum number of persons infected with *S. mansoni* was estimated to be about 57 million.[12]

Distribution

S. mansoni occurs in 53 countries. It is widespread in many African countries, Madagascar, and parts of the Middle East, South America (especially Brazil) and the West Indies as shown in Fig. 20.3. In several countries, *S. mansoni* occurs with *S. haematobium*.

As with *S. haematobium*, water development projects for water conservation, irrigation, and hydroelectric power have contributed to the spread of *S. mansoni* and changes in its distribution.

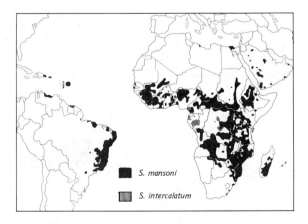

Fig. 20.3 Distribution of *S. mansoni* and *S. intercalatum. *Reproduced from WHO Technical Report Series No. 728, 1985.*

Transmission and life cycle

S. mansoni schistosomiasis is caused by persons passing faeces containing the eggs of the parasite into water which is used for bathing, washing clothes, agricultural purposes, fishing, and recreational purposes.

S. mansoni requires a species of aquatic snail belonging to the genus *Biomphalaria* in which to reproduce and develop to its infective cercarial stage. The snails are found among vegetation in lightly shaded slow to moderate flowing shallow water.

There is some evidence that rodents and possibly baboons may act as reservoir hosts of *S. mansoni* but humans, especially children, are the most important definitive hosts of the parasite.

Life cycle

The life cycle of *S. mansoni* is similar to that described for *S. haematobium* in 20:2 with a few exceptions.

After mating, the mature *S. mansoni* flukes migrate to the small tributary veins of the inferior mesenteric vein which drains the large intestine. Flukes can also be found in the portal venous system.

Mature S. mansoni flukes: The body surface of the male is covered with prominent tubercles. The male fluke is short and cylindrical, measuring 6-13 × 1 mm. There are 2 to 14 testes. The female is longer and thinner, measuring 7-17 × 0.25 mm and darker than the male due to blood pigment in the gut. The ovary is situated anteriorly and the short uterus contains only 1 or 2 eggs at a time.

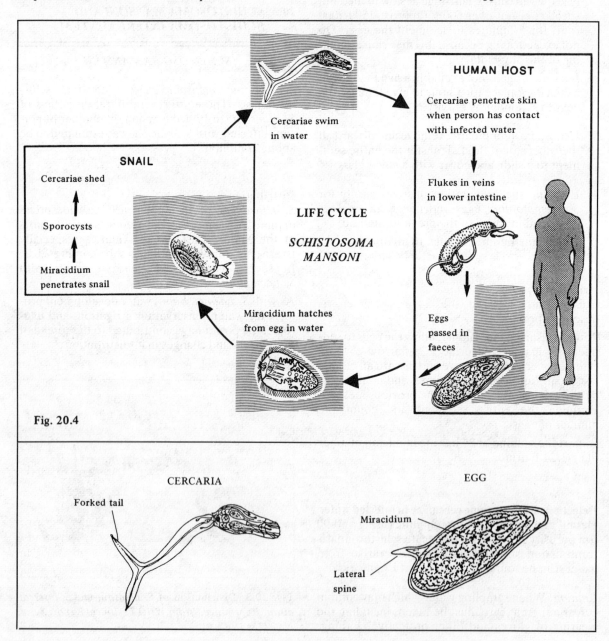

Cercariae swim in water

HUMAN HOST

Cercariae penetrate skin when person has contact with infected water

Flukes in veins in lower intestine

SNAIL

Cercariae shed

Sporocysts

Miracidium penetrates snail

LIFE CYCLE

SCHISTOSOMA MANSONI

Eggs passed in faeces

Miracidium hatches from egg in water

Fig. 20.4

CERCARIA

Forked tail

EGG

Miracidium

Lateral spine

Eggs are laid in the venules (small veins) and penetrate through to the lumen of the bowel to be excreted in the faeces. The estimated egg output of *S. mansoni* is 100-300 eggs per day. In the water, the miracidia hatch and infect *Biomphalaria* snails. In the snails the miracidia become sporocysts which reproduce and finally produce infective cercariae which are shed from the snails during daylight hours.

Biomphalaria snails: They are flat (discoid), without a spire and measure up to about 20 mm wide according to species (see Plate 20.7). *Biomphalaria* snails are aquatic and hermaphroditic (male and female).

The life cycle of *S. mansoni* is shown in Fig. 20.4.

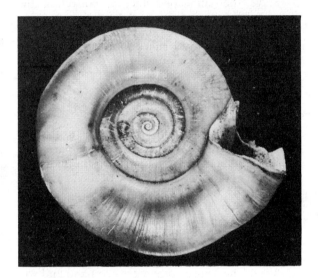

Plate 20.7 Shell of a *Biomphalaria* snail.
Courtesy of K. L. Frampton.

Clinical features and pathology

There may be irritation and a skin rash at the site of cercarial penetration ('swimmer's itch').

As in other forms of schistosomiasis, it is the eggs not the adult flukes which are responsible for the main features and pathology associated with *S. mansoni* infection. By acquiring host antigens, the flukes are protected from attack by host immune responses.

The majority of *S. mansoni* eggs penetrate through the intestinal wall and are excreted in the faeces often with blood and mucus. Host reaction to eggs lodged in the intestinal mucosa leads to the formation of granulomata, ulceration and thickening of the bowel wall. Large granulomata cause colonic and rectal polyps.

A proportion of the eggs reach the liver through the portal vein. In the liver, reaction to the eggs may eventually cause a thickening of the portal vessels known as claypipe-stem fibrosis. Prolonged heavy infection can lead to a marked enlargement of the liver with fibrosis, portal hypertension, and ascites. The spleen may also become enlarged. Death from haematemesis can occur following rupture of varicose veins in the oesophagus or stomach. The prevalence of liver disease associated with *Schistosoma mansoni* infection in endemic areas is only about 4% (see also laboratory findings in hepatic schistosomiasis, described under *Laboratory Diagnosis*).

Other complications can arise following the depositing of eggs in the spinal cord, lungs and other organs of the body.

Salmonella infections in patients with *S. mansoni* tend to become chronic and prolonged. There is also thought to be an association between hepatitis B infection and hepatic schistosomiasis.

Prevention and control

The measures described for *S. haematobium* in 20:2 also apply to the prevention and control of schistosomiasis caused by *S. mansoni*.

Note: Further information about the control of schistosomiasis can be found in:

World Health Organization 1985 report, *The Control of Schistosomiasis*.[13]

Findings of a 1982 *Symposium on Schistosomiasis Control in Brazil, Egypt and the People's Republic of China*.[4]

LABORATORY DIAGNOSIS

Laboratory confirmation of *S. mansoni* infection is by:

☐ Finding *S. mansoni* eggs in faeces.

  Occasionally *S. mansoni* eggs may also be found in urine (often following faecal contamination).

☐ Examining a rectal biopsy for eggs when they cannot be found in faeces, especially after a patient has been partially treated.

Other findings

— Mucus and blood are often present in faecal specimens.

— There is usually a blood eosinophilia and a raised erythrocyte sedimentation rate (ESR).

— Patients with hepatic schistosomiasis are anaemic and have raised serum aspartate aminotransferase (AST) activity, low serum albumin and a high serum total protein due to raised globulin.[14]

Other studies have reported rises in serum alkaline phosphatase and AST, both in patients with uncomplicated *S. mansoni* infection and those with hepatosplenic schistosomiasis.[15]

Examination of faeces for *S. mansoni* eggs

Because the eggs can be few in number, it is best to use a concentration technique. Several specimens may need to be examined to detect the eggs.

A quantitative technique should be used because the number of eggs excreted is an indication of the severity of infection. Heavily infected patients (i.e. over 100 eggs/g of faeces) are more likely to develop serious complications. A quantitative and reproducible technique is essential in epidemiology and control work (see later text).

The following concentration techniques are recommended:

- Formol detergent quantitative technique.
- Formol ether centrifuge technique (quantitative) as described in 13:4.

Note: Floatation techniques are not suitable for concentrating schistosome eggs because the eggs are too heavy to float.

Formol detergent sedimentation technique for counting schistosome eggs in faeces[16]

This technique is recommended because it is reproducible, inexpensive, simple, safe and hygienic to perform and gives good preservation of schistosome eggs. The principle of the technique is described in 13:5.

Required
— Formol detergent solution   Reagent No.38
— Universal container with a conical base and measuring spoon (Sterilin type)
— Sieve (strainer) with small holes, perferably 400-450 μm in size. The small plastic strainer available in most countries is suitable.

Faecal formol detergent kit
A kit containing all the equipment (reusable) required to carry out the formol detergent concentration technique, is available to developing countries from Tropical Health Technology (see Appendix IV, Faecal formol detergent Schisto kit). The kit contains:

- 12 reusable Sterilin Universal containers with conical base and measuring spoon.
- 1 rack to hold 12 Universal containers.
- 5 reusable plastic sieves.
- 1 wash bottle (500 ml) to dispense the formol detergent reagent (the reagent is not supplied).
- 10 reusable plastic bulb pipettes.
- 5 polypropylene beakers to receive filtrate.
- 50 cover glasses, 40 × 22 mm.

- 1 roll of 1000 self-adhesive (water-soluble) printed labels for Universal containers showing 10 ml volume.

Method
1. Dispense about 10 ml of formol detergent solution into the Universal container.

2. Using the spoon attached to the cap of the Universal container, transfer a *level* spoonful of faeces to the container (approx. 335 mg when using a Sterilin spoon), and mix well in the formol detergent solution to break up the faeces. Tighten the cap and shake for about 30 seconds.

3. Sieve the emulsified faeces, collecting the sieved suspension in a beaker.

4. Return the sieved suspension to the conical based Universal container.

5. Stand the container upright in a rack for 1 hour (do not centrifuge).

6. Using a plastic bulb pipette or a Pasteur pipette, remove and discard the supernatant fluid, taking care not to disturb the sediment which has formed in the base of the container.

7. Add about 10 ml of 10% formol detergent solution, and mix well for a minimum of 30 seconds.

   Leave to sediment for a further 1 hour. Further 'clearing' of the faecal debris will take place.

   Note: The schistosome eggs are fixed and will not overclear or become distorted.

8. Using a plastic bulb pipette, remove and discard the supernatant fluid. Take care not to remove the fine sediment that has collected in the conical base of the container.

9. Transfer the *entire* sediment to a slide and cover with a 22 × 40 mm cover glass or if unavailable with two smaller square cover glasses.

10. Systematically examine the entire sediment microscopically for schistosome eggs using the 10× objective with the condenser iris *closed sufficiently* to give good contrast.

    Count the number of eggs and multiply the number counted by 3 to give the approximate number per gram (g) of faeces.

Interpretation of faecal egg counts
The definition of a heavy infection is area-specific and may vary from 100/800 eggs per gram of faeces.[13]

The features which identify *S. mansoni* are as follows:

Egg of *Schistosoma mansoni*

- It is pale yellow-brown, large, and oval, measuring about $150 \times 60 \ \mu m$.

- Has a characteristic side (lateral) spine.

  Note: Sometimes the spine may appear terminal like that of an *S. haematobium* egg but if the egg is rolled over by pressing gently on the cover glass the spine will be seen to be lateral.

- Contains a fully developed miracidium.

- A viable egg (in fresh unpreserved faeces) shows flickering of the excretory flame cells. The position of flame cells in a schistosome egg is shown in Plate 20.5. Tests to demonstrate the viability of schistosome eggs are described in 20:2.

- A non-viable egg is dark-coloured and shows no structural detail or flame cell movement. It may be surrounded by fibrous cells.

- A calcified egg is usually smaller and appears black and often distorted with a less distinct spine.

Illustrations: See Plate 20.9 and colour Plate 15.

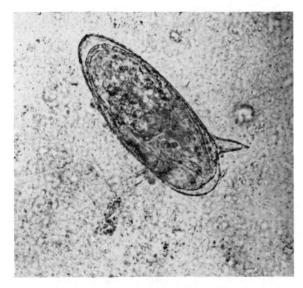

Plate 20.9 Egg of *Schistosoma mansoni* in faeces as seen with **40x objective.**
Courtesy of Wellcome Medical Museum of Science.

Note: *S. mansoni* eggs are sometimes found in urine and occasionally *S. haematobium* eggs are found in faeces (see Plate 20.5 in 20:2).

Intestinal schistosomiasis epidemiological and control techniques

In recent years several modified Kato techniques have been developed for detecting and counting schistosome eggs in faeces. Such techniques have been shown to be of value in schistosomiasis epidemiology and control work.[17, 18]

In these techniques faeces is pressed through a mesh screen to remove large particles. A portion of the sieved sample is then transferred to the hole of a template on a slide. After filling the hole, the template is removed and the remaining sample (approx. 10 mg, 20 mg, or 50 mg depending on size of template) is covered with a piece of cellophane soaked in glycerol (glycerine). The glycerol 'clears' the faecal material from around the eggs. The eggs are then counted and the number calculated per gram (g) of faeces. Kato kits are commercially available.[19]

Note: While the original Kato technique was a simple technique, the modified quantitative Kato techniques are more complex to perform and there is a risk of the operators' fingers and working area becoming contaminated. It is therefore to be hoped that the inexpensive, simpler, and safer formol detergent sedimentation technique described in this subunit may be of value to field workers engaged in schistosomiasis epidemiology and control. It also has the advantage that a larger amount of faeces can be tested.

Examination of a biopsy for schistosome eggs

When schistosome eggs cannot be found in faeces they can sometimes be found in a rectal biopsy. The eggs are often non-viable and calcified.

A biopsy is examined as follows:

1. Immediately after removal, place the tissue in physiological saline and soak it for 30-60 minutes.

2. Transfer the tissue to a slide and cover with a cover glass. With care, press on the cover glass to spread out the tissue and make a sufficiently thin preparation.

3. Examine the entire preparation microscopically for eggs using the $10\times$ objective with the condenser iris *closed sufficiently* to give good contrast. Constant focusing is necessary to detect the eggs.

   Note: If the preparation is too thick to examine well, add a drop of lactophenol solution (Reagent No. 48) and wait a few minutes for the tissue to clear sufficiently.

4. Identify the eggs and estimate the number of uncalcified eggs in the biopsy and the proportion that are calcified (black). Uncalcified and calcified eggs of *S. mansoni* in tissue are shown in Plate 20.10.

Note: A rectal biopsy may also contain (depending on geographical area) the eggs of *S. intercalatum* (see Plate 20.11), *S. japonicum* (see Plate 20.13), *S. mekongi* and *S. haematobium* (see plate 20.5).

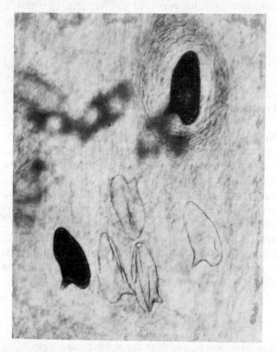

Plate 20.10 Uncalcified and calcified eggs of *S. mansoni* in rectal biopsy.
Reproduced from Medical Parasitology, courtesy of W. B. Saunders Company and Dr W. Jann Brown.

Serological diagnosis of schistosomiasis
Serological tests are of value in studying the epidemiology of schistosomiasis and in diagnosis when eggs cannot be found because they are being excreted in too few numbers or because the patient has been partially treated.

A wide range of serological tests have been developed for the diagnosis of *S. mansoni* and *S. japonicum* infections. Little work has been done with regard to *S. haematobium* because this species is more easily diagnosed parasitologically and because it is difficult to establish it in animals to obtain material to work with.

Among the *S. mansoni* and *S. japonicum* tests that have been developed, the following are considered the most promising:

- Circumoval precipitin (COP) test in which the patient's serum is incubated with viable schistosome eggs. A positive reaction is shown by an oval precipitate around the eggs at 24 h.

  Although this test is simple to perform, preparation and standardization of the antigen are difficult as also is the interpretation of the test. A technique has been described in which frozen *S. mansoni* eggs are used to facilitate standardization.[20]

- Indirect fluorescent antibody (IFA) test in which sections or whole organisms from different stages of the schistosome life cycle are used as antigen. This test however lacks specificity.

- Enzyme linked immunosorbent assay (ELISA), in which purified egg extracts are used as antigens. This technique is the most promising of the serological techniques.[21,22]. In epidemiological surveys blood can be collected in the field on filter paper, stored in a desiccator at room temperature, and the batch of papers sent to the laboratory for testing.[23]

  ELISA reagents are not yet (1986) available commercially but it is possible for interested workers to obtain supplies of *S. mansoni* antigen or ready-coated micro plates, other required reagents, and details of the ELISA technique from the London School of Hygiene and Tropical Medicine.[24]

SCHISTOSOMA INTERCALATUM

Schistosoma intercalatum causes intestinal schistosomiasis but compared with *S. mansoni*, *S. japonicum*, and *S. mekongi* it is less pathogenic.

Distribution
S. intercalatum has a high infectivity rate but is limited in its distribution mainly to West and Central Africa, i.e. Zaire, Chad, Congo, Central African Republic, Gabon, the Cameroons and Nigeria. Infections have also been reported from Tanzania.

Note: Natural hybrids between *S. intercalatum* and *S. haematobium* have been found in the Cameroons.

Transmission and life cycle
The transmission of *S. intercalatum* is similar to that of *S. mansoni*, i.e. contact with water contain-

ing cercariae. *S. intercalatum* cercariae are found near or at the surface of the water.

Life cycle
Eggs are passed in the faeces. The miracidia hatch in water and are taken up by *Bulinus* snails. In its snail host, the parasite multiplies and develops to its infective cercarial stage.

Humans are the main definitive hosts of *S. intercalatum* but animal reservoir hosts may also be important in some areas.

The mature flukes live in the mesenteric veins and portal venous system.

Mature S. intercalatum flukes: The body surface of the male is covered with tubercles and fine spines. The male fluke measures 11-14 × 0.3-0.4 mm. There are 4-6 testes. The female measures 10-14 × 0.15-0.18 mm and is darker than the male due to blood pigment in the gut. The uterus holds 5-50 eggs at a time.

Eggs are laid in the mesenteric venules. Most break through to the lumen of the intestine and are passed in the faeces.

Clinical features and pathology
S. intercalatum can cause abdominal pain, diarrhoea, and other symptoms but eggs trapped in the tissues cause less host immune reaction and damage than the eggs of other human schistosomes.

More severe and prolonged *Salmonella* infections are associated with *S. intercalatum* as with other human schistosomes.

Prevention and control
The control measures described in 20:2 for *S. haematobium* also apply to the prevention and control of schistosomiasis caused by *S. intercalatum*.

LABORATORY DIAGNOSIS

Laboratory confirmation of *S. intercalatum* infection is by:

☐ Finding eggs in faeces.

☐ Detecting eggs in a rectal biopsy.

Examination of faeces for *S. intercalatum* eggs
The eggs can be few in number and therefore a concentration technique should be used. The technique already described in this subunit for con-

centrating *S. mansoni* eggs is also suitable for detecting and counting *S. intercalatum* eggs in faeces.

Egg of *Schistosoma intercalatum*

- It is pale yellow-brown, large, and elongate, measuring about 175 × 60 μm.

- Has a characteristic long spine at one end (terminal spine) which often appears bent.

  Note: Because of its terminal spine, the egg of *S. intercalatum* can resemble that of *S. haematobium* but unlike *S. haematobium* the egg of *S. intercalatum* is usually found in faeces not in urine.

- Contains a fully developed miracidium which shows a central indentation.

- A viable egg (in fresh unpreserved faeces) shows flickering of the excretory flame cells. The position of flame cells in a schistosome egg is shown in Plate 20.5.

- A calcified egg appears black and often distorted.

- Unlike other terminally-spined schistosome eggs, the egg of *S. intercalatum* is acid fast (Ziehl-Neelsen staining).

Illustrations: See Plate 20.11.

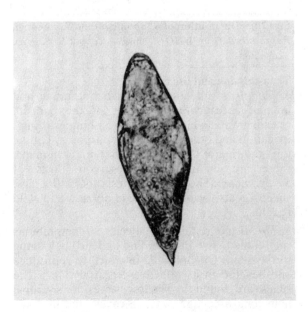

Plate 20.11   Egg of *Schistosoma intercalatum* with terminal spine.

Examination of a biopsy for *S. intercalatum* eggs
The technique already described for detecting *S. mansoni* eggs in tissue can also be used to examine a rectal biopsy for *S. intercalatum* eggs.

20:4 SCHISTOSOMA JAPONICUM AND SCHISTOSOMA MEKONGI

SCHISTOSOMA JAPONICUM

Schistosoma japonicum causes intestinal schistosomiasis. In 1982 it was estimated that some 5% of the world's population lived in S. japonicum endemic areas.[25]

Distribution

S. japonicum is found in China and also in parts of the Philippines and Western Indonesia. Its distribution is shown in Fig. 20.5.

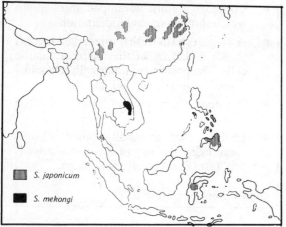

IIIII S. japonicum
■ S. mekongi

Fig. 20.5 Distribution of S. japonicum and S. mekongi. Reproduced from WHO Technical Report Series No. 728, 1985.

Transmission and life cycle

S. japonicum infection is caused by human and animal faeces containing eggs of the parasite reaching water which is used for bathing, washing, irrigation and other agricultural purposes. Unlike the other major schistosomes that infect humans, there are many animal reservoir hosts of S. japonicum. They include dogs, cats, cattle, pigs, sheep, goats, water-buffaloes, horses, and wild rodents.

S. japonicum requires a species of amphibious snail (able to live in water and on land) belonging to the genus Oncomelania in which to reproduce and develop to its infective cercarial stage. The snails are found in shallow water in swamps, marshland, seepage water in caves, and in moist soil along the banks of water courses and the edges of irrigation channels.

A person becomes infected by contact with cercariae in water or on water vegetation to which cercariae have become attached. Once shed by the snail, S. japonicum cercariae swim for only a short time in water. They rapidly become attached to vegetation or other objects in the water.

Life cycle

The life cycle of S. japonicum is similar to that described for S. haematobium in 20:2 with a few exceptions.

After mating, the mature S. japonicum flukes migrate to the capillaries of the superior mesenteric vein or its tributaries in the wall of the small intestine. Some flukes can also be found in the inferior mesenteric veins which drain the large intestine and in the portal venous system.

Mature S. japonicum flukes: The body surface of the male is covered with fine spines. The male fluke measures 12-20 × 0.5 mm. There are 6-8 testes. The female measures 12-28 × 0.3 mm and is darker than the male due to blood pigment in the gut. The ovary is situated mid-body and the uterus which is long and straight contains 50 or more eggs at a time.

Eggs are laid in the venules and penetrate through to the lumen of the intestine to be excreted in the faeces. The estimated egg output of S. japonicum is 1500-3500 eggs per day. In the water, the eggs hatch miracidia which are taken up by Oncomelania snails. In the snails the miracidia develop into sporocysts which reproduce and finally produce infective cercariae which are shed from the snail during night hours. The cercariae are able to survive for up to 24 hours.

Oncomelania snails: They are small, measuring under 10 mm, ovoid and operculated with a steep conical spine (see Plate 20.12). Oncomelania snails are unisexual and amphibious.

The life cycle of S. japonicum is shown in Fig. 20.6.

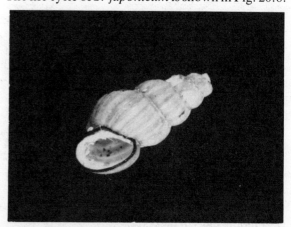

Plate 20.12 Shell of an Oncomelania snail. Courtesy of K. L. Frampton.

Clinical features and pathology

There is usually irritation and a skin rash at the site of cercarial penetration ('swimmer's itch').

About 20-60 days after infection a severe immune reaction to the products of young flukes and eggs may occur. It is known as Katayama reaction and takes the form of an acute illness with fever, muscular and abdominal pain, spleen enlargement, urticaria, and eosinophilia. Although this reaction is associated with *S. japonicum*, it can also occur with *S. haematobium* and *S. mansoni* infections.

The clinical features and pathology of *S. japonicum* infection are similar to those described for *S. mansoni* in 20.3. Reactions to eggs in the tissues can cause acute intestinal or hepatosplenic disease with dysentery, liver fibrosis, marked enlargement of the spleen and ascites. Complications arising from eggs deposited in the lungs, central nervous system and other parts of the body are more common in *S. japonicum* than *S. mansoni* infection.

Prevention and control

In the prevention and control of schistosomiasis caused by *S. japonicum*, a combination of some or all of the following methods is nearly always necessary.

- Destroying the snail intermediate hosts by:
  - Burying the snails in sufficient soil or water to kill them.[4]
  - Using molluscicides in water, along infested banks of water courses, and in trenches in which snails are buried.
  - Taking environmental measures to prevent seasonal flooding which results in an increase in snail numbers and transmission.

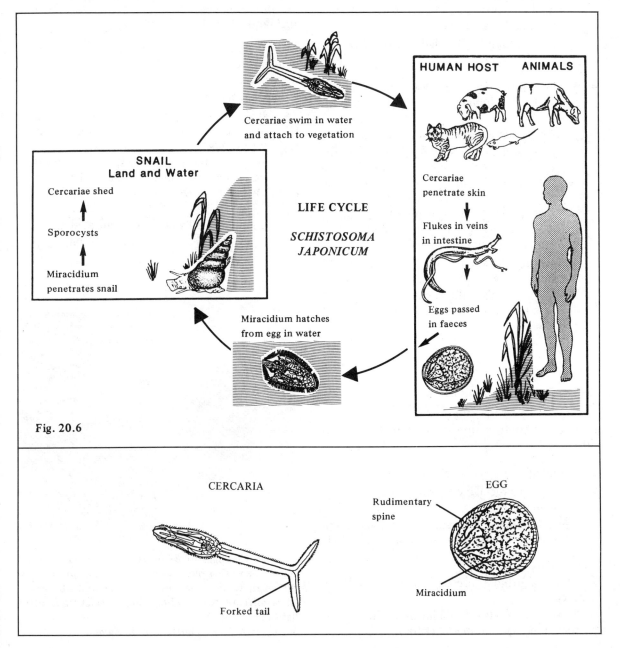

Fig. 20.6

LIFE CYCLE

SCHISTOSOMA JAPONICUM

HUMAN HOST   ANIMALS

Cercariae swim in water and attach to vegetation

Cercariae penetrate skin

Flukes in veins in intestine

Eggs passed in faeces

Miracidium hatches from egg in water

SNAIL Land and Water

Cercariae shed

Sporocysts

Miracidium penetrates snail

CERCARIA

Forked tail

EGG

Rudimentary spine

Miracidium

- Preventing water becoming contaminated with eggs by:
  - Health education and providing sanitation facilities.
  - Avoiding the use of untreated faeces as fertilizer.
  - Treating infected persons, especially in areas when humans are the only or main sources of water pollution.
  - Taking measures to prevent water sources becoming polluted from infected animals.

- Avoiding contact with water or vegetation known to contain cercariae by:
  - Providing safe water supplies to reduce as much as possible contact with infested water and vegetation.
  - Constructing footbridges across infested water courses.

- Minimising the risk of increased infection from new water development projects and irrigation schemes by:
  - Not employing infected workers.
  - Siting settlements away from canals, drains and irrigation channels, and providing latrines and sufficient safe water for domestic use.
  - When making new irrigation ditches, filling in completely formerly used ditches with clean soil to bury the snails.
  - Varying the water levels in the system and using molluscicides at regular intervals.
  - Lining canals with cement and keeping them free from silt and vegetation in which snails can live.

LABORATORY DIAGNOSIS

Laboratory confirmation of *S. japonicum* infection is by:

☐ Finding *S. japonicum* eggs in faeces.
☐ Examining a rectal biopsy when eggs cannot be found in faeces.

Note: Serological tests used in the diagnosis of intestinal schistosomiasis are described in 20:3.

Other findings
- Mucus and blood are often present in faecal specimens.
- There is a blood eosinophilia and raised erythrocyte sedimentation rate (ESR).

- In patients with hepatic disease, serum total protein is raised due to raised globulin, serum albumin is often low and serum alkaline phosphatase and aspartate aminotransferase (AST) activities are usually raised.

Examination of faeces for *S. japonicum* eggs

When only a few eggs are excreted they may not be detected in a direct saline preparation and therefore a concentration technique and the examination of more than one faecal specimen may be necessary to detect them. The formol detergent sedimentation technique described in 20:3 for concentrating and counting *S. mansoni* eggs in faeces is also suitable for the detection and quantifying of *S. japonicum* eggs. Alternatively the formol ether technique described in 13:4 may also be used.

The following features identify the egg of *S. japonicum*.

Egg of *Schistosoma japonicum*

- It is colourless or pale yellow-brown, large and round to oval, measuring about $90 \times 65 \mu m$.

- A very small hook-like spine (rudimentary spine) can sometimes be seen projecting from the egg wall but often it is hidden by faecal debris and red cells.

- Contains a fully developed miracidium.

- Calcified egg is usually smaller and appears black.

Ilustrations: See Plate 20.13 and colour Plate 16.

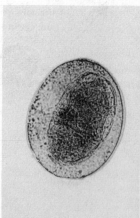 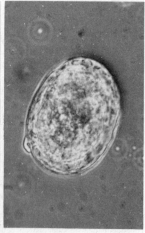

Plate 20.13 Eggs of *Schistosoma japonicum*. Right egg is seen using phase contrast microscopy to show the small spine projecting from the wall of the egg (it is difficult to see when using normal transmitted light microscopy).
Right photograph, courtesy of V. Zaman.

Note: Floatation techniques are not suitable because schistosome eggs are too heavy to float.

In the epidemiology and control of *S. japonicum* schistosomiasis, quantitative techniques are essential.

Examination of a rectal biopsy
The technique used to examine a rectal biopsy for schistosome eggs is described in 20:3.

SCHISTOSOMA MEKONGI

S. mekongi is a recently recognized species of *Schistosoma* that is closely related to *S. japonicum*. It causes intestinal schistosomiasis.

Distribution
S. mekongi is found in Laos, Kampuchea (Cambodia) and Thailand in the Mekong River Basin. Prevalence rates are estimated at 15-50% with children (up to 15y) being more commonly infected.

Transmission and life cycle
The transmission and life cycle of *S. mekongi* are similar to that of *S. japonicum* except that the snail vector of *S. mekongi* is *Lithoglyphopsis* (*Tricula*) *aperta* which is an aquatic not an amphibious snail. *L. aperta* lives in water on soil debris. Transmission occurs mostly in the dry season when the snails are mature enough to become hosts and the level of the river is low. Dogs have been identified as reservoir hosts of *S. mekongi*.

The adult flukes live in the mesenteric blood vessels and the female lays eggs in the venules.

Mature S. mekongi flukes: The body of the male is covered with spines. The male fluke measures about 15 × 0.4 mm. There are 6 or 7 testes. The female worm measures about 12 × 0.23 mm and is darker than the male due to blood in the gut.

Clinical features and pathology
Infection with *S. mekongi* produces features similar to those found with *S. japonicum* infection. The disease can be severe with hepatosplenomegaly and portal venous hypertension being common complications.

Prevention and control
The measures described for *S. haematobium* in 20:2 apply to the prevention and control of schistosomiasis caused by *S. mekongi*. Some of the control measures described for *S. japonicum* also apply but the snail hosts of *S. mekongi* live in water only and not on land like the amphibious snail vectors of *S. japonicum*.

LABORATORY DIAGNOSIS

Laboratory confirmation of *S. mekongi* infection is the same as that described for *S. japonicum*. As for *S. japonicum* infections, a concentration technique and examination of more than one faecal specimen may be required to detect the eggs of *S. mekongi*.

Identification of the egg of *S. mekongi* is as follows:

Egg of S. mekongi
• It is similar to but smaller and rounder than the egg of *S. japonicum*, measuring about 56 × 66 μm.
• Has a small knob-like spine similar to the egg of *S. japonicum*.

20:5 INFECTIONS CAUSED BY ANIMAL SCHISTOSOMES

Several *Schistosoma* species that are naturally parasitic in animals can infect humans and cause mild gastrointestinal symptoms but with the exception of *S. mattheei* such infections are rare.

Schistosoma mattheei
This species is a natural parasite of cattle, sheep, goats, zebras, and antelopes. It has been reported as infecting up to 30% of persons in parts of South Africa. It also occurs in Zimbabwe and Zaire.

The eggs of *S. mattheei* are usually found in those already infected with *S. haematobium* or *S. mansoni*. It is thought that hybridization occurs between *S. mattheei* and *S. haematobium*. *S. mattheei* is not thought to cause serious disease.

Eggs are excreted in urine or faeces and can be detected by the techniques described in 20:2 (urine) and 20:3 (faeces).

The following features identify the egg of *S. mattheei*:

Egg of S. mattheei

- It has a terminal spine and therefore requires differentiating from *S. haematobium* and *S. intercalatum*.

- It is larger than the egg of *S. haematobium*, measuring about 220 × 60 µm.

- The terminal spine is not as long as that of *S. intercalatum* (see Plate 20.11).

- Unlike *S. intercalatum* the shell of *S. mattheei* is not acid fast (Ziehl-Neelsen staining).

Illustration: See Fig. 20.7.

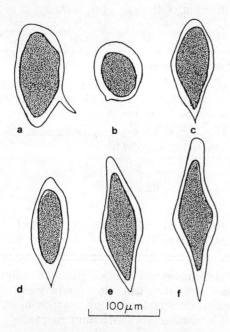

100µm

Fig. 20.7 Shapes and sizes of schistosome eggs.
a S. mansoni, b S. japonicum, c S. haematobium,
d S. intercalatum, e S. mattheei, f S. bovis.

References

1 World Health Organization. *Epidemiology and Control of Schistosomiasis*. WHO Technical Report Series, No. 643, 1980.

2 Iarotski, L. and Davis, A. The schistosomiasis problem in the world: results of a WHO questionnaire survey. *Bulletin of the World Health Organization*, **59,** pp 115-127, 1981.

3 World Health Organization. The prevention of bladder cancer: an integrated approach through the control of schistosomiasis. WHO/SCHISTO/83.73, WHO/CAN/83.10.

4 Cline, B. L. (Chairman and Editor) Symposium on schistosomiasis control. *American Journal of Tropical Medicine and Hygiene*, 31 (1), pp 75-127, 1982.

5 Peters, P. A., Warren, K. S., Mahmoud, A. A. F. Rapid accurate quantification of schistosome eggs via Nuclepore filters. *Journal of Parasitology*, **62**, pp 154-155, 1976.

6 Mott, K. E. A reusable polyamide filter for diagnosis of *S. haematobium* infection by urine filtration. *Bulletin de la Societe de Pathologic Exotique*, **76**, pp 101-104, 1983.

7 World Health Organization. Urine filtration techniques for *S. haematobium* infection. PDP/83.4, WHO, Geneva, 1983.

8 Feldmeier, H., Bienzle, U., Dietrich, M., and Sievertsen, H. J. Combination of a viability test and a quantification method for *Schistosoma haematobium* eggs. *Tropenmedizin und Parasitologie*, **30**, pp 417-422, 1979. (English translation available).

9 Mott, K. E., Dixon, H., Osei-Tutu, E., and England, E. C. Relationship between intensity of *Schistosoma haematobium* infection and clinical haematuria and proteinuria. *The Lancet*, May 7, pp 1005-1008, 1983.

10 Stephenson, L. S., Latham, M. C., Kinoti, S. N., Oduori, M. L. Sensitivity and specificity of reagent strips in screening of Kenyan children for *Schistosoma haematobium* infection. *American Journal of Tropical Medicine and Hygiene*, **33**, pp 862-871, 1984.

11 Prentice, M. A. A field-evolved differential filtration method for recovery of schistosome cercariae. *Annals of Tropical Medicine and Parasitology*, **78**, pp 117-127, 1984.

12 Peters, W., and Gilles, H. M. A colour Atlas of *Tropical Medicine and Parasitology*. Wolfe Medical Publications, 2nd Edition, 1981. ELBS edition, 1985, priced £9.

13 World Health Organization. *The Control of Schistosomiasis*, WHO, Technical Report Series, No. 728, 1985.

14 Mackenjee, M. K. R., Coovadia, H. M., and Chutte, C. H. J. Clinical recognition of mild hepatic schistosomiasis in an endemic area. *Transactions of the Royal Society of Tropical Medicine and Hygiene*, **78**, pp 13-15, 1984.

15 Mansour, M. M. *et al.* Serum enzyme tests in hepatosplenic schistosomiasis. *Transactions of the Royal Society of Tropical Medicine and Hygiene*, **76**, 1982.

16 The author is grateful to Mr Anthony Moody, Chief MLSO and MLSO colleagues of the laboratory, Hospital for Tropical Diseases, London for assisting in the development of the formol-detergent sedimentation technique and for carrying out the practical work involved.

17 Valencia, C. I., and Abear, R. F. A modification of the quantitative thick smear method for *Schistosoma japonicum*. *Acta Medica Philippina*, **17**, (3; Ser. 2), pp 91-94, 1981.

18 Peters, P. A., El Alamy, M., Warren, K. S., Mahmoud, A. A. F. Quick Kato smear for field quantification of *Schistosoma mansoni* eggs. *American Journal of Tropical Medicine and*

Hygiene, **29**, pp 217-219, 1980.

19 Kato kit tests are available from:

Japanese Association of Parasite Control, c/o Hokenkaikan, 1-1 Ichigaya-Sadohara, Shinjuku-ku, Tokyo, Japan.

Boehringer Mannheim Bioquimica, Rua Nair 170, Olaria, CEP21021, Rio de Janeiro, RJ, Brasil.

20 Ismail, S. A., Slek, M. J., and Leef, J. L. Circumoval precipitin (COP) test in schistosomiasis with frozen *Schistosoma mansoni* eggs. *Transactions of the Royal Society of Tropical Medicine and Hygiene*, **77**, pp 809-811, 1983.

21 Voller, A., and De Savigny, D. Diagnostic serology of tropical parasitic diseases, *Journal of Immunological Methods*, **46**, pp 1-29, 1981.

22 Voller, A. ELISA - a widely applicable diagnostic tool. *Medicine Digest*, **10**, pp 5-10, 1984.

23 Long, E. G., Lawrence, M. C., and Augustine, T. ELISA for *Schistosoma mansoni* infection: durability of blood spots on filter paper. *Transactions of the Royal Society of Tropical Medicine and Hygiene*, **75**, (5), pp 740-741, 1981.

24 Requests for *S. mansoni* ELISA reagents should be addressed for the attention of Dr. C. C. Draper, London School of Hygiene and Tropical Medicine, Keppel Street, London WC1E 7HT, England.

25 Mott, K. E. *S. japonicum* and *S. japonicum*-like infections. In *Schistosomiasis, Epidemiology Treatment and Control*, William Heinemann Medical Books, p 128, 1982.

26 Klumpp, R.K., Southgate, B.A. Nytrel filters not reusuable, *Transactions of the Royal Society of Tropical Medicine and Hygiene*, Correspondence, **80**, pp 494-495, 1986.

- Showing the effectivity of the syringe urine filtration technique.
- Quantitative epidemiological evaluation, chemotherapy, supplemental mollusciciding and follow-up of patients at predetermined intervals.
- Community education and integration of control operations into health care delivery systems.
- Continuing research into the biochemistry and physiology of schistosomes, and toxicity of antischistosomal agents.
- Use of monoclonal antibodies and other procedures in identifying protective antigens that might lead eventually to the development of vaccines.

Recommended Reading

Jordan, P., Webbe, G. *Schistosomiasis, Epidemiology Treatment and Control*, William Heinemann Medical Books Ltd, 1982. International edition, 1982, priced £12.95.

World Health Organization. *The Control of Schistosomiasis*. WHO Technical Report Series, No. 728, 1985. This publication describes the different species of schistosomes that infect humans and gives information on the epidemiology, distribution, disease features, diagnosis, treatment, control and prevention of schistosomiasis.

Peters, W., Gilles, H. M. A colour Atlas of *Tropical Medicine and Parasitology*. Wolfe Medical Publications, 2nd Edition, 1981. ELBS edition, 1985, priced £9.

Tropical Diseases Research Programme
SCHISTOSOMIASIS

Schistosomiasis is included in the *UNDP/World Bank/World Health Organization Special Programme for Research and Training in Tropical Diseases*.

Tropical Diseases Research (TDR) activities with regard to schistosomiasis as recorded in No. 5 of the 1985 *WHO Chronicle* include:

21 Intestinal Nematodes

21:1 CLASSIFICATION AND FEATURES OF INTESTINAL NEMATODES

The general characteristics of nematodes (roundworms) are described at the beginning of the Parasitology Section in 12:4.

Classification of intestinal nematodes of medical importance or common occurrence

Superfamily	ASCARIDOIDEA
Species	*Ascaris lumbricoides*

Superfamily	OXYUROIDEA
Species	*Enterobius vermicularis*

Superfamily	RHABDITOIDEA
Species	*Strongyloides stercoralis*

Superfamily	TRICHINELLOIDEA
Species	*Trichuris trichiura*

Note: The tissue nematode *Trichinella spiralis* also belongs to this superfamily. It is described with the other tissue nematodes in Chapter 22.

Superfamily	ANCYLOSTOMATOIDEA
Species	Hookworms:
	Ancylostoma duodenale
	Necator americanus

Animal intestinal nematodes of lesser medical importance or low occurrence

Superfamily	ASCARIDOIDEA
Species	*Toxocara canis*

Superfamily	RHABDITOIDEA
Species	*Strongyloides fuelleborni*

Superfamily	TRICHINELLOIDEA
Species	*Capillaria* species

Superfamily	ANCYLOSTOMATOIDEA
Species	*Ancylostoma caninum*
	Ancylostoma brasiliense

Superfamily	TRICHOSTRONGYLOIDEA
Species	*Trichostrongylus*

Features of intestinal nematodes that infect humans

- Adult worms live in the intestinal tract.

- Female worms are oviparous, i.e. lay eggs.

- Humans are the only or the most significant hosts of the intestinal nematodes of major medical importance.

- Most species are soil-transmitted, i.e. spread by faecal pollution of the soil. Under favourable climatic conditions the larva (free or in the egg) develops to its infective stage in the soil.

A person becomes infected by swallowing infective eggs (*A. lumbricoides*, *T. trichiura*, *E. vermicularis*) or by infective larvae penetrating the skin (hookworms, *S. stercoralis*).

- Before becoming adults in their human host, the larvae of *A. lumbricoides*, *S. stercoralis* and hookworms migrate through the heart and lungs for about 10 days as shown in Fig. 21.1. During their migration the larvae grow and develop.

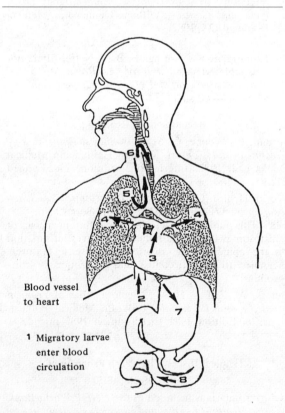

Blood vessel to heart

1 Migratory larvae enter blood circulation

Fig. 21.1 Diagram to show the migration of *Ascaris*, *Strongyloides* and hookworm larvae through the heart and lungs.

- The term filariform larva is used to describe the infective larva of those intestinal nematodes that cause infection by penetrating the skin, i.e. *S. stercoralis* and hookworms.

The term rhabditiform larva is used to describe the non-infective first stage larva that hatches from the egg in the intestine (*S. stercoralis*) or in the soil (hookworms).

Note: The eggs of *S. stercoralis* also hatch rhabditiform larvae in the soil because this nematode can live freely in the soil as well as parasitically.

- Laboratory confirmation of infection with *A. lumbricoides*, *T. trichiura*, and hookworms is by finding eggs in the faeces and with *S. stercoralis* by finding larvae in the faeces. *E. vermicularis* infection is confirmed by recovering eggs from the skin around the anus (perianal skin).

Occasionally the worms of *A. lumbricoides* and *E. vermicularis* can be recovered.

Note: The morphology of the medically important intestinal nematodes is shown in the life cycle figures contained in the subsequent subunits of this Chapter.

Intestinal Nematodes of Major Medical Importance
LIFE CYCLE SUMMARIES

T. trichuria	*A. lumbricoides*	*A. duodenale* / *N. americanus*	*S. stercoralis*	*E. vermicularis*
Transmitted by ingesting infective eggs in food or from contaminated hands	Transmitted by ingesting infective eggs in food or from contaminated hands	Transmitted by infective larvae penetrating skin	Transmitted by infective larvae penetrating skin	Transmitted by ingesting infective eggs mainly from contaminated fingers
	Heart-lung migration	Heart-lung migration	Heart-lung migration	
Adult worms in large intestine	Adult worms in small intestine	Adult worms in small intestine	Adult worms in small intestine	Adult worms in large intestine
EGGS IN FAECES	EGGS IN FAECES	EGGS IN FAECES	LARVAE IN FAECES	EGGS ON PERIANAL SKIN
Eggs become infective in the soil*	Eggs become infective in the soil*	Eggs hatch larvae. Become infective in the soil*	Larvae become infective in the soil*	Eggs become infective a few hours after exposure to air

Notes

* These soil-transmitted helminths are sometimes referred to as geohelminths.

With *S. stercoralis*, internal autoinfection (self-infection) can also occur when larvae become infective in the intestine.

With *E. vermicularis*, autoinfection can also occur when eggs hatch on the perianal skin and the infective larvae migrate through the anus to the intestine.

21:2 ASCARIS LUMBRICOIDES

Ascaris lumbricoides, also known as the large intestinal roundworm, causes ascariasis.

Distribution

A. lumbricoides has a world-wide distribution. It is one of the commonest and most widespread of all human parasites. It is particularly common in areas of inadequate sanitation and where untreated human faeces are used as fertilizer (night-soil).

Transmission and life cycle

A. lumbricoides is spread by faecal pollution of the soil. A person becomes infected by ingesting infective eggs in contaminated food or from hands that have become faecally contaminated.

Ascaris worms produce many eggs and these are surrounded by a strong protective coat which enables them to remain viable in soil and dust for several years. These factors contribute to the widespread and often heavy *Ascaris* infections which can be found in the rural areas of developing countries, especially among children of 3-8 years whose fingers become contaminated while playing on open ground.

Life cycle

— Following ingestion of infective eggs, the larvae hatch in the small intestine and penetrate blood vessels in the intestinal wall.

— In the circulation, the larvae follow a heart-lung migration during which they develop (see 21:1).

— After migrating up the trachea, the larvae are swallowed. They remain in the small intestine and grow into mature worms.

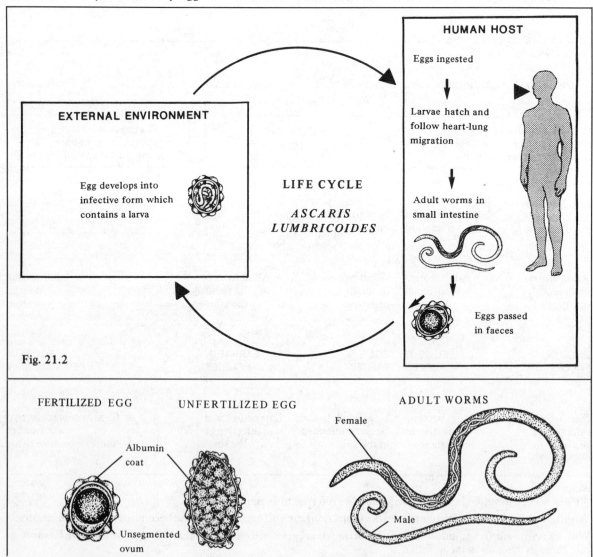

Fig. 21.2

Mature A. lumbricoides worms: Freshly expelled worms are pinkish in colour with an appearance similar to earthworms. There is a small mouth which is surrounded by three lips. They measure up to 35 cm in length with the male being shorter than the female. The male has a curved tail and two copulatory spicules of unequal length.

— After mating, the female produces large numbers of eggs which are passed in the faeces. Egg production commences about 2 months after infection.

— In shaded soil with a temperature of 20-40 °C and humidity of over 40%, the eggs develop and within 30-40 days of being passed each egg contains an infective larva. The larva does not hatch until the egg is swallowed.

Ascaris eggs are resistant to drying out but are killed by direct sunlight.

Note: The life cycle of *A. lumbricoides* is shown in Fig. 21.2.

Clinical features and pathology

During their heart-lung migration, *Ascaris* larvae can cause inflammatory and hypersensitive reactions including pneumonia-like symptoms, attacks of coughing, and bronchial asthma. Eosinophilia is common and often urticaria but these features are less marked after the larvae return to the intestine. Signs of toxaemia may develop and very occasionally neurological disorders.

Developing and mature worms in the intestine frequently cause abdominal pain, nausea, diarrhoea and vomiting. Occasionally intestinal muscle may become damaged and absorption impaired. The worms ingest protein and vitamins from their host and therefore heavy infections can contribute to malnutrition especially in children already malnourished.

Ascaris worms are large and in heavy infections, especially in children, worm masses can cause obstruction or perforation of the intestine and occasionally obstruction of the bile duct and pancreatic duct. These acute complications can be fatal. Other complications include liver abscesses and appendicitis caused by migrating worms. Worms can pass out through the anus or be vomited.

Prevention and control

- Preventing soil becoming faecally polluted by:
  — Providing and using adequate latrines.
  — Avoiding the use of untreated human faeces as fertilizer.
  — Treating infected individuals as part of a control programme, especially children.

- Preventing eggs being ingested by:
  — Washing the hands before eating.
  — Avoiding the eating of uncooked vegetables, green salads and fruits which may be contaminated with faeces containing *Ascaris* eggs from infected soil.

Caution: Laboratory staff wishing to store *Ascaris* eggs for teaching purpose should first treat faecal deposits containing the eggs with hot (70-80 °C) 10% formol saline. This will prevent the eggs from developing to an infective stage. Forceps should always be used when handling *Ascaris* worms because they can cause asthma and other allergic reactions.

LABORATORY DIAGNOSIS

Laboratory confirmation of ascariasis is by:

☐ Finding *A. lumbricoides* eggs in faeces.
☐ Identifying *A. lumbricoides* worms expelled through the anus or mouth.

Examination of faeces for *Ascaris* eggs

Most *Ascaris* infections can be detected by finding eggs in a direct saline preparation of faeces. Many eggs are produced and therefore concentration techniques are rarely required.

Direct saline preparation

The direct examination of a faecal specimen for helminth eggs is described in 13:2. The following features identify the eggs of *A. lumbricoides*:

Eggs of *Ascaris lumbricoides*

Usually fertilized eggs are found in the faeces but occasionally unfertilized eggs are passed when the worms in the intestine are mostly female.

FERTILIZED EGG
- It is yellow-brown and the shell is covered by an uneven albuminous coat.
- Oval or round and measures 60 x 40 μm.
- Contains a central granular mass which is the unsegmented fertilized ovum.

DECORTICATED EGG

This term is used to describe an egg that has no albuminous coat. A decorticated egg has a smooth shell and appears pale yellow or colourless.

Illustrations: See Plate 21.1 (left) and colour Plate 24.

UNFERTILIZED EGG

- It is darker in colour and has a more granular albuminous covering than a fertilized egg.
- More elongated than a fertilized egg, measuring about 90 × 45 μm.
- Contains a central mass of large refractile granules.

Illustrations: See Plate 21.1 (right) and colour Plate 24.

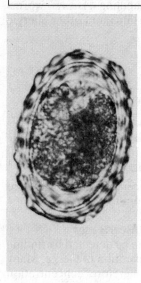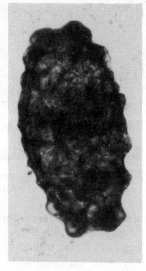

Plate 21.1 *Left* **Fertilized egg of** *A. lumbricoides.*
Right **Unfertilized eggs of** *A. lumbricoides.*
Courtesy of K. L. Frampton.

Identification of *Ascaris lumbricoides* worm

- It is large. This is a diagnostic feature if the worm is known to come from a human host. Adult female worms measure 20-35 cm long by 3-6 mm wide and male worms measure 15-30 cm long by 2-4 mm wide.

- Pink-brown (freshly expelled) or yellow-white in colour.

- Tail of the male is curved and has two small spicules (rod-like projections).

- When examined with a magnifying lens, three small lips can be seen surrounding a small mouth .

21:3 *ENTEROBIUS VERMICULARIS*

Enterobius vermicularis, also known as the pinworm or threadworm, causes enterobiasis.

Distribution
E. vermicularis has a world-wide distribution. Children are more commonly infected than adults.

Transmission and life cycle
E. vermicularis is transmitted by ingestion of infective eggs. The eggs are deposited on the anal skin usually during night hours and within a few hours of being laid they contain an infective larva. Infection is easily spread by way of clothing and bedding.

Autoinfection is common in children because the eggs cause intense irritation and scratching of the infected area leads to contamination of the fingers.

Airborne transmission of *E. vermicularis* eggs can also occur.

Life cycle
— Following ingestion of infective eggs, the larvae hatch in the intestine.

— The larvae develop into fully mature worms in the large intestine. Most worms inhabit the caecum and appendix.

  Mature E. vermicularis worms: They are small yellow-white worms. The female measures 8-13 mm in length and has a thin pointed tail. The male measures only 2-5 mm and has a coiled tail with a single spicule. Cervical alae (wing-like expansions) are present on each side of the head. This feature helps to identify the worm in transverse sections of tissue e.g. appendix. At the end of the oesophagus there is a bulbous enlargement.

— After mating, the female worms migrate to the rectum, pass out of the anus and lay their eggs on the perianal skin. Within about 6 hours each egg contains an infective larva. The eggs are produced about 6 weeks after infection.

— Depending on climatic conditions, the infective eggs can remain viable on clothing, household objects, and in dust for several weeks. Warm temperatures and high humidity favour survival.

  Occasionally larvae hatch from the eggs on the perianal skin and migrate back into the intestine where they grow into mature worms. This type of infection is called retroinfection.

Note: The life cycle of *E. vermicularis* is shown in Fig. 21.3.

Clinical features and pathology
Enterobiasis rarely causes serious symptoms. There is usually intense irritation around the anus and in females, infection of the urinary and genital

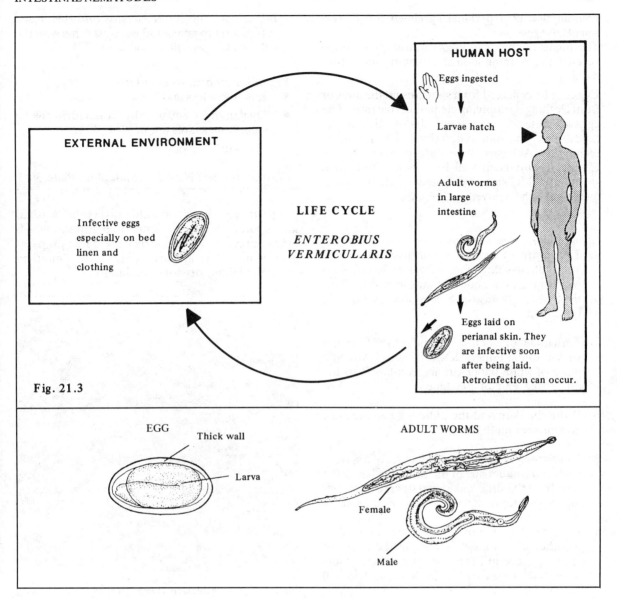

EXTERNAL ENVIRONMENT

Infective eggs especially on bed linen and clothing

HUMAN HOST

Eggs ingested

Larvae hatch

Adult worms in large intestine

Eggs laid on perianal skin. They are infective soon after being laid. Retroinfection can occur.

LIFE CYCLE

ENTEROBIUS VERMICULARIS

Fig. 21.3

EGG

Thick wall

Larva

ADULT WORMS

Female

Male

tract can occur. Worms in the appendix may be associated with appendicitis.

Prevention and control

Because *E. vermicularis* eggs are infective very soon after being laid, an entire family or community (e.g. in a school or institution) often becomes infected after handling bedding and other articles which have become contaminated. Control and preventive measures therefore include:

- Treating all members of a family in which infection has occurred.

- Washing of the anal skin each morning soon after waking.

- Washing of clothing worn at night.

LABORATORY DIAGNOSIS

Laboratory confirmation of enterobiasis is by:

☐ Finding *E. vermicularis* eggs in samples collected from perianal skin or recovered from clothing worn at night.

Note: Eggs (from perianal skin) may also be found in faeces and less commonly in urine specimens from females.

☐ Finding *E. vermicularis* worms in faeces or during a clinical examination.

Examination of a perianal specimen for *E. vermicularis* eggs

The highest number of eggs can usually be recovered in the morning soon after waking and before bathing.

Eggs can be collected from skin around the anus or from clothing by applying clear adhesive tape. The eggs are detected microscopically by sticking the tape directly on a slide as described in the following technique. Adhesive tape-slide preparations of *E. vermicularis* keep well for several days when stored at 2-8 °C should examination of the specimen need to be delayed.

Clear adhesive tape technique

1. Take a strip of about 20 cm of clear cellulose or vinyl adhesive tape (e.g. *Sellotape*, *Scotch tape*) which measures about 20 mm in width. Stick the tape lengthways on a clean slide as shown in Fig. 21.4 a.

2. Turn under one of the free ends of the tape and stick it to the underside of the slide. Attach a piece of white paper (to act as a label) to the other free end of the tape ·

    Write the date and the patient's name, ward, and number on the label.

3. Hold a tongue depressor (or handle of a spoon) against the underside of the slide. Peel back the tape from the slide and loop it over the projecting tongue depressor as shown in Fig. 21.4c.

4. Holding the tongue depressor and slide together, touch the skin around the anus (or clothing) several times with the adhesive surfaces of the tape (see Fig. 21.4e). The eggs will stick to the tape.

5. Loop back the tape and stick it down on the slide as before (see Fig. 21.4f).

6. Immediately before examining the preparation, lift up the tape and place a small drop of xylene in the centre of the slide. Stick down the tape again and smooth it out with a piece of cotton wool.

    Use of xylene: This is not essential but a drop of xylene will clear any debris and air bubbles and therefore make it easier to detect the eggs. Do not, however, add the xylene until ready to examine the preparation because prolonged contact with xylene may cause the eggs to collapse.

7. Examine the preparation microscopically using the 10× objective to detect the eggs and the 40× objective to identify them.

Important: The condenser iris *must* be closed sufficiently to give good contrast otherwise the colourless eggs will not be seen.

Egg of *Enterobius vermicularis*

- It is colourless and has a clear shell.

- Oval in shape and usually flattened on one side. It measures about 55 × 30 μm.

- Contains a larva.

Illustrations: See Plate 21.2 and colour Plate 30.

Caution: The hands should always be washed immediately after handling preparations which may contain *E. vermicularis* eggs. Most preparations will contain infective eggs by the time they reach the laboratory for examination.

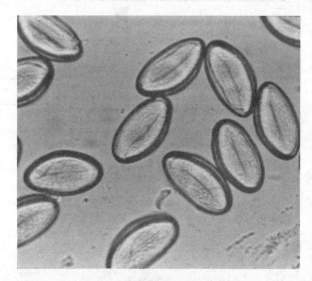

Plate 21.2   Adhesive tape preparation showing embryonated eggs of *Enterobius vermicularis*, as seen with the 40x objective. *Courtesy of H. Zaiman.*

Identification of an *Enterobius vermicularis* worm

Worms may be recovered during a clinical examination of the patient or occasionally in a faecal specimen. Only female worms will be found.

Features used to identify an *E. vermicularis* female worm are as follows:

- It is small, measuring only 8-13 mm in length and resembling a small piece of white thread (hence the name threadworm).

- When examined with a magnifying lens, the long pointed tail will be seen and also the characteristic shaped anterior end (see Fig. 21.3).

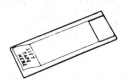

a Cellulose-tape slide
preparation

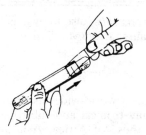

b Hold slide against tongue
depressor one inch from end
and lift long portion of tape
from slide

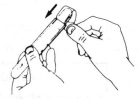

c Loop tape over end of
depressor to expose
gummed surface

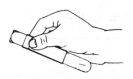

d Hold tape and slide against
tongue depressor

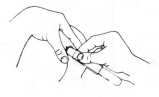

e Press gummed surfaces against
several areas of perianal region

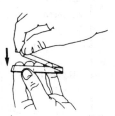

f Replace tape on slide

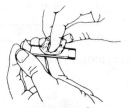

g Smooth tape with cotton
or gauze

Note: Specimens are best obtained
a few hours after the person has
retired, perhaps at 10 or 11P.M., or
the first thing in the morning before
a bowel movement or bath.

Fig. 21.4 Recovery of the eggs of *Enterobius vermicularis* from perianal skin using cellulose adhesive tape.
Reproduced with permission from US Air Force and the Army, Clinical Laboratory Procedures - Parasitology.
After Melvin and Brooke.

21:4 *STRONGYLOIDES STERCORALIS*

Strongyloides stercoralis, also known as the dwarf threadworm, causes strongyloidiasis.

Distribution

S. stercoralis has a world-wide distribution. It is endemic in many tropical and subtropical countries including those of Africa, Asia and South America.

Transmission and life cycle

Strongyloidiasis is transmitted in the following ways:

- By filariform (infective) larvae penetrating the skin.

- By autoinfection (self-infection) with rhabditiform larvae (first stage larvae) developing into filariform larvae (infective larvae) in faecal matter on perianal skin followed by penetration of the skin.

- By autoinfection with rhabditiform larvae developing into filariform larvae in the intestine followed by penetration of the gut wall.

Transmammary transmission of *Strongyloides* larvae can also occur, i.e. larvae are transmitted from mother to infant in breast milk.

Reservoir hosts for *S. stercoralis* include monkeys and dogs but human transmission is essentially from person to person.

Life cycle

— Following penetration, the larvae enter small blood vessels and follow a heart-lung migration during which they develop (see 21:1).

— After migrating up the trachea, the larvae are

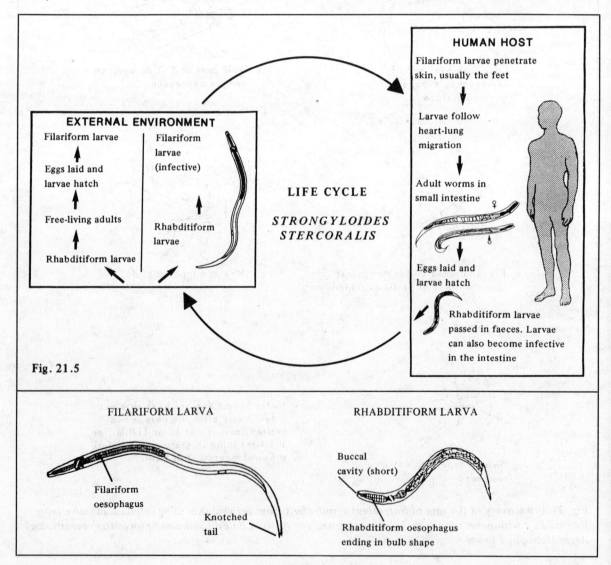

LIFE CYCLE

STRONGYLOIDES STERCORALIS

EXTERNAL ENVIRONMENT

Filariform larvae
↑
Eggs laid and larvae hatch
↑
Free-living adults
↑
Rhabditiform larvae

Filariform larvae (infective)
↑
Rhabditiform larvae

HUMAN HOST

Filariform larvae penetrate skin, usually the feet
↓
Larvae follow heart-lung migration
↓
Adult worms in small intestine
↓
Eggs laid and larvae hatch
↓
Rhabditiform larvae passed in faeces. Larvae can also become infective in the intestine

Fig. 21.5

FILARIFORM LARVA

Filariform oesophagus

Knotched tail

RHABDITIFORM LARVA

Buccal cavity (short)

Rhabditiform oesophagus ending in bulb shape

swallowed. They mature in the intestinal tract. Because male worms have rarely been found in humans, it is thought that mating between male and female worms is not essential for reproduction of the parasite.

Female worms become embedded in the wall of the small intestine and lay eggs. Male worms are expelled.

Mature S. stercoralis female worms: They are very small, measuring only about 2 mm in length. There is a small buccal cavity surrounded by four lips.

— Very soon after the eggs are laid the rhabditiform larvae hatch out in the intestine. They either develop in the intestine into infective larvae and penetrate the intestinal wall (causing autoinfection) or they are passed out in the faeces.

— Rhabditiform larvae which are expelled in the faeces are capable, under suitable conditions, of developing into infective larvae in the soil within 3-4 days.

The larvae can remain infective in the soil for several months. The life cycle is continued by the larvae penetrating human skin.

Free-living existence
Given favourable climatic conditions *S. stercoralis* can follow a free-living existence for several generations. Instead of the the rhabditiform larvae in the soil developing into filariform larvae they are able to develop directly into mature egg-producing worms in the soil. Rhabditiform larvae that hatch from eggs laid in the soil may grow into infective filariform larvae and require a human host in which to become mature worms.

Note: The life cycle of *S. stercoralis* is shown in Fig. 21.5.

Clinical features and pathology
When penetrating the skin, *S. stercoralis* larvae may cause an itchy dermatitis and rash. During the heart-lung migration of the larvae, allergic and respiratory symptoms may occur and there may be haemorrhages in the lung alveoli.

Mature worms can cause acute attacks of diarrhoea often with blood and mucus being passed. Damage to the intestinal mucosa by mature worms can develop into ulcerative enteritis, leading to anaemia and low plasma protein levels. Abdominal pain is common and symptoms can resemble those of a duodenal ulcer.

Heavy infections (especially common in children) may result in malabsorption, steatorrhoea, and dehydration with electrolyte disturbance. There is usually an eosinophilia.

Autoinfection with *S. stercoralis* can become overwhelming and sometimes fatal when the body's normal immune responses are reduced, e.g. by drugs, malnutrition, pregnancy or puerperium, or when other diseases are present which cause immune deficiency or immunosuppression. In such infections, larvae can be found in most tissues and serous cavities of the body. It is therefore important to check for strongyloidiasis in those at risk of developing serious widespread infection.

Prevention and control
- Preventing soil becoming faecally polluted by:
  — Providing and using adequate latrines.
  — Avoiding the use of untreated human faeces as fertilizer.

- Preventing the entry of larvae by wearing protective footware.

- Treating those infected.

LABORATORY DIAGNOSIS

Laboratory confirmation of strongyloidiasis is by:

☐ Finding *S. stercoralis* larvae in faeces.
☐ Finding *S. stercoralis* larvae in duodenal aspirates.

Note: In widespread infections, larvae can be found in most body fluids.

Examination of faeces for *Strongyloides stercoralis* larvae
Because *S. stercoralis* larvae tend to be excreted at intervals and can be few in number, concentration techniques should be used if infection is suspected

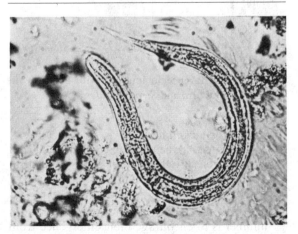

Plate 21.3 Larva of *Strongyloides stercoralis* as seen with the 40x objective. *Courtesy of A. C. Rijpstra and Royal Tropical Institute, Amsterdam.*

and the larvae are not detected in a direct physiological saline preparation.

Direct saline preparation

S. stercoralis larvae are often found in mucus passed with the faeces. Examination of a direct saline preparation is described in 13:2. The following features identify the larva of *S. stercoralis*:

Larva of *Strongyloides stercoralis*

- It is actively motile except in formalin preparations when the immobilized larva can be identified by its form.

- It is large, measuring 200-300 μm $\times$ 15 μm and is unsheathed.

- Shows a typical rhabditiform bulbed oesophagus (see Fig. 21.5).

- It can be distinguished from a hookworm larva (sometimes seen in faeces more than 24 h old) by its shorter buccal cavity (mouth cavity) as shown in Plate 21.4.

  To examine the buccal cavity of a motile larva, run a drop of Dobell's iodine under the cover glass to immobilize the larva. Examine using the 40× objective.

Illustrations: See Plate 21.3, 21.4 and colour Plate 27.

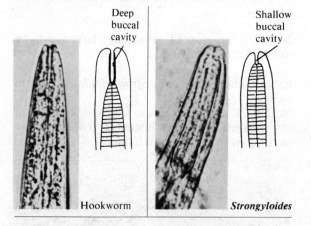

Plate 21.4 **Difference in buccal cavity between the larvae of hookworm and *Strongyloides*.**

Concentration techniques

- *S. stercoralis* larvae are well concentrated (but immobilized) by the formol ether concentration technique described in 13:4.

- Alternatively, a simple method of detecting *S. stercoralis* larvae when they are few in number is to encourage their emergence from faeces into water and then examine the water for the motile larvae as described in the following technique.

Water emergence technique for detecting Strongyloides stercoralis larvae

A *fresh* (not more than 2 hours old) formed or semiformed faecal specimen is required. The method is as follows:

1. Using a piece of stick, make a central deep depression in the specimen. Fill the depression with warm water (not over 37 °C).

2. Incubate the specimen in a 35-37 °C incubator or on a warm part of the bench for 1½-3 hours during which time the larvae will migrate out of the faeces into the warm water.

3. Using a plastic bulb or other pipette, transfer some of the water to a slide and cover with a cover glass. Alternatively, transfer all the water to a conical tube, centrifuge, and transfer the sediment to a slide.

4. Examine the preparation microscopically for motile larvae using the 10× objective with the condenser iris closed sufficiently to give good contrast.

Note: The examination of unformed specimens for motile *S. stercoralis* larvae using a modified Baermann water emergence technique is described in 13:12.

Examination of duodenal aspirates for *S. stercoralis* larvae

1. Transfer the specimen to a conical tube and centrifuge at medium to high speed for about 5 minutes.

2. Using a Pasteur pipette, remove and discard the supernatant fluid. Transfer the sediment to a slide and cover with a cover glass.

3. Examine microscopically for motile larvae using the 10× objective with the condenser iris closed sufficiently to give good contrast.

Note: The string capsule *Enterotest* (as used for diagnosing giardiasis) can also be used for recovering *Strongyloides* larvae from duodenal contents, (see 14:4).

STRONGYLOIDES FUELLEBORNI

S. fuelleborni is a natural parasite of monkeys and dogs but it can also infect humans.

Human *S. fuelleborni* and *S. fuelleborni*-like infections have been reported from tropical Africa and Papua New Guinea, especially in young children and infants.

In Papua New Guinea, *S. fuelleborni* infections are associated with an acute infantile disease known as 'Swollen Belly Syndrome'.

LABORATORY DIAGNOSIS

S. fuelleborni infection can be diagnosed by finding eggs in *fresh* faeces.

Egg of S. fuelleborni

- It is colourless.
- Oval in shape and measures about 50 × 35 μm.
- When passed, it contains a partially developed larva.

21:5 *TRICHURIS TRICHIURA*

Trichuris trichiura, also known as the whipworm, causes trichuriasis.

Distribution

T. trichiura has a world-wide distribution but is more commonly found in warm moist climates. It is the most prevalent helminth in the Caribbean and is also widespread in South East Asia and tropical Africa. It is rarely found in arid areas and at high altitudes.

Transmission and life cycle

T. trichiura is spread by faecal pollution of the soil. A person becomes infected by ingesting infective eggs in contaminated food or from contaminated fingers.

Children are more often infected than adults, often as a result of playing on faecally contaminated ground.

Life cycle

— Following ingestion of infective eggs the larvae hatch in the small intestine and penetrate villi.

— After about a week's development, the larvae leave the small intestine and migrate to the large intestine (caecum) where they develop into mature worms. The thin anterior part of the worms becomes embedded in the intestinal mucosa.

> *Mature T. trichiura worms*: They have a characteristic whip-like shape, being coiled and narrow at the anterior end and wide at the tail end (see Fig. 21.6).

The female worm measures up to 50 mm in length and the male up to 40 mm. The male has a coiled tail with a single spicule.

— After mating, the female worms lay eggs which are passed in the faeces.

— In damp warm soil the larvae develop and after 2-3 weeks each egg contains an infective larva.

  The eggs can remain infective for several months in moist warm soil but they are unable to withstand desiccation.

Note: The life cycle of *T. trichiura* is shown in Fig. 21.6.

Clinical features and pathology

Light *T. trichiura* infections produce few symptoms but heavy infections can cause abdominal pain and diarrhoea often with blood being passed. There is usually an eosinophilia.

In young children, severe infections can cause chronic diarrhoea, intestinal ulceration, anaemia, failure to develop at the normal rate, weight loss, and prolapse of the rectum. Massive infections can be fatal.

Severe trichuriasis is thought to increase the risk of infection with *Entamoeba histolytica* and pathogenic enterobacteria such as *Shigella* species. Migrating worms occasionally cause appendicitis.

Prevention and control

- Preventing soil becoming faecally polluted by:
  - Providing and using adequate latrines.
  - Avoiding the use of untreated human faeces as fertilizer.

- Treating individuals as part of a control programme.

LABORATORY DIAGNOSIS

Laboratory confirmation of trichuriasis is by:

☐ Finding *T. trichiura* eggs in faeces.

Note: Heavy infections can be diagnosed clinically by examining the rectum for worms using a proctoscope.

Examination of faeces for *T. trichiura* eggs

Many eggs are produced by the female worms and

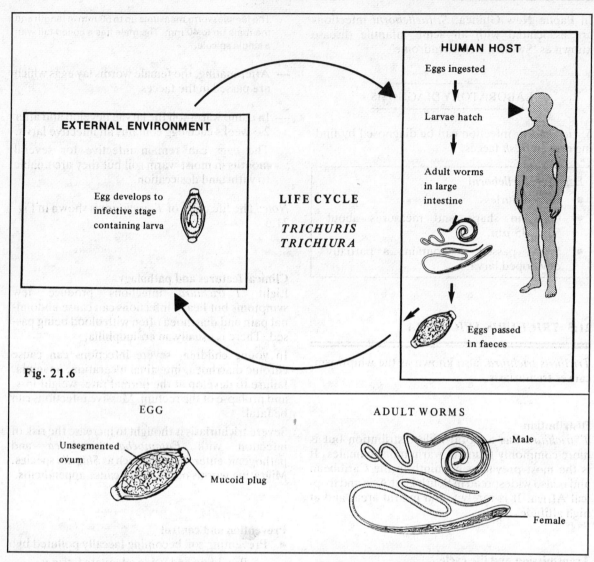

HUMAN HOST

Eggs ingested

Larvae hatch

Adult worms
in large
intestine

Eggs passed
in faeces

EXTERNAL ENVIRONMENT

Egg develops to
infective stage
containing larva

LIFE CYCLE

TRICHURIS
TRICHIURA

Fig. 21.6

EGG

Unsegmented
ovum

Mucoid plug

ADULT WORMS

Male

Female

therefore concentration techniques are not required to detect significant infections.

Direct saline preparation
The direct examination of faeces for helminth eggs is described in 13:2. The following features identify the egg of *T. trichiura*:

Egg of Trichuris trichiura

- It is yellow-brown and measures about 50 × 25 μm.
- Has a characteristic barrel shape with a colourless protruding mucoid plug at each end.
- Contains a central granular mass which is the unsegmented ovum.

Illustrations: See Plate 21.5 and colour Plate 26.

The laboratory report should include a semiquantitative estimation of the number of eggs (see 13:2) because heavy *T. trichiura* infections are associated with serious complications, especially in children.

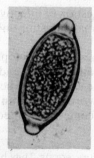

Plate 21.5 Egg of *Trichuris trichiura* as seen with the 40x objective. *Courtesy of K. L. Frampton.*

21:6 *CAPILLARIA PHILIPPINENSIS*

Capillaria philippinensis is a very small whipworm which is normally parasitic in fish-eating birds but can infect humans causing capillariasis.

Distribution
C. philippinensis as its name suggests is found in the Philippine Islands where it is fairly widely distributed in northern Luzon. It is also found in Thailand and more recently infections have been reported from Japan.

Transmission and life cycle
C. philippinensis is transmitted by the ingestion of infective eggs in raw, undercooked, or pickled fish. Occasionally infective larvae develop in the intestine and cause autoinfection.

Life cycle
— Following human ingestion, the larvae hatch and develop into mature worms in the small intestine. The worms become embedded in the jejunal mucosa.

   Mature C. philippinensis worms: They are similar in appearance to *T. trichiura* worms except that they are much smaller whipworms. The male worm measures 2.1-3.7 mm in length and the female 2.6-4.9 mm.

— Female worms produce eggs which are passed in the faeces.

— Fish-eating birds are thought to be the natural definitive hosts of *C. philippinensis*. Eggs passed by definitive hosts require a period of development in the environment before becoming infective. The larval stages of *C. philippinensis* have been found in several species of fresh and salt water fish.

Clinical features and pathology
Early and mild infections cause abdominal pain, intestinal 'gurgling', and chronic watery diarrhoea.

Heavy infections can lead to muscle wasting and oedema caused by loss of protein and severe malabsorption of fats and sugars. Plasma potassium, sodium and calcium are reduced.

Prevention and control
Capillariasis is prevented by cooking thoroughly fish which may contain infective larvae. Estuary fish in which *C. philippinensis* larvae have been found include the bacto, bagsit and bagsan. Crustaceans may act as carrier hosts.

Laboratory confirmation of *C. philippinensis* is by:

☐ Finding eggs in faeces.

Examination of faeces for *C. philippinensis* eggs
The eggs can be few in number and therefore if infection is suspected and the eggs are not found in direct preparations, a concentration technique should be used.

Direct saline preparation
Examination of a direct saline preparation for helminth eggs is described in 13:2. The following features identify the egg of *C. philippinensis*:

Egg of *Capillaria philippinensis*
Features used to identify the egg and differentiate it from *T. trichiura* are as follows:

● Smaller than *T. trichiura*, measuring about 45 × 21 μm.

● It is yellow-brown but less elliptical in shape than *T. trichiura*.

● The plugs (one at each end of the egg) are smaller and do not protrude like those of *T. trichiura*.

Illustrations: See Plate 21.6.

Concentration techniques
C. philippinensis eggs are well concentrated by the formol ether technique described in 13:4.

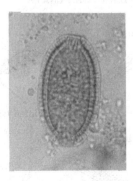

Plate 21.6 Egg of *Capillaria* as seen with the 40x objective. *Courtesy of H. Zaiman.*

21:7 HOOKWORMS

Hookworm infection is caused by *Necator americanus* and *Ancylostoma duodenale*.

Distribution

N. americanus is the more common hookworm infecting man in the Far East, South Asia, Pacific Islands, tropical Africa, Central and South America.

A. duodenale is found in the Middle East, in countries around the Mediterranean, and North China but can also be found with *N. americanus* in Africa, South East Asia, the Pacific Islands and South America.

Transmission and life cycle

Hookworm infection is spread by faecal pollution of the soil. Infection occurs when infective filariform larvae penetrate the skin, especially when a person is walking barefoot on infected ground.

A. duodenale can also be transmitted by ingesting infective larvae. Transmission of *A. duodenale* from mother to infant can occur when larvae are present in breast milk. The larvae can also cross the placenta. These methods of transmission are rare.

Life cycle

— Following penetration of the skin, the larvae enter small blood vessels and follow a heart-

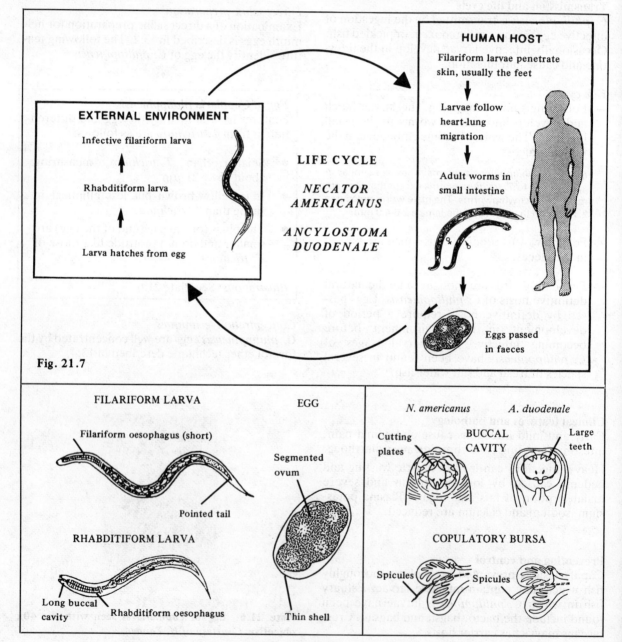

Fig. 21.7

lung migration during which they develop (see 21:1).

— After migrating up the trachea, the larvae are swallowed. They reach the small intestine where within about 6 weeks (or possibly longer for *A. duodenale*) they develop into mature worms and mate.

The worms become attached to the wall of the small intestine by sucking part of the mucosa into their mouth-parts. They ingest mucous membrane and blood from their host but much of the blood passes through the worm undigested. Some of the iron in the undigested red cells is reabsorbed by the host.

The worms, especially *A. duodenale*, migrate in the intestine in search of new sites from which to suck blood. The abandoned sites continue to bleed for some time.

Mature A. duodenale worms: Female worms measure up to 15 mm in length and male worms up to 10 mm. The male has two spicules and a characteristic bursa as shown in Fig. 21.7. The mouth is large and possesses teeth on its ventral surface and a smaller pair of teeth on its dorsal surface.

Mature N. americanus worms: They are slightly smaller than *A. duodenale* worms and bent more obviously anteriorly in the opposite direction to the body curve. The structure of the male bursa is different to that of *A. duodenale*. The mouth has two cutting plates on its ventral surface and two on its dorsal surface.

— Female worms lay eggs which are passed in the faeces. About twice as many eggs are produced by *A. duodenale* than *N. americanus*.

— Rhabditiform larvae hatch in damp, warm, well-oxygenated soil. It takes about a week for the first stage larvae to develop into infective filariform larvae.

Usually infective larvae do not live more than 2-6 weeks but in suitable surroundings the larvae can survive and remain infective for several months. They are, however, rapidly killed in dry sunlit soil.

Note: The life cycle of hookworms is shown in Fig. 21.7.

Clinical features and pathology

The first sign of hookworm infection is frequently a skin reaction at the site of larval penetration. This is known as 'ground itch' and is usually more intense in those previously infected. During the migration of the larvae through the heart and lungs, mild respiratory symptoms may develop and an eosinophilia.

Adult hookworms cause chronic blood loss. It has been estimated that a single *A. duodenale* worm ingests about 150 μl (0.15 ml) of blood per day and a *N. americanus* worm about 30 μl (0.03 ml). The test for occult blood in faeces is positive.

An iron deficiency anaemia usually develops with heavy prolonged infection, especially with *A. duodenale*. This may be severe and even fatal especially in those with inadequate iron stores and a low iron intake. Infected pregnant women are also at risk of becoming anaemic due to their increased need for iron. Loss of protein can lead to oedema.

Hookworms can live for up to 10 years in their hosts.

Cutaneous larva migrans

Penetration of the skin by filariform larvae of hookworms normally parasitic in animals can cause cutaneous larva migrans, also known as 'creeping eruption'. This condition is described in 21:8.

Prevention and control

- Preventing soil from becoming infected by:
  - Providing and using adequate latrines .
  - Avoiding the use of untreated human faeces as fertilizer.
  - Treating individuals as part of a control and health education programme.

- Preventing infective larvae penetrating the skin of the feet by wearing adequate protective footware. Open sandals are not effective barriers to infection.

LABORATORY DIAGNOSIS

Laboratory confirmation of hookworm infection is by:

□ Finding hookworm eggs in faeces.

Note: Hookworm infection is usually accompanied by a blood eosinophilia.

Examination of faeces for hookworm eggs

The direct examination of faeces is usually adequate to detect hookworm eggs. The number of eggs found in the entire preparation (approx. 2 mg faeces) should be reported because this gives an indication of the degree of infection.

Direct saline preparation

The direct examination of a faecal specimen for helminth eggs is described in 13:2.

Egg of Hookworm

Morphologically the eggs of *A. duodenale* and *N. americanus* are similar and the following features can be used to identify the egg of either species:

- It is colourless with a thin shell which appears as a black line around the ovum.

- Oval in shape, measuring about 65 × 40 μm.

- Contains an ovum which usually appears segmented. If the specimen is more than 12 hours old, a larva may be seen inside the egg. If the faeces is more than 24 hours old, the larva may hatch and must then be differentiated from a *Strongyloides* larva (see 21:4).

Note: Hookworm eggs need to be distinguished from the eggs of *Trichostrongylus* species and the eggs of *Ternidens deminutus* (hookworm-like nematodes normally parasitic in animals which can infect humans as described in 21:8).

Compared with a hookworm egg, the egg of *Trichostrongylus* is larger, more elongate and pointed at one or both ends (see Plate 21.7, right). The egg of *Ternidens deminutus* has a similar structure to a hookworm egg but is much larger, measuring about 85 μm in length.

Illustrations: See Plate 21.7 and colour Plate 25.

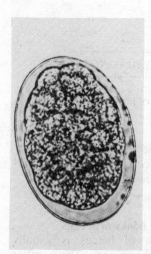 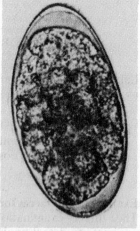

Plate 21.7 *Left* **Egg of hookworm.** *Right* **Egg of** *Trichostrongylus. Courtesy of K. L. Frampton.*

Differentiating A. duodenale and N. americanus
When examined microscopically, the eggs of *A. duodenale* and *N. americanus* look the same. If required, the two species can be differentiated by culturing the faeces at room temperature for 10 days. During this time the larvae will hatch from the eggs and develop into filariform larvae. Species identification is then possible. The technique is described in 13:13.

Concentration techniques
Hookworm eggs can be concentrated by the formol ether technique (see 13:13) or sodium chloride floatation technique (see 13:6) but significant hookworm infections can usually be detected using a direct technique.

21:8 INFECTIONS CAUSED BY ANIMAL INTESTINAL NEMATODES

TRICHOSTRONGYLUS SPECIES

Trichostrongylus nematodes, occasionally referred to as pseudo-hookworms, are mainly parasites of ruminants, equines, and rodents but several species can infect humans.

Infections have been reported from parts of Africa, Egypt, Indonesia, Iran, Iraq, South-East Asia, India, Japan, and Chile.

A person becomes infected by ingesting third stage larvae in contaminated food or drink. The adult worms live in the small intestine, with the head penetrating the mucosal wall. The head is without cutting teeth or plates. Eggs are produced which are passed in the faeces.

Like hookworms, *Trichostrongylus* worms also suck blood from their host. The clinical features of trichostrongyliasis, however, are less severe than those of hookworm infection and the treatment is different.

LABORATORY DIAGNOSIS

Laboratory confirmation of *Trichostrongylus* infection is by finding eggs in faecal specimens.

Trichostrongylus eggs are often mistaken for hookworm eggs. The features which differentiate *Trichostrongylus* eggs from those of hookworm are as follows:

Egg of Trichostrongylus
- It is longer and thinner than a hookworm egg, measuring 85-115 μm in length.

- It is more pointed at one or both ends as shown in Plate 21.7 (right).

TERNIDENS DEMINUTUS

T. deminutus is a nematode which resembles a hookworm. It is normally parasitic in monkeys and baboons but can infect man. Human infections have been reported mostly from South Africa and East Africa.

Transmission is probably by ingestion of third stage larvae. The worms are found in the large intestine. Like hookworms, *T. deminutus* worms also suck blood from their host and anaemia may develop in heavy infections.

LABORATORY DIAGNOSIS

T. deminutus eggs can be found in faeces. They have a similar structure to hookworm eggs except that they are longer, measuring up to 85 μm in length.

ANIMAL HOOKWORMS THAT CAUSE CUTANEOUS LARVA MIGRANS

Human infection with larvae of the cat and dog hookworm *Ancylostoma brasiliense* and less commonly with *Ancylostoma caninum* can cause cutaneous larva migrans.

The larvae are present in the soil and infection occurs when infective larvae penetrate the skin. In a human host the larvae are unable to develop into mature worms. Instead, they migrate in the superficial layers of the skin especially of the feet, legs, hands, thighs and back.

The wandering larvae cause allergic reactions. There is intense irritation of the inflamed larval tracks and scatching can lead to secondary infection. There is usually a marked eosinophilic leucocytosis. Most of the larvae die in the skin but occasionally they migrate to the lungs where they can cause respiratory disorders.

Note: Very occasionally, cutaneous larva migrans is caused by *Strongyloides* species or human hookworm larvae before they begin their heart-lung migration.

ROUNDWORMS THAT CAUSE VISCERAL LARVA MIGRANS

Human ingestion of the embryonated eggs of the dog roundworm *Toxocara canis* and the cat roundworm *Toxocara cati* can cause visceral larva migrans.

Infection is more common in children between 18 months and 3 years of age. The eggs are usually ingested from hands that have become contaminated when handling an infected puppy or from playing on ground contaminated with infective dog faeces.

In the human host the larvae hatch from the eggs but are unable to develop into mature worms. The larvae penetrate the intestinal wall and are carried in the blood to the liver and other organs of the body in which they become lodged and eventually die. The main organs affected are the liver, lungs, heart, brain, and eyes.

Antigens secreted by the larvae cause inflammatory host reactions with the formation of eosinophilic granulomata. Other complications depend on the sites affected. They include liver and occasionally spleen enlargement, eye damage which can lead to blindness, and disorders of the central nervous system.

LABORATORY DIAGNOSIS

With *Toxocara* infection there is an eosinophilic leucocytosis and hyperglobulinaemia. Ig M antibodies are raised with naturally occurring Anti-A and Anti-B titres of over 1 in 1000. Ig G and occasionally Ig E levels are also raised.

The best serological test to diagnose *Toxocara* infection is an ELISA which uses as antigen the secretions from *T. canis* larvae maintained in cultures. Details of this test can be obtained from the London School of Hygiene and Tropical Medicine*

* Attention of Dr C C Draper, Dept of Tropical Hygiene, London School of Hygiene and Tropical Medicine, Keppel Street, London WC1E 7HT, UK.

Recommended Reading

Bell, D. R. *Lecture Notes on Tropical Medicine*, Blackwell Scientific Publications, 2nd Ed, 1985. Paperback priced £9.80.

Peters, W., Gilles, H. M. *A Colour Atlas of Tropical Medicine and Parasitology*, Wolfe Medical Publications, 2nd Ed, 1981. ELBS edition priced £9.00

World Health Organization. *Intestinal Protozoan and Helminth Infections*. WHO, Technical Report Series, No. 666, 1981.

Knight, R. *Parasitic Disease in Man*. Churchill Livingstone, 1982. ELBS edition priced £4.50.

Filarial Worms
Other Tissue Nematodes

22:1 CLASSIFICATION AND FEATURES OF TISSUE NEMATODES

The general characteristics of nematodes (roundworms) are described at the beginning of the Parasitology Section in 12:4.

Classification of tissue nematodes of medical importance

Superfamily FILARIOIDEA (Filarial worms)
Species *Wuchereria bancrofti*
  Brugia malayi
  Brugia timori
  Loa loa
  Onchocerca volvulus

Less pathogenic or nonpathogenic filariae:
  Mansonella perstans†
  Mansonella ozzardi
  Mansonella streptocerca‡

  † Formerly called *Dipetalonema perstans* and *Acanthocheilonema perstans*.

  ‡ Formerly called *Dipetalonema streptocerca*

Superfamily DRACUNCULOIDEA
Species *Dracunculus medinensis*

Superfamily TRICHINELLOIDEA
Species *Trichinella* species

Note: The intestinal nematodes *Trichuris trichiura* and *Capillaria* species also belong to the superfamily Trichinelloidea. These species are described with the other intestinal nematodes in Chapter 21 (see 21:5 and 21:6).

Animal tissue nematodes that occasionally infect humans

Superfamily FILARIOIDEA
Species *Dirofilaria* species

Superfamily METASTRONGYLOIDEA
Species *Angiostrongylus cantonensis*

Superfamily SPIRUROIDEA
Species *Gnathostoma spinigerum*

General features of tissue nematodes that infect humans

- Adult worms (according to species) live in the lymphatics, subcutaneous tissue, connective tissue, muscle, or body cavities.

- Female worms are viviparous, i.e. produce live larvae.

- Humans are the only or most significant hosts of the tissue nematodes of major medical importance except for *T. spiralis* where the natural hosts are animals, especially wild and domestic pigs, bears and rats.

- Filarial worms are transmitted through the bite of an insect vector. *T. spiralis* is transmitted by ingestion of larvae in infected tissue and *D. medinensis* by ingestion of an infected intermediate host (*Cyclops*).

- The immature first stage larva of filarial worms is called a microfilaria.

  Microfilariae of pathogenic filarial worms that live in the blood show what is called periodicity, i.e. they are released periodically into the peripheral blood from lung blood and are therefore found in peripheral blood in greater numbers during certain hours (see later text).

  Nonpathogenic blood microfilariae and microfilariae that are found in the skin are nonperiodic.

Periodicity of pathogenic blood microfilariae
Periodicity is thought to be an adaptation by microfilariae to the biting habits of their insect vectors. The exact mechanism of periodicity is not fully understood. It is influenced by the sleeping, waking, and bodily activities of the host and may depend (according to species) on changes in temperature and chemical composition and differences in oxygen tension between venous and arterial blood. The different terms used to describe the periodicity of microfilariae are as follows:

Nocturnal periodicity
Microfilariae are present in greatest numbers in the peripheral blood during night hours, e.g. periodic *Wuchereria bancrofti*, *Brugia malayi* and *Brugia timori*.

Diurnal periodicity
Microfilariae are present in greatest numbers in the peripheral blood during day hours, e.g. *Loa loa*.

Nocturnal subperiodicity or diurnal subperiodicity
Microfilariae can be found in the peripheral blood throughout the 24 hours with only a slight increase in numbers during day or night hours e.g. subperiodic *W. bancrofti* and subperiodic *B. malayi*.

- Laboratory confirmation of infection with *W. bancrofti*, *Brugia* species and *L. loa* is by finding microfilariae in the blood and sometimes in urine and other body fluids and with *O. volvulus* by finding microfilariae in the skin. Infection with *D. medinensis* is confirmed by detecting larvae in water surrounding a ruptured ulcer and infection with *T. spiralis* is by finding encysted larvae in a muscle biopsy.

Serological tests are also available to assist in the diagnosis of trichinellosis.

Note: The morphology of the medically important tissue nematodes is shown in the life cycle figures contained in the subsequent subunits of this Chapter.

Tissue Nematodes of Major Medical Importance
LIFE CYCLE SUMMARIES

Wuchereria bancrofti *Brugia malayi* *Brugia timori*	*Loa loa*	*Onchocerca volvulus*	*Trichinella spiralis*	*Dracunculus medinensis*
Infective larvae penetrate skin through bite wound made by insect vector			Larvae ingested in undercooked pork or flesh of bush pig or bear	Ingested by drinking water containing infected *Cyclops*
Adult worms in lymphatic system	Adult worms in connective tissue	Adult worms in subcutaneous tissue	Adult worms in small intestine	Adult worms in connective tissue
MICROFILARIAE IN BLOOD	MICROFILARIAE IN BLOOD	MICROFILARIAE IN SKIN, BODY FLUIDS, OR URINE	LARVAE IN MUSCLE†	LARVAE IN WATER
Taken up by mosquito Larvae develop into infective forms	Taken up by *Chrysops* Larvae develop into infective forms	Taken up by *Simulium* Larvae develop into infective forms		Taken up by *Cyclops* Larvae develop into infective forms

† In nature the life cycle of *Trichinella spiralis* is maintained between rodents, domestic pigs, bush pigs, bears and other carnivores. Adult worms and larvae are found in the same host but a change of host is required to complete the life cycle. Infection occurs when a pig or other carnivore ingests an infected rodent or the flesh of another carnivore in which infective larvae are encysted. The larvae develop into adult worms. When mature, they produce larvae which are carried in the blood circulation to striated muscle where they encyst. The larvae are infective to other carnivores and to humans. Human infection is a zoonosis.

22:2 WUCHERERIA BANCROFTI

Wuchereria bancrofti causes lymphatic filariasis. The term bancroftian filariasis is often used to describe the form of filariasis caused by *W. bancrofti*.

Lymphatic filariasisis is also caused by Brugia *species which are described in 22:3.*

It has been estimated that 81.6 million people are infected with *W. bancrofti* and 8.6 million with *Brugia* species.[1] These numbers include both microfilaria positive people and those with filarial disease who are microfilaria negative.

Two variants of *W. bancrofti* are recognized:

- Periodic (nocturnal) *W. bancrofti*. This is the most widespread.
- Subperiodic (nocturnal and diurnal) *W. bancrofti*.

Note: Terms used to describe the periodicity of microfilariae are explained in 22:1 and collection times are given under *Laboratory Diagnosis*.

Distribution

W. bancrofti is the most widely distributed of the filarial worms with the most seriously affected areas being in India, South-East Asia, China, east coast of Africa, and the Pacific islands.

Periodic *W. bancrofti* is endemic in tropical America, Caribbean, tropical Africa, Egypt, the Middle East, South-East Asia, southern and eastern China, the Far East and New Guinea.

The diurnal subperiodic variant of *W. bancrofti* is found mainly in the eastern Pacific (Polynesia) and

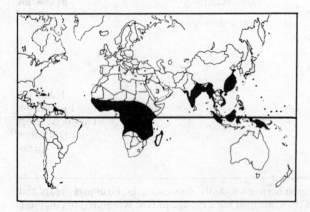

Fig. 22.1 Distribution of *Wuchereria bancrofti*. Subperiodic strains occur in South Asia and Polynesia.
Compiled from information in WHO Technical Report Series No. 702, 1984.

is often referred to as the Pacific form. The nocturnal subperiodic variant is found especially in Thailand and Viet Nam.

W. bancrofti is found with *B. malayi* in parts of South-East Asia and South India. The distribution of both periodic and subperiodic *W. bancrofti* is shown in Fig. 22.1.

Transmission and life cycle

Periodic *W. bancrofti* is transmitted by species of mosquitoes belonging to the genera *Culex*, *Anopheles*, and *Aedes*. Subperiodic *W. bancrofti* is transmitted by *Aedes* mosquitoes.

The appearance, breeding and biting habits of mosquitoes are described in 23:3.

Life cycle
— Infective larvae are deposited on human skin when an infected mosquito vector takes a blood meal. The larvae penetrate the skin through the bite wound.

— By way of peripheral blood vessels, the larvae reach lymphatic vessels and lymph nodes. Development takes place in the lymphatics.

— Within 3-15 months, the larvae become mature male and female worms.

Mature W. bancrofti *worms*: They appear creamy white with a smooth surface. The anterior end tapers to a rounded slightly swollen head. The male measures 23-40 × 0.1 mm. Its tail is sharply curved with two spicules.

The female measures about 50-65 × 0.16 mm, has a curved tail, and tapers towards the front end.

The worms can live for many years in their host depending in part on the extent of the host's immune response. Their mean lifetime is 4-6 years but they can survive up to 15 years or more.

— The adults mate and produce many sheathed larvae which enter the blood. These immature first-stage larvae are called microfilariae and can be found in the blood about 1 year after infection. When only a few worms are present, it may not be possible to detect microfilariae in the blood.

— The microfilariae are taken up by a mosquito vector when it sucks blood. Those microfilariae which are not ingested die within 6 months - 2 years.

— In the stomach of the mosquito the microfilariae lose their sheath and migrate from the midgut to the thorax of the vector where they develop into infective larvae.

Development in the mosquito takes 1-2 weeks and requires a temperature of 26 °C and a relative humidity of over 70%.

— Mature infective larvae migrate to the mouth-parts of the mosquito ready to be transmitted when the insect next takes a blood meal.

The life cycle of *W. bancrofti* is shown in Fig. 22.2 (that of *Brugia* species is similar).

Clinical features and pathology

Only a proportion of persons infected with *W. bancrofti* develop clinical symptoms. Lymphatic filariasis is characterized by recurrent attacks of fever with painful inflamed lymphatics. Damage to the lymphatics leads to thickening and eventual blockage of lymphatic vessels. The lymphatics involved are mainly those of the limbs, genital organs (especially those of the spermatic cord) and breasts. Obstruction to the flow of lymph causes swelling, fibrosis and eventually elephantiasis.

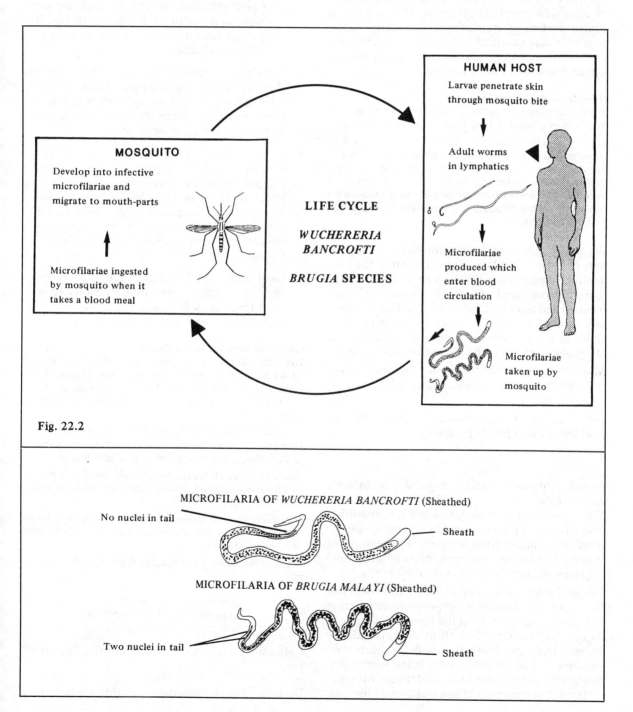

Fig. 22.2

The features and pathology of bancroftian filariasis depend on the sites occupied by developing and mature worms, the number of worms present, length of infection, and the immune responses of the host especially to damaged and dead worms. Symptoms of infection often differ from one endemic area to another.

In chronic lymphatic filariasis and usually after repeated infection, hydrocoele can occur. It is most commonly seen in East Africa, Japan and China. Microfilariae can occasionally be found in hydrocoele fluid. Elephantiasis is a complication of advanced lymphatic filariasis. It is seen as a coarse thickening, hardening and cracking of the skin overlying enlarged fibrosed tissues. The condition is more commonly seen in parts of Africa, China, India, and Pacific regions.

Non-filarial elephantiasis

In tropical countries, causes of elephantiasis other than filarial worms include tuberculosis and siliceous deposits.

Endemic elephantiasis of the lower legs associated with siliceous deposits has been reported from the highlands of Kenya, Tanzania, Ethiopia, Ruanda, Burundi, western Sudan, Cape Verde Islands, the Cameroons and Rajastan in India. Damage to local lymphatics with obstruction occurs when the deposits are absorbed from the soil through bare feet.

An uncommon complication of chronic bancroftian filariasis is chyluria. It occurs when the urogenital lymphatic vessels which are linked to those that transport chyle from the intestine become blocked and rupture. Chyle and occasionally blood and microfilariae can be found in the urine especially in early morning specimens. Microfilariae are usually present in the fibrin clots which form.

Most patients with lymphatic filariasis show reduced immune responses. Eosinophilia is usually present.

Infections with subperiodic *W. bancrofti* are associated with filarial abscesses.

Occult filariasis and tropical pulmonary eosinophilia[2]

The term occult filariasis refers to a rare condition which is thought to be caused by a hypersensitivity reaction to microfilarial antigens. The features of lymphatic filariasis are not present and microfilariae are not detected in the blood.

Tropical pulmonary eosinophilia is a form of occult filariasis in which there is a hypersensitive reaction to microfilariae present in the lung and lymphatic tissues. It is found particularly in filariasis endemic areas of India and South-East Asia. It affects both children and adults with males being more commonly affected than females. It interferes with breathing and can lead to chronic pulmonary fibrosis.

Symptoms are worse at night. There is a marked eosinophilia, raised erythrocyte sedimentation rate, and high levels of filarial antibody including high titres of Ig E. Eosinophils often appear vacuolated.

Prevention and control

- Control of mosquito vectors by:
  - Studying the ecology and behaviour of local vectors to reduce mosquito breeding and eradicate breeding sites.
  - Using effective insecticides but the most important vector of *W. bancrofti* is *Culex quinquefasciatus* and this is resistant to most insecticides.

- Avoiding mosquito bites by wearing suitable clothing, using mosquito nets, and as far as possible making houses mosquito-proof. The use of bed-netting impregnated with pyrethroids is proving successful in many areas.

- Treating infected individuals with diethylcarbamazine (DEC) as part of a mass control programme to prevent mosquitoes becoming infected. *W. bancrofti* has no known animal reservoir host. Community-administered DEC mass treatment (with careful monitoring of side effects) has been successful in East Africa and China.

- Informing those living in endemic areas about the cause, early symptoms, detection and control of lymphatic filariasis. Community participation is essential in the control of filariasis.

Further information about filariasis

The 1984 World Health Organization Technical Report Series No. 702, *Lymphatic Filariasis* gives detailed information about vectors, clinical features, pathology, treatment, control and the socioeconomic aspects of lymphatic filariasis.[1]

The 1984 Supplement, *Recent Advances in Research on Filariasis* covers treatment, immunological aspects, epidemiology, and the control of lymphatic filariasis.[3]

The 1984 review, *Filariasis* includes abstracts from papers on filariasis published between January 1983 and March 1984.[4]

The application of science and technology at primary health care level in filarial diseases is discussed in the 1985 WHO paper of Duke.[5]

See also *Recommended Reading* at the end of this Chapter.

LABORATORY DIAGNOSIS

Laboratory confirmation of bancroftian filariasis is by:

☐ Detecting *W. bancrofti* microfilariae in blood.

□ Occasionally *W. bancrofti* microfilariae can be found in chylous urine or hydrocoele fluid.

Note: A blood eosinophilia is found with *W. bancrofti* infection.

Examination of blood for *W. bancrofti* microfilariae

Microfilariae begin to appear in the blood a year or more after infection. They are rarely found when the lymphatics have become obstructed.

Blood must be collected at the correct time, i.e. during the hours when the greatest number of microfilariae are likely to be present in the blood as follows:

Collection times for W. bancrofti
— Periodic *W. bancrofti*: Collect blood between 22.00-0400 hours (time of peak density is 24.00 h).
— Subperiodic (nocturnal) *W. bancrofti*: Collect blood between 20.00-22.00 h (time of peak density is 21.00 h).
— Subperiodic (diurnal) *W. bancrofti*: Collect blood between 14.00-18.00 h (time of peak density is 16.00 h).

Outside of these times *W. bancrofti* microfilariae may still be present in the blood, especially the subperiodic type, but they will be more difficult to detect. The distribution of periodic and subperiodic *W. bancrofti* is shown in Fig. 22.1.

Use of DEC to detect nocturnal periodic W. bancrofti during day hours
The use of diethylcarbamazine (DEC) to stimulate the circulation of nocturnal periodic *W. bancrofti* microfilariae during day hours is not necessary or recommended especially when using a filtration technique.[5]
The DEC day test must *not* be used in areas where *Loa loa* or *Onchocera volvulus* is found, i.e. in tropical Africa and parts of South and Central America (see Figs. 22.1, 22.4, 22.8). This is because DEC can cause severe allergic and damaging reactions in persons with loiasis or onchocerciasis.[1]

Blood specimen
The amount of blood required and whether to collect capillary or venous blood will depend on the technique used. Full details of techniques that are used to detect and identify *W. bancrofti* microfilariae in blood, including concentration techniques, can be found in 22:6.

W. bancrofti microfilariae need to be distinguished from those of *Brugia* species, *L. loa*, and *Mansonella* species which can also be found in some of the areas where *W. bancrofti* occurs (see Chart 22.II at the end of 22:6).

Wuchereria bancrofti microfilaria
- It is large in size compared with *Mansonella* species, measuring 275-300 × 8-10 μm.
- Sheath is present.
- Body nuclei are fewer and more distinct than in other species.
- There are no nuclei in the end of the tail which is pointed.

Illustrations: See Plate 22.1, Plate 22.2, Plate 22.9 at the end of 22:6 and colour Plate 32.

Examination of urine for *W. bancrofti* microfilariae

In chronic bancroftian filariasis a condition called chyluria can occur, i.e. passing of chyle in urine.

Chyle consists of lymph and particles of digested fat (soluble in ether). Urine containing chyle appears creamy white. When blood is also present, the urine appears pinkish-white. Microfilariae can often be found in the fibrin clots which form.

Specimen: Collect 10-20 ml of early morning urine, i.e. first urine passed by the person after waking.

Method
1. Report the appearance of the urine. Add about 2 ml of ether and shake to dissolve the chyle.
   Caution: Ether is highly flammable, therefore use well away from an open flame and make sure the room is well-ventilated.

2. Centrifuge the specimen at slow to medium speed, (approx. 2000 rpm). High speed centrifugation may cause the microfilariae to lose their sheath.

3. Remove and discard the supernatant fluid.
   If the sediment contains blood, lyze the red cells by adding an equal volume of saponin-saline solution (Reagent No. 64) or if unavailable add an equal volume of water. Mix and centrifuge again. Discard the supernatant fluid.

4. Transfer the sediment to a slide and cover with a cover glass. Examine microscopically for motile microfilariae using the 10× objective with the condenser aperture closed sufficiently to give good contrast.

5. If microfilariae are seen, run a drop of 0.1% methylene blue – saline (Reagent No. 49) under the cover glass. This will stain the nuclei and show whether the microfilariae are sheathed.
   The identifying features of *W. bancrofti* mic-

rofilariae are summarized and illustrated in 22:6.

Note: O. volvulus microfilariae may also be found in urine in heavy infections and after treatment with diethylcarbamazine. Unlike *W. bancrofti*, the microfilariae of *O. volvulus* are unsheathed. Other identifying features of *O. volvulus* microfilariae are described and illustrated in 22:7.

Examination of aspirates for *W. bancrofti* microfilariae

The method described above for examining urine (omitting the addition of ether) can also be used to examine aspirates of hydrocele fluid or lymph gland fluid for *W. bancrofti* microfilariae.

Immunodiagnosis of bancroftian filariasis

Immunodiagnostic tests are of value because microfilariae are often difficult to find in the blood of patients with bancroftian filariasis. Such tests, however, are not widely used routinely because the antigens required are not as yet commercially available or sufficiently sensitive or specific.

Problems in developing serological tests for the immunodiagnosis of lymphatic filariasis include lack of laboratory models, the difficulty in obtaining adequate quantities of human filarioids from patients, and the cross-reactivity of all filarial antigens. A number of animal filarioids have been tried as antigens. The most promising tests are fluorescent antibody tests (FAT) and enzyme linked immunosorbent assays (ELISA) using *Brugia pahangi* antigen.

It is to be hoped that monoclonal antibodies will be developed to detect specific filarial antigens in blood or urine. The finding of circulating antigens is an indication of active infection but their absence does not exclude infection because the antigens may have become bound to antibodies, forming immune complexes.

Note: A 1984 review of the immunological aspects of lymphatic filariasis, including immunodiagnosis, can be found in the paper of Ottesen.[7]

22:3 *BRUGIA* SPECIES

Brugia malayi and *Brugia timori* cause lymphatic filariasis. That caused by *B. malayi* is often referred to as Malayan filariasis.

The most widespread cause of lymphatic filariasis is *Wuchereria bancrofti*. This species is described in 22:2.

Two variants of *B. malayi* are recognized:
- Periodic (nocturnal) *B. malayi*. This is the most widespread.
- Subperiodic (nocturnal) *B. malayi*.

B. timori shows a nocturnal periodicity.

Note: Terms used to describe the periodicity of microfilariae are explained in 22:1 and collection times are given under *Laboratory Diagnosis*

Brugia pahangi
This species is naturally parasitic in dogs and cats. It is found in Malaysia and occasionally infects humans. Special staining procedures are required to differentiate *B. pahangi* from *B. malayi*.

Distribution

B. malayi is endemic in parts of South-East Asia including many of the islands of the Malay Archipelago. It also occurs in South-west India, the Philippines, Viet Nam, China, and South Korea.

Periodic *B. malayi* is commonly found in open swamps and the rice-growing areas of coastal regions. The subperiodic variant is found mostly in fresh water swamps in forests along major rivers.

B. timori is found only in the Lesser Sunda Islands of Indonesia. The species takes its name from the island of Timor which forms part of the group in which *B. timori* is endemic. It is found in low lying riverine and coastal areas.

B. malayi occurs in many of the places where *W. bancrofti* is also found. The distribution of *Brugia* species is shown in Fig. 22.3.

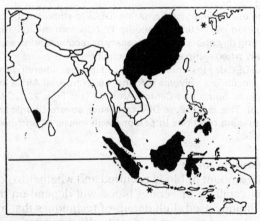

Fig. 22.3 Distribution of *Brugia malayi*. Areas where *Brugia timori* occurs are marked with an asterisk. *Compiled from information in WHO Technical Series No. 702, 1984.*

Transmission and life cycle

Nocturnal periodic *B. malayi* is transmitted mainly by species of mosquitoes belonging to the genera *Anopheles* and *Mansonia*.

Subperiodic *B. malayi* is transmitted by *Mansonia* and *Coquillettidia* mosquitoes. Monkeys are important reservoirs of subperiodic *B. malayi* in parts of Malaysia, Sumatra, and Kalimantan. Domestic cats, dogs and possibly other animals are also thought to be reservoir hosts of subperiodic *B. malayi*.

B. timori is transmitted by *Anopheles* mosquitoes.

Note: The appearance, breeding and biting habits of *Anopheles* and *Mansonia* mosquitoes are described in 23:3.

Life cycle

The life cycle of *Brugia* species is similar to that of *W. bancrofti* which is described in 22:2. It is illustrated in Fig. 22.2.

The mature worms of *Brugia* species are similar to but smaller than those of *W. bancrofti*.

Clinical features and pathology

Symptomless carriers are common among *Brugia* infected persons. There are only a few differences in the clinical features and pathology of lymphatic filariasis caused by *Brugia* species and that caused by *W. bancrofti*.

Compared with bancroftian filariasis, the symptoms of Malayan filariasis tend to develop more rapidly and children are often more affected than adults. Elephantiasis occurs less frequently and tends to involve only the lower limbs. The scrotum and spermatic cord are not usually affected and chyluria and hydrocele are rarely seen.

Filarial abscesses are common with *B. timori* infections.

Prevention and control

Control and preventive measures for *Brugia* species are similar to those described in 22:2 for *W. bancrofti*.

The use of selective weed killers has proved an effective control measure against *Mansonia* mosquitoes which are the important vectors of *Brugia malayi*.

In areas where monkeys are important reservoirs of infection, the clearing of trees around settlements is recommended.[1]

LABORATORY DIAGNOSIS

Laboratory confirmation of filariasis caused by *Brugia* species is by:

☐ Detecting *Brugia* microfilariae in blood.

Note: A blood eosinophilia can be found with *Brugia* infections.

Examination of blood for *Brugia* microfilariae

Microfilariae begin to appear in the blood about a year after infection or sometimes within a shorter period. They are rarely found when the lymphatics have become obstructed.

Blood must be collected at the correct time, i.e. during the hours when the greatest number of microfilariae are likely to be present in the blood as follows:

Collection times for Brugia species

— Periodic *Brugia malayi*: Collect blood between 22.00-04.00 hours (time of peak density is 24.00 h).

— Subperiodic *Brugia malayi*: Collect blood between 20.00-22.00 hours (time of peak density is 21.00 h).

— Periodic *Brugia timori:* Collect blood between 22.00-04.00 hours (time of peak density is 24.00 h).

Outside of these times *Brugia* microfilariae may still be present in the blood, especially subperiodic *B. malayi*, but they will be more difficult to detect.

Blood specimen

The amount of blood required and whether to collect capillary or venous blood will depend on the technique used. Full details of techniques that are used to detect and identify *Brugia* microfilariae in blood, including concentration techniques, can be found in 22:6.

Identification of Brugia microfilariae

The following are the important identifying features of *B malayi* and *B. timori* microfilariae:

Brugia malayi microfilaria
- Measures $200\text{-}275 \times 5\text{-}6\ \mu m$ (periodic variant is slightly larger).
- Stains more intensely than *W. bancrofti*. Body nuclei are dense and the body appears coiled and kinked with many small angular curves.
- Sheath is present and stains darkly.

  Loss of sheath
  In Malaysia and Indonesia the sheath of periodic *B. malayi* is often lost during drying of the blood prior to staining. Loss of the sheath has not been noticed with periodic *B. malayi* strains from other endemic areas.
- There are 2 nuclei in the end of the tail which tapers irregularly.

Illustrations: See Plate 22.3 and Plate 22.4 at the end of 22:6 and colour Plate 34.

Brugia timori microfilaria

The following features distinguish B. timori from B. malayi:

- It is longer, measuring 290-325 × 5-6 μm and less kinked.

- Sheath stains palely with Giemsa. Only about 50% of B. timori microfilariae lose their sheath.

- Body nuclei are less dense and the space at the head end (cephalic space) is longer.

Brugia microfilariae need to be distinguished from those of W. bancrofti which can also be found in some areas where Brugia species occur (see Chart 22.II in 22:6).

22:4 LOA LOA

Loa loa causes loiasis which is a subcutaneous filariasis. The disease is also known as Calabar swelling. L. loa is often referred to as the 'eye worm' because the adult worms sometimes migrate across the conjunctiva or eyelid.

Loa loa has a diurnal periodicity (see 22:1 and under Laboratory Diagnosis).

Distribution
The distribution of L. loa is restricted to the equatorial rain forest areas of West and Central Africa as shown in Fig. 22.4.

L. loa is endemic in many places where W. bancrofti also occurs.

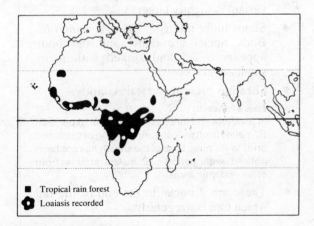

Tropical rain forest
Loaiasis recorded

Fig. 22.4 Distribution of loiasis.
Courtesy of Wolfe Medical Publications.

Transmission and life cycle
L. loa is transmitted by blood-sucking daytime biting tabanid flies of the genus Chrysops. They are often referred to as mangrove flies or horseflies. The appearance, breeding places and biting habits of Chrysops flies are described in 23:6.

Life cycle
— Infective larvae (often in large numbers) enter human skin through the deep wound made by an infected Chrysops fly when it sucks blood. The larvae penetrate subcutaneous connective tissues and within 6-12 months they develop into mature male and female worms.

Mature L. loa worms: They are white and their surface is covered with small knobs. The anterior end tapers to a narrow head. The female measures 50-70 × 0.5 mm and the male measures 30-34 × 0.4 mm. The tail of the male has two spicules of unequal length.

The worms may live for 4-12 years in their host. They wander in subcutaneous tissue and occasionally under the conjunctiva of the eye.

— Viviparous females produce sheathed microfilariae which can be found in the blood during day hours. They can also be found in the tissues.

— The microfilariae are taken up by a female Chrysops when sucking blood.

— In the stomach of the Chrysops the microfilariae lose their sheath. They pass through the stomach wall, penetrate thoracic muscles, and develop into infective larvae. Development in the insect vector takes about 10 days.

— Mature infective larvae migrate to the mouthparts of the insect ready to be transmitted when the Chrysops next takes a blood meal.

The life cycle of L. loa is shown in Fig. 22.5.

Clinical features and pathology
Many people infected with L. loa do not develop clinical symptoms. The disease is characterized by the formation of swellings known as Calabar swellings which may last from a few days up to 3 weeks and measure from 3-10 cm in diameter. The arms are most frequently affected. The inflamed areas are an allergic response to adult L. loa worms migrating in the subcutaneous tissue. Worms are not usually present in the swellings but they can occasionally be seen migrating below the skin surface.

Adult worms also migrate in subconjunctival tissues. They can be seen under the eyelids and occasionally slowly crossing the white of the eye. They can cause inflammation and irritation but not blindness.

The microfilariae do not seem to cause any serious symptoms although it has been reported that encephalitis can occur following treatment of heavy infections.

An eosinophilic leucocytosis and high titres of specific anti-filarial antibodies are found in patients with loiasis.

Prevention and control
- Avoiding the bites of *Chrysops* flies by:
    - Wearing protective clothing, e.g. long trousers.
    - Siting settlements, including adequate water supplies, away from forest areas.

- Destruction of *Chrysops* flies by:
    - Changing the character of breeding places wherever possible e.g. clearing vegetation to allow in sunlight to dry out muddy areas which were previously heavily shaded. The breeding habits of *Chrysops* flies are described in 23:6.
    - Using insecticides as part of a control programme where this is feasible.
- Treating infected individuals but with great care in areas where *O. volvulus* also occurs.[5]

Further information about loiasis
The application of science and technology at primary health care level in filarial diseases is discussed in the WHO paper of Duke.[5]

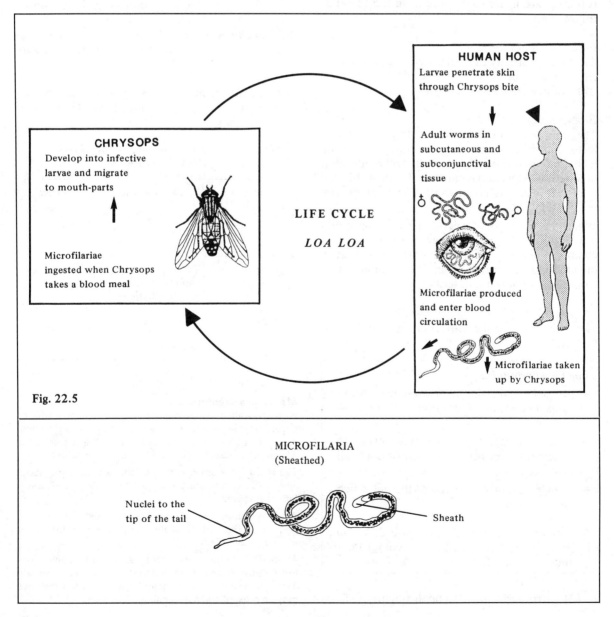

Fig. 22.5

LIFE CYCLE
LOA LOA

CHRYSOPS
Develop into infective larvae and migrate to mouth-parts

Microfilariae ingested when Chrysops takes a blood meal

HUMAN HOST
Larvae penetrate skin through Chrysops bite

Adult worms in subcutaneous and subconjunctival tissue

Microfilariae produced and enter blood circulation

Microfilariae taken up by Chrysops

MICROFILARIA
(Sheathed)

Nuclei to the tip of the tail

Sheath

LABORATORY DIAGNOSIS

Laboratory confirmation of loiasis is by:

☐ Detecting *L. loa* microfilariae in blood.

☐ Occasionally *L. loa* microfilariae can be found in joint fluid.

Note: Calabar swelling is accompanied by a marked eosinophilia.

Examination of blood for *L. loa* microfilariae

Microfilariae begin to appear in the blood from about 6 months onwards after infection.

Blood must be collected at the correct time, i.e. during the hours when the greatest number of microfilariae are likely to be present in the blood as follows:

Collection times for L. loa
L. loa has a strictly diurnal (daytime) periodicity. Blood should be collected between 10.00-15.00 h (time of peak density is 13.00 h).

Blood specimen
The amount of blood required and whether to collect capillary or venous blood will depend on the technique used. Full details of the techniques that are used to detect and identify *L. loa* microfilariae in blood, including concentration techniques, can be found in 22:6.

When the numbers of microfilariae in the blood are high, this should be reported because serious complications can occur when treating heavily infected persons (methods used to estimate microfilariae numbers are described in 22:6).

Identification of L. loa microfilariae
The following are the important identifying features:

Loa loa microfilaria

- It is large in size compared with *Mansonella perstans*, measuring 250-300 × 8-10 μm.

- Sheath is present and stains best with haematoxylin. It stains poorly or not at all with Giemsa.

- Nuclei extend to the end of the tail which is rounded.

Illustrations: See Plate 22.5, Plate 22.6, and Plate 22.7 at the end of 22:6, and colour Plates 33 and 36.

L. loa microfilariae need to be distinguished from those of *W. bancrofti* and *Mansonella* species which can also be found in some of the areas where *L. loa* occurs (see Chart 22.II at the end of 22:6).

22:5 *MANSONELLA* SPECIES

Although *Mansonella* species can cause allergic reactions, they rarely cause serious disease. They can be found, however, in areas where *W. bancrofti*, *L. loa*, and *O. volvulus* also occur.

Microfilariae of the following *Mansonella* species require differentiation from those of the major pathogenic filariae:

Mansonella streptocerca: Requires differentiation from *O. volvulus*.

Mansonella perstans: Requires differentiation from *W. bancrofti* and *L. loa*.

Mansonella ozzardi: Requires differentiation from *O. volvulus* and *W. bancrofti*.

Distribution and Occurrence of Microfilariae of Mansonella Species

Species	Distribution	Occurrence
M. streptocerca	Rain forests of Central and West Africa	Found in skin
M. perstans	Tropical Africa, Central America, South America	Found in blood
M. ozzardi	West Indies, Central America, South America	Found in blood and skin

Mansonella streptocerca

Formerly called *Dipetalonema streptocerca*, this species occurs only in the rain forests of Africa. It is found especially in Ghana, Nigeria, Zaire, and the Cameroons. *M. streptocerca* is transmitted by *Culicoides* midges.

The worms are small with the female measuring about 27 × 0.75 mm and the male about 17 × 0.05 mm. The surface is smooth.

Adult worms and microfilariae (see later text) can be found just below the surface of the skin, usually of the upper trunk and shoulders.

Although many *M. streptocerca* infections are asymptomatic, an itching dermatitis of infected areas is a common finding. Occasionally hypopigmented macules may be present and a thickening of the skin.

Mansonella perstans

Formerly called *Dipetalonema perstans* and *Acanthocheilonema perstans*, this species is widely distributed in tropical Africa and also occurs in Guatemala, Trinidad and parts of South America (Venezuela, Brazil, northern Argentina, Columbia). In some areas it is found with *M. ozzardi*.

M. perstans is transmitted by *Culicoides* midges which are often found in the rotting stems of banana trees.

The female measures up to 80 × 0.12 mm and is about twice the size of the male. The surface is smooth and in both sexes the tail is curved. The spicules of the male are rod-like and of unequal length.

Adult worms are rarely found in man. They are thought to live in the serous cavities of the abdomen and chest. The microfilariae are found in the peripheral blood and very occasionally in cerebrospinal fluid. They are nonperiodic.

M. perstans is not considered pathogenic although allergic reactions with eosinophilia have been reported.

Note: Although occasionally found in cerebrospinal fluid, *M. perstans* is not the cause of cerebral filariasis. This rare disease has been reported from Zimbabwe. The species responsible is *Meningonema peruzzii* which normally infects the meninges of monkeys. *M. peruzzii* microfilariae resemble those of *M. perstans*.

Mansonella ozzardi

This species is found in the West Indies, South America (Surinam, Guyana, Colombia, Brazil, northern Argentina), and Central America (Mexico, Panama).

M. ozzardi strains are transmitted by *Culicoides* midges and *Simulium* blackflies.

The female worm measures about 70 × 0.2 mm and is about twice the size of the male. The tail of the male is coiled and there is a single spicule. The surface is smooth.

The adult worms live in the mesenteric and subperitoneal tissues. The microfilariae are present in small blood vessels in the skin and outside of capillaries in subcutaneous tissue. They can be found therefore in skin snips as well as in the blood (see later text). *M. ozzardi* microfilariae can be found in blood collected both during the day and night.

Infections with *M. ozzardi* are usually nonpathogenic but can be associated with chronic arthritis, skin rashes, and other symptoms.

LABORATORY DIAGNOSIS

Full details of the techniques which are used to detect and differentiate microfilariae in blood can be found in 22:6. Techniques to detect and identify microfilariae in skin can be found in 22:7.

Mansonella streptocerca

M. streptocerca occurs only in West Africa and Central Africa.

The following are the main identifying features of *M. streptocerca* microfilariae:

Mansonella streptocerca microfilaria

- It is small compared with *O. volvulus*, measuring 180-240 × 4.5 μm.
- When immobile, the tail usually appears hooked and its tip is rounded. In fresh preparations the tip of the tail may appear forked (reported from West Africa).
- Nuclei extend to the end of the tail.
- No sheath.
- Found in skin.

Illustrations: See Plate 22.15 and 22.16 at the end of 22:7 and colour Plate 40.

Because *M. streptocerca* microfilariae are found in the skin they need to be differentiated from *O. volvulus* microfilariae (see Chart 22.IV in 22:7).

Mansonella perstans

M. perstans is found in tropical Africa and parts of the West Indies, tropical central America and South America.

The following are the main identifying features of *M. perstans* microfilariae:

Mansonella perstans microfilaria

- It is small compared with *W. bancrofti* and *L. loa*, measuring 190-240 × 4.5 μm.
- No sheath.
- Nuclei extend to the end of the tail and there is a large nucleus at the tip.
- Tip of the tail is rounded.
- Nonperiodic, i.e. found in day and night blood.

Illustrations: See Plate 22.7 and Plate 22.8 at the end of 22:6 and colour Plates 35 and 36.

Because *M. perstans* microfilariae are found in the blood they need to be differentiated from *W. bancrofti*, *L. loa*, and *M. ozzardi* microfilariae (see Chart 22.II in 22:6). Techniques used to examine blood for microfilariae are described in 22:6.

Mansonella ozzardi

M. ozzardi occurs only in the West Indies and tropical Central America and South America.

The following are the main identifying features of *M. ozzardi* microfilariae:

Mansonella ozzardi microfilaria

- It is small compared with *O. volvulus* and *W. bancrofti*, measuring 150-200 × 4.5 μm.
- No sheath.
- There are no nuclei in the end of the tail which is long and pointed.
- Found in blood (nonperiodic) and in skin.

Illustrations: See Plate 22.9 and Plate 22.10 at the end of 22:6, and colour Plate 37.

Because *M. ozzardi* microfilariae are found in the blood and occasionally in the skin they need to be differentiated from *W. bancrofti*, *M. perstans*, and *O. volvulus* (see Chart 22.II in 22:6 and Chart 22.IV in 22:7). Techniques used to examine blood for microfilariae are described in 22:6 and skin for microfilariae in 22:7.

22:6 EXAMINATION OF BLOOD FOR MICROFILARIAE

Microfilariae which may be Found in Blood

PATHOGENIC SPECIES	OTHER SPECIES
Wuchereria bancrofti	*Mansonella perstans*
Brugia malayi	*Mansonella ozzardi*
Brugia timori	
Loa loa	

Note: *Onchocerca volvulus*, normally found in skin (see 22:7), can also be found in blood and other body fluids in heavy infections and after treatment with diethylcarbamazine (DEC).

Distribution of Microfilariae which may be Found in Blood

AFRICA	INDIA
W. bancrofti	*W. bancrofti*
L. loa	*B. malayi*
O. volvulus	
M. perstans	SOUTH-EAST ASIA
M. streptocerca	PHILIPPINE ISLANDS
	W. bancrofti
CENTRAL AMERICA	*B. malayi*
SOUTH AMERICA	*B. timori* (Lesser
W. bancrofti	Sunda Is.)
O. volvulus	
M. perstans	CHINA
M. ozzardi	*W. bancrofti*
	B. malayi
PACIFIC REGION	
W. bancrofti	

Collection Times for Pathogenic Periodic Blood Microfilariae

SPECIES	COLLECTION TIME
Wuchereria bancrofti	
Periodic, nocturnal	22.00-04.00 h
(Asia, Africa, Caribbean, South America, west Pacific)	Peak 24.00 h
Subperiodic, nocturnal	20.00-22.00 h
(Thailand, Viet Nam)	Peak 21.00 h
Subperiodic, diurnal	14.00-18.00 h
(Southeast Pacific)	Peak 16.00 h
Brugia malayi	
Periodic, nocturnal	22.00-04.00 h
(South and east Asia)	Peak 24.00 h
Subperiodic, nocturnal	20.00-22.00 h
(South-East Asia)	Peak 21.00 h
Brugia timori, nocturnal	22.00-04.00 h
	Peak 24.00 h
Loa loa, diurnal	10.00-15.00 h
	Peak 13.00 h

Note: Mansonella microfilariae are nonperiodic, i.e. can be found in day and night blood.

Blood collection times depend on the periodicity of locally occurring *W. bancrofti, B. malayi, B. timori* and *L. loa*. Microfilariae of these filarial worms are released periodically from the blood in the lungs into the peripheral blood. Terms that are used to describe the periodicity of microfilariae are explained in 22:1.

Factors to be considered when examining blood for microfilariae

- The specimen must be collected at the correct time, i.e. during the hours when the numbers of microfilariae circulating in the peripheral blood are at their highest (see above).
- Even when specimens are collected at the correct time, the numbers of microfilariae in the blood are often few and therefore the larger the volume of blood examined the greater the possibility of detecting the parasites.
- In chronic infections, microfilariae are rarely found in the peripheral blood.
- In *W. bancrofti* and *Brugia* infections, microfilariae numbers are higher in capillary blood than in venous blood. Nathan and colleagues have shown that a similar number of *W. bancrofti* microfilariae can be recovered from 0.1 ml (100 μl) of ear lobe capillary blood as from 1 ml of venous blood.[8]
- More microfilariae can often be found in capillary blood collected from the ear lobe than from the finger.

- In some areas where *W. bancrofti* and *L. loa* occur, microfilariae of the nonpathogenic or less pathogenic *Mansonella* species can also be found in the blood.

Choice of techniques

Based on the above considerations, the following techniques are recommended to detect, quantify, and identify microfilariae in blood (full details of techniques are given later in this subunit).

☐ *Lyzed capillary blood technique*: In this, 100 μl (0.1 ml) of capillary (ear lobe) blood is haemolyzed in 1 ml of lyzing fluid. The microfilariae are concentrated by centrifugation or overnight sedimentation and the sediment examined microscopically for microfilariae. The addition of methylene blue helps to identify the species. The number of microfilariae counted multiplied by 10 gives the approximate number per ml of blood (mf/ml).

If no microfilariae are detected by this technique, a venous blood (10 ml) concentration technique should be carried out.

☐ *Venous blood filtration concentration technique*: In this, 10 ml of blood is collected into sodium citrate anticoagulant and the blood passed through a polycarbonate (clear) membrane filter of 5 μm porosity. The living microfilariae are retained and the membrane is examined microscopically.

This is the best method of detecting small numbers of microfilariae but it requires venous blood and is a more expensive technique than the lyzed capillary blood technique. It should be used therefore only when no microfilariae are detected by the capillary blood technique. The number of microfilariae counted divided by 10 gives the number per ml of blood (mf/ml).

☐ *Venous blood tube concentration technique*: When 5 μm polycarbonate filters are not available, 10 ml of lyzed blood can be centrifuged or left to sediment to recover the microfilariae. This technique is a modification of the Knott concentration method in which venous blood is lyzed in a weak formalin solution.

Other techniques used to detect microfilariae in blood

☐ *Thick stained smear technique*: In this, 20 μl (0.02 ml) of capillary blood is collected from the ear lobe, allowed to dry and stained by Field's or Giemsa stain. It is less sensitive than the lyzed capillary blood technique in which 100 μl of blood is examined but is of value in malaria endemic areas when the same smear can be used to detect both malaria parasites and microfilariae. Smears should be stained within 48 hours of collecting the blood to prevent shrinkage and distortion of the microfilariae.

Providing 20 μl of blood is used to make the smear, the number of microfilariae counted in the entire smear multipled by 50 will give an approximate number of microfilariae per ml of blood (mf/ml).

☐ *Wet slide preparation*: In this 20 μl (0.02 ml) of capillary blood is mixed with 2 drops of water (to lyze the red cells) on a slide. The preparation is covered with a cover glass and examined for motile microfilariae using the 10× objective, preferably by dark-field microscopy.

This technique is sometimes used as a screening test but it is not as reliable as techniques in which 100 μl of blood is examined.

☐ *Counting chamber technique*: This is similar to the lyzed capillary blood technique already described except that the 100 μl of blood is lyzed with water in a simple ruled chamber (prepared from strips of glass slides).

The technique is not as convenient as the lyzed capillary blood technique. In the counting chamber technique, microfilariae are more difficult to focus in such a large depth of red fluid. The preparation also takes longer to examine because the microfilariae are not concentrated and methylene blue cannot be added to assist in identifying the microfilariae.

☐ *Capillary tube centrifuge technique*: In this, capillary blood is collected into two heparinized capillary tubes (about 50 μl of blood in each tube). Alternatively, 100 μl of blood can be collected first into EDTA or sodium citrate anticoagulant, mixed, and then transferred to two plain (non-heparinized) capillary tubes. After sealing the tubes, the blood is centrifuged. The capillary tubes are then mounted on a glass slide as described in 16:2. The plasma above the buffy coat layer is examined for motile microfilariae.

This technique is reliable and simple to perform but it does require plain or heparinized capillary tubes, centrifuging is essential, and a stained preparation of the plasma is needed to identify the species. In areas where the species is known, this technique is a rapid reliable screening test for use in district laboratories able to obtain capillary tubes.

Lyzed Capillary Blood Technique

See previous text for an explanation of the principle of this technique.

Required
— Saponin-saline solution   Reagent No. 64
to lyze the red cells.

— Methylene blue-saline,   Reagent No. 49
1 g/l (0.1 w/v).
This will stain the nuclei and show whether the microfilariae are sheathed (the sheaths do not stain but can be seen as unstained extensions at the head and tail end).

Method
1. Collect 100 μl (0.1 ml) of capillary blood from

the ear lobe and dispense it into a centrifuge (conical) tube containing 1 ml of saponin-saline lyzing solution.

Note: If saponin-saline is not available, dispense the blood into 1 ml of water. When water is used, the microfilariae remain motile as in saponin-saline but the haemolysate is not as clear (contains red cell stroma).

Field surveys
Collect 0.1 ml of capillary blood into 3% v/v acetic acid (Reagent No. 1). This will fix and preserve the microfilariae, enabling the specimen to be examined several days or weeks later if necessary. In some cultures, local beliefs may make the collection of blood at night difficult.

2. Mix the blood gently in the lyzing solution and leave for about 2 minutes to allow time for all the red cells to lyze.

3. Centrifuge for 5 minutes at slow to medium speed, (approximately 2000 rpm). Do not centrifuge at high speed because this may cause the loss of sheaths from pathogenic microfilariae.

   If a centrifuge is not available, add a small drop of concentrated formaldehyde solution to kill the microfilariae (or collect the blood into 3% v/v acetic acid) and leave the haemolysate undisturbed for at least 4 h or preferably overnight to allow the microfilariae time to sediment by gravity.

4. Using a plastic bulb pipette or other suitable pipette, remove and discard the supernatant fluid. Transfer all the sediment to a slide, add a *small* drop of methylene blue-saline, and cover with a cover glass.

5. Examine the entire preparation microscopically for motile microfilariae (non-motile if acetic acid or formaldehyde has been used) using the 10× objective with the condenser iris *closed sufficiently* to give good contrast, or preferably examine by dark-field microscopy.

Value of dark-field microscopy
When using dark-field microscopy, the sheaths of the pathogenic microfilariae can be clearly seen when viewed with the 40× objective. The preparation must be sufficiently thin and the cover glass and slide completely clean.

Note: Simple kits to make condenser stops to give dark-field microscopy for use with the 10× and 40× objectives are provided with Volume II of the Manual.

The identifying features of microfilariae found in blood are summarized in Chart 22.I at the end of this subunit.

6. Count the number of microfilariae in the entire preparation. Multiply the number counted by 10 to give an approximate number of microfilariae per ml of blood (mf/ml).

Value of microfilaria count in routine diagnosis
In heavy infections, especially in loiasis, severe reactions can occur during treatment and therefore it is helpful for the medical officer to know whether the microfilaria concentration is high before starting treatment.

7. If unable to identify the species with certainty, examine a fixed stained preparation with the 100× objective as follows:

   — Remove the cover glass and add a *small* drop of plasma, serum, or albumin solution. Mix and spread thinly. Allow the preparation to dry completely.

   Note: The addition of albumin plasma, or serum (known to be microfilaria-free) will help to prevent the preparation from being washed from the slide during staining.

   — Fix, by covering the preparation with absolute methanol or ethanol for 2-3 minutes.

   — Stain using modified Field's stain and Delafield's haematoxylin (see p. 380), or Giemsa stain if not looking for *L. loa*, (see 13:14 for Giemsa staining technique).

Note: The identifying features of *W. bancrofti*, *B. malayi*, *B. timori*, *L. loa* and *Mansonella* microfilariae are described and illustrated in Chart 22.1 and in colour Plates 32-40.

Venous Blood Filtration Concentration Technique
See previous text for an explanation of the principle of this technique.

Required
— Nuclepore polycarbonate filter, 13 mm diameter 5 µm pore size.
   To prevent the filters from sticking to each other, they are usually packaged between white paper discs. The filters are the thin *transparent* discs. They are fairly strong but require handling with *blunt-ended* forceps to avoid damaging them.

Reuse of polycarbonate filters
With care polycarbonate filters can be disinfected, washed, and reused several times when no microfilariae are detected. The same procedure can be used as described for reusing polycarbonate filters in schistosomiasis work (see 20:2).

Note: Positive filters should not be reused because microfilariae become trapped in the small pores of the filter and are difficult to wash out.[9]

— Syringe filter holder (Swinnex type), 13 mm diameter

— Syringe, Luer, 10 ml capacity
— Sodium citrate anticoagulant,   Reagent No. 68
   38 g/l (3.8% w/v)
— Methylene blue-saline,   Reagent No. 49
   1 g/l (0.1% w/v)

Availability of filariasis filtration kit
A kit containing 20 polycarbonate membranes of 13 mm diameter and 5 μm pore size, 1 syringe filter holder of 13 mm diameter with spare gasket (washer), 1 blunt-ended forceps, 2 reusable 10 ml Luer syringes, is available to developing countries at low cost from Tropical Health Technology Laboratory Equipment Service (see Appendix IV, Filariasis filtration kit).

Method
1. Collect 10 ml of venous blood and dispense it into 1 ml of sodium citrate anticoagulant. Mix well but do not shake.

   Caution: Blood may contain highly infectious viruses and other pathogens, therefore handle the blood and the needles and syringes used to collect it with great care. Make sure the needles, syringes and other equipment used to test the specimens are soaked in a suitable disinfectant (e.g. domestic bleach diluted 1 in 5 in water) immediately after use. Leave soaking overnight.

2. Withdraw the plunger of a clean 10 ml Luer syringe.

3. Unscrew the filter holder, and using blunt-ended forceps, *carefully* position a polycarbonate filter (13 mm diameter, 5 μm pore size) on the filter support of the filter holder. Re-assemble the filter holder and attach it to the end of the syringe barrel.

   Mansonella species
   Although some *Mansonella* microfilariae are retained on a 5 μm porosity membrane, if blood needs to be examined specifically for *Mansonella* species, a 3 μm porosity membrane should be used to ensure the full retention of these smaller microfilariae.

4. Fill the syringe barrel with the anticoagulated blood, holding it over a beaker or other suitable container. Carefully replace the plunger of the syringe and slowly pass the citrated blood through the filter.

5. Remove the filter holder and attach a needle or small length of tubing to the syringe. Draw up about 10 ml of the methylene blue-saline solution, re-attach the filter holder, and pass the solution through the filter.

6. Remove the filter holder and draw air into the syringe. Re-attach the filter holder and pass the air through the filter. This will help to stick the microfilariae to the filter.

7. Detach the filter holder, unscrew it, and using blunt-ended forceps, carefully remove the filter and place it *face upwards* on a slide. Add a small drop of physiological saline, and cover with a cover glass.

8. Examine the entire filter microscopically for motile microfilariae using the 10× objective with the condenser iris *closed sufficiently* to give good contrast.

   Use the 40× objective to see whether the microfilariae are sheathed (seen as unstained extensions at the head and tail end of the microfilariae) and whether the pale blue stained nuclei extend into the tip of the tail. The identifying features of microfilariae can be found in Chart 22.I at the end of this subunit.

   Count the number of microfilariae in the entire preparation. Divide the number counted by 10 to give the approximate number of microfilariae per ml of blood (mf/ml).

9. If unable to identify with certainty the species of microfilariae, examine a fixed stained preparation with the 100× objective as follows:

   — Wash the filter off the slide (using a washbottle if available) into a bottle containing about 2 ml of physiological saline. Stopper and shake to dislodge the microfilariae from the filter.

   — Transfer the washings to a conical tube and centrifuge for 5 minutes at slow to medium speed.

   — Using a plastic bulb pipette or other suitable pipette, immediately remove and discard the supernatant fluid. Transfer the entire sediment to a slide, mix with a small drop of albumin, plasma or serum (known to be microfilariae-free) and spread thinly. Allow the preparation to dry completely.

   — Fix by covering the preparation with absolute methanol or ethanol for 2-3 minutes.

   — Stain using modified Field's stain and Delafield's haematoxylin (see p. 380), or Giemsa stain if not looking for *L. loa*, (see 13:14 for Giemsa staining technique).

Note: The identifying features of *W. bancrofti*, *B. malayi*, *B. timori*, *L. loa* and *Mansonella* microfilariae are described and illustrated in Chart 22.I and in colour Plates 32-40, and the differentiating features are summarized in Chart 22.II.

Venous Blood Tube Concentration Technique
See previous text for an explanation of the principle of this technique.

Required
— Saponin-saline solution   Reagent No. 64
— Methylene blue-saline   Reagent No. 49
  1 g/l (0.1% w/v)

Method
1. Collect 10 ml of venous blood and dispense it into 10 ml of saponin-saline lyzing solution.

   Note: If saponin-saline is not available, dispense the blood into 10 ml of distilled water.

2. Mix the blood gently in the lyzing solution and leave for 5 minutes to give time for all the red cells to lyze.

3. Centrifuge the haemolysate for 10 minutes at slow to medium speed (approx. 2000 rpm).

4. Using a plastic bulb pipette, immediately remove and discard the supernatant fluid. Transfer all the sediment to a slide and cover with a cover glass.

5. Examine the entire preparation microscopically for motile microfilariae using the 10× objective with the condenser iris *closed sufficiently* to give good contrast, or preferably examine by dark-field microscopy (see comment under *Lyzed Capillary Blood Technique*).

If using transmitted light and microfilariae are seen, run a drop of methylene blue-saline solution under the cover glass. This will stain the nuclei and show whether the microfilariae are sheathed. The identifying features of microfilariae found in blood are summarized in Chart 22.I at the end of this subunit.

Count the number of microfilariae in the entire preparation. Divide the number counted by 10 to give the approximate number of microfilariae per ml of blood (mf/ml).

6. If unable to identify the species with certainty, examine a fixed stained preparation with the 100× oil immersion objective as described under the Lyzed Capillary Blood Technique.

Chart 22.1 IDENTIFICATION OF BLOOD MICROFILARIAE IN STAINED PREPARATIONS

Wuchereria bancrofti (see 22:2)   Plates 22.1 22.2
- Measures 275-300 × 8-10 µm and is therefore larger than *Mansonella* microfilariae.
- Body curves are large and few (graceful).
- Has a sheath which stains pink with Giemsa and palely with haematoxylin.
- Body nuclei are fewer and more distinct than in other species.
- There are no nuclei in the end of the tail which is pointed.

Notes *W. bancrofti* microfilariae need to be distinguished from those of *B. malayi*, *L. loa* and *Mansonella* species which can also be found in some areas where *W. bancrofti* occurs. *W. bancrofti* microfilariae can also be found in chylous urine and in aspirates of hydrocele fluid.

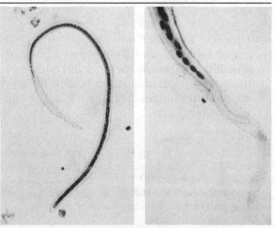

Colour Plate: See colour section, Plate 32.

Brugia malayi (see 22:3)   Plates 22.3 22.4
- Measures 200-275 × 5-6 µm (periodic variant is slightly larger than the subperiodic variant).
- Body is usually coiled and kinked, i.e. has many small angular curves.
- Has a sheath which stains dark pink with Giemsa and pink-mauve with haematoxylin.
- Body nuclei are dense and stain darkly.
- There are 2 nuclei in the end of the tail which tapers irregularly.

Notes In Malaysia and Indonesia, periodic *B. malayi* is often

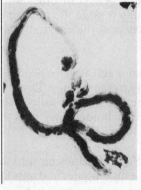
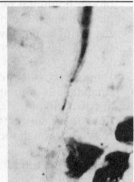

seen without its sheath. Loss of sheath has not been noticed with periodic *B. malayi* strains from other endemic areas. The sheath is rarely lost from subperiodic *B. malayi*.

B. malayi microfilariae need to be distinguished from those of *W. bancrofti* which can also be found in some areas where *B. malayi* occurs. *B. malayi* can also be found in aspirates of lymph gland fluid.

Colour Plate: See colour section, Plate 34.

Brugia timori (see 22:3)
- Measures 290-325 × 5-6 μm.
- Body is curved but not kinked like *B. malayi*.
- Has a sheath (sometimes lost) which does not stain as darkly as that of *B. malayi*.
- Body nuclei are less dense than those of *B. malayi*.
- There are 2 nuclei in the end of the tail which tapers irregularly.

Loa loa (see 22:4)   Plates 22.5 22.6
- Measures 250-300 × 8-10 μm and is therefore larger than *Mansonella* microfilariae.
- Body has several curves and kinks.
- Has a sheath which stains best with haematoxylin.
- Body nuclei are not distinct and appear more dense than those of *W. bancrofti*.
- Nuclei extend to the end of the tail which is rounded.

Notes *L. loa* microfilariae need to be distinguished from those of *W. bancrofti* and *M. perstans* which can also be found in areas where *L. loa* occurs.

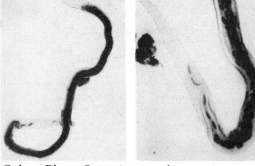

Colour Plates: See colour section, Plates 33 and 36.

Mansonella perstans (see 22:5)   Plates 22.7 22.8
- Measures 190-240 × 4.5 μm and is therefore much smaller than *W. bancrofti* and *L. loa*.
- No sheath.
- Body nuclei are irregular but fairly distinct.
- Nuclei extend to the end of the tail which is rounded. The tip contains a large nucleus.

Notes *M. perstans* can be found in areas where *W. bancrofti* and *L. loa* occur. Unlike *W. bancrofti* and *L. loa*, the microfilariae of *M. perstans* are nonperiodic.

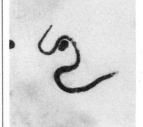

Colour Plate: See colour section, Plates 35 and 36.

Mansonella ozzardi (see 22:5)   Plates 22.9 22.10
- Measures 150-200 × 4.5 μm and is therefore much smaller and thinner than *W. bancrofti*.
- No sheath.
- Body nuclei are not distinct.
- There are no nuclei in the end of the tail which is long and pointed.

Notes *M. ozzardi* can be found in areas where *W. bancrofti* occurs. Unlike *W. bancrofti*, the microfilariae of *M. ozzardi* are nonperiodic.

M. ozzardi microfilariae can also be found in the skin and therefore they require differentiating from *O. volvulus* (see 22:7).

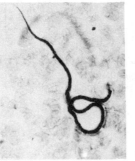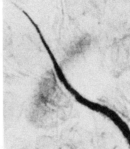

Colour Plate: See colour section, Plate 37.

Note: Onchocerca volvulus, normally found in skin, can be found in blood and urine in heavy infections and after treatment with diethylcarbamazine (DEC). An *O. volvulus* microfilaria is large and unsheathed with a slightly enlarged head and pointed tail which contains no nuclei (see Chart 22.III in 22:7).

Chart 22.II SUMMARY OF DIFFERENTIATING FEATURES OF MICROFILARIA FOUND IN BLOOD

Species	Size	Sheath	Body and Tail	Other Points
W. bancrofti [a]	Large and thick, 275 - 300 × 8 - 10 μm	+	Body curves are large and few. Body nuclei are fewer and more distinct than in other species. There are no nuclei in the end of the tail which is pointed.	Differentiated from *Brugia* species and *L. loa* mainly by its tail features. Differentiated from *Mansonella* species by its larger size and sheath.
B. malayi	Large and thick, 200 - 275 × 5-6 μm	+ [d]	Body and sheath stain darkly. Body is usually coiled and kinked. Nuclei are large and dense. There are 2 nuclei in the end of the tail which tapers irregularly.	Differentiated from *W. bancrofti* by its darker stained sheath and nuclei, kinked body, and tail features. Differentiated from *B. timori* by its shorter length, darker staining, and kinked body.
B. timori	Large and thick, 290 -325 × 5 - 6 μm	+	Does not stain darkly. There are 2 nuclei in the end of the tail which tapers irregularly.	Differentiated from *B. malayi* by its greater length, fewer body kinks, paler stained sheath, less dense nuclei, and longer space at head end.
L. loa [b]	Large and thick, 250 - 300 × 8 - 10 μm	+	Body has several curves and kinks. Nuclei are dense and stain darkly. Sheath stains best with haematoxylin. Nuclei extend to the end of the tail which is rounded.	Differentiated from *W. bancrofti* by its tail features, staining characteristics of its sheath, and diurnal periodicity. Differentiated from *M. perstans* by its larger size and sheath.
M. perstans	Small and thin, 190 - 240 × 4.5 μm	–	Body nuclei are irregular but fairly distinct. Nuclei extend to the end of the tail which is rounded. The tip contains a large nucleus.	Differentiated from *L. loa* and *W. bancrofti* by its smaller size, absence of sheath, tail features, and nonperiodicity.
M. ozzardi [c]	Small and thin, 150 - 200 × 4.5 μm	–	Body nuclei are not distinct. There are no nuclei in the end of the tail which is long and pointed	Differentiated from *W. bancrofti* by its smaller size, absence of sheath, and non-periodicity.

a   *W. bancrofti* can occasionally be found in chylous urine and hydrocele fluid.
b   *L. loa* can occasionally be found in joint (synovial) fluid.
c   *M. ozzardi* can also be found in skin.
d   Periodic *B. malayi* is often seen unsheathed.

Note: *O. volvulus*, usually detected in skin, can also be found in blood, urine and other body fluids and secretions especially in heavy infections and after treatment with DEC. It is described and illustrated in 22:7.

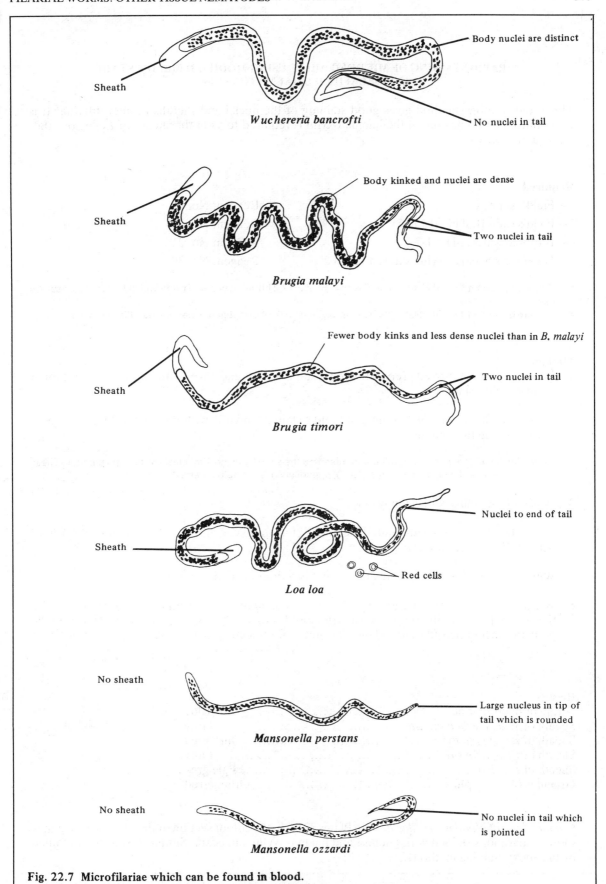

Fig. 22.7 Microfilariae which can be found in blood.

RAPID STAINING OF MICROFILARIAE USING MODIFIED FIELD'S STAIN AND DELAFIELD'S HAEMATOXYLIN [9]

This rapid staining method gives good staining of the nuclei and sheaths of microfilariae. It is economical and no heating of the haematoxylin is required to stain the sheath of *L. loa* or other pathogenic species.

Required

— Field's stain A	Reagent No. 35
— Field's stain B, diluted 1 in 5†	Reagent No. 36
— Buffered water, pH 7.1-7.2	Reagent No. 21
— Delafield's haematoxylin, diluted 1 in 10‡	Reagent No. 30

† Prepare by mixing 1 ml of Field's stain B with 4 ml of pH 7.2 buffered water. If preferred, 0.5% w/v eosin can be used.

‡ Prepare by mixing 1 ml of Delafield's haematoxylin with 9 ml of distilled water or clean filtered water.

Method

1. Place the methanol-fixed preparation on a staining rack and cover with approximately 1 ml of diluted Field's stain B.

2. Add immediately an equal volume of Field's stain A and mix with the diluted Field's stain B. Leave to stain for 1 minute.

    Note: The stains can be easily applied and mixed on the slide by using 1 ml plastic bulb type pipettes. These plastic pipettes can be used many times (see Appendix IV, Plastic bulb pipettes).

3. Wash off the stains with clean water.

4. Cover the preparation with diluted Delafield's haematoxylin and stain for 5 minutes. Wash off with pH 7.1-7.2 buffered water.

5. Wipe the back of the slide clean and place it in a draining rack.

6. When the smear is dry, spread a drop of immersion oil on it and examine microscopically. Use the 10× objective (with the condenser iris closed sufficiently to give good contrast) to scan the preparation for microfilariae and the 40× and 100× objectives to identify the species (see Chart 22.I).

Results

Nuclei of microfilariae	Blue
Sheath of *Wuchereria bancrofti*	Grey
Sheath of *Brugia malayi*	Dark grey
Sheath of *Brugia timori*	Grey
Sheath of *Loa loa*	Pale grey
Granules of eosinophils	Orange-red

Colour Plates of blood microfilariae: See Plates 32-37 in the colour section of the Manual (the plates show preparations stained with Giemsa and haematoxylin and eosin. Similar results are obtained by the above staining method).

22:7 ONCHOCERCA VOLVULUS

Onchocerca volvulus causes onchocerciasis which is a cutaneous filariasis. The disease is also referred to as river blindness because invasion of the eye can lead to loss of vision.

It is estimated that *O. volvulus* infects about 30 million people and has caused blindness in about 500 000 people.

Distribution

O. volvulus occurs most widely along the courses of fast running rivers in the rain forests and savannah areas of West and Central Africa. It is endemic from Senegal in the west to Uganda and Ethiopia in the east and as far south as Zambia (see Fig. 22.8).

Smaller endemic areas occur in the Yemen Arab Republic, Saudi Arabia and in central America (Mexico and Guatemala). In central America, the vectors of *O. volvulus* breed in slow running streams.

O. volvulus is also found in South America where the main focus of infection is in Ecuador with smaller foci in Brazil, Venezuela and Columbia.

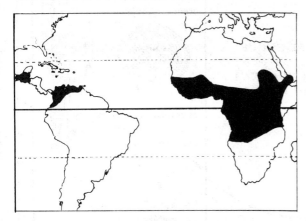

Fig. 22.8 Distribution of *Onchocerca volvulus*.
Courtesy of Wolfe Medical Publications.

Transmission and life cycle

O. volvulus is transmitted by *Simulium* blackflies. The commonest vectors belong to the *Simulium damnosum* complex. The appearance, biting and breeding habits of *Simulium* species are described in 23:5.

Life cycle
— Infective larvae are deposited on human skin when an infected blackfly takes a blood meal and enter through the bite wound.

— The larvae develop into male and female worms in subcutaneous tissue. Development takes several months.

Mature O. volvulus worms: They appear white with a surface which is ringed with raised ridges. The female measures 330-550 × 0.35 mm. The male is much smaller, measuring 25-40 mm in length. The tail of the male is curved, bulbous, and has two spicules of unequal length.

The adults live in subcutaneous tissue and in lymph spaces, occurring singly or in tangled masses. In the later stages of infection the worms become encapsulated in fibrous nodules. The worms can live up to 10 years or more in their host.

— Viviparous females produce many unsheathed microfilariae which can be found just below the surface of the skin in the lymph spaces and in connective tissue. They can also be found in the fluid of nodules. Microfilariae are thought to be present in the skin from about 7 months onwards after infection.

The microfilariae also migrate to the eye and other organs of the body.

— The microfilariae are ingested by a blackfly as it feeds.

After passing through the stomach wall of the fly, the microfilariae migrate to the thoracic muscles where they develop into infective larvae. Development in the blackfly vector takes about 10 days.

— Mature infective larvae migrate to the mouthparts of the blackfly ready to be transmitted when the fly next takes a blood meal.

The life cycle of *O. volvulus* is shown in Fig. 22.9.

Clinical features and pathology

The serious clinical features and pathology of onchocerciasis are caused mainly by the inflammatory reactions around damaged and dead microfilariae.

Clinical features and pathology vary from one area of infection to another and within a particular population. Variations are due to differences in parasitic strains, degree and frequency of infection, and host differences which include nutritional state and immune responses to parasite antigens. For example, in West Africa the form of disease found in savannah areas is more severe than that found in forest areas.

An inflammatory reaction causes the eventual encapsulation of adult worms in subcutaneous tissue. The resulting nodules are called onchocercomas. They are firm, smooth and rubbery, round or elongated and measure from 5 mm across up to 50 mm when found in clusters. They are freely mobile or attached to underlying tissue and may contain large numbers of microfilariae. In many endemic areas of Africa, nodules are commonly found on the lower part of the body around the pelvis. In Central America and the savannah areas of Africa, nodules are often found on the upper part of the body. In young children (below 9 y), the nodules are found mainly on the head. In Yemen the lower limbs are mainly affected.

There is an inflammatory dermatitis which may be accompanied by intense irritation, raised papules on the skin, and subsequently alteration in the pigmentation of the skin. The term 'sowda' (black disease) is used to describe a severe allergic response

usually affecting only one limb with darkening of the skin. The lymph nodes draining the limb become swollen and painful.

In chronic onchocerciasis, the skin loses its elasticity and becomes wrinkled which makes people look more aged than they are (known as 'elephant skin'). When the skin around the groin becomes affected 'hanging groin' develops. The term 'leopard skin' refers to a spotted depigmentation of the skin which is associated with chronic onchocerciasis.

The most serious complication of onchocerciasis (affecting mainly those that have lived in endemic areas for several years) is when microfilariae in the skin of the face migrate into the eye. In early ocular

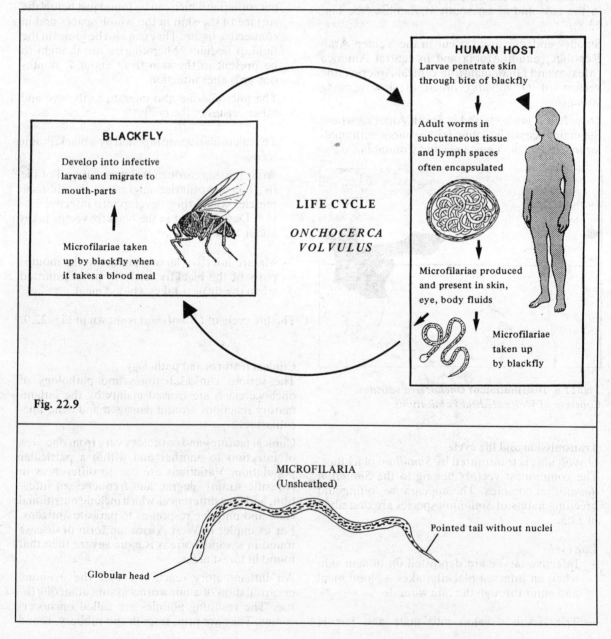

HUMAN HOST

Larvae penetrate skin through bite of blackfly

Adult worms in subcutaneous tissue and lymph spaces often encapsulated

Microfilariae produced and present in skin, eye, body fluids

Microfilariae taken up by blackfly

LIFE CYCLE

ONCHOCERCA VOLVULUS

BLACKFLY

Develop into infective larvae and migrate to mouth-parts

Microfilariae taken up by blackfly when it takes a blood meal

Fig. 22.9

MICROFILARIA
(Unsheathed)

Pointed tail without nuclei

Globular head

(eye) onchocerciasis, the microfilariae can be found in the cornea and in the anterior chamber. There is redness and irritation of the eye. Progressive changes caused by inflammatory reactions around damaged and dead microfilariae can cause sclerosing keratitis which can lead to blindness. Often the iris is also affected. Inflammation of the choroid and retina can also lead to blindness.

There is a slight to marked eosinophilia.

Prevention and control

- Destruction of *Simulium* larvae by:
    - Applying insecticides using simple drip feed methods in smaller rivers and aerial spraying of larger rivers.
    - Introducing other methods to reduce the breeding of blackflies in rivers. The breeding and biting habits of *Simulium* flies are described in 23:5.
- Avoiding *Simulium* bites by covering as far as possible those parts of the body most at risk.
- Identifying infected persons, especially those with nodules on the head or ocular symptoms which may lead to blindness. Drugs used to treat the disease can cause severe reactions.[6] There is no suitable drug for widespread use in control programmes and DEC should not be administered except under strict supervision. 'The dangers, particularly to the eye, of haphazard, unsupervised dosage with DEC in onchocerciasis, are far greater than previously thought'.[5]

Further information on onchocerciasis

The 1984 supplement *Recent Advances in Research on Filariasis*[3] gives further details on the treatment, immunological aspects, epidemiology, vectors and control of onchocerciasis.

Abstracts of papers on onchocerciasis published between January 1983 and March 1984 can be found in the review *Filariasis.*[4]

A review of the action of diethylcarbamazine (DEC) in onchocerciasis can be found in the 1985 paper of Mackenzie and Kron.[6]

The application of science and technology at primary health care level in filarial diseases is discussed in the 1985 WHO paper of Duke.[5]

A major Onchocerciasis Control Programme is operating in Benin, Burkina Faso, Ghana, Ivory Coast, Mali, Niger, and Togo. For information readers should write to WHO Onchocerciasis Control Programme, PO Box 549, Ouagadougou, Burkina Faso (formerly Upper Volta).

LABORATORY DIAGNOSIS

Laboratory diagnosis of onchocerciasis is by:

☐ Finding *O. volvulus* microfilariae in skin snips.

Note: In heavy infections and following treatment, *O. volvulus* microfilariae can also be found in urine, blood, and most body fluids.

Slide technique for detecting *O. volvulus* microfilariae in skin

Skin snips should be taken from those sites most likely to be heavily infected. In Africa and South America, the highest number of microfilariae can usually be found in skin snips taken from the buttocks, iliac crests or calves of the legs, in Mexico and Guatemala from behind the shoulders or trunk, and in Yemen from the lower limbs.

Skin specimen

A bloodless skin snip is required. It can be collected using a sterile needle and razor blade (or scalpel) as follows:

1. Cleanse the skin using a spirit swab. Allow the area to dry.

2. Insert a sterile fine needle almost horizontally into the skin. Raise the point of the needle, lifting with it a small piece of skin measuring about 2 mm in height and diameter.

3. Cut off the piece of skin with a sterile razor blade (or scalpel) as shown in Plate 22.11.

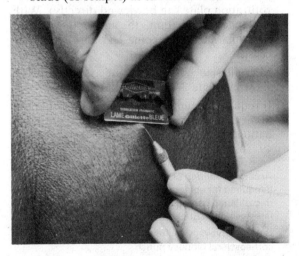

Plate 22.11 Taking a skin snipping for *Onchocerca volvulus* microfilariae.
Reproduced by permission of Tropical Doctor original: Drs B. O. L. Duke and J. Anderson.

---

4. Immerse the skin snip in physiological saline on a slide or in the well of a microtitration tray.

    Water can also be used but the microfilariae take longer to emerge from the skin.

5. Cover the preparation with a cover glass. Place the slide or tray on a piece of damp tissue in a petri dish or plastic box to prevent the preparation from drying out.

Note: Do not tease (pull apart) the skin because this makes the preparation more difficult to examine and damages the microfilariae.

6. Incubate the preparation at room temperature for the length of time needed for the microfilariae to emerge from the skin.

Incubation time and the emergence of microfilariae
In some areas it has been shown that after 1 hour up to 90% of microfilariae contained in a skin snip (saline preparation) will have emerged, whereas in other areas an incubation time of more than 4 hours is needed for most of the microfilariae to emerge. An overnight incubation period should be allowed before recording a negative test (see following text).

In practice most workers look at the preparation after 5 minutes of being incubated and if no microfilariae are detected, again at 15 minute intervals for up to 1 hour. If no microfilariae are seen, the preparation should be left overnight and examined the following day.

7. Examine the preparation microscopically for actively motile microfilariae using the 10× objective with the condenser iris *closed sufficiently* to give good contrast (the well of a microtitration plate can be viewed directly). With prolonged incubation, the movement of the microfilariae will become less and eventually cease.

Microfilariae emerging from a skin snip are shown in Plate 22.12 and colour Plate 39.

If required, count the number of microfilariae in the entire preparation (after overnight incubation) and report the number as 1-4, 5-14, 15-49, 50-100 or more than 100 per skin snip.

Accurate counting of microfilariae
If required for epidemiological surveys, the number of microfilariae per mg (or per mm^2) of skin can be calculated using the Brinkmann nomograph.[10]

During surveys, skin snips are best collected using a corneoscleral bioposy punch.

8. Confirm the species of microfilariae in a stained preparation as follows:

— Remove the cover glass and allow the preparation to dry *completely*.

— Fix the dried preparation with absolute methanol or ethanol for 2-3 minutes.

— Stain with Giemsa as described in 13:14. Cover the preparation with a drop of

immersion oil and examine it microscopically using the 40× and 100× objectives to identify the microfilariae.

Important: It is essential to confirm that the species of microfilaria seen is *O. volvulus* because microfilariae of the species *M. ozzardi* (found in West Indies, Central and South America) and *M. streptocerca* (found in West and Central Africa) can also be found in skin and can be confused with *O. volvulus* especially in wet preparations. Other microfilariae may also be found if the skin becomes contaminated with blood at the time it is collected.

The important identifying features of *O. volvulus* microfilariae and other microfilariae which can be found in skin can be found in Chart 22.III and the differentiating features are summarized in Chart 22.IV.

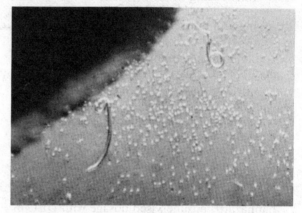

Plate 22.12 *O. volvulus* **microfilariae emerging from a skin snip.**
Courtesy of Wolfe Medical Publications.

Tube technique for detecting *O. volvulus* microfilariae in skin
The following technique is preferred by some workers for detecting *O. volvulus* in skin especially when microfilarial numbers are few. It can be performed when the slide preparation is negative (using the same skin snip).

1. Immerse the skin snip in 2 ml of physiological saline in a centrifuge tube. Incubate at room temperature overnight.

2. Using forceps, remove the skin snip, place it on a slide, and cover with a cover glass.

3. Centrifuge the contents of the tube at medium speed (approx. 2000 rpm) for 5-10 minutes. Remove and discard the supernatant fluid. Transfer the entire sediment to a slide.

4. Examine the skin and sediment microscopically for microfilariae using the 10× objective with the condenser iris closed sufficiently to give good contrast.

Chart 22.III IDENTIFICATION OF SKIN MICROFILARIAE IN STAINED PREPARATIONS

***Onchocerca volvulus* microfilaria**   Plates 22.13   22.14
- It measures 240-360 μm × 5-9 μm and is therefore large compared with *Mansonella* species.
- No sheath.
- Head end is slightly enlarged.
- Anterior nuclei are positioned side by side.
- There are no nuclei in the end of the tail which is long and pointed.

Notes *O. volvulus* microfilariae need to be distinguished from those of *M. ozzardi* and *M. streptocerca* which can also be found in some areas where *O. volvulus* occurs (see Chart 22.IV).

O. volvulus microfilariae can also be found in urine, blood and other body fluids and secretions in heavy infections and after treatment with DEC.

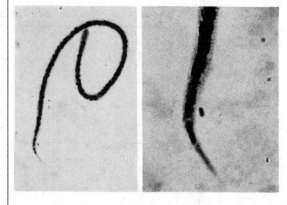

Colour Plate: See colour section, Plate 38.

***Mansonella streptocerca* microfilaria** Plates 22.15 22.16
- It is small compared with *O. volvulus*, measuring 180-240 × 4.5 μm.
- When immobile, the tail usually appears hooked and its tip is rounded or forked (reported from West Africa)
- Nuclei extend to the end of the tail.
- No sheath.

Notes *M. streptocerca* is found only in West Africa and Central Africa.

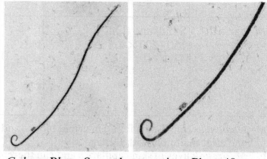

Colour Plate: See colour section, Plate 40.

***Mansonella ozzardi* microfilaria**   Plates 22.17   22.18
- It is small compared with *O. volvulus*, measuring 150-200 × 4.5 μm.
- No sheath.
- There are no nuclei in the end of the tail which is long and pointed.

Notes *M. ozzardi* is found only in the West Indies, Central America and South America.

M. ozzardi lives in skin capillaries and can be found also in capillary blood (nonperiodic).

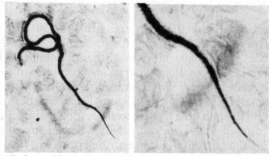

Colour Plate: See colour section, Plate 37.

---

5. Confirm the species of microfilariae in a stained preparation as described in step No. 8 of the previous method.

Onchocerciasis epidemiological and control techniques

For onchocerciasis epidemiological and control surveys, it is recommended that skin be collected using a corneoscleral biopsy punch and a microtitration plate technique be used. The technique is as follows:

— Place the skin biopsy in the well of a microtitration plate which contains 200 μl (0.2 ml) of physiological saline. Cover the plate and leave overnight.

— The following day, add 1 small drop of 20% v/v formalin to preserve the microfilariae.

— Seal the plate using *Parafilm*, *Filmoplast* or other similar material.

Once formalin-fixed, the preparation can be examined in the laboratory several days or even weeks later. The individual specimens can be weighed and the number of microfilariae (mf) counted can be expressed as mf/mg.

Alternatively a simple technique for field surveys developed by Kale[11] is to immerse each skin specimen in saline on a slide, incubate in a damp

**Chart 22.IV SUMMARY OF THE DIFFERENTIATING FEATURES OF MICROFILARIAE
WHICH CAN BE FOUND IN SKIN**

Species	Size	Sheath	Body and Tail	Other Points
O volvulus[a]	Large and thick 240 - 360 × 5 - 9 μm	—	Head is slightly enlarged. Anterior nuclei positioned side by side. There are no nuclei in the end of the tail which is long and pointed.	Differentiation is easy from M. streptocerca, but more difficult from M. ozzardi.
M. streptocerca	Small and thin, 180 - 240 × 4.5 μ m	—	Anterior nuclei are positioned in single file. Nuclei extend to the end of the tail which is rounded and usually hooked.	Differentiated from O. volvulus is by its smaller size, single file anterior nuclei, and tail features.[c]
M. ozzardi[b]	Small and thin, 150 - 200 × 4.5 μm	—	Anterior nuclei are positioned side by side. There are no nuclei in the end of the tail which is long and pointed.	Differentiated from O. volvulus is mainly by its smaller size and different shaped head.[c]

a O volvulus can also be found in urine, blood, and other body fluids and secretions, especially in heavy infections and after treatment with DEC.
b M. ozzardi lives in skin capillaries and can therefore be found also in *capillary* blood.
c In wet preparations, M. streptocerca and M. ozzardi are less motile than O. volvulus.

chamber, dry the preparation using gentle heat from a spirit lamp, and then transport the slides back to the laboratory in air-tight containers. In the laboratory the preparations are reconstituted by covering each dried area with a drop of distilled water. The Kale method is simple and inexpensive and the microfilariae are well-preserved and easily counted. A species confirmation is made by staining the microfilariae as described previously.

Fixation of filarial worms for identification
Fixation of worms for identification can be made by immersing the worms and tissue in an alcohol-glycerol fixative (80 ml absolute ethanol or methanol mixed with 20 ml of glycerol). The worms can then be sent to a Reference Laboratory for identification.

Immunodiagnosis of onchocerciasis
Although antibody and antigen tests are of value in diagnosing onchocerciasis particularly early and light infections, there are as yet no commercially available reagents to test for O. volvulus antibodies in serum or free antigen in blood or urine.

Note: Developments in onchocerciasis immunodiagnostic techniques can be found in the 1984

review *Filariasis*[4] and in the 1984 supplement *Recent Advances in Research on Filariasis*.[3]

Diethylcarbamazine (DEC) patch test
A simple and sensitive DEC localized skin test has been developed in Sudan to assist in the clinical diagnosis (but *not* treatment) of onchocerciasis and in survey work.[15]

The patch skin test consists of applying a small amount of 10% DEC in *Nivea* lanolin cream to an area of skin about 5 mm in diameter and covering the area with a dressing. The area is inspected 8, 12, 24, 48 and 72 h later. A positive test is shown by a papular eruption developing 8-24 hours after applying the DEC. The reaction is an allergic response to dead microfilariae at the site of application. Positive reactions cause the patient only limited itching. Several different sites can be tested.

The test is inexpensive, rapid, simple to perform and safer for the patient. Full details can be found in the paper of Stingl *et al*.[12]

Important: The DEC cream must *not* be used for the treatment of onchocerciasis because DEC can cause severe skin changes and damage to the eyes.[5]

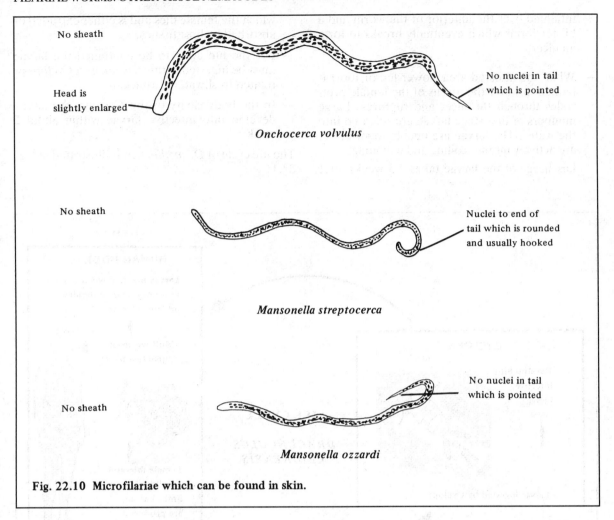

No sheath

Head is
slightly enlarged

No nuclei in tail
which is pointed

Onchocerca volvulus

No sheath

Nuclei to end of
tail which is rounded
and usually hooked

Mansonella streptocerca

No nuclei in tail
which is pointed

No sheath

Mansonella ozzardi

Fig. 22.10 Microfilariae which can be found in skin.

22:8 DRACUNCULUS MEDINENSIS

Dracunculus medinensis, (Guinea worm) causes guinea worm ulcers. Infection is referred to as dracontiasis or dracunculosis.

Distribution
D. medinensis is found in areas where communities use shallow ponds or walk-in open wells as sources of drinking water. It is particularly widespread in India and is also found in Pakistan, parts of South America, Africa (especially West Africa, Sudan, Kenya, Uganda), the Middle East (Saudi Arabia, Yemen, Iran) and Burma.

Transmission and life cycle
D. medinensis is transmitted by swallowing water containing infected crustaceans belonging to the genus *Cyclops* and other related genera (see 23:16).

Transmission is greatest during the dry season when water levels are low and the *Cyclops* are therefore at their most concentrated.

Dogs and possibly other animals may act as reservoir hosts for *D. medinensis*.

Life cycle
— A person swallows water which contains *Cyclops* crustaceans that are infected with *D. medinensis* larvae.

The larvae are freed and penetrate through the duodenal wall. After development and fertilization in the connective tissues, the female worm migrates to the subcutaneous tissues (usually of the lower limbs) where within about a year it becomes fully mature.

Mature D. medinensis worms: They are white and have a smooth surface. The female is very long, measuring up to one metre or more. The male measures only about 25 mm and is thought to die after fertilizing the female.

— The female worm buries its anterior end in the dermis of its host. The skin then becomes inflamed over the anterior of the worm and a blister forms which eventually breaks to form an ulcer.

— When the affected area (lower leg or foot) is bathed in water the uterus of the female protrudes through the ulcer and ruptures. Large numbers of first stage larvae are released into the water. The larvae are unable to swim but are actively motile, coiling and uncoiling.

Discharge of the larvae takes 2-3 weeks after which the female dies and is either extruded or absorbed by host tissues.

— For the life cycle to be continued the larvae must be ingested within a week by a *Cyclops* or related freshwater crustacean.

— In the body cavity of the *Cyclops*, the larvae develop into infective larvae within about 2 weeks.

The life cycle of *D. medinensis* is illustrated in Fig. 22.11.

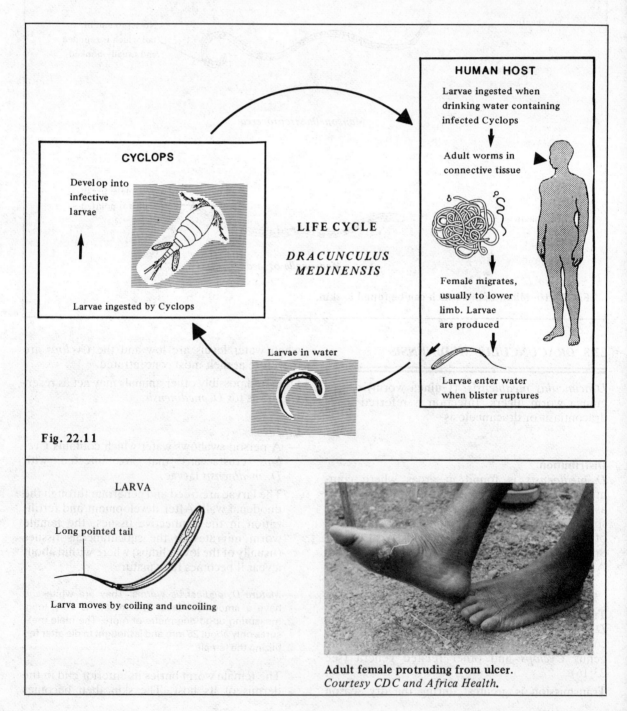

HUMAN HOST

Larvae ingested when drinking water containing infected Cyclops

Adult worms in connective tissue

Female migrates, usually to lower limb. Larvae are produced

Larvae enter water when blister ruptures

CYCLOPS

Develop into infective larvae

Larvae ingested by Cyclops

LIFE CYCLE

DRACUNCULUS MEDINENSIS

Larvae in water

Fig. 22.11

LARVA

Long pointed tail

Larva moves by coiling and uncoiling

Adult female protruding from ulcer.
Courtesy CDC and Africa Health.

Clinical features and pathology

Dracontiasis often causes serious clinical symptoms especially in heavy infections. The female worms cause severe pain and allergic reactions including urticaria, fever, nausea and vomiting. Damage to the worms in the skin can produce severe inflammation.

Secondary infection may also occur leading to cellulitis and occasionally septicaemia. Tetanus is a serious but rare complication.

If a joint is involved, arthritis may develop. The disease can have crippling effects preventing normal work activity with serious consequences when crops cannot be planted during the rainy season.

Prevention and control

Dracontiasis is one of the easiest parasitic diseases to prevent because the period of infectivity is usually only a few weeks and there is no important animal reservoir. Areas of transmission tend to be small and easily defined. Once transmission is interrupted in an area for a single rainy season, infection ceases entirely unless it is reintroduced from outside.[13]

Preventive and control measures include the following:

- As a community measure, preventing water sources becoming infected by:
  — Installing a piped water supply.
  — Filling in step-wells or replacing them with draw-wells.
  — Covering community water supplies and chlorinating when possible.
  — Providing wells which do not allow the return of water.
  — Providing health education including demonstrating *Cyclops* in community drinking water supplies.

- Avoiding drinking infected water by:
  — Filtering drinking water through nylon or muslin cloth (100 mesh to 1 cm) or other suitable filter to hold back the larvae.
  — Boiling all drinking water.

- Destroying the *Cyclops* intermediate host by using organophosphorus chemicals or chlorine in pot chlorinators.

- Covering with a waterproof dressing all exposed worms in infected persons.

Further information: The application of science and technology at primary health care level in guinea-worm infection (and filarial diseases) is discussed in the 1985 WHO paper of Duke.[5]

Laboratory tests to investigate dracontiasis are limited because the larvae of *D. medinensis* are normally washed into water. A diagnosis is usually made when the blister has ruptured and the anterior end of the female worm can be seen.

If required, laboratory confirmation of the diagnosis can be made as follows:

1. Place a few drops of water on the ulcer to encourage discharge of the larvae.
2. After a few minutes collect the water in a plastic bulb pipette or other suitable pipette
3. Transfer the water to a slide and examine microscopically for motile larvae using the 10× objective with the iris diaphragm closed sufficiently to give good contrast.

The following are the main identifying features of *D. medinensis* larvae:

***Dracunculus medinensis* larva**

- It is large, measuring 500-700 μm in length.

- Anterior end is rounded.

- Tail is long and pointed. In wet preparations the tail can be seen coiling and uncoiling.

Illustrations: See Plate 22.19 and colour Plate 29.

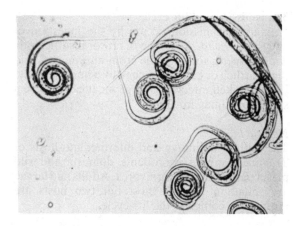

Plate 22.19 Larvae of *Dracunculus medinensis* as seen with the 10x objective. *Courtesy of A. Moody.*

Note: Serological techniques have been developed to assist in the diagnosis of dracontiasis but not all of these have been found to be reliable. Details of a visually read ELISA which has been reported as being of value in the early serodiagnosis of dracontiasis can be found in the paper of Kliks and Rao.[14]

22:9 *TRICHINELLA SPECIES*

Trichinella species are common parasites of domestic and wild pigs, rats, and many carnivores. Human infection with *Trichinella* is called trichinellosis (trichinosis, trichiniasis) and is a zoonosis.

Species classification
Based on differences in the biological, enzymatic, and genetic characteristics of *Trichinella*, it has been proposed that four distinct species of *Trichinella* should be recognized. Three of the species are associated with human infections as follows:

- *Trichinella spiralis*: This is the species which is maintained in domestic pigs in developed parts of the world and also infects rats, cats, and dogs.

- *Trichinella nativa*: This is the species which infects carnivores and marine mammals in the Arctic.

- *Trichinella nelsoni*: This is the species which naturally infects carnivores and wild pigs in the tropics and subtropics.

Note: Morphologically, the different species are indistinguishable.

Distribution
Trichinella species can be found in parts of Africa, Asia and South America. They are also widely distributed in the northern hemisphere including the Arctic.

Transmission and life cycle
Human transmission occurs by the ingestion of encysted *Trichinella* larvae in raw or insufficiently cooked meat, for example from an infected wild pig, warthog or bear barbecued by a hunting party. Undercooked infected sausage meat can also be a source of human infection.

Natural life cycle
The natural definitive and intermediate hosts of *Trichinella* species are rodents, domestic and wild pigs, bears and other carnivores. Adults and larvae are found in a single host but two hosts are required to complete the life cycle.

- When an infected rodent or the flesh of another carnivore containing infective larvae is ingested by a pig or other carnivore, the larvae are freed and become mature worms in the small intestine.

  Mature Trichinella worms: They are white and very small. The female measures up to 4 mm in length and the male up to 1.5 mm. The adults live for only a few weeks after which they are passed in faeces.

- Following fertilization, the viviparous females produce many larvae which are carried in the blood circulation to striated muscles where they encyst.

- The natural cycle is completed when the flesh of an infected carnivore is eaten by another carnivore.

  Among wild pigs and wild carnivores the life cycle is maintained by scavenging and cannibalism among carnivores. Domestic pigs are commonly infected by ingesting larvae in pork products, offal or garbage, or by eating infected rodents.

Development in a human host
Human infection with *Trichinella* is a zoonosis. When man becomes a host, the life cycle ends 'blindly'. There is no transfer of the parasite to a secondary host except by cannibalism or where carnivores such as dogs, jackals or hyaenas are able to feed on human remains. Encysted larvae can remain viable for many years.

Following ingestion of *Trichinella* larvae, development of the parasite in a human host is similar to that in an animal host. The ingested larvae become mature worms in the small intestine. The adults produce larvae which enter the lymphatics and pass into the blood circulation. They are carried to skeletal muscles where they encyst and often become calcified.

The life cycle of *Trichinella* is illustrated in Fig. 22.12.

Clinical features and pathology
Within 48 hours of ingesting *Trichinella* larvae, intestinal disturbances may occur. These can include abdominal pain, nausea and vomiting.

During migration of the larvae, allergic symptoms develop including fever, oedema of the face, headache, and eosinophilia. Encystment of the larvae often causes muscle pain.

Heavy infections with widespread migration of larvae may cause neurological disorders and occasionally a fatal myocarditis.

Prevention and control
- Avoiding the eating of raw or undercooked pork or the flesh of wild animals such as bush pig or warthog which may be infected with *Trichinella* larvae.

To avoid infection, meat should be cooked right through to a temperature of at least 60 °C.

Trichinella larvae can also be killed by deep-freezing meat (not more than 15 cm thick) at −25 °C for 10 days. Smoking, curing, or drying of meat are not reliable methods of destroying the larvae.

- Inspecting meat for infective larvae. Encysted larvae can remain infective for many years.

- By not feeding raw garbage to pigs (where transmission is through domestic pigs).

LABORATORY DIAGNOSIS

Laboratory confirmation of trichinellosis is by:

- ☐ Detecting *Trichinella* larvae in striated muscle.
- ☐ Testing serum for *Trichinella* antibodies.

Note: An eosinophilic leucocytosis is found in the acute stage of the disease and serum amino-transferases are often raised.

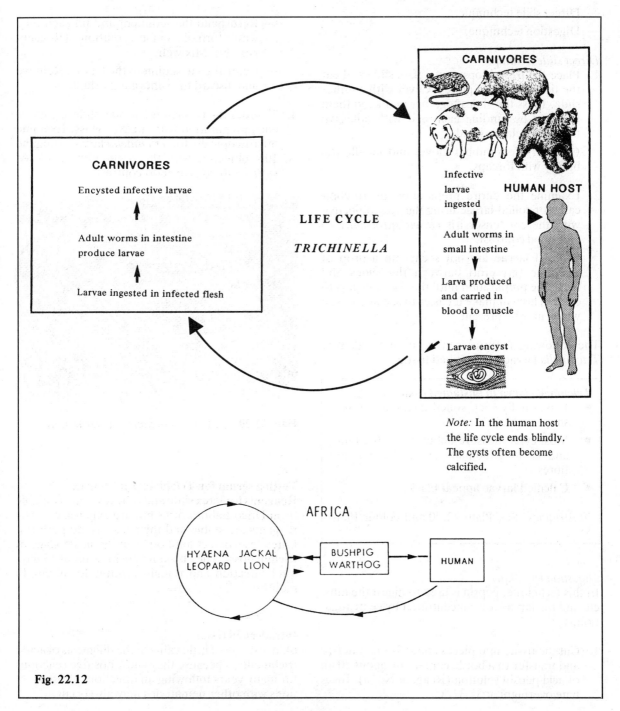

CARNIVORES

Encysted infective larvae

↑

Adult worms in intestine produce larvae

↑

Larvae ingested in infected flesh

LIFE CYCLE

TRICHINELLA

CARNIVORES

Infective larvae ingested

HUMAN HOST

Adult worms in small intestine

↓

Larva produced and carried in blood to muscle

↓

Larvae encyst

Note: In the human host the life cycle ends blindly. The cysts often become calcified.

AFRICA

HYAENA JACKAL
LEOPARD LION
→ BUSHPIG WARTHOG →
HUMAN

Fig. 22.12

Examination of muscle for *Trichinella* larvae
The larvae can be found in muscle tissue from the second or third week after infection.

Specimen: A striated muscle biopsy (collected under local anaesthesia) is required. Suitable sites to biopsy include the muscles of the shoulder, outer thigh, or calf of the leg. A biopsy measuring about 20 × 10 mm is adequate.

Techniques used to detect *Trichinella* larvae in muscle include:
— Direct slide technique.
— Digestion technique.

Direct slide technique
1. Place the fresh biopsy on a glass slide and cut the tissue into thin pieces. Cover with another slide. Press the slides together and keep them together by binding each end with adhesive tape or an elastic band.
   Caution: Wear rubber gloves and handle the biopsy with forceps.

2. Examine the entire preparation microscopically for coiled larvae using the 10× objective with the condenser iris *closed sufficiently* to give good contrast.
   Note: If larvae are not seen, run a drop of glycerine (glycerol) between the slides and leave the preparation until the tissue begins to clear. This will make it easier to see any larvae which may be present.

The following features can be used to identify *Trichinella* larvae in unstained tissue:

> **_Trichinella larva in unstained tissue_**
> - It is usually seen coiled inside a lemon-shaped cyst.
> - Most cysts measure about 0.5 × 0.2 mm and lie longitudinally along the muscle fibres.
> - Calcified larvae appear black.
>
> *Illustrations*: See Plate 22.20 and colour Plate 31.

Digestion technique
In this technique, pepsin is used to digest the muscle and the larvae are concentrated by centrifugation.

1. Cut the tissue into pieces about 2-3 mm in size and transfer to a bottle containing about 20 ml of acid pepsin solution (Reagent No. 5). Incubate overnight at 35-37 °C.

Caution: Wear rubber gloves and use forceps to handle the tissue.

2. Mix well and transfer the contents of the bottle to two conical tubes. Centrifuge at medium speed (approx. 2000 rpm) for 2-5 minutes to sediment the larvae.

3. Using a plastic bulb pipette or other suitable pipette, remove and discard the supernatant fluid from each tube. Wash and fix the sediments as follows:

   — Resuspend the sediment and fill each tube with formol saline solution (Reagent No. 39). Mix well.
   — Centrifuge to sediment the larvae. Remove and discard the supernatant fluid.

4. Transfer the two sediments to a slide and cover each preparation with a cover glass. Examine microscopically for *Trichinella* larvae using the 10× objective with the condenser iris *closed sufficiently* to give good contrast.

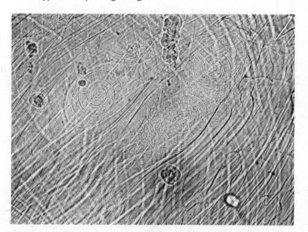

Plate 22.20 Unstained *Trichinella* larvae in muscle.

Testing serum for *Trichinella* antibodies
Reagents for latex slide and tube tests are available from Difco Laboratories but are expensive.[15] The reagents are stable and the tests easy to perform. Latex tests detect antibodies in the acute stage of trichinellosis. They become positive about 15 days after infection and remain positive for about 10 months.

Intradermal tests
Skin tests are of little value in the diagnosis of acute trichinellosis because they show positive reactions for many years following an infection. Cross-reactions with other nematodes may also occur.

22:10 INFECTIONS CAUSED BY ANIMAL TISSUE NEMATODES

DIROFILARIA SPECIES

Filarial worms of the genus *Dirofilaria* are normally parasitic in dogs and racoons. Infection in humans can occur but is rare. Species which have been reported as causing pulmonary or subcutaneous disease in humans include:

Dirofilaria immitis (dog heartworm)
Dirofilaria tenuis (racoon parasite)
Dirofilaria repens (dog parasite)

Distribution
D. immitis infections have been reported from Japan, Australia, southern and eastern USA, and parts of South America. *D. tenuis* infections have occurred in southern USA. *D. repens* infections have been reported from India, Asia, and Europe.

Transmission and life cycle
Dirofilarial worms are transmitted from animal hosts to humans by various species of mosquito. In humans, the larvae may develop but they do not produce microfilariae.

In their natural animal hosts the worms mature and produce microfilariae which circulate in the blood and are taken up by mosquitoes.

Clinical features and pathology
D. immitis can cause pulmonary dirofilariasis with fever, chest pain, cough, and occasionally haemoptysis. There is not usually a blood eosinophilia. The presence of the worm in the lung stimulates inflammation and eventually the dead worm becomes surrounded by a fibrous wall. Calcification can occur.

D. tenuis and *D. repens* can cause subcutaneous dirofilariasis with the formation of painful erythematous subcutaneous nodules especially in and around the eyes. Occasionally other parts of the body are affected such as the scrotum, breasts, arms and legs.

LABORATORY DIAGNOSIS

Laboratory confirmation of dirofilariasis is by identifying the worms in tissue sections. Formalin fixed biopsies should be sent to a Histology Laboratory.

Note: With pulmonary dirofilariasis, what is known as a 'coin lesion' can sometimes be seen on a chest X-ray.

ANGIOSTRONGYLUS SPECIES

Angiostrongylus cantonensis is a natural parasite of rodents and is often referred to as the rat lungworm. In humans it can cause eosinophilic meningoencephalitis.

Angiostrongylus costaricensis also infects rodents. It has been identified as causing intestinal disease in humans.

Distribution
A. cantonensis has been reported from many of the Pacific Islands, the Philippines, Sumatra, and parts of South-East Asia especially Thailand.

A. costaricensis has been reported from Costa Rica and South America.

Transmission and life cycle
Humans become infected by ingesting *Angiostrongylus* larvae in snails (second intermediate hosts) or in freshwater prawns or crabs (carrier hosts). The parasite is unable to develop to its egg-producing stage and dies in the central nervous system of its human host.

In their natural rodent hosts, *Angiostrongylus* larvae migrate to the brain where they develop into adult worms. Eggs are laid in the lungs and the hatched larvae migrate up the trachea and are swallowed and finally excreted in the faeces. The life cycle is continued by a slug or land snail ingesting the larvae and the cycle is completed by a rodent swallowing the infected slug or snail.

Crabs and freshwater prawns can act as carrier hosts.

Clinical features and pathology
The main feature of human infection is an eosinophilic meningoencephalitis which develops in response to toxins released from dead and degenerating worms. Other reported symptoms include pain, weakness of the limbs, and partial facial palsy. Fever is not a common finding.

Infection with *A. costaricensis* is associated with intestinal eosinophilic granulomata and obstruction of the intestinal tract.

Prevention and control
This is by avoiding eating raw or insufficiently cooked molluscs, crabs, or prawns that may be infected. The larvae can be killed by being boiled or frozen at −15 °C for 12 hours.

LABORATORY DIAGNOSIS

The commonest laboratory findings in angiostrongyliasis are as follows:

Cerebrospinal fluid
- Cell count is usually over 500 cells /μl with 50-75% of the cells being eosinophils (there is also a blood eosinophilia).
- Protein is raised.
- Glucose is reduced.
- Very occasionally larvae are found.

GNATHOSTOMA SPINIGERUM

Gnathostoma spinigerum is normally found in the stomach wall of cats, tigers, lions, leopards, dogs and other animals where it causes tumours. The larvae of the parasite can infect humans.

Distribution
Human infections have been reported from South-East Asia especially Thailand and also from the Philippines, Bangladesh, India, Japan, and China.

Transmission and life cycle
Humans become infected by ingesting third stage larvae in a second intermediate host (freshwater fish) or less commonly in a carrier host (e.g. reptile, frog, chicken).

The larvae cannot develop to egg-producing worms in a human host. They usually develop to young adults and migrate through the organs of the body and subcutaneous tissues.

In their animal host, the larvae reach maturity and eggs are laid and pushed out into the stomach to be passed in the faeces. In water the eggs hatch larvae which are ingested by a *Cyclops*. The life cycle is continued by a second intermediate host (fish) ingesting the infected *Cyclops* and the cycle is completed by an animal definitive host ingesting the infected fish.

Clinical features and pathology
Migration of the larvae in cutaneous tissues causes recurring allergic swellings. The inflamed swellings are often painful and itchy.

Occasionally, worms enter the eye, mucous membranes, respiratory tract, central nervous system, or abdominal organs where they can cause serious inflammatory reactions, haemorrhages, and fibrosis.

Prevention and control
Infection can be prevented by boiling fish which may be infected. Alternatively the fish can be immersed in vinegar for 5-6 hours which will also kill any larvae present.

LABORATORY DIAGNOSIS

Laboratory confirmation of gnathostomiasis is limited. Most infections are diagnosed by a skin test. Details of this can be found in the 1980 SEA-MIC *Monograph on the genus Gnathostoma and Gnathostomiasis in Thailand*[16] and in the paper of Miyazaki.[17]

Note: The SEAMIC Monograph also contains detailed descriptions of human infections, the definitive and intermediate hosts of *G. spinigerum*, and also photomicrographs of the eggs, larvae and adult worms of the parasite.

Infection with *G. spinigerum* is frequently accompanied by an eosinophilic leucocytosis.

Identification of helminth parasites in tissue sections
For details of the identification of helminth parasites in tissue sections, readers are referred to the paper of Chitwood, M., and Lichtenfeld, J. R.[18]

References
1 World Health Organization. *Lymphatic filariasis*, WHO Technical Report Series **702**, 1984.

2 Ismail, M. M. *Occult Filariasis - Tropical pulmonary eosinophilia and other obscure syndromes associated with lymphatic filarial parasites*. WHO/FIL/84.173.

3 Goodwin, L. G., Ottesen, E. A., Southgate, B. A., Lucas, A. O. Recent advances in research on filariasis. *Transactions of the Royal Society of Tropical Medicine and Hygiene*, **78**, (supplement), pp 1-28 1984.

4 Taylor, A. E. R. Filariasis, a review of recent abstracts (January 1983 - March 1984). *Tropical Diseases Bulletin*, **81**, 9, R1 - R24, 1984.

5 Duke, B. O. L. The application of science and technology at the primary health care level in filarial diseases and guinea-worm infection. World Health Organization, WHO/FIL/85.179, WHO/ONCHO/ 85.164, WHO/VBC/85.921, 1985. This document is available from WHO, Filariasis Unit, 1211 Geneva-27, Switzerland.

6 Mackenzie, C. D., Kron, M. A. Diethylcarbamazine. A review of its action in onchocerciasis, lymphatic filariasis and inflammation. *Tropical Diseases Bulletin*, **82**, R1 - R37 (supplement), 1985.

7 Ottesen, E. A. Immunological aspects of lymphatic filariasis and onchocerciasis in man. *Transactions of the Royal Society of Tropical Medicine and Hygiene*, **18**, (supplement), pp 9-18, 1984.

8 Nathan, M. B., Lambourne, A., Monteil. *Annals of Tropical Medicine and Parasitology*, **76**, pp 339-345, 1982.

9 Personal communication from Mr. A. H. Moody, Senior Chief MLSO, Pathology Department, Hospital for Tropical Diseases, 4 St Pancras Way, London NW1 0PE, UK.

10 Brinkmann, U. K. The assessment of microfilarial densities in skin snips from onchocerciasis patients under field conditions. *Tropenmedizin und Parasitologie*, **25**, pp 160-166, 1974.

11 Kale, O. O. A simplified technique for counting onchocercal microfilariae in skin snips. *Bulletin of the World Health Organization*, **56**, pp 133-137, 1978.

12 Stingl, P., *et al*. A diagnostic 'patch test' for onchocerciasis using tropical diethylcarbamazine. *Transactions of the Royal Society of Tropical Medicine and Hygiene*, **78**, pp 254-258, 1984.

13 Muller, R. Guinea worm disease: epidemiology, control and treatment. *Bulletin of the World Health Organization*, **57**, pp 683-689, 1979.

14 Kliks, M. M., Rao, C. K. Development of rapid ELISA for early serodiagnosis of dracunculiasis. *Journal of Communicable Diseases*, **16**, 4, pp 287-294, 1984.

15 The Difco latex test requires Bacto-*Trichinella* antigen (1 ml, code 2375-50-2), Bacto-Latex 0.81 (5 ml, code 3102-56-4) and RA Buffer which is a buffer (available pack 10 × 1 litre, code 3103-37-7). Difco also provide a positive *Trichinella* control serum (1 ml, code 2376-50-1). The costs (1986) of the reagents are £23.30 for antigen, £45.40 for latex, £29.95 for buffer and £24.35 for the control antiserum.

16 Daengsvang, S. A. *Monograph on the Genus Gnathostoma and Gnathostomiasis in Thailand*. SEAMIC, 1980. Copies available from 6th Toyokaiji Bldg, 7-2 Shimbashi 4-chome, Minato-ku, Tokyo, Japan.

17 Migatzaki, I. On the genus Gnathostoma and human gnathostomiasis, with special reference to Japan. *Experimental Parasitology*, **9**, 338, 1960.

18 Chitwood, M. and Lichtenfeld, J. R. Parasitological Review: Identification of parasitic metazoa in tissue sections. *Experimental Parasitology*, **32**, pp 407-519, 1972.

Recommended Reading

World Health Organization. *Lymphatic Filariasis*. WHO, Technical Report Series, No. **702**, 1984.

Bell, D. R. Lecture *Notes on Tropical Medicine*, Blackwell Scientific Publications, 2nd Ed, 1985. Paperback priced £9.80.

Knight, R. *Parasitic Disease in Man*, Churchill Livingstone, 1982. ELBS edition priced £4.50.

Peters, W., Gilles, H. M. *A Colour Atlas of Tropical Medicine and Parasitology*, Wolfe Medical Publications, 2nd Ed, 1981. ELBS edition priced £9.00.

Duke, B. O. L. The application of science and technology at the primary health care level in filarial diseases and guinea-worm infection. World Health Organization, WHO/FIL/85.179, WHO/ONCHO/85.164, WHO/VBC/85.921., 1985. Available from TDR Filariasis Programme., WHO, 1211 Geneva-27, Switzerland.

UNDP/World Bank/WHO-TDR Programme. *Lymphatic Pathology and Immunopathology in Filariasis. Report of the Twelfth Meeting of the Scientific Working Group on Filariasis*. TDR/FIL-SWG (12) /85.3, 1985. Available from TDR Filariasis Programme, WHO, 1211 Geneva-27 Switzerland.

Tropical Diseases Research Programme
FILARIASIS

Filariasis is included in the *UNDP/World Bank/World Health Organization Special Programme for Research and Training in Tropical Diseases*.

Tropical Diseases Research (TDR) activities with regard to filariasis as recorded in No. 5 of the 1985 *WHO Chronicle* are as follows:

- Research into new drugs active against *Onchocerca volvulus*.

- Development of specific immunodiagnostic test for filarial infection in man. New techniques using DNA probes are being devised to differentiate the larvae of the human parasites from those of related filarial species that are parasites of animals.

- Development of effective vector control measures for use in endemic onchocerciasis areas.

23 Insects and Arachnids of Medical Importance

23:1 INTRODUCTION TO INSECTS AND ARACHNIDS AND THE DISEASES THEY CAUSE

Insects and arachnids belong to the phylum Arthropoda which contains those segmented invertebrate animals that are supported by a rigid framework known as an exoskeleton.

Insects and arachnids are associated with many parasitic infections and other tropical diseases and therefore a knowledge of their characteristics, breeding, and feeding habits is essential for the successful prevention and control of the diseases they cause.

INSECTS
The class Insecta includes flies, fleas, bugs, lice, ants, and bees.

The body of an insect is divided into a head, thorax, and abdomen. The head bears mouth-parts and a single pair of antennae. In the adult insect there are three pairs of legs attached to the thorax. Many insects are equipped with two pairs of wings, one or both of which may be vestigial.

Some diseases are transmitted simply by the insect carrying the organism mechanically from one subject to another. Such insects are therefore known as carriers. Other diseases require the organism to pass through a more or less complicated development in the insect, such as the malaria parasite in the mosquito, so that the insect is a necessary stage in the life cycle of the disease. Such insects are called vectors.

Insects of medical importance
- Diptera (true flies) which includes:
  - Mosquitoes which transmit malaria, dengue fever, filariasis, yellow fever, and viruses.
  - Sandflies which transmit leishmaniasis, sandfly fever, and Oroya fever.
  - Blackflies which transmit onchocerciasis.
  - Horseflies which transmit loiasis.
  - Tsetse flies which transmit African trypanosomiasis.
  - Blowflies which cause myiasis.

- Siphonaptera (fleas) which includes:
  - *Xenopsylla* species which carry plague and typhus.
  - *Pulex* and other species which cause discomfort and irritation.
  - *Tunga* species which cause a painful irritation.

- Hemiptera (bugs) which includes:
  - Triatomine (cone-nose) bugs which transmit South American trypanosomiasis.
  - Cimicidae bugs (bed-bugs) which cause discomfort and irritation.

- Anoplura (lice) which includes:
  - *Pediculus* species which transmit relapsing fever, epidemic typhus, and trench fever.
  - *Phthirus* species which cause discomfort and irritation in the pubic region.

- Dictyoptera which includes:
  - Cockroaches which act as mechanical vectors and reservoirs of disease.

ARACHNIDS
The class Arachnida includes ticks, mites, spiders, and scorpions.

Adult arachnids have four pairs of legs. In some species the body appears undivided while in others it is segmented into a cephalothorax and abdomen. The cephalothorax has mouth-parts, simple eyes, but no antennae.

Not all arachnids transmit disease. Some by their bites and stings cause pain, discomfort, irritation, and more serious conditions.

Arachnids of medical importance
- Ticks which include:
  - Hard ticks which transmit rickettsial fevers, viruses, and tularaemia.
  - Soft ticks which transmit relapsing fever.

- Mites which include:
  - *Sarcoptes* species which cause scabies.
  - *Trombicula* species which transmit scrub typhus.

23:2 DIPTERA

The body of a dipteran insect is divided into:

- A head, which bears a pair of antennae, a pair

of compound eyes, and mouth-parts adapted for piercing and sucking or sponging.

— A thorax, consisting of fused segments and one pair of wings. The hind pair of wings are replaced by a pair of club-shaped organs, known as halteres, which are used for balancing. There are three pair of legs (fore, mid, and hind).

— An abdomen, which is segmented.

The life cycle is one of complete metamorphosis in which there is usually an egg, a larval, and a pupal stage from which the adult emerges,

Mosquitoes: *Anopheles, Culex, Aedes, Mansonia* species

Sandflies: *Phlebotomus, Lutzomyia* species

Blackflies: *Simulium* species

Horseflies: *Chrysops* species

Midges: *Culicoides* species

Tsetse flies: *Glossina* species

Houseflies: *Musca* species

Blowflies: *Chrysomya, Cochliomyia, Cordylobia, Wohlfahrtia, Dermatobia* species

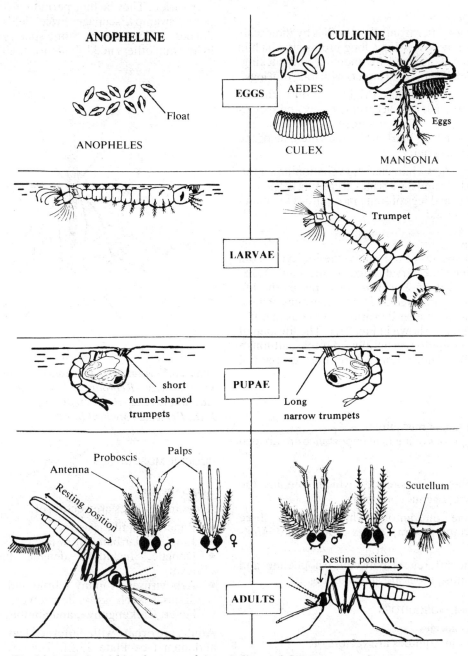

Fig. 23.1 Distinguishing features of Anopheline and Culicine mosquitoes.

23:3 MOSQUITOES

Mosquitoes are the most widespread of the medically important insects. The tropical diseases they transmit are responsible for much illhealth and loss of human life. By frequenting human dwellings, some species are serious pests of man. Many species of mosquito, however, are more attracted to animals and do not feed from humans.

Female mosquitoes, by needing blood for egg production, are responsible for transmitting disease. Male mosquitoes do not bite and therefore they do not transmit disease. They live on plant juices.

Appearance
Mosquitoes differ from all other flies by their scaly wings and by possessing a long proboscis which in the female is adapted for piercing and sucking. They are delicate, small insects with long thin legs.

The long proboscis has a rigid palp on each side which varies in length according to sex and species (see Fig. 23.1). The antennae in the male are covered with long hairs, while the antennae of the female are less hairy.

The wings show characteristic venation and spotting with light and dark scales according to species. The thorax and legs of some mosquitoes are beautifully patterned.

Life cycle
For most species of mosquito, the life cycle from egg through the larval stage to the adult takes about 10-14 days. For *Mansonia* species the life cycle takes up to 3 weeks. Different groups of mosquitoes lay their eggs by various methods in different patterns as shown in Fig. 23.1. The lifespan of an adult mosquito is generally 3-4 weeks, although it may be reduced in nature due to natural enemies.

Classification of mosquitoes
The mosquitoes of medical importance are divided into:

☐ Anopheline mosquitoes which contains the important genus *Anopheles*.
☐ Culicine mosquitoes which contain three important genera, *Aedes, Culex*, and *Mansonia*.

The main differences between Anopheline and Culicine mosquitoes are shown in Fig. 23.1.

ANOPHELINE MOSQUITOES

Anopheles species
Anopheles mosquitoes are vectors of:
● Malaria

● Bancroftian and Brugian filariasis.
● Arboviruses of a few febrile and encephalitic diseases.

Feeding habits
Most *Anopheles* mosquitoes are twilight or night feeders although a few are also day feeders. Some species of *Anopheles* feed and rest indoors, some feed out of doors, while others feed indoors and rest out of doors. Anopheline mosquitoes rest with the body sloping forwards (see Fig. 23.1).

Breeding sites
The breeding sites of *Anopheles* mosquitoes are very varied. They include permanent or temporary pools, swamps, seepages, rice fields, tree-holes, ditches, and reservoirs. Some species require sunlight while others need shade for their breeding.

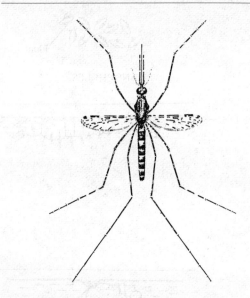

Plate 23.1 *Anopheles* **mosquito** *(A. gambiae).* **About x5 true size.** *Reproduced from Common African Mosquitoes and their Medical Importance, Gillett, J. D., Heineman Medical Books.*

CULICINE MOSQUITOES

Aedes species
Aedes mosquitoes are vectors of:

● Bancroftian filariasis.
● Jungle and urban yellow fever.
● Dengue, including dengue haemorrhagic fever.
● Arboviruses of many febrile and encephalitic diseases such as yellow fever, Rift Valley Fever, Chikungunya, and Sindbis.

Adults are ornate with patterned legs, thorax, and abdomen (see Plate 23.2). Their wings are not spotted.

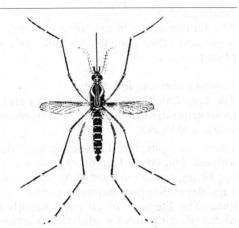

Plate 23.2 *Aedes* mosquito *(A. aegypti).* **About x4 true size.** *Reproduced from Common African Mosquitoes and their Medical Importance, Gillett, J. D., Heineman Medical Books.*

Feeding habits
Aedes mosquitoes feed during the day or night, indoors and out of doors.

Breeding sites
The breeding sites of *Aedes* mosquitoes include stagnant water in dark tree holes, coconut shells, old tins, bamboos, pots, axils of leaves of banana trees, or in mud holes made by land crabs. Forest mosquitoes breed high up in the trees, in holes, or in bamboos.

Culex species
Culex mosquitoes are vectors of:
- Bancroftian filariasis.

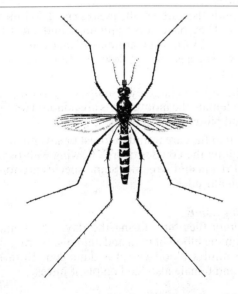

Plate 23.3 *Culex* mosquito *(C. fatigans).* **About x4 true size.** *Reproduced from Common African Mosquitoes and their Medical Importance, Gillett, J. D., Heineman Medical Books.*

- Arboviruses of several febrile and encephalitic diseases such as Sindbis, Spondweni, West Nile fever, Western Equine and Japanese encephalitis.

Adults are not ornate.

Feeding habits
Many *Culex* mosquitoes are attracted to animals. They are mostly indoor night feeders.

Breeding sites
Culex mosquitoes breed in latrines and in waste water containing organic material, including natural collections of water around houses, in swamps, water tanks, and in temporary muddy pools and ponds.

Mansonia species
Mansonia mosquitoes are vectors of:
- Brugian filariasis
- Bancroftian filariasis

Adults are of moderate size and strongly built.

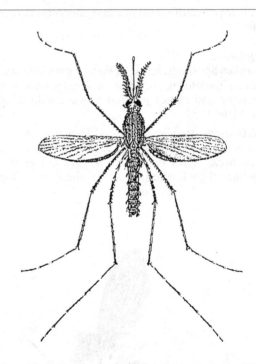

Plate 23.4 *Mansonia* mosquito *(M. uniformis).* **About x5 true size.** *Reproduced from Common African Mosquitoes and their Medical Importance, Gillett, J. D., Heineman Medical Books.*

They are black-brown and yellowish with a characteristic speckled appearance due to the broad asymmetrical light and dark scales which clothe their wings (see Plate 23.4). The legs show pale markings and white bands.

Feeding habits
Mansonia mosquitoes feed at night, indoors or out of doors, and during the day in swamp forests.

Breeding sites
The breeding sites of *Mansonia* mosquitoes are swamps, neglected paddy fields, ponds or other collections of water containing water plants or swamp grass. The siphon of the larva is short, conically shaped, and modified for piercing submerged stems and roots of plants to obtain oxygen.

23:4 PHLEBOTOMINE FLIES (SANDFLIES)

Phlebotomus sandflies are vectors of:

- Visceral leishmaniasis
- Cutaneous leishmaniasis
- Mucocutaneous leishmaniasis
- Sandfly fever
- Oroya fever (Carrion's disease)

The bites of sandflies often cause allergic skin reactions.

Appearance
Sandflies are small, hairy, yellow or grey-coloured insects, measuring 3-5 mm in length with long antennae and rather pointed upward-held wings (see Plate 23.5).

Phlebotomus species are found in warm and hot climates, in dry desert-like regions or in humid forest areas. They fly near to the ground in short hop-like flights often near to their breedings places.

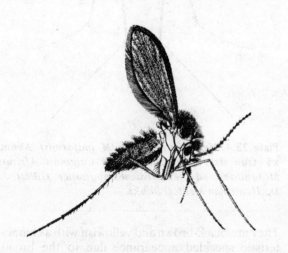

Plate 23.5 Adult female *Phlebotomus*. **True size 2-3 mm.** *Reproduced with permission of the British Museum (Natural History).*

Feeding habits
The female sucks blood from humans, rodents, dogs, and other animals, and the male feeds on plant juices.

Breeding sites and life cycle
The eggs (50-100) are laid in cracks and holes in moist ground, including animal burrows and under stones and bricks.

There are four larval stages before pupae are formed. The larvae feed on organic matter. From egg-laying to the emergence of adults takes 35-60 days, depending on temperature and availability of food. The life-span of an adult sandfly is a few weeks. Resting sites for adults include tree trunks, tree-holes, walls of buildings, and in cracks and crevices.

23.5 *SIMULIUM* FLIES (BLACKFLIES)

Simulium flies, also known as biting blackflies, are the vectors of human onchocerciasis. They can also transmit bovine onchocerciasis and mansonelliasis.

The species which transmit African onchocerciasis belong to the *Simulium damnosum* complex. The important vector in central America is *S. ochraceum*. In South America the main vectors are *S. metallicum* and the *S. amazonicum* complex.

Sandfly bites are painful and often cause allergic reactions.

Appearance
Simulium flies are small, measuring 1.5-4 mm in length. They have short antennae and short legs (see Plate 23.6). They are mostly black and white (a few species are yellow or less commonly orange).

The head bears large eyes and short mouth-parts. In the female the mouth-parts are adapted for tearing and piercing the skin.

Simulium flies are found in forest or savannah regions along the courses of free flowing well-oxygenated rivers and streams. Some species are found at high altitudes.

Feeding habits
Simulium flies bite during the day. The females feed on the blood of man and animals, tearing skin tissue until a blood vessel is damaged. Both the male and female also feed on plant juices.

Breeding sites and life cycle
The eggs are laid on rocks just below the surface of flowing water or on vegetation dipping into the water. The larvae and pupae remain attached to

rocks and dead leaves, feeding on small organic particles filtered from the water. There are six to nine larval stages.

Breeding is greatly increased in the rainy season. The life-span of the adult is a few weeks.

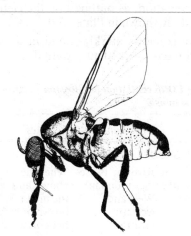

Plate 23.6 *Simulium* **(blackfly). True size 1.5-4 mm.** *Reproduced with permission of the British Museum (Natural History).*

23:6 *CHRYSOPS* FLIES (HORSEFLIES)

Chrysops flies, also known as horseflies, clegs, or gad flies, are members of the family Tabanidae. They are vectors of loiasis.

Chrysops flies can also act as mechanical carriers of bacteria and some protozoa.

The bites of the flies are often severe and painful.

Appearance
Chrysops flies are easily seen, measuring 9-10 mm in length. They have broad-banded wings and a wide triangular head bearing long antennae and large eyes (see Plate 23.7). The mouth-parts are well adapted for piercing.

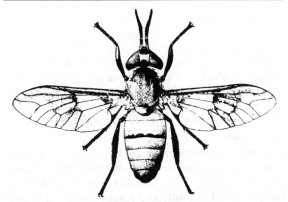

Plate 23.7 *Chrysops* **(horsefly or gad fly). True size 9-10 mm.** *Reproduced with permission of the British Museum (Natural History).*

The abdomen is yellow or orange and often patterned with black stripes or other markings. The abdomen, thorax, and legs are covered with small hairs.

Feeding habits
Chrysops species which transmit loiasis live in the African equatorial rain forest. Attracted by smoke or human activity in forest clearings, the flies bite often in late afternoon or early morning. Some species also bite indoors. The female feeds on blood and plant juices and the male on plant juices only.

Breeding sites and life cycle
Chrysops breed in muddy, heavily shaded swampy areas. Eggs are laid on plants growing in mud, covered by shallow slow-flowing water in the beds of drying streams. The larvae hatch and drop into the mud where they live for several months, feeding on small organisms. After growing and moulting they pupate on drier ground. Development takes several months.

23:7 *CULICOIDES* FLIES (MIDGES)

Culicoides flies, also known as biting midges, transmit the less pathogenic filarial worms *Mansonella perstans*, *Mansonella streptocerca*, and *Mansonella ozzardi*.

The bites of midges are painful, and frequently cause irritation which may last for several days. In some coastal areas, dark midges with milky white wings, of the genus *Leptoconops*, may be extremely annoying by their bites.

Appearance
Culicoides flies are small, measuring less than 2 mm in length. They are dark coloured with a humped thorax and small spotted wings. The antennae are long and the mouth-parts of the female are adapted for sucking blood as shown in Plate 23.8.

Feeding habits
Culicoides species live in swampy areas along the banks of rivers and pools, in mud and sand soaked by sea water, and around decaying trees and vegetation, including rotten banana tree stumps. Midges often swarm and bite in the early morning and during the evening, especially in overcast weather. Only the female sucks blood. The male feeds on plant juices.

Breeding sites and life cycle
The eggs are laid on plants in the water or on mud

and development takes a few weeks. There are four larval stages. The larvae have a pigmented head.

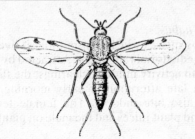

Plate 23.8 *Culicoides* **(midge). True size 1-2 mm.** *Reproduced with permission of the British Museum (Natural History).*

23:8 GLOSSINIDAE (TSETSE FLIES)

Tsetse flies belong to the family Glossinidae, and the genus *Glossina*. They are vectors of African trypanosomiasis.

Tsetse flies are divided into two main groups:

☐ *Morsitans* savannah group which are associated mainly with gambiense trypanosomiasis.

☐ *Palpalis* riverine group which are mainly the vectors of rhodesiense trypanosomiasis.

The differences between the *Morsitans* and *Palpalis* groups of tsetse flies and the medically important vectors in each group are listed in Chart 23.I.

In a trypanosomiasis endemic area only a small proportion of tsetse flies actually become infected with trypanosomes (1 in 2 000 to 1 in 10 000). Both *Morsitans* and *Palpalis* tsetse flies can transmit *T. b. gambiense* and *T. b. rhodesiense*.

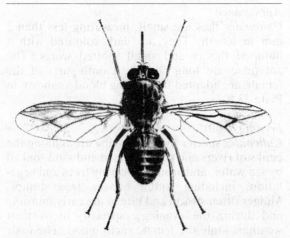

Plate 23.9　Tsetse fly. Note the axe-shaped venation, as outlined on the right wing. True size 6-15 mm. *Reproduced with permission of the British Museum (Natural History).*

Appearance
Tsetse flies are large yellow-brown or brown-black flies, measuring 6-15 mm in length. They have a long proboscis and short antennae.

The wings of a tsetse fly show a characteristic axe-shaped venation, as outlined on the right wing of the tsetse fly shown in Plate 23.9.

The thorax shows markings and in some species the abdomen is striped and spotted.

Chart 23.I Differentiation of Glossina Vectors of Trypanosomiasis

	Distribution	Features
PALPALIS GROUP		
G. palpalis G. tachinoides G. fuscipes	Riverine tsetse flies found in West and western Central Africa	When viewed from above, all segments of the hind tarsi are dark brown or black. The back of the abdomen is generally uniformly brown without distinct transverse dark bands.
MORSITANS GROUP		
G. morsitans G. pallidipes G. swynner-toni	Savannah tsetse flies found in East Africa, Ruanda, Burundi, and Botswana	When viewed from above, only the distal segments of the hind tarsi are dark coloured, with the remaining segments appearing pale in colour. The back of the abdomen generally shows distinct dark bands on a pale background.

Feeding habits
Both the male and female tsetse flies suck blood. They feed from humans, other mammals, and reptiles. The flies usually feed every 4-5 days, out-of-doors in open spaces. They are attracted by movement and smell, and readily become attached to moving vehicles on open roads.

Breeding sites and life cycle
When breeding, tsetse flies prefer shade to direct sunlight. Species of the *palpalis* group of flies live in vegetation bordering rivers, lakes, and other water places, whereas tsetse flies of the *morsitans* group prefer thinly wooded savannah areas away from water.

A tsetse fly does not lay eggs but produces a single fully developed larva, which on leaving the female, pupates in an area of shaded vegetation just below the surface of the soil. The adult emerges after several weeks. The flies are more numerous in the rainy season. The life-span of a tsetse fly is 2-3 months.

23:9 HOUSEFLIES

One of the commonest houseflies is *Musca domestica* which belongs to the family Muscidae.

Although *M. domestica* is a non-blood sucking muscid, it is important medically because it can ingest and transfer parasitic eggs and cysts, bacteria, and viruses from infected faeces to human food. Pathogenic organisms are easily transmitted because the feeding habits of the fly involve regurgitation of its crop contents and defaecation while feeding.

Diseases which *M. domestica* can transmit mechanically include:

- typhoid
- bacillary dysentery
- cholera
- brucellosis
- plague
- tetanus
- streptococcal infections
- amoebic dysentery
- poliomyelitis, hepatitis, and other viral diseases.

Appearance
M. domestica is about 8 mm in length, greyish-black with four dark stripes on its thorax and a variable amount of orange marking on its abdomen (see Plate 23.10). The antennae are short and the proboscis is retractable.

Feeding habits
Houseflies feed during the daytime, in and around human dwellings.

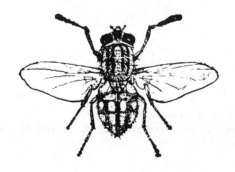

Plate 23.10 *Musca domestica*. **True size 8 mm.**

Breeding sites and life cycle
M. domestica lays its eggs in masses in manure and other decaying refuse. In warm conditions, the larvae (maggots) hatch within 24 hours and pupate after about 5 days. Adults emerge after about 3 days and live for about 1 month.

23:10 BLOWFLIES

Blowfies of medical importance belong to the genera:

Chrysomya
Cochliomyia
Cordylobia
Wohlfahrtia
Dermatobia

Medically, blowflies are important because their larvae, known as maggots, invade the skin, mucous membranes or conjunctiva. The invasion of tissues by maggots is called myiasis.

The larvae obtain their oxygen through small air holes known as spiracles. These are situated at the end of the maggot which lies in contact with the surface. The spiracles of different blowflies show a characteristic morphology when examined microscopically.

Note: Details of the preparation of posterior spiracles for examination and species identification may be found in textbooks of entomology.[1]

After about a week or more, the larvae leave their host and pupate in the ground to continue their development.

The prevention of myiasis is mainly by reducing the numbers of flies, by sanitary measures, and the use of insecticides. It may also be necesary to use repellants, screening, and protective clothing.

***Chrysomya* species**
Chrysomya flies are found throughout South East Asia, India, and Africa. They are a metallic green or green-blue colour. A medically important species is *C. bezziana*.

Myiasis caused by *Chrysomya* larvae can be serious because the maggots burrow deeply into tissues producing ulcers, especially around the eyes, ears, nose, and mouth. Frequently the larvae require surgical removal. *Chrysomya* flies are often referred to as 'Old World screw-worms'.

Infection is by the female fly laying eggs on the edges of wounds and other damaged tissue.

***Cochliomyia* species**
Cochliomyia flies are found in South America and the Caribbean region. They are similar to *Chrysomya* flies being a metallic blue-green colour.

The larvae cause deep ulceration. *Cochliomyia* flies are often referred to as 'New World screwworms'.

Infection is by the female laying eggs on damaged tissue.

Cordylobia species

Cordylobia flies are found in tropical Africa, where they are known as mango flies or tumbu flies. They are a non-metallic yellow-brown colour.

The larvae cause cutaneous myiasis in humans and in a variety of domesticated and wild animals. Rats and dogs are important reservoir hosts.

The eggs are laid on the ground or on clothing, particularly that which has been contaminated with sweat or urine. The larvae have small spines to enable them to penetrate the skin. A maggot can often be removed by pouring water on the skin which causes the spiracles to the surface. The maggot can then be squeezed out.

Wohlfahrtia species

Wohlfahrtia flies are found in Asia and elsewhere. They are large, measuring 10-24 mm in length, and of a non-metallic grey colour. The thorax is striped and the abdomen is usually marked with distinctive rows of black spots.

Myiasis is caused by the female discharging larvae on open wounds and other damaged tissue. Some species can cause serious ulceration with disfigurement.

Dermatobia species

Dermatobia flies, also known as botflies, are found in Central and South America. They are of a metallic purple-colour.

The larvae can cause painful swellings and allergic reactions. The maggots take several weeks to develop in the subcutaneous tissues.

Infection is usually by way of a blood-sucking insect acting as a carrier of the eggs. The newly hatched larvae penetrate through the wound made by the insect.

Auchmeromyia luteola

A. luteola has a widespread distribution in tropical and subtropical Africa.

The larvae of *A. luteola*, also known as Congo floor maggots, do not cause a true myiasis. They penetrate the skin only to obtain a blood meal after which they leave and continue their development in the cracks of the floors of mud huts.

The larvae are nocturnal feeders and their bites cause discomfort and irritation.

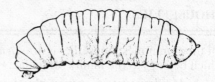

Plate 23.11　　Larva of *Auchmeromyia luteola* (Congo floor maggot). True size 10-12 mm.
Reproduced with permission of the British Museum (Natural History).

23:11 SIPHONAPTERA (FLEAS)

The medically important fleas belong to the following genera:

- □ *Pulex*
- □ *Xenopsylla*
- □ *Tunga*

Appearance
Fleas are small wingless insects, usually brown in colour, and easily recognized because they are greatly flattened laterally, with long hind legs that are well-developed for jumping (see Plate 23.12). The body is covered with backward pointing spines which give easy forward movement in the fur of animals. The mouth-parts are adapted for piercing and sucking blood. The thorax, as in all insects, is divided into 3 segments, and the abdomen has 10-12 segments.

The presence or absence of genal and pronotal combs is used in the identification of fleas.

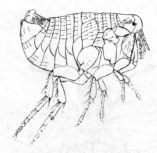

Plate 23.12　*Xenopsylla* (rat flea).
Reproduced with permission of the British Museum (Natural History).

Feeding and life cycle
Adult fleas feed on the blood of mammals and birds. The female ingests more blood than the male. An unfed flea can live up to a year, and a fed flea can live up to 5 years, which makes the insect an efficient reservoir for infection.

The life cycle of a flea is one of complete metamorphosis as described for dipteran insects.

Pulex species
P. irritans is the human flea and has a worldwide distribution. By its frequent and prolonged feeding on the blood of its host, it causes discomfort and irritation. The fleas reach their host usually by jumping, attracted by the warmth of their host's body.

Xenopsylla species
In the genus *Xenopsylla*, the rat fleas *X. cheopis*, *X. astia*, and *X. brasiliensis* are medically important species because they are carriers of:

- Bubonic plague
- Flea-borne murine typhus (endemic typhus)

X. cheopis has a wide distribution between latitudes 35 °N and 35 °S, naturally infesting rats in cities, rural areas, ports, and on ships.

X. brasiliensis occurs in Africa, South America, and India, infesting rats mostly in villages and also in ports.

X. astia is found in South East Asia and Indonesia. It naturally infests rats in fields, villages, and ports.

Other rat fleas which can carry plague and can live on humans include *X. vexabilis*, found in the Pacific Islands and infesting rats mainly in fields, and the rat flea *Nosopsyllus fasciatus* which has a worldwide distribution and is found mainly in the ports of cool temperate countries. When the rats are killed by plague, the fleas leave the rats and can become parasitic on humans.

Infection with plague or typhus occurs by the infected faeces or contents of a crushed flea entering the skin which has become damaged by scratching. Transmission of plague can also occur by regurgitation of the plague bacilli when the flea is feeding or by direct mechanical contamination from the mouth-parts of the flea.

The female *Xenopsylla* flea lays its eggs in batches in or near the dwelling of its host. There are three larval stages and a pupal stage. In suitable climatic conditions development from the egg to the adult stage takes 2-3 weeks. *X. cheopis* prefers a moderately warm moist climate in which to develop. *X. brasiliensis* does not exist well in hot temperatures. *X. astia* is affected by low temperatures.

Tunga species
T. penetrans, also known as the jigger flea, or chigoe, can be found in South America, Africa, and India.

It is the female jigger flea which is medically important because it requires an endoparasitic existence for egg development. The pregnant female burrows into the skin of its host, often around the toes, fingers, or other parts of the body. The greatly enlarged flea (see Plate 23.13) produces an irritating and often painful swelling just under the skin. Over a period of several days the eggs are discharged through the skin, after which the female dies. Irritation causes tissue damage which may lead to secondary bacterial infection.

Control of tungiasis is difficult. In endemic areas, preventive measures include the wearing of shoes and the use of insecticides.

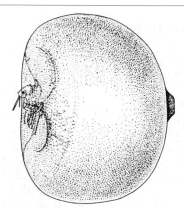

Plate 23.13 Female gravid *Tunga penetrans* (jigger flea). True size about 5 mm in diameter (five-fold increase in size. *Reproduced with permission of the British Museum (Natural History).*

Ctenocephalides species (fleas of cats and dogs)
These fleas are medically important because they serve as hosts for the tapeworms *D. caninum*, *H. diminuta*, and *H. nana* (see Chapter 18). When ingested by flea larvae, the eggs develop into the infective cysticercoid larval forms. Humans become infected by accidently swallowing a flea which contains these cysticercoid larvae.

The cat fleas, *Ctenocephalides felis felis* and *C. f. orientis* can also cause intense allergic reactions in humans. They are found in areas of high humidity. The larvae breed in carpets and their numbers greatly increase in the hot and humid season.

23:12 HEMIPTERA (BUGS)

Bugs vary greatly in size and morphology. Their life cycle is one of incomplete metamorphosis, i.e. the larva which hatches from the egg has the appearance of a small adult and maturity is reached through a series of moults. The young developing bugs are known as nymphs.

There are two medically important families of bugs:

Cimicidae
Reduviidae

CIMICIDAE BUGS
Cimicidae bugs are wingless, oval to round in

shape, and flattened from above. The body is divided into:

— A head, which is small and bears a pair of long thin antennae, large eyes, and mouth-parts adapted for piercing and sucking.

— A thorax which bears no wings.

— An abdomen which consists of several segments.

The Cimicidae family of bugs includes the bedbugs:

☐ *Cimex lectularius*
☐ *Cimex rotundatus*.

Bed bugs

Although there is no direct evidence that *Cimex* bugs are carriers of human disease, their bites are irritating and the bugs may become infected with bacteria and viruses. Hepatitis B has been reported in bedbugs from West Africa, Ethiopia, South America, and elsewhere and there is growing evidence that bedbugs can transmit hepatitis.

Bedbugs are small, brown in colour, and give out a characteristic smell from glands in their thorax. The appearance of a *Cimex* bug is shown in Plate 23.14.

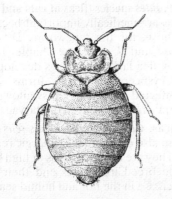

Plate 23.14 *Cimex lectularius* (bedbug). True size 4–5 mm. *Reproduced with permission of the British Museum (Natural History).*

Bedbugs live in the cracks of walls, floors, and wood-work and in the furniture of human dwellings. They emerge at night in search of hosts from which to feed. The bugs suck blood from humans and other warm-blooded animals. They lay their eggs in dark cracks and it takes several weeks for the nymphs to emerge and develop into mature bugs.

REDUVIID BUGS

Reduviid bugs are winged with a body which is basically divided into:

— A head which is long and bears a pair of slender antennae, large eyes, and a proboscis containing mouth-parts adapted for biting and sucking.

— A thorax with two pairs of wings.

— An abdomen which is large and oval.

The family Reduviidae contains an important subfamily, the Triatominae.

Triatomine bugs

Triatomine bugs are known as cone-nose bugs or kissing bugs because they often bite around the mouth. They measure up to 35 mm in length, are dark coloured, and may show red and yellow banding (see Plate 23.15).

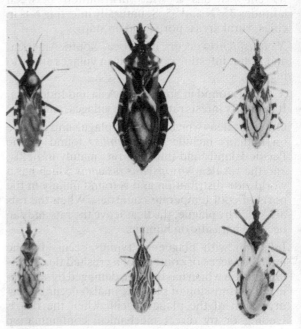

Plate 23.15 Principal domestic vectors (adults) of Chagas' disease in South and Central America: above (from left to right) *Triatoma infestans* **(Argentina, Bolivia, Brazil, Chile, Paraguay, Peru, Uruguay):** *Panstrongylus megistus* **(Brazil):** *Triatoma brasiliensis* **(north eastern Brazil) and, below** *Triatoma sordida* **(Brazil):** *Rhodnius prolixus* **(Colombia, Venezuela):** *Triatoma dimidiata* **(Ecuador and Central America). Scale: the specimen of** *P. megistus* **is approximately 30 mm long.**
Courtesy of Dr. Habib Fraiha and Dr. M. A. Miles.

The life cycle of a triatomine bug involves five nymphal stages, each stage requiring a blood meal for its development. The wings are formed during the last two stages. Adults are long lived and can survive for several weeks without a blood meal.

There are three medically important genera:

☐ *Triatoma*
☐ *Rhodnius*
☐ *Panstrongylus*

Triatomine bugs are vectors of South American trypanosomiasis (Chagas' disease) which is caused by *Trypanosoma cruzi*.

The most widespread species is *Triatoma infestans* which inhabits human dwellings throughout Argentina, Bolivia, Brazil, Chile, Paraguay, Peru and Uruguay. *Panstrongylus megistus* is an important vector in Brazil and *Rhodnius prolixus* is found in Colombia, Ecuador and Venezuela.

Human infection with *T. cruzi* occurs when infected bug faeces enter the wound made by the bite of the bug or are rubbed in as a result of irritation.

Triatomine bugs feed from humans mainly at night. They bite mainly on the face around the mouth and eyes. Triatomine bugs also feed on many wild and domestic animals.

The bugs invade houses by flight, often attracted to light. They can also enter human dwellings when the leaves of trees in which bugs (*R. prolixus*) are living are used for roofing. The bugs colonize badly made mud houses, living in the cracks of floors and walls, and also in roofing, behind pictures, and in and between furniture. New houses can also become infested when bugs are transferred with the personal belongings from a previous bug infested house.

☐ *Pediculus*
☐ *Phthirus*

Pediculus species

Species include:

— *P. humanus var. capitis*, the head louse which lives in the hair of the head.

— *P. humanus var. corporis*, the body louse.

Pediculus species transmit:

● Relapsing (louse-borne) fever

● Epidemic (louse-borne) typhus

● Trench fever

Louse bites also cause irritation and scratching which may lead to secondary infection.

Louse-borne relapsing fever is caused by *Borrelia recurrentis*. Infection occurs when the borreliae enter damaged skin following the crushing of an infected *Pediculus* body louse. The organisms live in the blood of the louse and are not passed in the faeces.

Typhus is caused by rickettsial organisms, which are found in the faeces of the louse. Infection occurs when infected louse faeces are deposited on the skin during or after feeding. Irriration causes the organisms to be rubbed in.

23:13 ANOPLURA (LICE)

Lice are host-specific permanent ectoparasites of humans and animals. Animal lice rarely transfer to humans and human lice do not infest animals. They have a leathery surface and are flattened from above (dorsoventrally). The body is divided into:

— A head, which is small and bears a pair of short antennae, small eyes, and mouth-parts adapted for sucking.

— A thorax without wings. The legs are well-developed for gripping.

— An abdomen, the tip of which in the female is divided.

The life cycle is one of incomplete metamorphosis as described for the bugs. The eggs are laid on hair or clothing and fixed firmly to the host or to clothing by a glue-like substance secreted around the eggs by the female. Development takes 2-3 weeks. Both sexes feed on blood. Lice are affected by temperature changes with a fever or death of their host causing them to seek a new host.

The medically important lice belong to the genera:

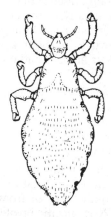

Plate 23.16 *Pediculus humanus* **(head louse). True size 2-3 mm.** *Reproduced with permission of the British Museum (Natural History).*

Phthirus species

Species include *P. pubis*, the pubic louse, also known as the crab louse.

P. pubis lives in the hair of the pubic region, axillae, and other parts, but not on the head. Its bite causes irritation and discomfort.

Phthirus lice are shorter and rounder than *Pediculus* lice, as shown in Plate 23.17.

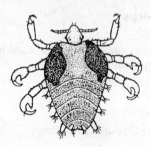

Plate 23.17   *Phthirus pubis* **(crab-louse). True size about 2 mm.**

23:14 COCKROACHES

Cockroaches are insects that belong to the order Dictyoptera. Included in the same order are the mantes to which cockroaches are closely related.

There are nearly 4 000 species of cockroach, distributed throughout most parts of the world. Species which are common pests in tropical countries include:

□   *Periplaneta americana*
□   *Periplaneta australasiae*

There is increasing evidence that cockroaches may act as mechanical carriers and efficient reservoirs of pathogenic organisms. Domestic cockroaches have been shown to harbour a wide variety of pathogens in their hindgut and on their body surface, including:

●   major pathogenic enterobacteria
●   polioviruses
●   hepatitis viruses
●   *Entamoeba histolytica*
●   several nematodes.[2]

Cockroaches can transmit pathogens by walking over and defaecating on food or by transmitting pathogens in vomit drops or from their legs and body surfaces. Non-specific involvement of cockroaches in outbreaks of human disease, particularly of the excremental group, have been reported.

Appearance
Cockroaches vary greatly in size from 5 mm to 9 cm in length. They have three pairs of legs and most species have two pairs of wings (see Plate 23.18). The body is divided into:

— A clearly defined head which bears a pair of long antennae.
— A thorax which has a large pronotal area.
— A large elongated abdomen.

Feeding, breeding and life cycle
Cockroaches are exopterygote, i.e. some time after mating the female lays an egg-case or oötheca which contains 12 to 48 eggs according to species. The eggs hatch nymphal insects which look like adults except they are much smaller and have no wings. The nymphs become adults by passing through as many as twelve moults and therefore may take as long as 18 months to reach maturity.

Cockroaches can often be found infesting kitchens, store-rooms, eating places, badly built human dwellings, drains, sewers and refuse containers. They feed at night. During the day, cockroaches hide in any enclosed space such as behind walls, doors, window frames, cupboards, lockers, ovens, refrigerators, shelving, loose tiling and in flooring.

Infestation is encouraged by positioning equipment too near to walls which makes access for regular cleaning difficult or impossible. Infested places will show dark blots or smears of faeces from the insects.

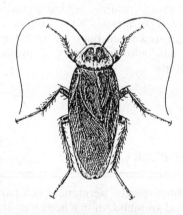

Plate 23.18   **Adult cockroach** *(Periplaneta americana).* **True size about 25 mm.**   *Reproduced from Insects and other Arthropods of Medical Importance. Courtesy of the British Museum.*

23:15 TICKS AND MITES

Ticks and mites are not insects but belong to the class Arachnida and order Acarina, the basic features of which are described in 23:1.

TICKS
Two families of ticks are medically important:

□   Argasidae, or soft ticks
□   Ixodidae, or hard ticks

Soft ticks (argasid ticks)
Among the soft ticks, the species *Ornithodoros moubata* is important because it sucks blood from

man and can transmit the borreliae of relapsing fever.

Once infected with *Borrelia duttoni*, a tick remains infected for life and can also transmit the borreliae to new generations of ticks. Human infection occurs when the borreliae are deposited on the skin in fluid from the coxal gland when the tick bites or following crushing of the tick on the skin.

O. moubata is oval in shape with short legs, and from above no mouth-parts are visible (see Plate 23.19).

Although ectoparasitic, soft ticks can survive for long periods without a host. The eggs are laid in batches in the cracks and crevices of walls. The life cycle takes 6-12 months, with up to eight nymphal stages usually spent on the same host. Soft ticks survive best in dry climates. Both sexes feed on blood.

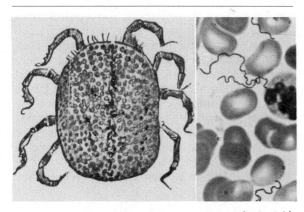

Plate 23.19 *Left* ***Ornithodoros moubata*** **(soft tick). True size of unfed female about 5 mm.** *Right* **Borreliae of relapsing fever in blood.**

Hard ticks (ixodid ticks)

Among the hard ticks the genera *Dermacentor* and *Amblyomma* are medically important as follows:

- *Dermacentor* and *Amblyomma* ticks transmit tick-borne typhus.
- *Dermacentor* ticks transmit tick-borne encephalitis.

A type of temporary paralysis can result from a toxin inoculated through the bite of a female hard tick. Q fever and tularaemia are also thought to be transmitted by hard ticks.

Unlike soft ticks, hard ticks have a hard dorsal covering and mouth-parts which can be seen from above (see Plate 23.20). Hard ticks may be dark or brightly coloured with metallic markings.

Hard ticks parasitize humans and animals with both sexes feeding on blood. The eggs are laid in a single batch after which the female dies.

There is only one larval and one nymphal stage from which the adult emerges. Each stage of

development may be spent on a different host. A blood meal is required for each stage.

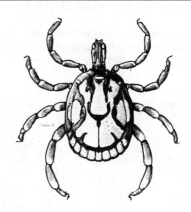

Plate 23.20 *Amblyomma* **tick (hard tick). True size of unfed female 4-5 mm.** *Reproduced with permission of the British Museum (Natural History).*

MITES

Mites also belong to the Acarina group of arachnids. Two genera are medically important:

- *Sarcoptes*
- *Trombicula*

Sarcoptes species

The species *Sarcoptes scabiei* (itch mite) has a worldwide distribution and is medically important because it causes scabies when the female mite burrows into the skin to lay its eggs. This usually occurs where the skin is thin, for example around the elbows, or wrists, or between the fingers, axillae, male genital organs or breasts. With children, the feet, face, and neck may be affected. Penetration of the mite causes severe irritation and a rash. Scratching often leads to secondary infection.

The eggs hatch larvae which become adults within a few days. The whole life cycle is completed under the skin.

Laboratory diagnosis of scabies: This is by finding mites or their eggs in skin scrapings. The mites are very small, measuring only about 0.3 mm in diameter and therefore a microscopical examination of the scraping is required. The surface of the skin should be examined first with a hand lens to detect fresh mite burrows.

A scraping of a suspect area is best made after applying a drop of mineral oil directly to the skin. The scraping in the oil can then be transferred to a slide, covered with a cover glass, and examined for mites and eggs using the 10× objective with the condenser iris closed sufficiently to give good contrast. Mounting in oil enables the movement of mites to be seen.

A *Sarcoptes* mite is shown in Plate 23.21. The eggs are oval and measure about $150 \times 100 \, \mu m$. Mature eggs contain a fully developed larva, as seen with the 40× objective (see Plate 23.21 left).

Note: Some workers prefer to take a dry scraping and mount this in potassium hydroxide (20% w/v) but this may damage the mites and by killing them make them more difficult to detect.

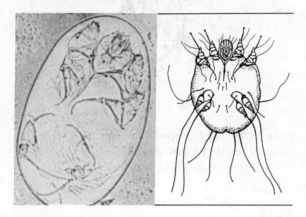

Plate 23.21 *Right* **Ventral view of a female *Sarcoptes* mite.** *Left* **Egg of *Sarcoptes* mite containing a larva.**

Trombicula species

Trombiculid mites transmit scrub typhus, especially in South East Asia. The rickettsial organisms which cause scrub typhus can be passed through several generations of mites. The bite of an infected trombiculid mite larva can also cause severe allergic dermatitis known as scrub itch.

Nymphs and adults of trombiculid mites are not parasitic but live in the soil in areas of selected scrub vegetation. The larvae are ectoparasitic on humans and warm-blooded animals, sucking lymph and tissue fluids from their hosts. The larvae can often be found around the waist under a belt, on the abdomen, or under a wrist or shoe strap. After several weeks the larvae drop off and continue their development in the soil.

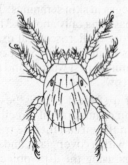

Plate 23.22 *Trombicula* **mite. True size about 0.55 mm.** *Reproduced with permission of the British Museum (Natural History).*

23:16 WATER FLEAS (*CYCLOPS* AND *DIAPOTOMUS*)

Water fleas belong to the class Crustacea, which also includes crabs, prawns and other sea and freshwater creatures.

Species of the genera *Diaptomus*, *Cyclops* (see Plate 23.23) and related genera are medically important because they are intermediate hosts of:

— *Diphyllobothrium latum*

— *Dracunculus medinensis*

In the life cycle of *D. latum*, *Cyclops* and *Diaptomus* species are hosts of the procercoid larvae. Following ingestion of an infected flea by a suitable freshwater fish, the procercoids develop into infective plerocercoids (see 18:8). Humans become infected by ingesting a fish containing plerocercoids.

The life cycle of *D. medinensis* also requires water fleas. The first stage parasitic larvae are discharged into the water by the female Guinea worm. They are ingested by species belonging to the genera *Cyclops*, *Mesocyclops*, *Tropocyclops*, or *Thermocyclops*. Inside the water flea, the larvae develop into infective forms. Humans become infected by accidentally swallowing a water flea containing infective larvae. Transmission is more frequent in the dry season when the water level in wells and other sources of drinking water is reduced. Infection can be easily prevented (see 22:16).

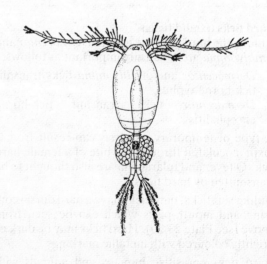

Plate 23.23 *Cyclops* **(water flea). True size about 0.5 mm.** *Reproduced from Practical Invertebrate Anatomy, courtesy of Macmillan .*

References

1 Zumpt, F. *Myiasis in Man and Animals in the Old World*. Butterworth, London, 1965.
2 Burgess, N. R. H. Hospital design and cockroach control. *Transactions of the Royal Society of Tropical Medicine and Hygiene*, **78**, pp 293-294, 1984.

Recommended Reading

Abushama, F. T. E. *Flies, Mosquitoes and Disease in the Sudan*. Univ. of Khartoum, 1974.

Bahmanyar, M., and Cavanaugh, D. C. *Plague Manual*. World Health Organization, 1975.

Burgess, N. R. H. *Grundy's Arthropods of Medical Importance*. Noble books, 1981.

Davies, H. *Tsetse Flies in Nigeria*. Oxford University Press, 1977.

Gillett, J. D. *Common African Mosquitoes and their Medical Importance*. Heineman Medical Books Ltd., 1972.

Gordon, R. M. and Lavoipierre, M. M. J. *Entomology for Students of Medicine*. Blackwell, Oxford, 1962.

Mattingly, P. F. *The Biology of Mosquito-Borne Disease*. Allen and Unwin, 1969.

Nash, T. A. M. *Africa's Bane, the Tsetse Fly*. Collins, 1969.

Service, M. W. A. *A Guide to Medical Entomology*. Macmillan, London, 1980.

Smith, K. G. V. (Ed.) *Insects and other Arthropods of Medical Importance*. British Museum (Nat. Hist.). 1973.

Snow, K. R. *The Arachnids: An Introduction*. Routledge and Kegan Paul, 1970.

Snow, K. R. *Insects and Disease*. Routledge and Kegan, 1974.

World Health Organization. *Chemical Methods for the Control of Arthropod Vectors and Pests of Public Health Importance*. WHO, Geneva, 1984.

Rishikesh, N. New methods of vector control. *Postgraduate Doctor*, Vol. 8, No. 10, p 299-304, 1986.

SECTION IV

CLINICAL CHEMISTRY

24 Introduction to Clinical Chemistry

24:1 CLINICAL CHEMISTRY AND ANALYTICAL METHODS

The discipline of clinical chemistry is sometimes called clinical biochemistry or chemical pathology. It integrates medical knowledge, physiology, statistics, electronics and other specialities to provide analyses of a wide variety of body fluids and to assist clinicians in the logical requesting of tests and in the interpretation of test results.

Applications of test results
Test results are used in a number of clinical situations including:

— establishing a diagnosis
— following the course of disease
— assessing prognosis
— monitoring therapy
— screening healthy individuals to assist in the prevention of disease.

Analytical methods
The examination, or analysis, of body fluids can be:

■ qualitative
■ semiquantitative
■ quantitative

Qualitative analysis
A qualitative test is one in which the presence or absence of a substance (analyte) is detected in a mixture by chemical means, for example Fouchet's test to detect bilirubin in urine.

Semiquantitative analysis
The speed and, or, intensity of a reaction such as the degree of colour generated in some qualitative tests is often a good indication of the quantity of analyte present. Such tests may be used therefore in a semiquantitative way.

Quantitative analysis
A quantitative test is one in which the quantity of an analyte is measured. Many substances of medical importance are examined in this way.

The following quantitative analytical techniques are used to perform the tests described in this manual:

☐ Spectrophotometric techniques: In these an analyte is reacted with a reagent(s) to give a coloured product, the absorbance of which can be measured using a colorimeter or spectrophotometer (principle described more fully in Chapter 25).

Colorimeters and spectrophotometers
In this Manual the term colorimeter is used to describe an instrument such as the WPA CO700D Colorimeter (see 25:3) in which coloured filters are used to provide the colours (wavelength ranges) of light absorbed by a test solution. Other terms used to describe a filter colorimeter include filter absorption spectrometer, absorptiometer, and filterphotometer.† A colorimeter is adequate for all the assays described in this Manual. The operation of a colorimeter is described in Chapter 25.

The term spectrophotometer refers to an instrument in which a diffraction grating or prism is used to provide a continuous spectrum of colours from which individual wavelengths can be selected. Some clinical chemists prefer to use the term absorption spectrometer.† The use of a costly spectrophotometer is rarely required for routine clinical chemistry tests (see 25:3).

†Colorimeter and spectrophotometer are the terms commonly used by manufacturers.

☐ Flame emission spectrometry: This is one of the methods used to determine the concentration of sodium and potassium in serum or plasma. Flame emission spectrometry and the operation of a flame photometer are explained in 29:2.

Note: Flame emission spectrometry was formerly referred to as flame photometry.

☐ Volumetric analysis: In this a substance in solution is measured by titration, for example the titrimetric method used to measure bicarbonate in serum or plasma as described in 29:14.

24:2 PRINCIPLES OF CHEMICAL REACTIONS

To understand the principles of clinical chemistry tests it is helpful to have a basic knowledge of chemical reactions.

Atoms
Atoms are the smallest particles of which any substance is composed that can take part in a chemical reaction.

An atom consists of a central compact nucleus which contains both positively charged particles called protons and particles with no electrical charge called neutrons. Very small negatively charged particles called electrons surround the nucleus.

Because the numbers of positively charged protons equal the numbers of negatively charged electrons, an atom is electrically neutral. Atoms of different elements differ from one another by the number of protons and neutrons in the nucleus of each. An element is a substance made up of only one kind of atom.

The chemical properties of an atom are controlled by its electrons, with the chemical combination of electrons taking place by the transfer or sharing of outer electrons between combining atoms. The nuclei of atoms remain unchanged during such reactions.

Atomic numbers and atomic masses of elements
The number of protons in the nuclei of atoms determines what is known as the atomic number of an element. For example, the number of protons in a carbon atom is 6, therefore the atomic number of the element carbon is 6.

The sum of the number of protons and neutrons determines what is called the atomic mass (weight) of an element. This does not represent an actual weighed mass but is a relative amount. It indicates how much heavier or lighter an atom of one element is than another based on the atomic weight of an isotope of carbon which has been assigned an atomic mass of 12 units.

Isotopes
Almost all the elements have what are called isotopes. These are atoms of the same element that have the same number of protons in their nuclei but a different number of neutrons, i.e. they have the same atomic number but different atomic masses. For example, the three isotopes of the element hydrogen (tritium, deuterium, protium) each have 1 proton and 1 electron but tritium has 2 neutrons, deuterium has 1 neutron, and protium has no neutron.

Isotopes of elements are shown by writing the atomic mass of the element followed by the symbol of the element, for example one isotope of carbon is written ^{12}C.

Not all isotopes remain in a stable physical state; some are unstable and radioactive. Such isotopes emit rays (alpha, beta, and gamma) due to their nuclei disintegrating in order to become stable. Such rays, although lethal to living cells, can be used in a controlled way in radiotherapy units to kill malignant cells in the body.

Molecules and relative molecular masses
Whereas an element is composed of only one kind of atom, a compound contains two or more different kinds of atom. A molecule is the smallest particle of an element or compound that can normally exist separately. For example, 2 atoms of hydrogen combine with 1 atom of oxygen to form 1 molecule of water.

The relative molecular mass of a molecule (previously called molecular weight) is the ratio of the average of a molecule to $\frac{1}{12}$ of the mass of the isotope of carbon (^{12}C). In mathematical terms the relative mass of a molecule is the sum of all the atomic weights of which it is composed.

Of all the 104 elements known, 80 of these are metals. The atomic weights of common elements are listed in Appendix III at the back of the book.

Valence
The way in which elements combine to form compounds by the transfer or sharing of electrons between atoms is known as valence. The valence of an element can be defined as the number of hydrogen atoms which will combine with, or replace, one atom of the element. For example, the valence of oxygen in water (H_2O) is 2.

Some elements have more than one valence number. The valence numbers of the common elements are listed in Appendix III.

The process of forming a compound through the transfer of electrons is called electrovalency. The atom that loses an electron becomes a positive ion and the atom that gains an electron becomes a negative ion.

Elements which give up 1, 2, or 3 electrons to form positive ions such as sodium (Na^+), calcium (Ca^{++}), or aluminium (Al^{+++}), are said to exhibit positive valence.

Elements which accept 3, 2, or 1 electrons to form negative ions, such as nitrogen (N^{---}), oxygen (O^{--}), or chlorine (Cl^-), are said to exhibit negative valence.

Oxidation and reduction reactions
In general terms, any reaction in which an atom loses electrons is referred to as oxidation. In more specific terms, oxidation can be the combination of oxygen with a substance or the removal of hydrogen from it. Any reaction in which an atom gains electrons is referred to as reduction, or more specifically, reduction can be the removal of oxygen from a substance or the addition of hydrogen to it.

A reducing agent can be described therefore as a substance that donates electrons, removes oxygen from, or adds hydrogen to another substance. An oxidizing agent is a substance that removes electrons, adds oxygen, or removes hydrogen from another substance.

In any reaction involving a valence change, both oxidation and reduction must be present with the total number of electrons gained being equal to the number of electrons being lost. Such reactions are referred to as redox reactions.

An ionic redox reaction is said to be balanced when both the number of atoms and the net charge are equal on both sides of an equation so that electrical neutrality is achieved.

Electrolytes and electrolysis

Electrolytes are acids, bases, or salts which, when dissolved in water, conduct an electric current. The passage of an electric current through an electrolyte solution is called electrolysis, and dissociates the electrolyte into its ions. Positively charged ions are known as cations and negatively charged ions as anions.

In an electrolytic system such as a battery, the negative anions migrate to the positive electrode (anode) and the positive cations migrate to the negative electrode (cathode). Chemical reactions of the oxido-reduction type take place at the electrodes with the ions giving up their electrical charges. Oxidation reactions take place at the anode and reduction reactions take place at the cathode.

Equivalent weights of elements and compounds

What is referred to as the equivalent weight of an element or compound is that weight of the substance which will combine with or displace 1 part by weight of hydrogen or 8 parts by weight of oxygen.

Mathematically the equivalent weight can be expressed as:

$$\text{For an element: } \frac{\text{Atomic mass (weight)}}{\text{valence}}$$

$$\text{For a compound: } \frac{\text{Molecular mass (weight)}}{\text{valence}}$$

Radicles

Certain groups of atoms when combined together in compounds behave as a single atom. Such units are called radicles. Each has an electrical charge and can combine with another atom or another radicle to form a compound. Some of the most important radicle ions and their valencies are as follows:

Radicles	Symbol	Valence Number
Ammonium	NH_4^+	+1
Acetate	CH_3COO^-	−1
Bicarbonate	HCO_3^-	−1
Chlorate	ClO_3^-	−1
Hydroxide	OH^-	−1
Cyanide	CN^-	−1
Nitrate	NO_3^-	−1
Nitrite	NO_2^-	−1
Permanganate	MnO_4^-	−1
Carbonate	CO_3^{--}	−2
Chromate	CrO_4^{--}	−2
Sulphate	SO_4^{--}	−2
Sulphite	SO_3^{--}	−2
Phosphate	PO_4^{---}	−3

24:3 ACIDS, BASES AND ACID-BASE REACTIONS

Acids

An acid is a substance that liberates hydrogen ions in solution and acts as a proton donor (donating H^+).

Acids have a sour taste, turn litmus red, and react with carbonates to produce the gas carbon dioxide. When reacted with a base, an acid produces a salt and water. Most acids are corrosive.

Sulphuric acid, nitric acid, and hydrochloric acid are referred to as strong acids because they ionize almost completely in solution with very few intact molecules of the acid remaining. Ionization is the dissociation of a substance in solution into electrically charged atoms known as ions. Lactic acid and glacial acetic acid are referred to as weak acids, because they ionize very little in solution.

The properties of the commonly used acids are as follows:

Sulphuric acid (H_2SO_4): Has a relative density of 1.840, molecular mass 98.08, and concentration 95-97% by weight.

It is very corrosive, viscous, oily, and *reacts violently with water* (hygroscopic). See also 2:5.

Hydrochloric acid (HCl): Has a relative density of 1.190 and molecular mass 36.46. The concentrated acid contains 37% by weight of the gas hydrogen chloride.

It is fuming and corrosive. See also 2:5.

Nitric acid (HNO_3): Has a relative density of 1.510, molecular mass 63.01, and concentration about 99% by weight.

It is fuming, corrosive, stains the skin yellow-brown, and is a powerful oxidizing agent. See also 2:5.

Bases

A base is a substance that liberates hydroxide ions in solution and can accept a proton.

Alkaline solutions have a soapy feel, turn litmus blue, and react with an acid to form a salt and water.

The common bases include oxides and hydroxides of metals such as sodium, potassium, calcium, lead, iron, and copper. The oxides of potassium, sodium, and calcium dissolve in water to form alkalis.

Sodium hydroxide and potassium hydroxide are referred to as strong alkalis because they dissociate completely into cations and hydroxide ions in water.

Acid-base reactions

Examples of chemical reactions involving acids and bases include:

Acid		Base		Salt		Water
H^+Cl^-	+	Na^+OH^-	$\longrightarrow$	Na^+Cl^-	+	H_2O
Hydrochoric acid		Sodium hydroxide		Sodium choride		Water
$CH_3COO^-H^+$	+	Na^+OH^-	$\longrightarrow$	$CH_3COO^-Na^+$	+	H_2O
Acetic acid		Sodium hydroxide		Sodium acetate		Water

pK of acids and bases

The strength of an acid or base is determined by its pK which is defined as the negative logarithm (to the base 10) of the ionization constant (K):

$$pK = \log_{10}K$$

For example, a strong acid has a low pK value whereas a weak acid has a high pK. The higher the pK value the weaker the acid.

Neutralization reactions

The process of adding an acid to a base, or a base to an acid, to give a neutral solution consisting of a salt and water, is known as neutralization. The neutral solution contains equal numbers of hydroxide and hydrogen ions.

Hydrolysis

Hydrolysis is the chemical decomposition of a substance by water, with the water also being decomposed. Salts of weak acids, weak bases, or both, are partially hydrolyzed to form molecules of weak electrolytes in solution. An ester may be hydrolyzed to form an alcohol and an acid.

24:4 pH OF SOLUTIONS

Neutral solutions have equal concentrations of hydrogen ions and hydroxide ions. Pure water is neutral because it ionizes very slightly to give one hydrogen ion and one hydroxide ion for each molecule ionized.

Whether a solution is acidic or alkaline, there are always both H^+ and OH^- ions present. It is the predominance of one type of ion over the other that determines the degree of acidity or alkalinity. When referring to the acidity and alkalinity of solutions it is usual to refer only to the hydrogen ion concentration.

Pure water at 25 °C contains 0.000 000 1 g, or 10^{-7} g, of hydrogen ions per litre.

Because the molecular mass of a hydrogen ion is 1, the hydrogen ion concentration of pure water can be expressed as follows:

$$[H^+] \text{ (Pure water)} = 1 \times 10^{-7} \text{ mol/l}$$

There is however no SI unit prefix for 10^{-7} (see 1:5) and therefore the prefix nano (n) which means 10^{-9} is used. The SI unit formula is written:

$$[H^+] \text{ (Pure water)} = 100 \times 10^{-9} \text{ mol/l}$$
$$= 100 \text{ nmol/l}$$

Normal blood, being slightly alkaline (pH about 7.4), contains fewer hydrogen ions than pure water:

$$[H^+] \text{ (Blood)} \simeq 40 \text{ nmol/l}$$

Expressing hydrogen ion concentration

As a convenient way of expressing hydrogen ion concentration, the symbol pH was introduced by Sorensen in 1909. pH is defined as the negative value of the logarithm to the base 10 of the hydrogen ion concentration:

$$pH = -\log_{10}[H^+]$$

The pH of pure water can be expressed as follows:

$$pH \text{ (pure water)} = \log \frac{1}{10^{-7}}$$
$$= 7 \text{ (neutral)}$$

The pH scale is usually expressed from 0 to 14 units, with a pH of less than 7 indicating acidity and a pH above 7 indicating alkalinity:

Acidity	Neutral	Alkalinity
$\longleftarrow$		$\longrightarrow$
pH 0	pH 7	pH 14

pH can be measured using pH papers which give an

approximate pH value, or by using a colorimeter with indicators and a series of coloured standards, or a pH meter which provides the most accurate method of determining pH. The use of pH meters is described in Chapter 3:11.

Buffer solutions
Buffer solutions contain a mixture of a weak acid and a salt of a strong base, or a weak base and its salt with a strong acid.

Due to their composition, buffers are able to resist changes in pH. For example, if a small amount of hydrochloric acid is added to a buffer solution the hydrogen ion content does not increase very much because it combines with the weak base of the buffer resulting in only a slight decrease in pH.

A buffer has its highest buffering ability when its pH is equal to its pK.

Buffers are used in clinical chemistry when the pH needs to be carefully controlled, e.g. when measuring enzyme activity.

Indicators
Indicators are substances that give different col-

ours or shades of colour at different pH values. For example, phenol red changes from yellow at pH 6.8 to a deep red at pH 8.4.

Indicators are used to determine the pH of liquids and the 'end-point' of acid-base titrations. When titrating a strong or a weak acid with a strong base, an indicator is selected which changes colour at an alkaline pH, e.g. phenolphthalein. When titrating a strong or weak base with a strong acid, an indicator is used which changes colour at an acid pH, e.g. methyl orange.

The pH ranges, colour changes, and preparation of the commonly used indicators are shown in Chart 24.1.

24:5 EXPRESSING THE CONCENTRATION OF SOLUTIONS

A solution is composed of a solvent which is the dissolving medium and a solute which is the substance dissolved. In a solution there is an even distribution of the molecules or ions of the solute throughout the solvent.

Chart 24.1   **Commonly Used Indicators**

Indicator	pH Range	Colour Change	Preparation
Topfer's reagent	2.9 - 4.2	Red to yellow	Dissolve 0.5 g dimethylaminoazobenzene in 100 ml 95% v/v ethanol
Methyl orange	3.0 - 4.4	Red to yellow	Dissolve 0.1 g indicator in 100 ml distilled water
Bromocresol green	3.8 - 5.4	Yellow to green	Dissolve 0.1 g indicator in 2.9 ml of 0.05 mol/l (0.05 N) sodium hydroxide. Make up to 250 ml with distilled water
Bromothymol blue	6.0 - 7.6	Yellow to blue	Dissolve 0.1 g indicator in 3.2 ml of 0.05 mol/l sodium hydroxide. Make up to 250 ml with distilled water
Methyl red	4.4 - 6.2	Red to yellow	Dissolve 0.05 g indicator in 100 ml 50% v/v ethanol
Neutral red	6.8 - 8.0	Yellow to red	Dissolve 0.1 g indicator in 100 ml 80% v/v ethanol
Phenol red	6.8 - 8.4	Yellow to red	Dissolve 0.1 g indicator in 5.7 ml of 0.05 mol/l (0.05 N) sodium hydroxide. Make up to 250 ml with distilled water
Phenolphthalein	8.3 - 10.0	Colourless to red	Dissolve 0.1 g indicator in 100 ml 50% v/v ethanol

Formerly, the concentration of a solute in a solution has been expressed in many ways, e.g. as a percentage solution (weight for volume (w/v) or volume for volume (v/v)), as a normal (N) solution, or as a molar (M) solution.

In considering the ways of expressing the concentration of solutions, it should be remembered that in chemical reactions it is 1 mole not 1 gram of a substance that reacts with 1 mole of another substance.

Based therefore on the fact that chemicals interact in relation to their molecular masses it is recommended that the concentration of solutions be expressed in terms of the number of moles of solute per litre of solution.

Only when the relative molecular mass of a substance is not known, should the concentration of such a substance in solution be expressed in terms of mass (weight) concentration, i.e. grams or milligrams per *litre* (per 100 ml should be discontinued).

Mole per litre solutions

A mole per litre (mol/l) solution contains one mole of solute dissolved in and made up to 1 litre with solvent.

Mole

A mole is defined as the amount of substance of a system which contains as many elementary units (atoms, molecules, or ions) as there are carbon atoms in 0.012 kg of the pure nuclide carbon–12 (^{12}C).

To avoid confusion, mole per litre solutions should not be referred to as molar or M solutions. The internationally agreed meaning of the word molar as used in chemistry is 'divided by amount of substance', i.e. divided by mole. Molar cannot be applied therefore to mole per litre solutions as these refer to mole divided by litre (mol/l). The use of the term molarity should be discontinued.

Preparation of mol/l solutions

To prepare a mol/l solution, use the following formula:

Required mol/l solution × Molecular mass of substance = Number of grams to be dissolved in 1 litre of solution.

Examples
■ To make 1 litre of sodium chloride (NaCl), 1 mol/l:

Required mol/l concentration = 1
Molecular mass of NaCl = 58.44

Therefore 1 litre NaCl, 1 mol/l contains:
1 × 58.44 = 58.44 g of the chemical dissolved in 1 litre of solvent.

Note: When writing mol/l solutions, the concentration is written after the name of the substance.

■ To make 1 litre of sodium chloride (NaCl), 0.15 mol/l (physiological saline):

Required mol/l concentration = 0.15
Molecular mass of NaCl = 58.44

Therefore 1 litre NaCl, 0.15 mol/l contains:
0.15 × 58.44 = 8.77 g of the chemical dissolved in 1 litre of solvent.

■ To make 50 ml of sodium chloride (NaCl), 0.15 mol/l (physiological saline):

Required mol/l concentration = 0.15
Molecular mass of NaCl = 58.44

Therefore 50 ml NaCl, 0.15 mol/l contains:
$$\frac{0.15 \times 58.44 \times 50}{1000} = 0.438 \text{ g of the chemical dissolved in 50 ml of solvent.}$$

Note: In some publications the decimal point is written as a comma, eg 0.15 would be written as 0,15.

Formula to convert a percentage solution into a mol/l solution

To change a percentage solution into a mol/l solution use the formula:

$$\text{mol/l solution} = \frac{g\% \text{ (w/v) solution} \times 10}{\text{molecular mass of substance}}$$

Examples
■ To convert a 4% w/v sodium hydroxide (NaOH) solution into a mol/l solution:

Gram % solution = 4
Molecular mass of NaOH = 40

Conversion to mol/l : $\dfrac{4 \times 10}{40} = 1$

Therefore 4% w/v NaOH is equivalent to NaOH, 1 mol/l solution.

■ To convert a 0.9% w/v sodium chloride (NaCl) into a mol/l solution:

Gram % solution = 0.9
Molecular mass of NaCl = 58.44

Conversion to mol/l : $\dfrac{0.9 \times 10}{58.44} = 0.15$

Therefore 0.9% w/v NaCl is equivalent to NaCl, 0.15 mol/l solution.

Conversion of a normal solution into a mol/l solution

To change a normal solution into a mol/l solution use the formula:

$$\text{mol/l solution} = \frac{\text{Normality of solution}}{\text{Valence of substance}}$$

Examples
- To convert 0.1 N (N/10) hydrochloric acid (HCl) into a mol/l solution:

  Normality of solution = 0.1

  Valence of Cl (in HCl) = 1

  Conversion to mol/l: $\dfrac{0.1}{1}$ = 0.1

  Therefore 0.1 N HCl is equivalent to HCl, 0.1 mol/l solution.

- To convert 1 N sodium carbonate (Na_2CO_3) into a mol/l solution:

  Normality of solution = 1

  Valence of CO_3^{--} (in Na_2CO_3) = 2

  Conversion to mol/l: $\dfrac{1}{2}$ = 0.5

  Therefore 1 N Na_2CO_3 is equivalent to Na_2CO_3, 0.5 mol/l solution.

Note: The relative molecular masses (molecular weights) of some of the more commonly used substances and the atomic masses and valencies of some of the elements, are listed in Appendix III.

24:6 HOW TO DILUTE SOLUTIONS AND BODY FLUIDS

In the laboratory it is frequently necessary to dilute solutions and body fluids. To dilute a solution or body fluid means to reduce its concentration.

Diluting solutions
A weaker solution can be made from a stronger solution by using the following formula:

Volume (ml) of stronger solution required

$= \dfrac{C \times V}{S}$

where:

C = Concentration of solution required
V = Volume of solution required
S = Strength of the stronger solution

Examples
- To make 500 ml sodium hydroxide (NaOH), 0.25 mol/l from a 0.4 mol/l solution:

  C = 0.25 mol/l V = 500 ml S = 0.4 mol/l

  ml of stronger solution required:

  $\dfrac{0.25 \times 500}{0.4}$ = 312.5

  Therefore, measure 312.5 ml NaOH, 0.4 mol/l,

and make up to 500 ml with distilled water.

- To make 1 litre hydrochloric acid (HCl), 0.01 mol/l from a 1 mol/l solution:

  C = 0.01 mol/l V = 1 litre S = 1 mol/l

  ml of stronger solution required:

  $\dfrac{0.01 \times 1000}{1}$ = 10

  Therefore, measure 10 ml HCl, 1 mol/l, and make up to 1 litre with distilled water.

- To make 100 ml glucose, 3 mmol/l in 1 g/l benzoic acid from glucose 100 mmol/l solution:

  C = 3 mmol/l V = 100 ml S = 100 mmol/l

  ml of stronger solution required:

  $\dfrac{3 \times 100}{100}$ = 3

  Therefore, measure 3 ml of glucose, 100 mmol/l, and make up to 100 ml with 1 g/l benzoic acid.

- To make 500 ml sulphuric acid (H_2SO_4), 0.33 mol/l from concentrated sulphuric acid which has an approximate substance concentration of 18 mol/l:

  C = 0.33 mol/l V = 500 ml S = 18 mol/l

  ml of stronger solution required:

  $\dfrac{0.33 \times 500}{18}$ = 9.2

  Therefore, measure 9.2 ml concentrated H_2SO_4, and slowly add it to about 250 ml of distilled water in a volumetric flask. Make up to 500 ml with distilled water.

Diluting body fluids and calculating dilutions
— To prepare a dilution or series of dilutions of a body fluid:

Examples
- To make 8 ml of a 1 in 20 dilution of blood:

  Volume of blood required: $\dfrac{8}{20}$ = 0.4ml

  Therefore, to prepare 8 ml of a 1 in 20 dilution, add 0.4 ml of blood to 7.6 ml of diluting fluid.

- To make 4 ml of a 1 in 2 dilution of serum in physiological saline:

  Volume of serum required: $\dfrac{4}{2}$ = 2.0 ml

  Therefore, to prepare 4 ml of a 1 in 2 dilution, add 2 ml of serum to 2 ml of physiological saline.

— To calculate the dilution of a body fluid:

Examples

■ Calculate the dilution of blood when using 50 μl (0.05 ml) of blood and 950 μl (0.95 ml) of diluting fluid:

Total volume of body fluid and diluting fluid: 50 + 950 = 1000 μl

Therefore, dilution of blood: $\dfrac{1000}{50}$ = 20

i.e. 1 in 20 dilution.

■ Calculate the dilution of urine using 0.5 ml of urine and 8.5 ml of diluting fluid (physiological saline):

Total volume of urine and diluting fluid: 8.5 + 0.5 = 9.0 ml

Therefore, dilution of urine: $\dfrac{9.0}{0.5}$ = 18

i.e. 1 in 18 dilution.

24:7 SATURATED SOLUTIONS AND DELIQUESCENT CHEMICALS HYDRATED AND ANHYDROUS SALTS

Saturated solutions

Saturated solutions contain the maximum amount of solute that can normally be dissolved at a given temperature and pressure. The concentration of a solute in a saturated solution is referred to as the solubility of the solute at a given temperature. For example, the solubility of copper sulphate is 143 g in 1 litre at 0 °C. Usually the solubility of a solid in a liquid increases as the temperature increases.

Deliquescent chemicals

Chemicals such as calcium chloride, potassium carbonate, and sodium hydroxide are very soluble in water and become moist when exposed to damp air. They become dissolved in the moisture and go on taking in moisture until the vapour pressure of the solution equals the pressure of the water in the atmosphere. Such chemicals are said to be deliquescent and can be used as drying agents (desiccants) in desiccators.

A substance which absorbs water from the air but does not dissolve in the water it absorbs is referred to as hygroscopic, e.g. sodium carbonate.

Supersaturated solutions

A solution which contains more solute than a saturated solution is said to be supersaturated. If such a solution is shaken, comes in contact with dust particles, is cooled, or is 'seeded' with a small crystal of the solute, it will precipitate the excess solute and revert back to being a saturated solution.

Hydrated and anhydrous salts

Salts which contain water of crystallization are said to be hydrated. Those which do not contain water of crystallization are referred to as anhydrous. Hydrated substances contain a definite amount of water, as shown in their formulae. For example, hydrated copper sulphate (blue) has a formula of $CuSO_4 \cdot 5H_2O$, which means it contains 5 molecules of water per molecule.

When calculating the molecular mass of a chemical it is *important* to check whether it contains water of crystallization. The molecular masses of some hydrated and anhydrous chemicals are listed in Appendix III.

24:8 TECHNIQUES FOR PREPARING SOLUTIONS

When preparing a solution decide whether the solution requires an accurate volumetric preparation, e.g. a standard (calibrant), or a less accurate method of preparation, e.g. a stain.

Guidelines for preparing accurate solutions

■ Use a balance of sufficient sensitivity.

Weigh the chemical as accurately as possible. The chemical should be of an analytical reagent grade. Hygroscopic and deliquescent chemicals need to be weighed rapidly.

■ Use calibrated, chemically clean glassware.

Read carefully the graduation marks and other information on flasks and pipettes, for example check whether a pipette is of the containing (rinsing-out) type or of the delivery (non-rinsing-out) type. It is best to use a delivery type.

■ Use a funnel to transfer the chemical from the weighing container to a volumetric flask. Wash any chemical remaining in the container into the flask with a little of the solvent.

■ Make the solution up to its final volume only when it has cooled to the temperature used to graduate the flask (this temperature is written on the flask).

■ To avoid over-shooting the graduation mark, use a Pasteur pipette or wash-bottle to add the final volume of solvent to the flask.

■ Make sure the bottom of the meniscus of the fluid is on the graduation mark when viewed at eye level (see Fig. 24.1).

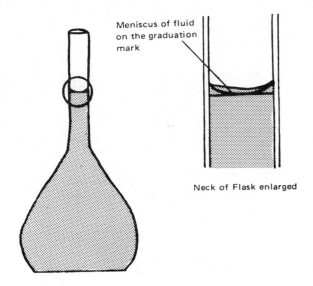

Fig. 24.1 How to read the level of a fluid.

■ Mix the solution well by inverting the flask at least twenty times.

■ Before transferring a solution to its storage container, first rinse out the container with a little of the solution.

Standard solutions

When preparing standard solutions the following are also important:

— Always use pure chemicals. The use of impure low grade chemicals can lead to serious errors in test results.
Chemicals labelled *AR, Analar, GR, PA,* or *Univar* are of suitable quality from which to prepare standards.

— Use an analytical balance of adequate sensitivity. Avoid weighing a very small quantity of a standard substance. Instead, prepare a concentrated stock solution which can be diluted to make working standard solutions.

— Use good quality distilled water. Electrolyte standard solutions require deionized water.

— Use calibrated glassware and a volumetric technique as described previously.

— Store standard solutions correctly as described in the method of preparation. Do not use the solutions beyond their working life.

Note: Whenever possible, standard solutions should be prepared and standardized in a regional or central laboratory and distributed with instructions for use to district laboratories.

Preparation of stains

To avoid staining flasks and other glassware, transfer the weighed dye direct to its leak-proof storage container. Add the correct volume of solvent and mix well. Before mixing, add a few glass beads to help the stain to dissolve.

Most stains are best stored in dark coloured bottles out of direct sunlight.

Instead of using a measuring cylinder each time a stain is prepared, mark the storage bottle with the level of solvent required.

Guidelines for handling chemicals and reagents

■ Handle chemicals and reagents with care particularly those that are flammable, poisonous, irritating or corrosive. The safe use of chemicals and reagents is described in 2:5.

■ *Do not* mouth-pipette reagents, especially acids, alkalis or irritating and poisonous chemicals. Instead, use a pipette filler or dispenser as described in 2:5.

■ Label all chemicals and reagents fully and if harmful, mark the container with an appropriate warning symbol (see 2:5). Record the date of preparation.

■ Always check that an opened bottle of chemical is completely finished before starting a new one.

■ Do not return excess chemical to the stock bottle. Always make sure a stock bottle of chemical is tightly stoppered before returning it to the shelf, particularly if the chemical is hygroscopic or deliquescent (see 24:7).

24:9 PREPARATION OF PROTEIN-FREE FLUIDS

Because protein is present in blood and other body fluids in large concentration it can interfere with the measurement of substances that are present in small amounts.

Proteins may cause turbidity, react with the reagents used in some tests, or form a precipitate which may interfere with the reading of a test. For some tests therefore a protein precipitation stage is included. It is recommended that the standard solutions should be treated with the precipitating reagents in the same way as the test samples and controls.

Protein precipitation

Proteins can be precipitated in body fluids in a

number of ways, e.g. by using certain acids or the salts of heavy metals. The precipitated proteins are then removed by filtration or sedimented by centrifugation.

The correct preparation of a protein-free fluid is essential. Protein precipitation is incomplete if the filtrate or supernatant fluid appears cloudy. The precipitating reagent must be prepared accurately and the correct volume of it must be used.

Choice of protein precipitant

The choice of protein precipitant depends on the test method being used. It is essential that the chemicals contained in the precipitating reagent do not interfere with the substance being measured and that the filtrate or supernatant fluid is of the correct pH for the assay.

The commonly used protein precipitants are acid reagents, such as tungstic acid or trichloroacetic acid.

Recommended Reading

World Health Organization. *The SI for the Health Professions*, WHO, Geneva, 1977.

World Health Organization. *Manual of Basic Techniques for a Health Laboratory*, WHO, Geneva, 1980.

Baker, F. J., Silverton, R. E. *Introduction to Medical Laboratory Technology*, Ch. 5. Butterworths, 6th Ed, 1985

25

Colorimetry

25:1 PRINCIPLES OF COLORIMETRIC TESTS

Most of the clinical chemistry quantitative methods described in this manual which measure substances in blood and other body fluids are colorimetric.

The principles of colorimetric analysis are based on the following:

- That many substances are coloured in solution or can be made to produce a coloured derivative in solution.

- That the intensity of colour in these coloured solutions is related to the amount of substance in the solution. A solution which contains a low concentration of a substance will appear pale in colour whereas one which contains a high concentration will appear dark in colour.

- That these coloured solutions absorb light at given wavelengths in the visible spectrum. The extent to which a solution absorbs light depends on the intensity of its colour. Only a small amount of light is absorbed by a pale coloured solution whereas a lot of light is absorbed by a dark coloured solution.

Wavelengths and the electromagnetic spectrum
Light waves are emitted in waves of varying length. The number of vibrations of wave motion per second is known as frequency and is measured in Hertz (Hz). A wavelength of light can be expressed in the following formula:

Wavelength (λ) of light =

$$\frac{\text{Velocity of light (distance travelled by light/second)}}{\text{Frequency (Hz)}}$$

The lower the wave frequencies, the longer the wavelengths. The lowest frequencies (i.e. longest wavelengths) are radio waves, followed by infrared heat radiation, visible light radiation, ultra violet radiation, X-rays and finally gamma-rays which have the highest frequencies (i.e. shortest wavelengths). The range of frequencies over which electromagnetic radiation is transmitted is referred to as the electromagnetic spectrum.

Visible light spectrum
Wavelengths between about 400 nm and 700 nm form the visible light band of the electromagnetic spectrum, referred to as the visible light spectrum (see Fig. 25.1). Wavelengths of about 700 nm are seen by the eye as red colours while those of progressively shorter wavelengths give rise in turn to the colours orange, yellow, green, blue, and finally violet which is produced by short wavelengths of 400 nm.

Vibrations with wavelengths greater than 700 nm are known as infrared or heat waves and these cannot be seen by the eye, while vibrations with wavelengths of less than 400 nm, that is beyond that of violet light, are known as ultraviolet light and these also cannot be seen by the eye.

What is known as white light is composed of all the wavelengths of visible colour. When two colours combine together to give the effect of white light such colours are said to be complementary. White light can be dispersed into its constituent wavelengths by being refracted through a glass prism or a diffraction grating. A natural dispersion of light occurs when a rainbow is formed with the light from the sun being dispersed into its various colours by the raindrops from a cloud.

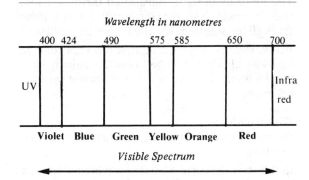

Fig. 25.1 The visible part of the electromagnetic spectrum. The colours of the spectrum are not separate blocks of colour, but merge into one another as in a rainbow.

Colour and light absorption
When light falls on a coloured solution in a tube, the light may be absorbed, reflected, or transmitted. A coloured solution appears coloured because it transmits a particular wavelength of light from the visible spectrum while selectively absorbing other wavelengths, e.g. a red solution is red because it transmits light from the red part of the visible spectrum and absorbs light from the green-blue end of the spectrum.

Pure water is colourless because instead of absorbing specific wavelengths of light it transmits all the visible wavelengths. The ability of a substance to selectively absorb certain wavelengths of light while transmitting others is determined by its molecular and atomic structure.

The Beer-Lambert law of light absorption

Beer and Lambert showed that under suitable conditions the amount of light absorbed by a coloured solution when illuminated with light of a suitable wavelength, is directly proportional to the concentration of the coloured solution and the length of the lightpath through the solution.

In colorimetric tests, the Beer-Lambert law can be applied to find the concentration of a substance in solution. Using a standard, the concentration of a substance in an unknown (test) solution can be determined as follows:

Concentration of test =

$$\frac{\text{Absorbance (A) of test}}{\text{Absorbance (A) of standard}} \times \frac{\text{Concentration of}}{\text{standard}}$$

The amount of light absorbed by a coloured solution i.e. absorbance (formerly referred to as optical density, or OD) is dependent on:

☐ Lightpath distance
☐ Wavelength or band of wavelengths used

Lightpath

The intensity of light transmitted through a solution becomes less the further it has to travel through the solution, i.e. the longer the lightpath.

In colorimetric tests, the lightpath is kept constant by using optically matched cuvettes usually of 10 mm lightpath distance or tubes of known lightpath distance.

Wavelength(s)

Substances absorb light at given wavelengths in the spectrum.

In selecting the correct band of wavelengths to use, both the maximum absorbance and selectivity of the wavelengths for a particular substance need to be considered. The means by which wavelengths are selected in colorimetric analytical tests are described in 25:3.

Application of the Beer-Lambert law

For most of the clinical chemistry quantitative tests described in Chapters 28 and 30 to 32, the Beer-Lambert law can be applied, i.e. a linear relationship can be shown to exist between the concentration of the substance being measured and its absorbance.

To determine whether the method and instrument used to measure a particular substance obey the Beer-Lambert law it is essential to prepare what is called a calibration graph. Calibration of a test method and the conditions which must exist to apply the Beer-Lambert law are explained in subunit 25:2. Instruments used to measure the absorbances of solutions are described in 25:3.

25:2 CALIBRATION OF COLORIMETRIC TESTS

As explained in 25:1, most colorimetric analytical tests are based on the Beer-Lambert law which states that the absorbance of a solution when measured at the correct wavelength is directly proportional to its concentration and the length of the lightpath through the solution.

For this law to hold true, both the solution being tested and the instrument used to measure the absorbance must meet certain requirements.

Solution requirements

■ The solution must be the same throughout (homogeneous) and the molecules of which it is composed must not associate or dissociate at the time absorbance is being measured.

■ The substance being measured in the solution should not react with the solvent.

■ Reagent blanks must be used to correct for any absorption of light by solvents. A reagent blank solution contains all the reagents and chemicals used in the chemical development of the colour but lacks the substance being assayed. Alternatively, a reagent blank may contain all components except a vital reagent.

■ Solutions must be prepared correctly using reliable chemicals and a good technique.

Instrument requirements

■ Instrument must show satisfactory accuracy, sensitivity, reproducibility and linearity at the different wavelengths used.

■ Cuvettes used in the instrument must be optically matched, free from scratches, clean and of the correct lightpath distance. A 10 mm lightpath distance is recommended for the tests described in this manual.

Importance of calibration

Calibration of a test method is necessary to establish whether the Beer-Lambert law and formula can be applied, i.e. whether the absorbance of the substance being measured increases in a linear way with its concentration.

Calibration of a test method involves:

— Testing a series of dilutions of the substance being assayed, i.e. standards.

— Reading the absorbance of each standard at the appropriate wavelength.

— Plotting the absorbance reading of each standard against its concentration.

— Drawing a line through the points plotted.

— Examining whether a linear (straight line) or a

non-linear (curved line) calibration is obtained.

Linear calibration

If a straight line can be drawn through the points plotted as shown in Fig. 25.2, then absorbance is directly proportional to concentration. The Beer-Lambert law applies and the following formula can be used:

Concentration of test (CT) =

$$\frac{\text{Absorbance of test (AT)}}{\text{Absorbance of standard (AS)}} \times \frac{\text{Concentration of}}{\text{standard (CS)}}$$

or in the abbreviated form: $CT = \dfrac{AT}{AS} \times CS$

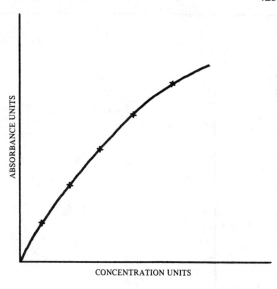

Fig. 25.3   Non-linear calibration showing a curved line joining the points plotted.

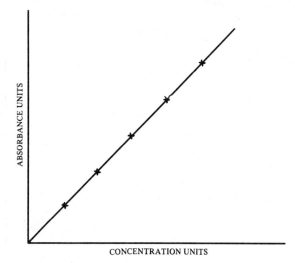

Fig. 25.2   Linear calibration showing a straight line joining the points plotted.

Non-linear calibration

If a straight line cannot be drawn through the points and a curved line is obtained as shown in Fig. 25.3, then absorbance is not directly proportional to concentration. The Beer-Lambert law and its formula cannot be applied. The concentration of the test solution must be obtained from the calibration curve (see later text).

Note: An analytical method where the Beer-Lambert law applies will have better performance characteristics than a method where the law cannot be applied.

Technique of calibrating a test method

General guidelines

☐ Use a minimum of 5 standards (instructions for preparing standard solutions are provided in test methods).

☐ Follow exactly the same method used to measure the patients' and control samples.

☐ Whenever resources permit, measure the standards in duplicate for greater accuracy and precission.

Drawing a calibration graph

1. Take a sheet of graph paper and rule the vertical axis and the horizontal axis. Mark the vertical axis *Absorbance*. Mark the horizontal axis *Concentration* and give the units of measurement (see Fig. 25.4).

   The graph paper can be turned any way round to obtain the best results as long as the point of origin is in the bottom left hand corner.

2. Depending on the range of concentrations and absorbance readings, divide each axis into the most suitable units for easiest reading. Use as much of the graph paper as possible.

   Example
   For glucose calibration graph, each square of the horizontal axis can be taken to represent 2 mmol/l and each of the vertical axis to represent 0.1 absorbance units as shown in Fig. 25.4.

3. Plot the absorbance of each standard solution against its concentration, marking each point with a small neat cross (see Fig. 25.4).

4. Join each cross, making sure that the line passes through the point of origin (equivalent to the reagent blank).

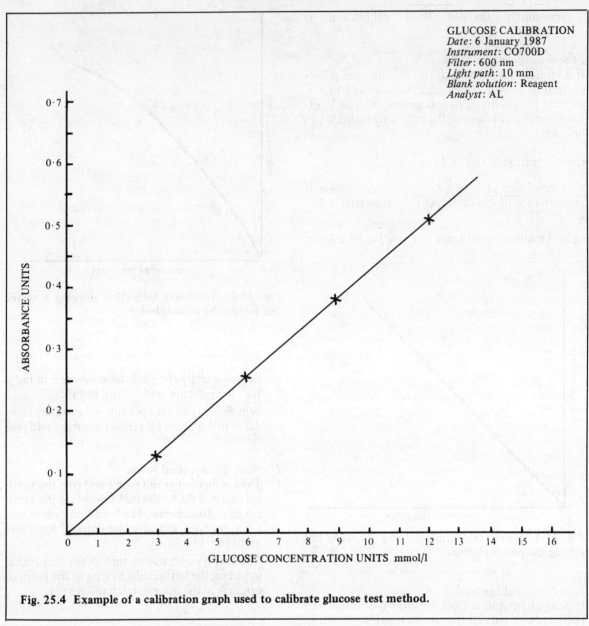

GLUCOSE CALIBRATION
Date: 6 January 1987
Instrument: CO700D
Filter: 600 nm
Light path: 10 mm
Blank solution: Reagent
Analyst: AL

Fig. 25.4 Example of a calibration graph used to calibrate glucose test method.

Linear calibration
If the line obviously looks as though it should be a straight line but one or two points are slightly off the line, this usually indicates inaccurate pipetting. A line of 'best fit' can be drawn if only one or two points are off the line. If a line of 'best fit' cannot be drawn, the calibration must be repeated.

If only one point is off the line this should be disregarded and the straight line drawn through the origin and all the other points.

Ideally the line passing through zero should be at an angle of 45 °. If this is not so and the curve is too steep or too flat, repeat the readings using the filter or wavelength near to maximum absorption.

Non-linear calibration
When the calibration is non-linear, the points will follow a curve, not a straight line. The curved line should be drawn smoothly and pass through the point of origin as shown in Fig. 25.3.

5. Write in the top right-hand corner of the graph:
   — date
   — instrument used
   — filter or wavelength at which the absorbances were measured
   — lightpath distance of the cuvette (usually 10 mm)
   — blank solution used to zero the instrument, i.e. water or a reagent blank solution
   — initials of analyst (person who performed calibration).

Using a calibration graph

Quality control samples must be carried through at the time of calibration and with each batch of tests. Only if the control samples give correct results can a calibration graph be used to determine patients' samples.

Control samples

A control sample contains a known amount of the substance being assayed. It is carried through every stage of the procedure in exactly the same way as the patients' samples. It is the best indication that a method, reagents, and instrument are functioning well and that the patients' results are correct.

The preparation of control sera and the practice of quality control in clinical chemistry work are fully covered in Chapter 27.

When determining the concentration of unknown samples, the instrument, the method, and the reagents must be the same as those used for determining the absorbances of the standard solutions.

At least one of the standards used to prepare the calibration graph should be included in each batch of tests carried through. The amount of analyte in this standard solution should be carefully chosen to give the best performance possible. Best performance is required at concentrations where clinical decisions are made.

The reagent blank must be treated in exactly the same way as the standards.

The procedures for determining the concentration of test and control samples depends on whether the calibration is linear or non-linear.

Using a linear calibration graph

When the calibration graph is linear, the Beer-Lambert formula can be used to calculate the concentration of unknown samples:

$$CT = \frac{AT}{AS} \times CS$$

Alternatively, a chart covering the appropriate range of values can be prepared from the calibration graph. Results can be read from the chart providing the reading of the standard (put through with each batch of tests) agrees with the chart and the control result is correct.

If the reading of the test solution is beyond the limits of the graph or the range of the instrument, the final coloured solution can be diluted with an appropriate diluent and the absorbance of the diluted fluid read. The result is multiplied by the dilution factor. It is better practice however to dilute the specimens and repeat the complete analytical procedure.

Using a non-linear calibration graph

When a test method produces a non-linear calibration, the values of the test and control samples must be read from the calibration graph. The formula based on the Beer-Lambert law *cannot* be used. A chart covering the appropriate range of values can be prepared from the calibration graph.

The reading of the standard must be checked to make sure it agrees with the calibration graph and the control result must be correct.

If the reading of the test solution is beyond the limits of the graph or the range of the instrument, the specimen must be diluted and the test repeated (the final coloured solution must not be diluted). The result is multiplied by the dilution factor used to dilute the specimen.

25:3 MEASUREMENT OF ABSORBANCY USING A COLORIMETER

Two types of instrument can be used to measure absorbance:

☐ Colorimeter,† or more correctly termed a filter absorption spectrometer (sometimes referred to as an absorptiometer or filterphotometer).

☐ Spectrophotometer,† or more correctly termed an absorption spectrometer.

† Colorimeter and spectrophotometer are the terms used by manufacturers.

The main difference between a colorimeter and a spectrophotometer is that with a colorimeter, absorbance can be measured only within certain wavelength ranges whereas with a spectrophotometer measurements can be made at specific wavelengths. This is because a spectrophotometer has a diffraction grating or prism which disperses white light into a continuous spectrum. This enables wavelengths of monochromatic (one colour) light to be selected. A colorimeter, however, is equipped with coloured filters which cover wavelength ranges e.g. an Ilford blue filter (No. 602) covers the wavelength range 450 to 480 nm, a green filter (No. 604) the range 505 to 535 nm, etc. The wavelength ranges and peak transmissions of all ten Ilford Spectrum Filters are shown in Table 25.1.

Selecting the correct type of instrument

For all the clinical chemistry tests described in this manual and also for many others, a modern colorimeter such as the battery/mains WPA CO700D Medical Colorimeter can be used (see later text). There is little if any advantage in using a spectrophotometer.

A spectrophotometer is much more expensive to buy and maintain than a colorimeter and usually far less rugged and more complex to use. Few spectrophotometers can be operated from a battery as well as from a mains electricity supply. A stable electricity supply is required for the reliable performance of a spectrophotometer. A spectrophotometer is required for tests which require reading in the ultra violet (UV) part of the spectrum or for tests which need to be read at specific wavelengths to reduce interference from unwanted chromogens.

Seaton in his paper *Measuring Absorbance on a Limited Budget*[1] comments, 'The absorption spectra of many of the chromogens used in routine clinical chemistry assays resemble not so much the steep mountain peaks and valleys but the gently undulating sand-dune. There are of course exceptions but it would be wrong to assume that all assays which instruct, measure the absorbancy at 525 nm, could not equally well be performed by the use of a wide range of wavelengths (such as 450-600 nm) with only marginal if any, loss of accuracy.' Seaton concludes 'True technical excellence is demonstrated by the ability to equip one's laboratory not with the most expensive but with the most appropriate instruments.'

Structure of a colorimeter (based on WPA CO700D Colorimeter)

The basic components of a colorimeter based on the Walden Precision Apparatus (WPA) CO700D Medical Colorimeter[2] are as follows:

- Light source
- Filters
- Photosensitive detector system
- Cells (cuvettes) to hold solutions

Light source

The WPA CO700D Colorimeter uses a 6 volt tungsten lamp which provides a good source of white light. With use, the 'burnt-off' tungsten atoms from the lamp's filament become deposited on the surface of the glass bulb forming a silvery-black coating. When this is sufficient to cause a reduction of light intensity the lamp must be replaced.Replacement is usually indicated when it is not possible to zero the colorimeter.

Replacement of the WPA lamp unit is easily achieved because the lamp in its mounting is replaced to ensure correct focusing of the new lamp. Instructions are supplied in the clearly written and well illustrated *Operations and Maintenance Manual* which accompanies the CO700D Colorimeter.

Filters

Ten Ilford Spectrum filters (No. 600-609) are supplied with the CO700D Colorimeter. These have an average bandwidth of 40 nm and enable absorbance to be read over the wavelength range 400 nm to 700 nm. Details of these filters are shown in Table 25.1.

The filters are glass mounted and sealed in a special filter wheel which is an integral part of the CO700D instrument. This avoids loss of any of the filters, protects them against finger marks and dust and helps to minimize the growth of moulds on the filters in hot humid climates. The required filter is moved into place by turning a *Filter Selector Knob* and the filter number and colour are shown in the *Filter Window* (see Plate 25.1 and Fig. 25.6) In the CO700D, the filter is positioned between the test solution in the cuvette and the photodiode which detects the filtered light (see Fig. 25.7).

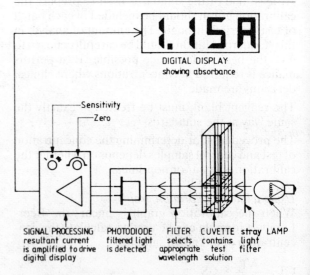

Fig. 25.7 Operation of a CO700D Colorimeter.

The correct filter to use in a particular colorimetric test is usually specified in the test method. It will be the one which transmits the most light over the range in which the solution absorbs the maximum light, i.e. the filter whose spectral transmission is opposite (complementary) to that of the colour of

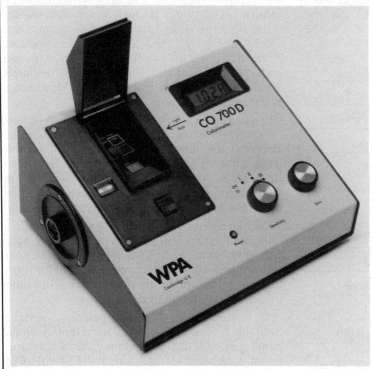

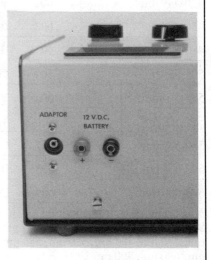

Plate 25.1 WPA mains and battery operated digital colorimeter.
Courtesy of Walden Precision Apparatus.

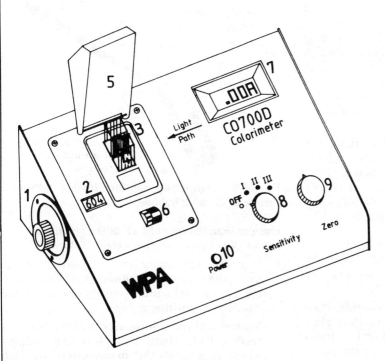

PARTS OF COLORIMETER

1 Filter selection knob
2 Filter window
3 Cuvette holder
4 Cuvettes (10 mm lightpath)
5 Cuvette cover
6 Cuvette movement switch
7 Absorbance display
8 On off and Sensitivity knob
9 Zero knob
10 Power indicator

Fig. 25.6 Components of the WPA CO700D Colorimeter.

the solution being measured. If the filter to use is not specified in the test method but only the wavelength, the correct filter to use can be obtained by referring to Table 25.1.

Table 25.1 Use of Filters

Wavelength Required	Ilford Filter to Use	
400-419 nm	No. 600	Deep violet
420-449 nm	601	Violet
450-479 nm	602	Blue
480-504 nm	603	Blue-green
505-534 nm	604	Green
535-564 nm	605	Yellow-green
565-589 nm	606	Yellow
590-639 nm	607	Orange
640-689 nm	608	Red
690-700 nm	609	Deep red

Note: The peak transmissions of the above Ilford Spectrum filters (No. 600 to 609) are 408 nm, 430 nm, 470 nm, 490 nm, 520 nm, 550 nm, 580 nm, 600 nm, 680 nm, 700 nm.

Photosensitive detector system
The photosensitive detector system in the WPA CO700D Colorimeter is a modern solid state silicon photodiode. This detects the filtered light which emerges from the solution in the cuvette and converts it to an electrical signal. The resultant current is proportional to the intensity of the emerging light. It is amplified to drive a digital display which shows absorbance units. As shown in Plate 25.1 and Fig. 25.6 the absorbance units are clearly displayed to two decimal places. The symbol **A** which appears to the right of the figures is a digital A (indicating Absorbance).

Note: Being digital, the CO700D Colorimeter is more rugged than analogue colorimeters which use a meter for reading results. It can be operated from a 12 v acid battery or from mains electricity through an adaptor (110 v or 240 v). Battery leads and adaptor are supplied with the instrument.[2]

Cells to hold solutions
For routine clinical chemistry work, optically matched cuvettes of 10 mm lightpath distance (see Fig. 25.8) are recommended.

Both glass and plastic cuvettes are available. Plastic cuvettes are much less expensive than glass cuvettes and with care can be used several times before they become scratched and unfit for use.

Cuvettes should be handled carefully by their ground glass sides (glass cuvettes) or lined opaque sides (plastic cuvettes). The optical surfaces of the cuvettes (clear sides through which light passes) must be kept clean, dry, and free from finger marks. Each day a mild detergent should be used to clean cuvettes followed by several rinses in clean water with a final rinse in distilled or deionized water. A soft clean cloth or tissue should be used to dry the optical surfaces.

The minimum volume of fluid which must be used in a cuvette when measuring the absorbance of samples varies according to the type of colorimeter used. The CO700D Colorimeter has been designed to read fluid volumes as low as 1.6 ml which enables semi-micro methods to be used for most tests which helps to keep costs to a minimum.

When transferring a solution to a cuvette it is important to avoid air bubbles forming. An incorrect absorbance reading will be obtained if a solution contains bubbles. To avoid air bubbles forming, a solution should be poured down the inner side wall of a cuvette (see Fig. 25.8).

A flow-through cell (pour in - suck out cuvette) is available for use with most colorimeters. A simple hand-operated suction system is available (optional accessory) for use with the CO700D Colorimeter. Although a flow-through cell reduces the number of cuvettes required and enables tests to be read more quickly because solutions are automatically sucked out of the cuvette, a flow-through cell does not allow a rechecking of sample readings.

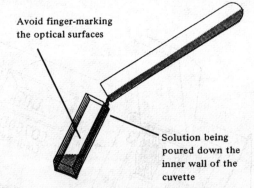

Avoid finger-marking the optical surfaces

Solution being poured down the inner wall of the cuvette

Fig. 25.8 Transferring solution from a tube to a cuvette to avoid air bubbles.

Use and maintenance of CO700D Colorimeter
A CO700D Colorimeter is used as follows:

1. Place the colorimeter on a solid surface that is free from mechanical vibration. Do not place the instrument in direct sunlight or on the same bench as a centrifuge.

2. Ensure that the colorimeter is connected correctly to its 12 v battery supply or to its adaptor which plugs into the mains electricity (full details can be found in the CO700D *Operations and Maintenance Manual*).

3. Turn on the colorimeter by moving the *Sensitivity Knob* from the OFF position to *Setting I*. The green *Power Indicator* lamp will come on. Allow at least 2 minutes for the instrument to stabilize sufficiently.

4. Turn the Filter Selector Knob until the required filter No. is shown in the *Filter Window* (see Plate 25.1 and Fig. 25.6).

5. Transfer at least 1.6 ml of the reagent blank solution or distilled water (as specified in the test method) to one of the cuvettes supplied with the instrument or to a glass cuvette of 10 mm lightpath distance (see Fig. 25.8).

   Important: Do not finger mark the clear optical sides of the cuvette and avoid air bubbles forming when transferring the solution to the cuvette (see Fig. 25.8).

6. Insert the blank solution in the rear cuvette holding, making sure that the clear sides of the cuvette are facing sideways.

7. Transfer at least 1.6 ml of the sample solution (standard, control or patient's) to another cuvette taking the same precautions as described in step 5.

8. Insert the sample solution in the front cuvette holder.

9. Move the *Cuvette Movement Switch* to the white position to bring the blank solution into the arrowed *Light Path* position. Close the *Cuvette Cover*.

10. Adjust the *Zero Knob* to give .00 Ħ reading on the display (Ħ indicates Absorbance units). If it is not possible to zero on setting I, move the *Sensitivity Knob* to setting II and if necessary to setting III. The lowest setting should always be used to zero the colorimeter.

    If the display does not show Ħ on the end of the reading, turn the zero knob to the right.

11. When the display reads .00 Ħ , move the *Cuvette Switch* to the red position to bring the sample solution into the *Light Path* position. Record the absorbance reading of the sample as shown in the display.

12. Return the blank solution to the *Light Path* position by moving the *Cuvette Switch* back to its white position. Check that the display still reads .00 Ħ . If the display does not read zero, adjust to .00 Ħ and read again the absorbance of the sample solution. The blank solution should continue to read zero each time it is returned to the *Light Path*.

13. Calculate the concentration of the control and test samples as instructed in the test method.

Maintenance of CO700D Colorimeter
The model CO700D Colorimeter is a rugged instrument which requires very little maintenance except for good laboratory practices when handling and transferring solutions, keeping battery terminals clean (when using battery power), and replacing the lamp when this becomes necessary. Each lamp has a long life.

At the beginning of each day's work, check that the cuvettes are completely clean and free from scratches (see previous text). At the end of the day's work, make sure the colorimeter is switched off (including from the mains). Cover the instrument with its protective dust cover.

At least 2 spare lamps should be kept with the Colorimeter.[2] The lamp is easily replaced when this becomes necessary. Detailed illustrated instructions for replacing the lamp (supplied prefocused in its mount) are given in the *Applications, Operation and Maintenance Manual* which accompanies the CO700D Colorimeter.

References

1 Seaton, B. Measuring absorbance on a very limited budget. *The Medical Technologist*, December, 1984.

2 WPA Model CO700D Colorimeter is available from Walden Precision Apparatus Ltd (for address, see Appendix II). The cost of the instrument is £197 (1986) which *includes* the complete range of 10 Ilford filters (400-700 nm), mounted prefocused lamp and 1 spare lamp, cuvette holder, 10 plastic cuvettes (10 mm lightpath distance), battery leads (2 metres), mains adaptor for 110-125 v or 220-240 v (*must specify which type when ordering*), dust cover, and *Applications, Operation and Maintenance Manual*.

A Pour in/Syphon out cuvette (No. 151M-OS) is available as an accessory at approximately £45.

Additional mounted prefocused lamps (No. CO55L) can be purchased at £4.50 per packet of 3 lamps.

Note: Glass and plastic cuvettes are available to developing countries from Tropical Health Technology Equipment Services (see Appendix IV, Cuvettes).

Recommended Reading

Baker, F. J.; Silverton, R. E. *Introduction to Medical Laboratory Technology*, Butterworth and Co Ltd., 6th edition, 1985.

26 Planning a Clinical Chemistry Laboratory Collection and Transport of Specimens

26:1 SELECTION OF CLINICAL CHEMISTRY TESTS AND METHODS

The clinical chemistry tests included in this manual are those that have been requested by the district and regional hospitals in tropical and developing countries. The tests included follow closely those that have been identified by a 1986 World Health Organization Working Group as essential clinical chemistry tests for intermediate hospital laboratories.[1]

Test methods have been selected from a consideration of:

- Reliability
- Cost
- Simplicity
- Availability of reagents
- Stability of reagents in tropical countries
- Suitability for use with a colorimeter

Standardization of methods

As far as possible there should be standardization of test methods between regional and district laboratories. This will increase the reliability of test results and lower the cost of tests. To achieve standardization the regional clinical chemistry laboratory should prepare and distribute essential reagents, standards, and control sera to district laboratories and ensure the adequate training, supervision, and updating of staff working in peripheral laboratories.

Micro methods

A further way to reduce costs is to use smaller quantities of reagents and control sera by following a micro or semi-micro method.

For most of the tests included in this manual, semi-micro methods are described. To follow these methods a colorimeter is required which can read small volumes such as the WPA CO700D Medical Colorimeter described in 25:3. Alternatively, an instrument must be used which can be adapted to read a minimum volume of about 1.5 ml.†

† *Adaption of Corning Model 252 Colorimeter to read small volumes of fluid*
Place a small block of wood (or other solid material) measuring 12 mm × 12 mm by 7.5 mm high in the bottom of the cuvette holder. This will raise the cuvette (4.5 ml capacity) to the correct height for the light to pass through a solution of 1.5 ml minimum volume.

The use of micro methods also reduces the volumes of specimens required. This is of particular value when only a small amount of sample is available, for example from a child.

Use of commercially produced reagent test kits

Although a wide range of clinical chemistry test kits are commercially available only a small number are manual colorimetric techniques suitable for use in district laboratories in developing countries.

Many kits have been developed for specific continuous flow systems, discrete analyzers or centrifugal analyzers that are used in large clinical chemistry laboratories.

Some kits are designated 'UV' which means that they can be used only with instruments that measure in the ultraviolet (UV) range, i.e. wavelengths less than 400 nm.

In the case of enzyme determinations, the terms 'kinetic' and 'optimized' (Opt) are used. These kits are for use with kinetic enzyme analyzers and require training in kinetic techniques.†

† Kinetic technique
A kinetic technique determines enzyme activity by measuring the rate of product formation (or substrate used) during the early linear part of the reaction. The term 'optimized' is used by some manufacturers to describe kinetic enzyme kits in which substrates, buffers, coenzymes, activators and other reagents have been selected to give the highest enzyme activity and therefore the greatest sensitivity.

The decision to use test kits in district laboratories will depend on:

- Availability of manual colorimetric kits that can be used with instruments that measure within the wavelength range 400-700 nm with a bandwidth of about 40 nm, e.g. WPA CO700D Medical Colorimeter or Corning 252 Colorimeter.

- Cost of using kits. In general it will be more expensive for district laboratories to use kits than to prepare their own reagents for clinical chemistry assays.

Although most test kits have at least a two year shelf-life from manufacture, some may reach a district laboratory within only a few months of their expiry date.

It is also important to note that the stability of diluted *working* reagents (prepared from stock solutions) may be much shorter than the stability of the stock reagents. The workload of a district laboratory may be insufficient to use the amount of working reagent supplied within its stated shelf-life.

It should also be noted whether *all* the reagents and standard solutions needed are provided in the kit. Extra reagents may sometimes be required. Control sera will also need to be ordered separately (see 27:5).

■ Whether the training and experience of the laboratory staff are adequate, especially with regard to preparing reagents and standards and performing clinical chemistry tests.

Kits that use *established technologies and that are known to work well in tropical countries* may make it possible for a laboratory to obtain better results because the kits contain ready-made reliable reagents and standards. Kits are particularly useful when the test reagents are complex and difficult to make in district laboratories, e.g. kits to measure the enzyme alkaline phosphatase (see 30:8) and aspartate aminotransferase (see 30:7) activities.

The method details that accompany some kits, however, are not always adequate. Calibration details may not be given and often there are no specific instructions regarding the use of controls. It is essential to include at least one control serum in every batch of tests. This is particularly important when using a test kit to ensure that the reagents have not deteriorated in transit to the laboratory due to incorrect storage, e.g. being left in high temperatures for a prolonged period.

Recommendations when considering purchasing test kits
Before purchasing clinical chemistry test kits, obtain from several manufacturers the following details:

□ Prices and local availability. Try to find out whether there is more than one local agent and whether prices of kits vary between suppliers.

□ Sizes of kits and pack presentations, i.e. how many tests can be performed and are the reagents packaged in small or large amounts.

□ Expiry dates of reagents (stock and *working*) and standards both from their date of manufacture and from when they are opened.

□ References and evaluations of kit methods.

Insert leaflet
Before purchasing a kit, *always* obtain a copy of the insert leaflet which accompanies it. This will describe the method and reagents used. It should also suggest a quality control serum to use. Read this sheet carefully:

— Confirm that the method is a *manual colorimetric* one and that it measures within the wavelength range 400-700 nm (see Filter Table in 25:3) with an endpoint reaction (not kinetic).

— Note whether the test method is easy to follow and gives sufficient detail, e.g. regarding calibration and details of reagents including how they should be stored and whether they are corrosive, toxic, flammable, etc. If the information supplied is insufficient, request further details.

— Check whether a control serum is suggested for use with the kit. At least one control must be used with each batch of tests.

— Note the reference ranges. These may vary from one kit to another for the same substance being measured depending on the test method used. Check whether SI units are being used.

— Look to see whether details are given of the useful working limit of the technique (linearity).

— Note whether there is a recommended OCV or RCV for the method (see 27:3).

Note: In some instances instead of buying entire kits it may be more economical to consider purchasing (when available) individual ready-made stable products for the more complex reagents and for some standards. Reagents and standards that are sold separately are listed under the different tests in Chapters 28, 30 and 31. When purchasing ready-made reagents it is important to check that the reagents are suitable for use with manual tests and not for use only with analyzers.

Dry reagent chemical analysis using reflectance spectroscopy
Recent advances in the application of dry reagent (solid phase) technology combined with the development of microprocessor controlled meters for measuring reflected light (reflectometers) have lead to the production of rapid easy to use systems for the measurement of substances in blood.

Depending on the manufacturer's system, the stable dry reagents are layered on slides or strips and the reflectometer is calibrated for the different tests from the information coded on the slides or strips or by inserting calibrating modules into the meter. The control or patient's sample is dispensed on the strip or slide and within a few minutes (or even 30 seconds for some tests) the result is displayed or produced on tape (depending on the system).

Three manufacturers have produced dry reagent technology systems for measuring substances in blood:

□ Eastman Kodak Company has produced the *Ektachem DT 60* analyzer. It uses a bar-coded slide for test recognition. Electrolyte tests require a special electrode module. Serum or plasma (10 μl) is required, an incubation stage at 37 °C is required, and results are recorded on tape about 6 minutes after inserting a test slide.

□ Ames Division Miles Laboratories Ltd has produced the *Seralyzer System*. It uses reagent strips and the reflectance meter is calibrated using single or *Multi-Component Calibrators*. Measurements are carried out using diluted serum or plasma. Reaction times range from 30-240 seconds. A buzzer sounds at the end of the reaction and the result is displayed digitally.

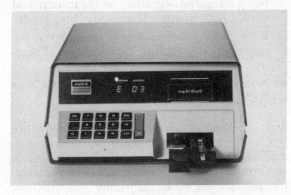

Plate 26.1 Ames Seralyzer system.
Courtesy of Ames division of Miles Laboratories.

□ Boehringer Mannheim has produced the *Reflotron System*. It is the most recently developed system and has the advantage that undiluted whole blood, plasma, or serum can be used. All the information needed by the reflectometer to measure the different substances is coded on each strip. No separate test modules or calibrators are required. Reaction times for the different tests are about 3 minutes and the results are displayed digitally.

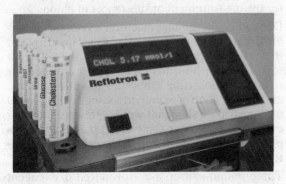

Plate 26.2 Boehringer Reflotron reflectance meter.
Courtesy Boehringer Mannheim.

Costs and availability

At the time of this manual going to press (late 1986), all three systems are still being developed with more tests becoming available including the measurement of electrolytes.

The cost of the *Ektachem DT 60* analyzer is about US$ 5500. The cost of the Ames *Seralyzer* is about £3600 with an additional cost for test modules. The Boehringer *Reflotron* system costs about £2600. These prices are current for 1985-1986 but can alter depending on the country in which the product is being sold. The price of test slides and test strips varies depending on the test and system. Most tests work out at about 25p to 50p each (1986). Some tests may be priced lower and some higher depending also on the country of purchase.

Important: Readers should write to the different manufacturers for up to date information about their systems, including local costs and availability, servicing, tests currently available and in development, packaging and stability of test slides or test strips, and the results of clinical evaluations and assessments. The addresses of Eastman Kodak Company, Ames Division Miles Laboratories Ltd, and Boehringer Mannheim can be found in Appendix II.

26:2 ORGANIZATION OF A CLINICAL CHEMISTRY LABORATORY

The careful organization of a clinical chemistry laboratory is essential if investigations are to be reliably and efficiently performed and reported.

Layout of a clinical chemistry laboratory

A bench or table should be set aside for the reception, checking and recording of specimens. A separate area close to the reception area should be organized for separating plasma or serum from whole blood specimens. It should be equipped with a centrifuge, racks, sample containers, Pasteur pipettes, disposal containers and marking pens. A refrigerator is necessary for storing specimens and reagents.

Pipettes, tubes, and other glassware used in the analysis of specimens should be conveniently situated as also containers of disinfectant in which to soak used pipettes and glassware. A hypochlorite (bleach) disinfectant should be used (see 2:3).

The colorimeter or spectrophotometer should be situated in an accessible, vibration-free place in the laboratory. It should not be positioned on the same bench as a centrifuge.

Reagents should be dated and clearly labelled. They should be placed on shelves above or near to where tests are being performed. Those requiring refrigeration should be assigned a place in the fridge where they can be easily found. Chemicals should be stored observing the safety measures recommended in 2:5.

In many tropical countries it may be necessary to use a separate air-conditioned room in which to store reagents and even to perform certain tests during the hot season.

As far as possible, reagents, standards (calibrants), and control sera should be prepared and standardized in a regional or central laboratory and distributed at regular intervals to district hospital laboratories. This will increase reliability and reduce the cost of clinical chemistry work.

Frequency of performing tests

Depending on the size of the hospital, prevalent diseases, and other local circumstances, certain biochemical tests will need to be performed daily, while others can be assayed in batches twice or three times a week as follows:

Investigations	Suggested frequency of tests
Serum or plasma: Urea Electrolytes Glucose	Daily
Serum or plasma: Total protein Albumin Liver function tests	Usually twice or three times a week
Serum or plasma: Amylase Calcium (serum) Urate Creatinine Cholesterol	As required
Urine tests Faecal tests Cerebrospinal fluid tests	As required

Important: When ever possible, tests should be performed in batches. It is costly to analyze specimens individually because expensive control sera and standards are required even when a single specimen is tested.

Staffing a clinical chemistry laboratory

A person appointed as head of a clinical chemistry laboratory must have sufficient knowledge and experience to manage a department on a daily basis, ensuring that:

- Staff are adequately trained.
- Test methods are followed correctly.
- Quality control is adequate.
- Test results are checked before being sent out.
- Chemicals and reagents are ordered in good time and prepared correctly.
- Safety measures are followed.

Depending on the workload of the laboratory, two or three staff members may be required. Although each member of staff is usually responsible for a group of tests, he or she should be capable of carrying out the full range of routine tests. Duties should be rotated on a weekly or monthly basis. This will make the work interesting and enable all staff members to perform emergency out of hours ('on call') investigations with confidence and efficiency.

Emergency service

An agreed system for testing urgent specimens should be understood and circulated to all those concerned. Only those tests that are essential for the immediate care of a patient should be requested urgently.

Emergency tests usually include serum or plasma electrolytes and glucose. Other tests such as urea and amylase may also need to be included depending on the clinical need and resources of the laboratory.

To minimize delay, the ward staff should collect the specimen and deliver it to the laboratory as quickly as possible. The specimen must be recorded by the technician, assayed and the result immediately phoned or taken to the ward for the attention of the medical officer treating the patient. If the result is phoned, the recipient of the result should repeat back the result to ensure that it has been recorded correctly. A written report should be issued as soon as possible.

Safety in the clinical chemistry laboratory

The practice of safety in a clinical chemistry laboratory as in other units of the laboratory is the responsibility of all those working in the department. The senior technologist or designated safety officer should ensure that a Code of Safety exists and that safety measures are followed.

Safety in the design and organization of a laboratory, safe use and storage of chemicals, safe handling of specimens, and safe methods of pipetting and dispensing, are described in Chapter 2.

26:3 SPECIMENS FOR BIOCHEMICAL ANALYSIS

The correct collection of specimens is essential for reliable test results. A summary of the collection and dispatch of specimens for biochemical analysis is given in chart form in 26:7.

Abnormal appearance of a specimen

Any abnormal appearance of a specimen should be reported and investigated if indicated. Such action on the part of a technician may lead to a condition being diagnosed more rapidly and a patient receiving the appropriate treatment at an earlier stage.

The following are examples of abnormal specimen appearances and their possible significance:

☐ A dark coloured urine may be positive for bilirubin or blood.

☐ A urine that contains whole blood may contain *S. haematobium* eggs.

☐ A black faecal specimen may contain occult blood due to gastrointestinal bleeding.

☐ A dark brown serum may indicate intravascular haemolysis due to sickle cell disease, severe malaria, or an incompatible blood transfusion.

☐ A lipaemic (fatty) serum may be associated with raised triglycerides.

☐ An icteric serum indicates that a patient is jaundiced. Such a specimen should be marked with a HIGH RISK warning symbol because it may contain infectious hepatitis viruses.

☐ A serum sample that is abnormally viscous (thick) may contain paraproteins.

☐ A serum that becomes markedly turbid after being refrigerated may contain cryoglobulins.

☐ A blood sample that contains a high concentration of red cells from which little serum or plasma can be obtained indicates severe dehydration or a blood disorder.

Request form for biochemical investigations

The request form should be as simple and clear as possible. It should provide essential information concerning the patient and a clinical note regarding diagnosis and treatment.

It is particularly important that details of drug therapy are supplied. Several drugs are known to interfere with the chemical reactions of certain test methods and a change of method may have to be considered if the interfering drug cannot be withheld.

The form must specify the actual tests required and avoid general requests such as 'liver function tests'.

The form must also state the date and time of specimen collection.

Before specimens reach the laboratory, those responsible for collecting samples must check that every specimen is labelled clearly with the patient's name and hospital number and that the name and number agree with what is written on the request form. Clerical mistakes can lead to serious errors and cause delays in the testing of specimens and subsequent treatment of patients.

Reporting of clinical chemistry results

It is *important* that all results be reported to the correct number of decimal places. The tables of reference ranges (27:8) show the number of decimal places that should be used for the tests detailed in this manual.

Each result reported should include the following:

■ Matrix (blood, serum, plasma, urine, cerebrospinal fluid or faeces)
■ Analyte (substance measured)
■ Result clearly presented in SI units
■ Reference range

26:4 COLLECTION OF BLOOD SPECIMENS

Factors regarding the collection of blood specimens that can affect the correctness of test results include:

■ Incorrect venepuncture technique
■ Haemolysis of red cells
■ Collection of a specimen into the wrong container
■ Instability of some chemical substances in whole blood, serum, and plasma

Venepuncture technique

Special precautions to be followed regarding the collection of venous blood are as follows:

☐ Do not apply the tourniquet too tightly or for too long a period because this will cause venous stasis leading to a concentration of substances in the blood such as haemoglobin, plasma proteins, and calcium.

☐ Do not collect the blood from an arm into which an intravenous (IV) infusion is being given.

☐ If an anticoagulated specimen is required, add the correct amount of blood to the tube or bottle and mix the blood with the anticoagulant by gently inverting the container several times. Do not shake the specimen.

Note: A vein which can be felt is usually easier to enter than one which can only be seen.

Avoiding haemolysis

The haemolysis (rupture) of red cells can be a serious source of unreliable test results. If red cells are haemolyzed, substances from the cells are released into the serum or plasma leading to a false increase in the concentration of analytes such as potassium. Haemolysis also interferes with many chemical reactions.

Haemolysis can be avoided by:

☐ Checking that the syringe and needle are dry and that the barrel and plunger of the syringe fit well.

☐ Not using a needle with too fine a bore.

☐ Not withdrawing the blood too rapidly or moving the needle once it is in the vein. Frothing of the blood must be avoided.

☐ Removing the needle from the syringe before dispensing the blood into the specimen container. Allow the blood to run gently down the inside wall of the container.

☐ Adding the correct amount of blood to anticoagulant. Do not shake the blood but gently mix it with the anticoagulant.

☐ Using clean dry glass tubes or bottles for the collection of blood from which serum is required and by allowing sufficient time for the blood to clot *and* clot retraction to take place. Red cells are very easily haemolyzed by the rough use of an applicator stick to dislodge a clot.

☐ Centrifuging blood samples for a minimum period of time. Centrifuging for 5 minutes at medium speed (about 700 g) is adequate to obtain sufficient serum or plasma from a whole blood sample.

☐ Not storing whole blood samples in, or next to, the freezing compartment of a refrigerator.

Specimen containers and anticoagulants

Specimen containers for clinical chemistry tests must be leakproof and chemically clean. They should be well washed with detergent, rinsed in several changes of clean water, and finally rinsed in distilled or deionised water before being allowed to dry. Syringes and needles used for collecting blood samples must also be chemically clean and *dry*.

To avoid the confusion which often arises from the use of several different types of container, the following system is recommended:

Non-urgent blood tests (excluding glucose)
Dispense about 5 ml of blood (see chart in 26:7) into a dry glass tube or bottle and allow to clot.† When the clot has retracted, centrifuge the specimen and transfer the serum to a labelled container. Tightly cap the container to avoid water evaporating from the specimen.

† Avoid collecting blood into a plastic container if serum is

required. Blood takes much longer to clot and clot retraction is poorer in a plastic tube or bottle than in a glass one.

Urgent blood tests (excluding glucose) and paediatric blood tests
Dispense the correct amount of blood into a tube containing lithium heparin anticoagulant.‡ *Gently* mix the blood with the anticoagulant. Centrifuge the specimen and transfer the plasma to a labelled container.

‡ Lithium heparin does not interfere with most chemical reactions and helps to minimize haemolysis. It does not contain sodium or potassium. Anticoagulants such as EDTA and fluoride-oxalate contain sodium or potassium salts and therefore these cannot be used when electrolytes are to be measured. Prior to analysis, stored plasma samples from heparinised blood often require re-centrifuging to remove clots.

Blood glucose (Non-urgent or urgent)
Dispense the correct amount of blood into a tube containing fluoride-oxalate.* *Gently* mix the blood with the anticoagulant. Centrifuge the specimen to obtain plasma.

* Fluoride is an enzyme inhibitor. It prevents the break down of glucose to lactic acid by enzyme action (glycolysis). Blood collected into fluoride-oxalate (Reagent No. 37) can also be used for measuring protein, urea and bilirubin but not for electrolytes or enzymes.

Note: The regional or central clinical chemistry laboratory should detail the exact collection procedures required for the tests referred to it for analysis.

Stability of chemical substances in blood specimens

Biochemical substances in blood are found in both plasma and cells but not necessarily in equal concentrations:

More concentrated in cells	Potassium Phosphate Aspartate amino- transferase Lactate dehydrogenase
More concentrated in plasma	Sodium Chloride Carbon dioxide
Concentration about equal in cells and plasma	Creatinine Glucose Urea Urate

Some of the chemical changes which may occur in blood specimens within a few hours of being collected include:

☐ Diffusion of potassium and some enzymes

through the red cell membrane into the serum or plasma.

□ Diffusion of carbon dioxide off the surface of the blood, leading to a lowering in the concentration of bicarbonate with a compensatory increase in plasma chloride (the 'chloride shift').

□ Decrease in the concentration of glucose by glycolysis (when fluoride-oxalate is not used).

□ Reduction or loss in the activity of certain enzymes, for example acid phosphatase.

□ Decomposition of bilirubin in daylight or fluorescent light.

Some of these changes can be prevented by separating the plasma or serum from the red cells as soon as possible (within 1 hour) after the blood has been collected. The blood should not be refrigerated before the serum or plasma is separated because this can lead to falsely raised potassium values. Glycolysis can be prevented by using fluoride-oxalate anticoagulant (see previous text). The decomposition of bilirubin can be avoided by protecting specimens from light.

Details regarding the stability of substances in whole blood and serum at room temperature (20-28 °C) and at 2-8 °C are summarized in the chart in 26:7.

To minimize any alteration in the concentration of substances due to the ingestion of food or daytime variation, most blood specimens are best collected at the beginning of the day before a patient takes food.

26:5 COLLECTION OF URINE SPECIMENS

Depending on the type of investigation, a single specimen of urine may be adequate or it may be necessary to collect urine over a 24 hour period.

A fresh, cleanly collected midstream 10-20 ml urine sample is required to test for protein, glucose, ketones, urobilinogen, and bilirubin. The container should be clean, dry, leak-proof, and sufficiently wide-necked for the patient to use. It must be free from all traces of disinfectants.

Whenever possible, the sample should be the first urine passed by the patient at the beginning of the day because this will generally contain the highest concentrations of substances to be tested.

Collection of a 24 hour urine
A 24 hour urine specimen is required for the quantitative analysis of substances such as hormones, steroids, phosphate, calcium, and protein. The successful collection of a 24 hour urine depends on explaining the procedure fully to the patient.

Procedure
1. At a specified time, usually 08.00 hours, instruct the patient to empty his or her bladder. *Discard* this urine. This should not form part of the collection.

2. Give the patient a large (2 litre capacity) bottle containing a preservative or stabiliser as required (see later text).

3. Instruct the patient to collect into the bottle all the urine he or she passes in the next 24 hours, up to and *including* the urine passed at 08.00 hours the following morning.

A 24 hour urine should reach the laboratory as soon after collection as possible. If a delay is unavoidable, the specimen must be refrigerated at 2-8 °C until it can be delivered to the laboratory. The bottle must be labelled with the patient's name, hospital number, and the date and time when the collection was started and completed. The appropriate request form must accompany the specimen.

Stability of chemical substances in urine
The chemical changes which may occur in urine specimens stored at room temperature include:

■ Breakdown of urea to ammonia by bacteria, leading to an increase in the pH of the urine. This may cause the precipitation of calcium and phosphates.

■ Oxidation of urobilinogen to urobilin.

■ Destruction of glucose by bacteria.

■ Precipitation of urate crystals in acidic urine.

These chemical changes can be slowed down by refrigerating the urine at 2-8 °C. Chemicals can also be added to urine to preserve it, especially to 24 hour specimens.

Urine preservatives and stabilizers
□ Hydrochloric acid: This can be used to preserve urine for determinations such as amino acids, inorganic phosphate, calcium and catecholamines. It must not be used to preserve urine for the measurement of protein or urate.

15-20 ml of 6 mol/l hydrochloric acid is required to preserve a 24 hour urine specimen.

□ Thymol (few crystals): This can be used to preserve a 24 hour urine specimen for measurements such as total protein and creatinine.

Important: Urine which contains preservatives or stabilizers must not be used for bacteriological culture.

26:6 COLLECTION OF FAECES, CEREBROSPINAL FLUID, AND ASPIRATES

Collection of faeces for occult blood testing

Instruct the patient to collect a small amount of faeces into a clean, dry, wide-necked container such as a waxed carton. It is usual to collect three specimens on different days. The patient should be on a diet free from meat and vegetables containing peroxidases for at least 1 day before collecting the specimen (see 30:12).

The specimen should be tested as soon after collection as possible. If a delay is unavoidable, the specimen should be refrigerated at 2-8 °C. No preservative should be added to the faeces.

Collection of cerebrospinal fluid

The biochemical analysis of cerebrospinal fluid (c.s.f.) usually includes the measurement of glucose and total protein. To prevent the breakdown of glucose in the c.s.f. (leading to a falsely low value), collect 0.5-1.0 ml of the fluid into fluoride-oxalate preservative (Reagent No. 37).

For total protein, collect 1 ml of fluid into a dry tube or bottle. Total protein can be measured using the supernatant fluid which remains after the bacteriological tests have been completed.

Great care must be taken when handling c.s.f. because the specimen is obtained by lumbar puncture. Only a limited amount of fluid can be withdrawn from a patient at any one time.

Collection of gastric and duodenal secretions

Aspirates of gastric secretions for the determination of pH and duodenal secretions for the estimation of trypsin activity should be collected into clean screw-cap containers of 20-30 ml capacity. Bottles of the Universal or McCartney type are suitable.

26:7 SUMMARY CHART FOR THE COLLECTION AND DISPATCH OF SPECIMENS FOR BIOCHEMICAL TESTS

The following chart gives information regarding the collection of specimens and minimum stability of substances for biochemical analysis. Although guidelines are also provided regarding the referral and dispatch of specimens, each laboratory must obtain detailed instructions from its own referral centre. If special specimen containers are required, these should also be obtained from the referral laboratory.

Notes
- 'Room temperature' refers to 20-28 °C.
- The term 'kept cool' refers to the transportation of specimens in an insulated flask or box that contains an ice pack or ice cubes.
- If a blood specimen is likely to take longer than 24 h to reach its destination, to reduce the risk of bacterial contamination, collect the specimen into a sterile container. Aseptically transfer the plasma or serum to a sterile tube or bottle for transport.

COLLECTION AND DISPATCH OF BLOOD SPECIMENS

Tests	Specimen	Container	Stability and Referral
Acid phosphatase	see Phosphatase, acid		
Alanine aminotransferase (previously SGPT)	3-5 ml clotted blood Haemolysis interferes with test (see 26:4)	Dry glass container	Stable in whole blood at room temperature up to 3 h or at 2-8 °C up to 12 h. Stable in serum at 2-8 °C up to 36 h. *Referral*: Send 1 ml serum, kept cool, to reach destination within 24 h.

Tests	Specimen	Container	Stability and Referral
Albumin	2 ml clotted blood Haemolysis interferes with test (see 26:4)	Dry glass container	Stable in whole blood at room temperature or at 2-8 °C up to 8 h. Stable in serum at 2-8 °C, for up to 4 days. *Referral*: Send 0.5 ml serum to reach destination within 72 h.
Alcohol (Ethanol)	2.5 ml anticoagulated blood	Fluoride-oxalate container	Stable in whole blood at room temperature or at 2-8 °C up to 3 h. *Referral*: Send whole blood kept cool, to reach destination within 3 h.
Alkaline phosphatase	see Phosphatase, alkaline		
alpha Fetoprotein	see Protein electrophoresis		
Amylase	3-5 ml clotted blood	Dry glass container	Good stability in whole blood. Stable in serum at 2-8 °C for up to 72 h (longer if frozen). *Referral*: Send 1-2 ml serum kept cool, to reach destination within 24 h.
Aspartate aminotransferase (previously SGOT)	3-5 ml clotted blood Haemolysis interferes with test (see 26:4)	Dry glass container	As for alanine aminotransferase
Bicarbonate	see Carbon dioxide		
Bilirubin, total	3-5 ml clotted blood *Infants*: 1-2 ml anticoagulated Haemolysis interferes with test (see 26:4)	Dry glass container *Infants*: Lithium heparin or EDTA container.	Protect from light Stable in whole blood at room temperature or at 2-8 °C up to 3 h. Stable in serum or plasma at 2-8 °C up to 12 h. *Referral*: Send 0.5-1.0 ml serum or plasma, kept cool and protected from light, to reach destination within 6 h.
Calcium	1-2 ml clotted blood Collect fasting blood and avoid venous stasis (see 26:4) Patient must not be receiving EDTA therapy	Dry glass container. Must be chemically clean	Stable in whole blood at room temperature or at 2-8 °C for up to 3 h. Stable in serum at 2-8 °C up to 72 h. *Referral*: Send 0.5 ml serum kept cool, to reach destination within 48 h.

Tests	Specimen	Container	Stability and Referral
Cholesterol	3-5 ml clotted blood *Also*: 2.5 ml of blood into EDTA	Dry glass container	Stable in whole blood at room temperature or at 2-8 °C up to 12 h. Stable in serum at 2-8 °C up to 72 h. *Referral*: Send 0.5-1.0 ml serum and 2.5 ml EDTA blood to reach destination within 72 h.
Cholinesterase	1-2 ml clotted blood or capillary blood collected into two plain capillaries	Dry glass container or plain capillaries	Stable in whole blood at room temperature or at 2-8 °C up to 3 h. Stable in serum at 2-8 °C up to 3 h. *Referral*: Send 0.2-0.5 ml serum to reach destination within 24 h. Whole blood in capillaries should reach laboratory within 3 h.
Carbon dioxide (bicarbonate) Blood pH PCO_2	5 ml anticoagulated blood Perform venepuncture with great care. Avoid introducing air bubbles into sample (make sure barrel and plunger of syringe fit well)	Lithium heparin container	Very poor stability. Plasma must be separated from cells and analyzed as soon as possible. *Referral*: Collect 5 ml blood into a sterile plastic syringe containing heparin anticoagulant. Gently rotate syringe to mix blood with the heparin. Send the syringe, with needle holder securely in place, to reach destination within 3 h.
Creatinine	2-3 ml clotted blood Haemolysis interferes with test (see 26:4)	Dry glass container	Stable in whole blood at room temperature or at 2-8 °C up to 12 h. Stable in serum at 2-8 °C up to 24 h. *Referral*: Send 0.5-1.0 ml serum kept cool, to reach destination within 18 h.
Electrolytes: Sodium Potassium Chloride	5-7 ml clotted blood or 5 ml anticoagulated blood Haemolyzed blood cannot be used (see 26:4) Do not collect blood from an arm receiving an I.V. infusion	Dry glass container or lithium heparin container	Stable in whole blood at room temperature up to 1 h. Do not refrigerate sample before removing serum or plasma Stable in serum or plasma at 2-8 °C up to 24 h. *Referral*: Send about 1 ml serum or plasma, kept cool, to reach destination within 12 h.

Tests	Specimen	Container	Stability and Referral
Glucose	1 ml anticoagulated blood (fasting, post-prandial, or random specimen) Do not collect blood from an arm receiving an I.V. infusion	Fluoride-oxalate container	Stable in fluoride/oxalated blood at room temperature up to 3 h. Stable in plasma at 2-8 °C up to 48 h. *Referral*: Send 0.5 ml plasma from fluoride/oxalated blood, kept cool, to reach destination within 36 h.
Iron Total iron-binding capacity (TIBC)	10-12 ml clotted blood Collect at the beginning of the day Markedly haemolyzed samples should not be used (see 26:4)	Dry glass container. Must be chemically clean	Stable in whole blood at room temperature up to 3 h or at 2-8 °C up to 24h. *Referral*: Send at least 4 ml serum, kept cool, to reach destination within 18 h.
Lactate dehydrogenase (LDH)	3-5 ml clotted blood. Blood which is haemolyzed (even slightly) must not be used (see 26:4)	Dry glass container	Stable in whole blood at room temperature or at 2-8 °C up to 3 h. Stable in serum at 2-8 °C for up to 48 h. *Referral*: Send 1-2 ml serum to reach destination within 48 h.
Magnesium	3-5 ml clotted blood Haemolysis interferes with test (see 26:4)	Dry glass container	As for alanine aminotransferase
Phosphatase, acid	3-5 ml clotted blood Haemolyzed blood must not be used (see 26:4)	Dry glass container	Poor stability in whole blood. Separate serum from cells as soon as possible. Assay within 1 h or store frozen. *Referral*: Add 10 mg disodium citrate per ml of serum, or if unavailable add one drop of glacial acetic acid. Send 1 ml of sample, kept cool, to reach destination within 24 h.
Phosphatase, alkaline	3-5 ml clotted blood Haemolysis interferes with test (see 26:4)	Dry glass container	Stable in whole blood at room temperature up to 12 h. Stable in serum at 2-8 °C up to 24 h or at room temperature up to 48 h. *Referral*: Send 1 ml serum to reach destination within 48 h.

Tests	Specimen	Container	Stability and Referral
Phosphate, inorganic (Phosphorus)	3-5 ml clotted blood Haemolyzed blood must not be used (see 26:4)	Dry glass container	Stable in whole blood at room temperature or at 2-8 °C up to 3 h. Stable in serum at room temperature up to 48 h or at 2-8 °C up to 5 days. *Referral*: send 1 ml serum to reach destination within 48 h.
Potassium	see Electrolytes		
Protein, total	3 ml clotted blood Avoid venous stasis (see 26:4) Haemolysis interferes with test (see 26:4)	Dry glass container	Stable in whole blood at room temperature or at 2-8 °C up to 8 h. Stable in serum or at 2-8 °C for up to 4 days. *Referral*: Send 0.5 ml serum to reach destination within 72 h.
Protein, electrophoresis: *alpha* Fetoprotein Paraproteins	3-5 ml clotted blood	Dry glass container	Separate serum from cells and store frozen until analysed. *Referral*: Send 1 ml serum, kept cool, to reach destination within 8 h.
Sodium	see Electrolytes		
Thyroxine (T$_4$)	5 ml clotted blood	Dry glass container	As for alanine aminotransferase
Triglycerides	3-5 ml clotted blood (fasting specimen) *Also*: 2.5 ml of blood into EDTA anticoagulant	Dry glass container	Stable in whole blood at room temperature or at 2-8 °C up to 3 h. Stable in serum at 2-8 °C up to 72 h. *Referral*: Send 1 ml serum and 2.5 ml EDTA blood, kept cool, to reach destination within 48 h.
Urate (Uric acid)	5 ml clotted blood	Dry glass container	Protect from daylight. Stable in whole blood at room temperature or at 2-8 °C up to 12 h. Stable in serum at 2-8 °C for up to 72 h. *Referral*: Send 1-2 ml serum to reach destination within 72 h.

Tests	Specimen	Container	Stability and Referral
Urea	1-2 ml clotted blood Plasma from EDTA or fluoride/oxalate blood can also be used.	Dry glass container	Stable in whole blood at room temperature or at 2-8 °C up to 12 h. Stable in serum at 2-8 °C for up to 48 h. *Referral*: Send 0.2-0.5 ml serum to reach destination within 48 h.

COLLECTION AND DISPATCH OF URINE SPECIMENS

Tests	Specimen	Container	Stability and Referral
Amino acids	*Adults*: 24 hour urine *Infants*: First morning urine	Large bottle containing 5 ml HCl, 6 mol/l Dry container	Stable for several hours at 2-8 °C. *Referral*: Measure volume of urine, mix, and send 20 ml aliquot kept cool to reach destination within 24 h.
delta Aminolaevulinic acid (ALA)	24 hour urine	Large bottle containing 10 ml glacial acetic acid	As for amino acids
Bence Jones protein	10-20 ml midstream first morning urine	Dry container	Stable at 2-8 °C for several hours. *Referral*: For protein electrophoresis, send urine (and serum sample) kept cool, to reach destination within 6 h.
Bilirubin	5-10 midstream urine	Dry container	Stable for a few hours at room temperature if protected from light.
Calcium	24 hour urine	Large bottle containing 20 ml HCl, 6 mol/l	Stable at 2-8 °C for several hours. *Referral*: Measure volume of urine, mix, and send 5 ml aliquot, kept cool, to reach destination within 6 h.
Chloroquine	20-30 ml midstream first morning urine	Dry container	Stable at 2-8 °C for a few hours. *Referral*: Send urine, kept cool to reach destination within 6 h.
Creatinine	24 hour urine	Large container without preservative	As for calcium
Glucose	5-10 ml midstream urine	Dry container	If not tested immediately, store at 2-8 °C to prevent glycolysis.

Tests	Specimen	Container	Stability and Referral
Haemoglobin	5-10 ml midstream urine	Dry container	Stable at room temperature for a few hours. *Referral*: Send urine, kept cool, to reach destination within 6 h.
11-Hydroxycorticosteroids (free)	24 hour urine	Large brown bottle containing 10 ml chloroform	As for calcium
5-Hydroxy indoles	24 hour urine	Large brown bottle containing 50 ml 50% v/v acetic acid	As for calcium
Ketones	5-10 ml midstream urine	Dry container	Test as soon as possible after collection
3-Methoxy-4-hydroxy mandelic acid (HMMA), (VMA)	24 hour urine	Large brown bottle containing 10 ml glacial acetic acid	As for calcium
Morphine and other opium-containing compounds	20-30 ml urine	Dry container	*Referral*: Send urine, kept cool to reach destination within 6 h
pH	3-5 ml midstream urine	Dry container	Test as soon as possible after collection
Phosphate, inorganic	24 hour urine	Large bottle containing 20 ml HCl, 6 mol/l	As for amino acids
Protein semi-quantitative	10-20 ml midstream urine	Dry container	Stable at 2-8 °C for several hours
quantitative	24 hour urine	Large dry container	Measure volume of urine *Referral*: Send 50 ml well-mixed aliquot, kept cool to reach destination within 6 h
Relative mass density (specific gravity)	50-60 ml if using a urinometer or 1 ml if using a refractometer Midstream, first morning urine	Dry container	Test as soon as possible after collection
Urea	10-20 ml midstream urine	Dry container	Test specimen as soon after collection as possible (urea is rapidly broken down to ammonia)
Urobilinogen	5-10 ml midstream urine	Dry container	Test as soon as possible after collection
Vanillyl mandelic acid (VMA)	see 3-Methoxy-4-hydroxy mandelic acid		
Xylose absorption test	Contact the Referral Laboratory for details		

COLLECTION AND DISPATCH OF FAECAL SPECIMENS

Tests	Specimen	Container	Stability and Referral
Lactose	5-10 ml *fluid* faecal specimen	Dry container	Test as soon as possible after collection
Occult blood	Collect a small sample each day for 3 days Patient should not eat meat or vegetables containing peroxidases for 1 day before the test	Dry wide-necked container, e.g. a waxed carton	Test as soon as possible after collection. If a delay is inevitable the sample can be preserved by storing at 2-8 °C.

COLLECTION AND DISPATCH OF CEREBROSPINAL FLUID SPECIMENS

Tests	Specimen	Container	Stability and Referral
Glucose	0.5 ml c.s.f.	Fluoride-oxalate container	Stable at room temperature up to 3 h, or at 2-8 °C up to 24 h. *Referral*: Send c.s.f. kept cool, to reach destination within 18 h.
Protein, total	1 ml c.s.f.	Dry container (sterile, if c.s.f. for culture also) Fluorixe-oxalate container can also be used (unsuitable for culture)	Stable at room temperature up to 3 h, or at 2-8 °C up to 48 h. *Referral*: Send c.s.f. to reach destination within 24 h.

COLLECTION OF GASTRIC AND DUODENAL SECRETIONS

Tests	Specimen	Container	Stability and Referral
pH of gastric juice	Fasting (12 h) specimen (i.e. resting juice)	Dry container	Test as soon as possible after collection
Trypsin activity of duodenal secretion	1 ml aspirate	Dry container	Test as soon as possible after collection

Postal regulations for transport of specimens

In most countries there are regulations regarding the sending of pathological specimens through the post. Each laboratory should therefore obtain a copy of these postal regulations from its local post office. The regulations usually state that:

- A specimen must be sent in a completely sealed container and this must be placed in another container sufficiently strong to withstand knocks and pressure.

- Each specimen must be surrounded with sufficient absorbent packing material to absorb completely a fluid specimen should leakage or breakage occur.

- All specimen packages must be clearly addressed and marked with the words 'FRAGILE WITH CARE - PATHOLOGICAL SPECIMEN

References

1   World Health Organization *Working Group on Assessment of Clinical Technologies. LAB/86.2*, 1986. Available from Health Laboratory Unit, WHO 1211-Geneva, 27 Switzerland.

Recommended Reading

WHO Methods for Essential Clinical Chemical and Haematological Tests for Intermediate Hospital Laboratories, 1986, WHO, Geneva.

WHO, LAB./83.1, obtainable from Health Laboratory Unit, WHO, 1211-Geneva, 27 Switzerland.

Zilva, J. F. Collection and preservation of specimens for chemical pathology. *British Journal of Hospital Medicine*, **4**, p 845, 1970.

27 Quality Assurance in Clinical Chemistry SI Units and Reference Ranges

27:1 WHAT IS MEANT BY QUALITY ASSURANCE

Although medical laboratory workers understand the importance of providing correct results, many find the subjects of quality assurance (QA) and quality control (QC) difficult to understand and are therefore unable to introduce effective control procedures into their laboratory.

Quality Assurance (QA)
This describes all the steps taken both in and outside the laboratory to achieve reliable results,starting with the preparation of the patient and collection of a specimen and ending with the correct interpretation of results.

Quality Control (QC)
This describes the steps taken by the laboratory to ensure that tests are performed correctly.

QA and QC are largely matters of common sense. In fact anyone who goes to their local store to buy items such as sugar or potatoes already understands much about QA and QC as the following story will show.

Story of storekeepers Messrs *Smith, Jones* and *Brown*
The story is about the owners of three village stores (the storekeepers have English names but you may like to substitute your own local names):

- ■ *Mr Smith*: He was a jolly man but unfortunately very careless.
- ■ *Mr Jones*: He was a helpful man but always so inefficient and disorganized.
- ■ *Mr Brown*: He was a friendly man who was both careful and efficient.

All three shopkeepers stocked sugar and sold it in 1 kg bags but whereas the service given by *Mr Brown* was of a high quality that given by *Mr Smith* and *Mr Jones* was not all it should have been.

— The bags of sugar sold by *Mr Brown* always contained the same amount of sugar and as near to the correct weight as *Mr Brown* could make them. *Mr Brown* checked regularly the equipment he was using and kept a careful eye on his assistant to make sure he was not getting careless in the amount of sugar he was putting into each bag.

— The bags of sugar from *Mr Smith's* store contained different amounts of sugar due to the careless way *Mr Smith* and his assistant worked.

— The bags of sugar from *Mr Jones'* shop all contained the same amount of sugar (his assistant weighed the sugar carefully) but they were underweight. *Mr Jones* never checked his scales.

Fig. 27.1 shows the weights of sugar in 10 of the bags sold from the three different stores.

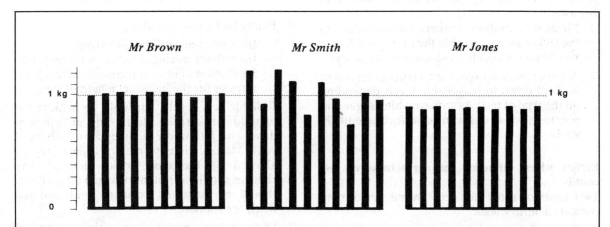

Fig. 27.1 Weights of individual 1 kg bags of sugar sold by Messrs *Brown*, *Smith* and *Jones*. The dotted line represents the correct weight of 1 kg. It can be seen that whereas Mr Jones' customers received a high standard of service, those customers of Mr Smith and Mr Jones received a poor service.
Courtesy of B. J. Seaton.

One day *Mr Smith* and *Mr Jones* had occasion to visit *Mr Brown* (they had run out of a few essential supplies) and after seeing the way he worked they resolved to improve the quality of service they gave to their customers. The way *Mr Smith* went about it is described in 27:3 and the action *Mr Jones* took is described in 27:5 (read the text in the boxes).

After improving their way of working and introducing various checks, the service given by *Mr Smith* and *Mr Jones* to their customers became very much better. They noticed however, that even with careful weighing and using equipment now known to be reliable, it was much more difficult to provide customers with exactly 1 kg of potatoes than 1 kg of sugar. Even *Mr Brown* experienced the same difficulty (see Fig. 27.2). The customers, however, understood that it was not easy to weigh such large items and were not surprised to find quite large variations in weights at different times.

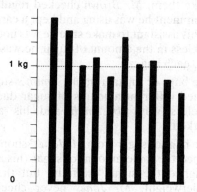

Fig. 27.2 Weights of individual 1 kg bags of potatoes achieved by Mr Brown.
Courtesy of B. J. Seaton.

Applying the story of Messrs Smith Jones and Brown

☐ Medical laboratory workers (storekeepers in the story) want to provide the best possible service to their patients (customers in the story).

☐ 'Customers' will expect any errors in results to be kept down to reasonable levels depending on the type of test. As with weighing sugar and potatoes, not all tests can be performed equally well.

Errors which influence the correctness of test results

Two types of error can occur when performing clinical chemistry tests:

■ Errors of scatter, i.e. imprecision.
■ Errors of bias, i.e. inaccuracy.

Errors of scatter (imprecision)
These are irregular or random errors. Results differ from the correct result by varying amounts (like *Mr Smith's* bags of sugar).

Compare *Mr Smith's* large scatter with *Mr Brown's* small scatter as shown in Fig. 27.1 and summarized in Table 27.1

Table 27.1 Actual Weights of '1 kg' Bags of Sugar Sold by Messrs Smith, Jones and Brown

BAGS	WEIGHTS (kg)		
	Mr Smith	*Mr Jones*	*Mr Brown*
1	1.069	0.952	0.991
2	0.955	0.947	1.000
3	1.076	0.954	1.002
4	1.031	0.947	0.995
5	0.920	0.951	1.004
6	1.031	0.952	1.006
7	0.978	0.949	1.002
8	0.883	0.954	0.990
9	0.997	0.948	0.999
10	0.971	0.959	1.002
Total weight	9.911 kg	9.513 kg	9.991 kg
Average weight:*	0.991 kg	0.951 kg	0.999 kg
Bias:†	−0.009	−0.049	−0.001
Scatter:‡	0.062	0.003	0.005

*   Calculated by dividing the total weight of all the bags by their number, i.e. by 10.

†   Bias is the difference between the average weights of the bags of sugar and their correct weight, i.e. 1 kg.

‡   Scatter is calculated as the standard deviation (SD) of the weights as described in 27:3 (see Fig. 27.3).

The commonest causes of scatter (imprecision) in clinical chemistry work are as follows:

☐ Faulty technique including:

— Incorrect and variable pipetting.
— Inadequate mixing of sample with reagents.
— Incubation of tests at inconsistent temperatures or for the incorrect length of time.

Reliable test results can only be achieved if methods are written clearly and in sufficient detail and followed *exactly* by all members of staff. Modifications to methods must only be allowed by the most senior person. Any changes should be put in writing. Test methods should be reviewed regularly and updated when appropriate.

☐ Dirty tubes, pipettes or other items of glassware used in tests.

☐ Too heavy a workload resulting in faulty technique, mistakes being made, or short cuts being taken.

□ Too low a workload resulting in loss of concentration and errors being made.

□ Fluctuating (erratic) colorimeter or spectrophotometer readings due to an unreliable mains voltage supply.

□ Use of dirty or finger marked cuvettes or reading samples when they contain air bubbles.

□ Incomplete removal of interfering substances in serum, e.g. red blood cells or proteins.

Note: The ways used to detect and measure scatter and keep it to a minimum when performing tests are described in 27:3.

Errors of bias (inaccuracy)

These are consistent or regular errors. All results differ from the correct result by approximately the same amount (like *Mr Jones'* bags of sugar).

Compare *Mr Jones'* high bias with *Mr Brown's* low bias as shown in Fig. 27.1 and summarized in Table 27.1.

The commonest causes of bias (inaccuracy) in clinical chemistry work are as follows:

□ Use of unsatisfactory reagents because they contain impure chemicals, have been prepared wrongly, stored incorrectly, or used after their stated expiry date or known working life.

Errors due to the use of impure chemicals can be avoided by purchasing chemicals that are labelled *Analar*, *Univar*, *AR* (*Analytical Reagent*), or *GR* (*Guaranteed Reagent*). *LR* (*Laboratory Grade*) reagents are of lower purity but may be suitable for some purposes. *Technical* and *Industrial* grade chemicals, although less expensive, must not be used to prepare standards or any reagent which requires a pure chemical.

When preparing standards and reagents, an analytical balance of sufficient sensitivity must be used and the chemicals must be weighed carefully (see 3:6). Good quality distilled water must be used and calibrated volumetric glassware is required when making standards and other accurate reagents.

□ Incorrect or infrequent calibration of a test method.

For the tests included in this manual, details of calibration can be found at the beginning of each test method.

□ Use of control sera that has been wrongly prepared, incorrectly stored, or has expired (see 27:5).

□ Tests being read at an incorrect wavelength (incorrect filter being used).

Note: The ways used to detect and measure bias and keep it as low as possible when performing tests are described in 27:5.

Occurrence of scatter and bias

Although both significant scatter and bias may and often do occur together when carrying out a test method, it is possible for only one type of error to be present.

In the story of the storekeepers, *Mr Brown's* bags of sugar were acceptable (consistently near to 1 kg) because his precise and accurate way of working produced *both* small scatter and a low bias. *Mr Smith's* bags of sugar were unacceptable because of large scatter even though his bias was low. *Mr Jones'* bags of sugar were unacceptable because of high bias even though his amount of scatter was small.

Laboratory test results will only be acceptable if both scatter (imprecision) and bias (inaccuracy) are kept to a minimum. If results are charted *regularly* as described in 27:4, it will be easy to see whether errors are being kept to reasonable levels.

Acceptable error for different tests

As mentioned previously, some tests will be easy to perform with minimal error (like weighing 1 kg bags of sugar) while other tests will inevitably be subject to quite large errors (like weighing 1 kg of potatoes).

Note the amount of scatter and bias recorded from the 1 kg bags of potatoes prepared by careful *Mr Brown* as shown in Table 27.2.

Table 27.2 Actual Weights of '1 kg' Bags of Potatoes Sold by Mr Brown

BAGS	WEIGHTS (kg)
1	1.169
2	1.126
3	1.007
4	1.032
5	0.962
6	1.102
7	1.007
8	1.029
9	0.961
10	0.918
Total weight:	10.310 kg
Average weight:*	1.031 kg
Bias:†	+0.031
Scatter:‡	0.079

* Calculated by dividing the total weight of all the bags by their number, i.e. by 10.

† Bias is the difference between the average weights of the bags of sugar and their correct weight, i.e. 1 kg.

‡ Scatter is calculated as the standard deviation (SD) of the weights as described in 27:3 (see Fig. 27.3)

When first introducing a test it is necessary to find out how well it can be performed. The method for doing this is described in 27:3.

Once an assay is put into routine use, a good laboratory worker will want to strive to improve his or her technique so as to achieve the best possible standard of performance for the method.

Summary

QA and QC, both why they are necessary and how they are carried out, are as readily understandable as selling sugar or potatoes in the local grocery store. They only *seem* to be more complicated than they are because some medical laboratory workers have made them very 'scientific' and 'technical'. It is true that a few statistical calculations have to be used to measure the amount of scatter and bias and how well an assay can be performed but having understood this subunit these terms should now be easy to understand.

Providing the best possible service to patients means checking continually for *both* bias and scatter in results. It is necessary to guard particularly against careless work which is one of the main causes of large scatter and against unsatisfactory reagents, controls, standards, and faulty equipment which are the commonest causes of high bias.

Messrs *Smith*, *Jones* and *Brown* will continue to be used as examples in the subsequent subunits of this Chapter to show that it is actually very easy to introduce control procedures in every district laboratory. Only then will patients receive the highest possible standard of medical laboratory service.

27:2 QUALITY ASSURANCE IN CLINICAL CHEMISTRY

As mentioned in 27:1, quality assurance (QA) is an overall term which covers those procedures which take place both outside and inside the laboratory to ensure the reliability of test results.

Quality assurance outside the laboratory

This includes:

- Selection of appropriate investigations .
- Preparation of a patient where this is necessary for a particular test, e.g. fasting blood glucose.
- Correct collection, labelling, storage, and transport of specimens.
- Correct filling in of a request form.
- Careful recording of results.
- Correct interpretation of test results.

In all of these areas of control the laboratory should assist medical officers and ward staff as much as possible.

Collection of specimens

The laboratory should circulate written instructions regarding:

- Collection methods, including advice on how to avoid haemolysis and venous stasis when collecting blood samples (see 26:4).
- Types of container to use, e.g. whether to use a bottle or tube which contains an anticoagulant, preservative, or stabilizer (see 26:4-26:7). The number of different containers should be kept to a minimum.
- Stability of different substances in samples and the time within which a specimen should reach the laboratory (see 26:7).
- Special precautions which need to be taken for certain specimens, e.g. protecting blood specimens against light and heat particularly when testing for bilirubin, urate, or enzymes. It is advisable however, to protect all samples from extremes of heat and light. Many samples are best refrigerated at 2-8 °C until analyzed or at least kept in a cool dark place (see 26:7).

Filling in of request forms

Details which the laboratory needs to know about a patient to perform clinical chemistry tests reliably are listed in 26:3.

Labelling of specimens

If errors and delays are to be avoided the clear labelling of specimen containers is of great importance (see 26:3).

Interpretation of test results

To assist in the interpretation of results the laboratory should provide reference (normal) ranges for each of the tests it performs (see 27:8).

Quality control in the laboratory (internal quality control)

The purpose of quality control (QC) in the laboratory is to ensure that tests are performed reliably, reported correctly and the results reach those treating patients at an early enough stage to influence clinical decision making.

QC in the laboratory includes:

- Training laboratory workers to perform tests correctly.
- Establishing performance standards for each test method.
- Using control samples to check for bias, charting results regularly to check for scatter and

taking action when a test is becoming unreliable.

■ Whenever possible, taking part in external quality assessment schemes.

■ Reporting results clearly and with the minimum of delay.

■ Making sure that equipment such as analytical balances, colorimeters, heat-blocks (or water baths), etc are being used correctly and maintained adequately.

Training and work experience
Those performing clinical assays *must* have sufficient knowledge and practical experience. There should be a rotation of duties between members of staff.

For district laboratory staff with limited experience, support and supervision should come from the nearest referral laboratory. Such support should include the supply of standard solutions, control sera, and test reagents and advice regarding the performance and control of test methods. Supervision of the work performed in district laboratories is essential (see also Chapter 1).

Opportunities should be made available for further education and training and the attendance of refresher courses.

Performance standards
Procedures should be established to determine the acceptable and best performance standards for each test method as described in 27:3.

Use of control charts
As explained in 27:1 (with the help of Messrs *Smith*, *Jones*, and *Brown*), it is essential to check regularly for scatter and bias in tests and to detect at an early stage when errors are being introduced that are going to lead to incorrect results.

When errors of scatter and bias are found it is essential to identify their cause and take the necessary action.

The commonest causes of scatter and bias in clinical chemistry tests are described in 27:1.

External quality assessment
Although steps may be taken to ensure that results are reliable, a system of assessing a laboratory's ability to do this to a satisfactory standard is desirable. Such a system of checking using an organization outside the laboratory is called external quality assessment (formerly called external quality control).

Participation in external quality assessment schemes should always be regarded as additional to internal quality control which is an essential part of the routine of a well-run laboratory. External quality assessment must *never* be a substitute for internal quality control because it can only assess past performance when test results have already been reported and acted on.

Reporting results
Test results should be reported carefully. The writing should be clear, particularly figures, and decimal points must be correctly placed. References (normal) ranges should be stated (see 27:8) to enable results to be interpreted correctly.

When reports are given verbally, a written report should always follow.

27:3 ESTABLISHING PERFORMANCE STANDARDS (OCV AND RCV)

Before any test method is used for patients, the laboratory must *first* ensure that the method is working reliably and that it can be performed with acceptable limits of variability. After a test has been introduced it must be constantly and adequately controlled as described in 27:4 and 27:5.

Assessing reliability and performance
As explained in 27:1, some tests will be easier than others to perform reliably (like weighing 1 kg of sugar compared with weighing 1 kg of potatoes). For example, serum total protein can be measured (Biuret method) with less variability than serum aspartate aminotransferase (Reitman Frankel method) using a manual colorimetric technique.

The following procedure is used to assess reliability and degree of variability under optimal (best possible) conditions. Once the optimal conditions variance (OCV) is known this can be compared with that which should be possible for the test method when put into routine use, i.e. routine conditions variance (RCV).

Establishing the optimal conditions variance (OCV)
1. Obtain a sufficient quantity of a control serum that contains a known amount of the substance being measured. The concentration of the substance should be similar to the amounts expected in patients' samples.

   Note: The preparation of control sera is described in 27:5.

2. Under optimal conditions, perform 20 measurements on the same sample of control serum. Follow the method as carefully as possible using the same reagents and equipment for each of the 20 measurements.

Note: The analyst should be well-trained, experienced and reliable. He or she should not be assigned any other task at the time.

3. Read off the values from the calibration graph (details of calibration are given at the beginning of each test method).

4. List the values for each of the 20 estimations as shown in the example in Table 27.3.

5. Calculate the mean (average value) by adding up all the results and dividing the total by 20.

6. For each result, work out the difference in value from the mean, entering the differences in the second column of the chart.

7. Multiply each difference value by itself to give the squared difference values, entering these figures in the third column of the chart.

8. Add up the figures in column three, to give the sum of the squared differences (see Table 27.3).

9. Calculate what is called the standard deviation (SD) using the formula:

$$SD = \sqrt{\frac{\text{Sum of the squared difference}}{n-1}}$$

Where n is the number of results, i.e. 20.

Example: Follow the SD calculation in Table 27.3

10. Calculate the OCV using the formula:

$$OCV = \frac{SD}{Mean} \times 100$$

Example: Follow the OCV calculation in Table 27.3

Note: In correct statistical terms, the formula $\frac{SD}{Mean} \times 100$ gives what is called the coefficient of variation (CV). It is simply expressing the SD (which is given in substance units) as a percentage of the mean.

Check whether the OCV is less than the maximum allowed for the particular test (given at the end of each test method).

Important: If the OCV is more than the maximum acceptable figure, the test must *not* be put into routine use. The standards, calibration graph, reagents, and other possible sources of error must be investigated. The commonest causes of scatter are listed in 27:1.

11. Chart the results as follows:

— Take a sheet of graph paper and draw on it three horizontal lines corresponding to the mean, +2 SD and −2 SD as shown in Fig. 27.3.

— Work out the values for +2 SD and −2 SD as follows:

+2 SD = Mean + 2 SD
−2 SD = Mean − 2 SD

Example
Using the mean of 0.15 mmol/l and SD of 6.7 mmol/l as shown in Table 27.3:

+2 SD = 6.7 + 0.3
     = 7.0 mmol/l

−2 SD = 6.7 - 0.3
     = 6.4 mmol/l

— Enter the mean, +2 SD, −2 SD, and other values on the left hand side of the chart.

— Mark the horizontal axis 'Control' and number it 1 to 20.

— Chart the result of each test as shown in the example chart (Fig. 27.3).

12. Examine the chart for the distribution of values around the mean. The chart should show a fairly even distribution of values on each side of the mean within +2 SD and −2 SD (see Fig. 27.3).

Messrs Smith Jones and Brown

As mentioned in the story in 27:1, *Mr Smith* after visiting *Mr Brown* wanted to improve the reliability of his 1 kg bags of sugar and decided to find out just how good he could be if he really tried. So he chose a time when he was not usually busy with customers, closed his shop, cleaned and adjusted his scales and weighed out 20 bags of sugar.

Mr Smith knows that he will not always be able to weigh the sugar so well when the shop is busy with customers but the exercise has shown him what he is capable of under optimal (ideal) conditions and gives him a standard to strive for.

Establishing the routine conditions variance (RCV)

When a test is performed under routine conditions of work the degree of variability i.e. routine conditions variance (RCV) will inevitably be higher than the OCV and therefore the range of acceptable values will be wider.

Although the OCV can be determined in a single experiment it takes some time to accumulate enough information from routine tests to calculate the RCV. When, therefore, a new test is first introduced, it is usual to set up the first control chart using twice the optimal conditions SD and OCV, as explained in 27:4.

Table 27.3 Example of How to Calculate the OCV for a Glucose Assay

27 MARCH 1986		GLUCOSE		ANALYST: SB
Test No.	*Test Results in mmol/l*	*Differences from mean*	*Squared differences*	*Calculations*
1	6.5	−0.2	0.04	
2	6.7	0.0	0.00	$SD = \dfrac{0.44}{20\text{-}1}$
3	6.5	−0.2	0.04	
4	6.6	−0.1	0.01	
5	6.8	+0.1	0.01	$= \sqrt{0.023}$
6	6.9	+0.2	0.04	
7	6.5	−0.2	0.04	$= 0.15\ mmol/l$
8	6.5	−0.2	0.04	
9	6.7	0.0	0.00	
10	6.8	+0.1	0.01	
11	6.7	0.0	0.00	$OCV = \dfrac{0.15}{6.7} \times 100$
12	6.8	+0.1	0.01	
13	6.4	−0.3	0.09	
14	6.8	+0.1	0.01	$= 2.2\%$
15	6.5	−0.2	0.04	
16	6.7	0.0	0.00	
17	6.9	+0.2	0.04	
18	6.6	−0.1	0.01	
19	6.8	+0.1	0.01	
20	6.7	0.0	0.00	

Total = 133.4 Total = 0.44

Mean = 133.4 ÷ 20
     ≑ 6.7 mmol/l

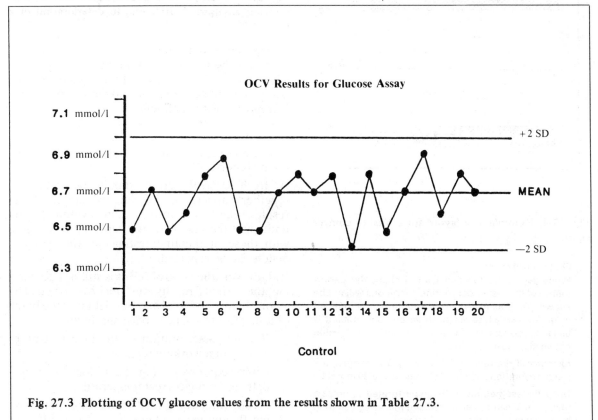

Fig. 27.3 Plotting of OCV glucose values from the results shown in Table 27.3.

27:4 HOW TO USE A QUALITY CONTROL CHART

Having established that a test method is reliable and has an acceptable OCV, it can be put into routine use providing it can be controlled adequately. A control serum must be used with *every* batch of tests.

The use of a control chart will enable most faults to be identified and corrected at an early stage before patients' results are affected and reporting has to be delayed.

Setting up a daily quality control chart

The daily control chart is similar to the OCV control chart illustrated in Fig. 27.3 except that the horizontal axis is numbered for the days of the month as shown in Fig. 27.4, and the ±2 SD are calculated from the routine conditions standard deviation.

1. Calculate the +2 SD and −2 SD values for the assay (see 27:3) and prepare a control chart as shown in Fig. 27.4.

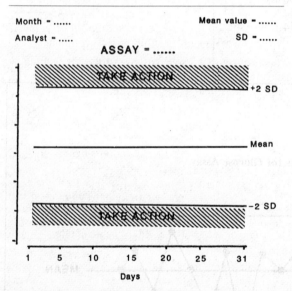

Fig. 27.4 Example of a layout for a quality control chart.

First control chart

When setting up the first control chart, the performance of the test under routine conditions will not be known. To obtain a realistic routine conditions SD value from which to establish acceptable limits, it is usual to double the optimal conditions SD value obtained as described in 27:3.

Example: If the optimal SD value is 0.15 mmol/l, the routine conditions SD should be taken as 0.30 mmol/l.

Once the test method has been performed 20 times a revised RCV can be calculated and this value can then be used instead of the 2 × OCV value.

2. Using the same control serum for each batch of tests, plot the values on the daily control chart as shown for the OCV chart in Fig. 27.3.

3. Each day after charting the control value, check that it is within the acceptable limits of ±2 SD and that there is no marked change in the distribution of results above or below the mean or a movement (drift) towards the TAKE ACTION zones.

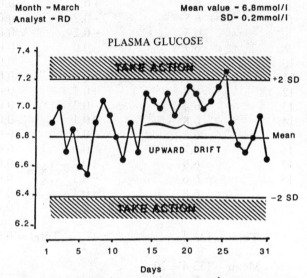

Fig. 27.5 Example of a daily quality control chart showing an upward drift due to deterioration of a reagent.

Interpretation of results

Control value within ±2 SD limits

This is a good sign. It can be assumed that the patients' results are reliable and therefore they can be reported with confidence.

Control value outside ±2 SD limits

This is unacceptable and the patients' results must *not* be reported.

A fresh control serum should be measured together with a few of the patients' samples. If the result of the fresh control serum is within ±2 SD limits and the results of the repeated tests agree with those of the first testing, all the patients' results can be reported.

If, however, the control result is still not acceptable, the patients' results must *not* be reported. The error(s) must be found and put right and the batch of tests repeated. Check particularly for:

— Reagent deterioration or the incorrect preparation of a working reagent.

— Faulty equipment, e.g. heat-block or water-bath not at the correct temperature.

— Wrong filter being used or the colorimeter giving fluctuating readings or readings different from those given previously for the control or standard solutions.

Control value moving towards TAKE ACTION zone
The patient's results can be reported but a drift of values upwards or downwards is a warning that the test is becoming unreliable and the cause(s) must be investigated before the next batch of tests is performed (see Fig. 27.5).

Note: The commonest causes of errors in tests are listed in 27:1.

Preparation of a new quality control chart
When the first quality control chart is almost completed, prepare a new one using the most recent 20 control results to re-calculate the RCV. The RCV is calculated in the same way as the OCV (see 27:3).

If, as is to be hoped, the test is being performed better, i.e. with less scatter, then the new RCV will be lower than the previous one.

Re-calculate the +2 SD and −2 SD values using the new SD value.

Improving the control of a test method
Whenever possible, introduce a second control serum into the batch of tests. The person performing the tests should not know its value.

If a second control serum is not available, the serum from one of the routine tests can be divided to provide an 'unknown' sample. Agreement between the two results can be checked when the batch of tests is completed.

Alternatively, dilute the control serum with a known volume of distilled water and calculate the values of the diluted serum.

Note: The preparation and calibration of control sera are described in 27:5.

27:5 QUALITY CONTROL SERA

A control sample is necessary to check for bias (inaccuracy) in tests, i.e. to check that the results being obtained are sufficiently close to their correct values. For blood assays, the most economical way of doing this is to use analyzed pooled sera which can be prepared and calibrated in the laboratory as described in this subunit.

Analyzed sera are also available commercially but are expensive for the daily quality control of tests.

A commercially prepared control serum is however useful for calibrating a pooled serum if a reference serum from a Quality Control Laboratory is not available (see later text).

Use of sera in quality control
Whenever a batch of tests or even a single test is analyzed, a control sample must be included. It should be assayed in exactly the same way as the test specimens, e.g. the same reagents, instrument, and calibration graph must be used.

A control will detect errors in reagents and standards but not individual pipetting or calculating errors in one or more of the patients' specimens unless the same errors have occurred in the entire batch of tests including the control.

When using a commercially prepared control or reference material, always check that the substance being measured is included in the material.

Always select the range of values (in the appropriate units) which apply to the test method which is being used. Different test methods will often give slightly different values even when the same substance is measured in the same sample. This is usual and is due to the various interfering substances which are usually present in blood samples affecting different methods in different ways.

The charts supplied by the manufacturer must be carefully kept because values change from one batch of control sera to another.

Chart 27.1 lists some of the commercially available control sera that give values for the manual colorimetric methods described in this manual.

Ranges of assay values supplied with commercially prepared control sera
These are based on the mean values found when the sera were analyzed in a number of different laboratories. Such ranges are *not* therefore the same as the ±2 SD acceptable ranges which should be established in each laboratory once the OCV and RCV have been found to be satisfactory (see 27:3).

Neither are the commercially supplied ranges of values the same as reference (normal) ranges. Reference ranges reflect the biological variations which occur between patients (guidelines for these are given at the end of test methods).

Controls for enzyme tests should always be stored frozen at −20 °C or lower, in the amounts required because serum enzymes are unstable. Bilirubin controls should also be stored in the amounts required because bilirubin is destroyed by light.

Preparation and use of pooled sera
The use of a pooled control serum for the routine daily quality control of tests is recommended because such a serum can be prepared locally at low cost.

Method of preparing a pooled serum

1. At the end of a morning's or afternoon's work collect any unused tested sera.

2. Transfer those sera that have given normal results to a screw-cap container. Exclude from the pool any sera which are not fresh or appear:
   — icteric (jaundiced)
   — cloudy (e.g. lipaemic)
   — pink coloured due to haemolysis
   — abnormally coloured due to dyes

Caution: When a control serum is prepared from a large pool of human sera, there is always the danger that this pool may be positive for hepatitis antigens. Every effort must be made therefore to exclude from the pool any sera from patients with hepatitis or with a known history of the disease. Before a pool of serum is put into routine use, a sample must be tested for hepatitis antigens. If found positive the serum must be discarded in a safe manner.

Use of animal sera

For most tests a perfectly satisfactory pooled serum can be prepared from bovine or equine serum. Animal sera is hepatitis-free and therefore safer to use than human sera.

3. Freeze the pooled sera. Continue to save and freeze the serum samples until about 1 litre has been collected or sufficient to last for 4-6 months.

   Note: For laboratories performing only a few tests each day it may be necessary to request blood from a few volunteer donors to obtain enough serum for the pool.

4. After sufficient sera has been collected, allow the frozen sera to thaw completely to room temperature. Transfer all the sera to a large screw-cap bottle and mix well but gently.

   Send a sample of the pooled sera for hepatitis antigen testing (see previous text).

5. Add the following preservatives to the pooled sera:
   — 100 mg sodium fluoride per 100 ml of serum.

   — 1 ml of sodium borate merthiolate reagent* per 100 ml of serum.

   * Prepare by dissolving 0.7 g sodium borate and 0.5 g merthiolate in 25 ml of distilled water.

6. Mix well but gently.

7. Check the glucose value. If necessary, add an appropriate amount of pure glucose to give a concentration of about 6.7 mmol/l.

8. Centrifuge at medium speed (about 700 g) for about 30 minutes to sediment any fibrin and other debris. Carefully remove the supernatant serum. If lipid is present on the surface, filter the serum through glass wool or cotton gauze.

9. Dispense the serum in about 1 ml amounts into small containers (such as penicillin vials). Immediately seal, label, and freeze at −20 °C or below.

10. For use, remove one container (or more if required) of the pooled serum and allow to thaw to room temperature. Gently mix the pooled serum by inverting the container several times.

Important: Adequate mixing of the serum is essential because separation occurs when serum is frozen and thawed. The serum should be used only *on the day that it is thawed*. Any serum that is left at the end of the day should be thrown away.

Update: A method of preparing stabilized liquid quality control serum using ethylene glycol has been developed by the World Health Organization, Details can be found in a 1986 WHO document called *Preparation of Stabilized Liquid Quality Control Serum to be Used in Clinical Chemistry* Lab /86.4. Copies can be obtained from the Health Laboratory Unit, WHO, 1211 Geneva, 27-Switzerland.

Establishing the values and acceptable assay limits of a pooled serum

1. Establish the OCV for each of the relevant substances in the control serum measuring 20 samples of the pooled serum (see 27:3). At the same time measure the relevant substances in a suitable commercially prepared control serum (see Chart 27.1) or analyzed reference serum from a Quality Control Reference Laboratory. Use fresh reagents and freshly prepared standards.

   If the values obtained for the commercially prepared or reference control serum are correct, it can be assumed that the values obtained for the pooled serum are also correct and can be assigned to the batch.

2. Record the results from the pooled serum as shown in Fig. 27.3 (see 27:3) and calculate the mean value, SD and OCV for each substance.

   If the OCV for each substance tested is satisfactory (see below), then the pooled serum is suitable for routine use.

Test	Suggested OCV %
Albumin	3%
Alkaline phosphatase	10%
Amylase	6%
Aspartate aminotransferase	8%
Bilirubin (total)	6%
Calcium	1.5%
Cholesterol	7%
Creatinine	4%
Glucose	2%
Total protein	2%
Urate	5%
Urea	3%

Note: If an OCV is higher than that quoted for a test method, the reason(s) must be investigated. The commonest causes of scatter (imprecision) are listed in 27:1.

Use of commercially prepared control sera

Commercially prepared control sera are available in two forms:

☐ Freeze-dried (lyophilized) sera
☐ Liquid synthetically manufactured sera

Freeze-dried control sera

When stored at 2-8 °C, unopened freeze-dried sera can usually be kept for up to 2 years or longer without showing signs of deterioration. An exact expiry date is usually printed on the bottle label.

The length of time that a reconstituted control serum can be kept when stored at 2-8 °C and −20 °C is specified by the manufacturer. Substances such as bilirubin and some enzymes have only a short life.

When reconstituting a dried serum the following precautions are necessary:

— Read carefully the manufacturer's instructions.

— Open the bottle slowly to avoid any loss of material (the serum is often vacuum packed).

— Reconstitute with good quality glass-distilled water or with the special diluent supplied by the manufacturer. Pipette accurately using a chemically clean pipette.

— After adding the water or diluent, stopper the container and gently *swirl* the contents. Allow to stand for 10 minutes and then swirl again. Repeat the process until the main solid 'plug' of serum has dissolved. Invert gently three or four times to ensure that any remaining powder on the stopper will be washed into the solution. Stand for 2-3 minutes and then invert again three or four times.

— Allow reconstituted serum to stand at room temperature (20-28 °C) for the time specified by the manufacturer (usually 30-60 minutes). After the waiting period, *gently* remix the serum.

— Dispense the serum in 0.5-1 ml amounts, or as required, into small sterile containers. To reduce the risk of contamination, it is advisable to transfer the serum by pouring, not by pipetting.

— Label each container with the date and Lot No. (Batch No.) of the serum. Freeze immediately and store at −20 °C or below until required.

For use, allow the serum to warm to room temperature. When completely thawed, mix gently but well.

Liquid control sera

Most liquid synthetic control sera must be stored at 2-8 °C. Unopened bottles can normally be kept for up to about 1 year but when opened a liquid serum is usually stable for only a few days. If therefore a laboratory performs only a few tests it should not buy this type of serum or buy it only in small quantities.

Messrs Smith, Jones and Brown

In the story told in 27:1, *Mr Jones* after visiting *Mr Brown* realized that if he were to obtain an exact 1 kg weight then he too would be able to make sure that his customers received the correct amount of sugar.

His assistant was pleased when the new 1 kg weight was obtained because although he had always weighed the sugar carefully he had never had a way of checking that he was in fact weighing exactly 1 kg.

Chart 27.1 Some Commercially Available Lyophilized Control Sera

With values for colorimetric manual methods described in this manual

Serum Test	Suggested Control Serum
Albumin	*Biotrol-33 Plus* [a] *Biotrol-33 Plus Pathologique* [a] *Wellcomtrol Normal BC 40* [b] *Wellcomtrol Abnormal BC 50* [b] *Lyotrol* [c]
Alkaline phosphatase	*Precipath E* [d]
Amylase	Caraway, starch-iodine: *Biotrol-33 Plus* [a] *Biotrol-33 Plus Pathologique* [a] Phadebas test kit: *Wellcomtrol Normal BC 40* [b] *Wellcomtrol Abnormal BC 50* [b]
Aspartate aminotransferase (Transaminase, GOT)	*Biotrol-33 Plus* [a] *Biotrol-33 Plus Pathologique* [a] *Lyotrol N* [c] *Zymotrol* [c]

Bilirubin	*Seronorm Bilirubin Paediatric*[e] *Biotrol-33 Plus Pathologique*[a] *Precibil*[d]
Calcium	*Wellcomtrol Normal BC 40*[b] *Wellcomtrol Abnormal BC 50*[b]
Cholesterol, total	*Biotrol-33 Plus*[a] *Biotrol-33 Plus Pathologique*[a]
Glucose	*Biotrol-33 Plus*[a] *Biotrol-33 Plus Pathologique*[a]
Protein, total	*Wellcomtrol Normal BC 40*[b] *Wellcomtrol Abnormal BC 50*[b]
Urea	*Biotrol-33 Plus*[a] *Biotrol-33 Plus Pathologique*[a]

a   Manufactured by Laboratoires Biotrol (see Appendix II). *Biotrol-33 Plus* gives medium levels and *Biotrol-33 Plus Pathologique* gives raised levels of analyte. 5 × 5 ml costs about £14 and 30 × 5 ml about £58 (1985-1986).

b   Manufactured by Wellcome Diagnostics (see Appendix II). *Wellcomtrol Normal BC 40* gives medium levels and *Wellcomtrol Abnormal BC 50* gives raised levels of analyte. 10 × 5 ml costs about £20 (1985-1986).

c   Manufactured by bioMérieux (see Appendix II). *Lyotrol N* gives medium values and *Zymotrol* gives raised values of enzyme activity. 6 × 5 ml *Lyotrol N* costs about £23 and 4 × 3 ml *Zymotrol* costs about £18 (1985-1986).

d   Manufactured by Boehringer (see Appendix (II). *Precipath E* gives raised values of enzyme activity. 4 × 3 ml costs about £9.50 (1985-1986). *Precibil* gives raised levels of analyte. 4 × 2 ml costs about £12 (1985-1986).

e   Manufactured by Nyegaard (see Appendix II). *Seronorm Bilirubin Paediatric* gives raised levels of analyte. 6 × 3 ml costs about £18.50 (1985-1986).

Recommendation: Before purchasing an expensive control serum it is advisable to write to the different manufacturers and request details of local availability and prices and a sample data sheet which accompanies the control. This sheet will give the stability of the different substances in the control *once it is reconstituted*. The values given will differ for each batch (Lot No.) of the control serum.

27:6   MEASUREMENT OF ENZYME ACTIVITY

To measure serum or plasma enzymes reliably, it is important to know what enzymes are and how they function. Enzymes are proteins produced by living cells. They have special catalytic functions, i.e. they are able in very small amounts to accelerate or modify a chemical reaction in the body without becoming involved in the reaction or changed by it.

An enzyme produced by more than one type of body tissue or one subcellular particle can be separated into its various isoenzymes by electrophoresis. Isoenzymes have identical functional features but differ in some physical properties.

Catalytic activities of enzymes
Enzymes act specifically on certain substances or closely related substances, i.e. they will catalyze only one type of reaction or a small range of reactions. For example, urease acts specifically on urea, protease on protein, amylase on starch, uricase on urate, and lactase on lactose (the names of many enzymes end in the suffix -ase).

The substance upon which an enzyme acts is called a substrate.

Enzymes such as dehydrogenases catalyze oxidation-reduction reactions. Aminotransferases catalyze the transfer of functional groups from one compound to another. The hydrolytic group of enzymes such as phosphatases break down a substrate by introducing water.

The reactions catalyzed by enzymes are often reversible with the direction of the reaction being determined by the conditions in the cell.

Many enzymes will work only with the assistance of an activator or a co-enzyme. An activator is a simple inorganic salt or ion and a co-enzyme is a complex organic compound.

Every enzyme has an optimal (most favourable) temperature activity. It is the point at which there is a balance between the increasing activity of the enzyme and its rate of destruction.

For every enzyme there is an optimal pH value at which the enzyme is most efficient as a catalyst. At extremes of pH, enzymes are irreversibly denatured. Variation of activity with pH is due to the change of state in ionization of the enzyme. Many enzymes have their maximum activity between pH 6 and 8. Important exceptions are alkaline phosphatase which has an optimal activity of around pH 9, and acid phosphatase which has an optimal activity of around pH 5.

Measurement of enzymes
Because enzymes are usually present in very small amounts in plasma or serum they cannot be measured directly like other substances. They are assayed indirectly by measuring either the reduction in concentration of the substrate upon which the enzyme acts or the amount of product formed from the substrate. It is therefore enzyme activity that is being measured.

Units for measuring enzyme activity have in the past been given the names of the persons who developed the different techniques, e.g. Somogyi, King-Armstrong, Bessey-Lowry, Reitman-Frankel, and Karmen. In an attempt to standardize the reporting of enzyme activity a unit of measurement has been introduced called the International Unit (U).

International Unit
An International Unit of enzyme activity is that amount of enzyme which under defined assay conditions will catalyze the conversion of 1 μmol of substrate per minute. Results are expressed in International Units per litre (U/l).

In accordance with this definition the assay conditions for enzyme analysis must be specified. These include:

- Substrate used, including its concentration.
- pH and buffer system.
- Time of incubation.
- Temperature of the reaction.
- Presence of activators or inhibitors.
- Direction in which the reaction proceeds.

Katal unit
The reporting of enzyme activity in katals is preferred by some clinical chemists because the katal refers to the conversion of 1 mol of substrate per *second* whereas the International Unit refers to the conversion of 1 μmol of substrate per *minute*. The second (s) is the SI unit of time (the minute is a non-SI unit).

The relationship between katals and International Units is 1 nkatal = 16.7 U

Factors influencing enzyme tests
There are many factors that influence enzyme activity. Small errors of technique may lead to grossly unreliable and misleading test results.

The following are the most important factors that can affect enzyme tests:

Temperature
Reaction rate increases with temperature. The majority of enzymes show their optimal activity between 30 °C and 50 °C. Above 60 °C, enzyme denaturation occurs. The incubation temperatures in test methods must be strictly followed.

Time
The substrate concentration falls with time as the product concentration increases. Timing is therefore important because substrate and product concentrations are changing all the time and it is one of these that is being measured. An accurate timer must be used to measure the incubation time of an enzyme and its substrate.

pH
Any increase or decrease in pH away from the optimum will cause a decrease in enzyme activity.

A marked change in pH can lead to the denaturation of an enzyme. The pH of buffers and substrates used in enzyme tests must therefore be correct.

Light rays
Ultraviolet light tends to inhibit enzyme activity while blue or red light tends to increase it. Samples for enzyme analysis must therefore be protected from direct light.

Enzyme stability
Many enzymes do not have good stability, e.g. acid phosphatase has very poor stability even at 4 °C. Specimens for enzyme analysis should not be left at room temperature for long periods (see also 26:7).

Serum should be separated from cells as soon as possible after the blood has clotted and the clot retracted. With the loss of carbon dioxide the pH of fresh blood rises rapidly. This leads to enzyme inactivation.

Haemolyzed specimens are generally unsuitable for enzyme analysis.

Glassware
Glassware contaminated with traces of heavy metals or detergents can inhibit enzyme activity. The use of chemically clean glassware is essential. Cuvettes must be clean and their optical surfaces dry and free from scratches and finger marks.

Reagents
Test results can be seriously affected if reagents, particularly substrates and buffers, are not prepared correctly. Precautions should be taken to avoid bacterial contamination of reagents.

27:7 SI UNITS IN CLINICAL CHEMISTRY

The system of International (SI) units is explained in 1:5. The following are the main changes involved in applying SI units in clinical chemistry work:

Changing the reporting of substances of known molecular mass
From units such as micrograms, milligrams or grams per 100 ml (μg%, mg%, g%) *to* nanomoles, micromoles, or millimoles per litre (nmol/l, μmol/l, mmol/l). For a definition of mole, see 24:5.

Substances now expressed in nmol/l, μmol/l and mmol/l include:

- [ ] nmol/l: Thyroxine
- [ ] μmol/l: Bilirubin, creatinine, urate, iron
- [ ] mmol/l: Calcium, cholesterol, glucose, phosphate, urea

Conversion from one unit to another involves multiplying or dividing by a factor. Conversion factors for the different substances are listed in 27:9.

Changing the reporting of substances of uncertain or unknown molecular mass
From units such as milligrams or grams per 100 ml (mg%, g%) to milligrams or grams per litre (mg/l, g/l).

Substances now expressed in g/l include:

☐ Albumin
☐ Total protein

Conversion from one unit to another requires only a change in the place of the decimal point as indicated in 27:9.

Changing the reporting of electrolytes
From milliequivalents per litre (mEq/l) to millimoles per litre (mmol/l).

Electrolytes now expressed in mmol/l include:

☐ Sodium
☐ Potassium
☐ Chloride

Conversion to the SI units is simple because 1 mEq is numerically the same as 1 mmol/l for monovalent ions.

Changing the reporting of enzyme activities
From named units such as King Armstrong units (phosphatases), Reitman-Frankel units (aminotransferases) or Karmen units (lactate dehydrogenase) to International Units per litre (U/l), see 27:6.

Enzyme activities now expressed in U/l include:

☐ Acid and alkaline phosphatases
☐ Aspartate aminotransferase
☐ Lactate dehydrogenase

Conversion from the former units to U/l depends on the method used to measure the enzymes, particularly the incubation temperature.

27:8 REFERENCE RANGES

The laboratory worker should know the accepted reference (normal) ranges and clinical significance of routine biochemical tests. This will ensure that significantly abnormal results are detected, checked, and reported as soon as possible. Such prompt action in the laboratory may prevent loss of life or lead to the earlier more effective treatment of a patient. The clinical significance of abnormal results is explained at the end of test methods.

Test results are affected by both biological and laboratory factors and these need to be considered when deciding the reference range for a particular test.

Biological factors
The following are among the biological factors that contribute to differences in test results among healthy people:

☐ *Age*: e.g. higher plasma urea concentrations are found in the elderly or higher alkaline phosphatase activity in growing children compared with adults.

☐ *Sex*: e.g. higher values of plasma creatinine, urate, and urea are found in men compared with women during the reproductive phase of life.

☐ *Diet and nutritional state*: e.g. plasma cholesterol and calcium are affected by diet.

☐ *Time of the day (diurnal variation)*: e.g. serum iron levels rise as the day progresses.

☐ *Posture*: e.g. plasma protein levels are lower in samples collected from patients when they are lying down.

☐ *Muscular activity*: e.g. the concentration of plasma creatinine rises following exercise.

Reference ranges are also affected by weight, phase of menstrual cycle, emotional state, geographical location, rural or city life, climate, genetic factors, cultural habits, and intrinsic homeostatic variation.

Laboratory factors
Among the analytical factors that influence reference ranges the most significant are:

☐ *Type of sample*: e.g. the concentration of glucose is 12-13% higher in plasma than in whole blood. Small variations also occur between serum and plasma samples for potassium and some other substances.

☐ *Test method*: e.g. a glucose oxidase enzyme method will give a narrower reference range for blood glucose than a Folin-Wu technique because the enzyme method is specific for glucose (Folin-Wu technique measures not only glucose but also other reducing substances).

☐ *Performance*: As mentioned in 27:1, some tests can be performed with less variation than others. The reference ranges for such tests will therefore be narrower than those with greater performance variation.

How reference ranges are established
The reference range for a particular substance is

worked out by testing a large number of healthy people and plotting a graph of frequency of value against concentration. For some assays (see later text) the graph produced is symmetrical in shape showing the highest number of people having values around the mean (average) with a gradual decrease in frequency on each side of the mean as shown in Fig.27.6.

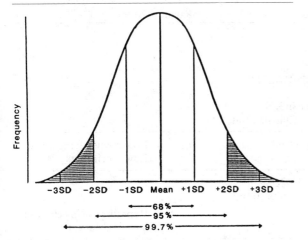

Fig. 27.6 Symmetrical distribution (Gaussian) graph.

In statistical terms the distribution of values around the mean can be expressed as standard deviation (SD). Calculation of the SD is described in 27:3.

When the results of a particular test show a symmetrical (Gaussian) type curve, the reference range for the substance being measured is defined by a plus or minus 2 SD from the mean (see Fig. 27.7). This covers 95% of the 'healthy' population (±1 SD covers 68% of the population, and ±3 SD covers 99.7% of the population).

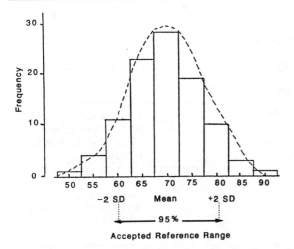

Fig. 27.7 Example of Gaussian distribution of plasma total protein giving a reference range of 60-81 g/l.

Assessing reference (normal) ranges
Because reference ranges are affected by a variety of biological and analytical factors, the ranges quoted in this manual, other publications, and test kit literature should not be assumed to be correct until they have been checked locally. They should be regarded only as *approximate interim reference ranges* to be assessed by clinicians and laboratory staff at a later stage when sufficient data becomes available.

Reference range for a new method
A practical approach to checking the reference range of a test under local conditions (when there is no previously locally established range with which it can be compared) is to use the interim range until a sufficient number of healthy adults in the community can be tested.

In a district laboratory, samples from healthy adults can be obtained from the clotted blood samples collected routinely from all blood donors (for antibody screening). When at least 100 samples have been collected and tested, the results can be compared with the interim reference range. If the local values do not correspond to the interim reference range a new range should be determined with the assistance of the Regional Laboratory. When established, the medical staff should be notified of the change in reference range.

Reference range when a method is changed
If wishing to introduce a new method, e.g. a kit test, the reference range quoted for the kit must be checked. The simplest way of doing this is to check whether there is agreement in the interpretation of values obtained by the new method with those of the previous test method (providing the reference range for the former method was checked).

This involves performing the previous method alongside the new one and noting whether both agree as to which results are 'normal' and which are 'abnormal'.

Interpretation of results outside the reference range
If a patient's result is outside of the accepted reference range this does not necessarily indicate ill health. The patient may be in the 5% minority healthy group outside the Mean ±2 SD range.

There can be no clear dividing line between 'normal' and 'abnormal' values. This is one of the reasons why the term *reference range* is preferred to normal range.

27:9 APPROXIMATE REFERENCE RANGES FOR CLINICAL CHEMISTRY TESTS

The reference ranges given in this manual have been compiled from accepted Western values and those received by the author from a small number of tropical countries. They should be used *only* as a guideline. Individual clinical chemistry laboratories must check that the reference ranges given below agree with their local findings, taking into consideration the biological and laboratory variation factors mentioned in 27:8.

Tests	SI Units	Old Units	Factor	Notes
To convert from SI units to old units, *multiply* by the factor				
To convert from old units to SI units, *divide* by the factor				
BLOOD BIOCHEMICAL TESTS				
Acid phosphatase	0-0.3 U/l	Expressed in King Armstrong units/100 ml		
Albumin	30-45 g/l	3.0-4.5 g/100 ml	0.1	Lower when lying down Lower in infants
Alkaline phosphatase	*Adults* 20-90 U/l	Expressed in King Armstrong units/100 ml		
	Children Up to 350 U/l			Rapidly growing children have highest values
alpha Fetoprotein	<1.0 µg/l	<1.0 ng/ml	1	
Amylase	70-340 U/l	Expressed in Caraway units per 100 ml		
Aspartate amino-transferase (AST)	Up to 42 U/l at 37 °C	Expressed in Reitman-Frankel units/ml		
Bicarbonate	23-31 mmol/l	23-31 mEq/l	1	
Bilirubin, total	*Adults* 3-21 µmol/l	0.2-1.3 mg/100 ml	0.06	
	Newborns 8-67 µmol/l	0.5-4.0 mg/100 ml	0.06	Highest values in first 3-5 days of life
Calcium	*Adults* 2.25-2.60 mmol/l	9.0-10.4 mg/100 ml	4	Lower when lying down
	Newborns 1.85-3.45 mmol/l	7.4-13.8 mg/100 ml	4	Values influenced by diet
PCO_2	4.6-6.1 kPa	35-46 mm Hg	7.5	SI units not often used
Chloride	96-107 mmol/l	96-107 mEq/l	1	
Cholesterol	3.0-7.8 mmol/l	116-300 mg/100 ml	38.7	Influenced by age and diet. Female values slightly higher than those of males
Cholinesterase	*Males* 2.60-5.53 U/l			Acylcholine acyl-hydrolase method (BDH Kit)
	Females 1.93-4.60 U/l			

Tests	SI Units	Old Units	Factor	Notes
Creatinine	*Males* 60-130 μmol/l	0.7-1.5 mg/100 ml	0.011	Lower in children depending on muscle mass
	Females 40-110 μmol/l	0.4-1.2 mg/100 ml		
Glucose	*Adults* - fasting (plasma) <6.4 mmol/l	<115 mg%	18	Whole blood values are about 15% lower than those of plasma
	- intermediate (plasma) <11.1 mmol/l	<199 mg%	18	Capillary blood values are slightly higher than those of venous blood (post-prandial)
	Newborns 1.1-4.4 mmol/l	20-80 mg%	18	
	Children - fasting (plasma) 2.4-5.3 mmol/l	43-95 mg%	18	
Iron (serum)	11-27 μmol/l	61-150 μg/100 ml	5.58	Take sample at 09.00 h
Iron binding capacity (TIBC)	41-74 μmol/l	229-413 μg/100 ml	5.58	Take sample at 09.00 h
Lactate dehydro-genase (LDH)	120-365 U/l	Expressed in Karmen units/ml		
Magnesium	0.7-1.3 mmol/l	1.8-3.1 mg/100 ml	2.43	
pH	7.36-7.42	7.36-7.42	1	
Phosphate, inorganic	*Adults* 0.8-1.5 mmol/l	2.5-4.7 mg/100 ml	3.1	
	Children 1.3-2.2 mmol/l	4.1-7.0 mg/100 ml	3.1	Highest value when fed on cows milk
Potassium	*Adults* 3.6-5.0 mmol/l	3.6-5.0 mEq/l	1	
	Newborns 4.0-5.9 mmol/l	4.0-5.9 mEq/l	1	Highest levels immediately after birth
Protein, total	60-81 g/l	6.0-8.1 g/100 ml	0.1	Lower when lying down
Sodium	134-146 mmol/l	134-146 mEq/l	1	
Thyroxine (T$_4$)	60-145 nmol/l	4.7-11.2 μg/100 ml	0.077	
Triglycerides	*Fasting* 0.4-2.0 mmol/l	35-175 mg/100 ml	87.5	Take sample after 12-16 h fast
Urate (Uric acid)	*Males* 206-460 μmol/l	3.5-7.8 mg/100 ml	0.017	
	Females 135-382 μmol/l	2.3-6.5 mg/100 ml	0.017	
	Children 60-290 μmol/l	1.0-4.9 mg/100 ml	0.017	

Tests	SI Units	Old Units	Factor	Notes
Urea	*Adults* 3.0-8.0 mmol/l	18-48 mg/100 ml	6.01	Values are higher in the elderly and slightly lower in females
	Infants 1.3-5.8 mmol/l	8-35 mg/100 ml	6.01	

URINE BIOCHEMICAL TESTS

Amino acids	*Adults* 12-38.0 μmol/24 h	0.9-2.8 μg/24 h	0.075	As glycine
	Infants 2.0-36.5 μmol/24 h	0.1-2.7 μg/24 h		
delta Aminolaevul-inic acid (ALA)	9.1-42.0 μmol/24 h	1.2-5.5 mg/24 h	0.13	
Calcium, total	1.6-7.0 mmol/24 h	65-280 mg/24 h	40	
Creatinine	7-16 mmol/24 h	0.8-1.8 g/24 h	0.113	Lower in children. Values depend on muscle mass
5-Hydroxy-indoles	<105 μmol/24 h	<20 mg/24 h	0.191	
3-Methoxy-4-hydroxy mandelic acid (HMMA) (VMA)	<50 μmol/24 h	<10 mg/24 h	0.198	
Protein	<0.15 g/24 h			

Note: There is very great variation in the accepted range of reference values for urine tests.

CEREBROSPINAL FLUID BIOCHEMICAL TESTS

Glucose	2.5-4.0 mmol/l	45-72 mg/100 ml	18	c.s.f. (lumbar) glucose is usually 60-80% of blood glucose
Protein	0.1-0.4 g/l	10-40 mg/100 ml	100	

Recommended Reading

Whitby, L. G., Percy-Robb, I. W., Smith, A. F. *Lecture Notes on Clinical Chemistry*, Blackwell Scientific Publications, 3rd Ed., 1984.

Whitehead, T. P. *Quality Control in Clinical Chemistry*, John Wiley and Sons, 1977.

Walmsley, R. N., White, G. H. *A Guide to Diagnostic Clinical Chemistry*, Blackwell Scientific Publications, 1983.

IFCC Expert Panel on Nomenclature and Principles of Quality Control in Clinical Chemistry: Part 1, General principles and terminology. *Clinica Chimica Acta*, **98**, F129-143, 1979.
Part 2, Assessment of analytical methods for routine use. *Clinica Chimica Acta*, **98**, F145-162, 1979.
Part 4, Internal quality control. *Clinica Chimica Acta*, **106**, F104-120, 1980.

World Health Organization. *Principles of Quality Control*. Lab 76/1, 1976.

World Health Organization. *Quality Assurance in Health Laboratories*. Report of a Working Group, 1979.

World Health Organization. *Practical Guidelines for the Preparation of Quality Control Sera for Use in Clinical Chemistry*. Lab 81/4, 1981.

World Health Organization. *Chemistry and Quality Control for District Laboratories*, Lab 83/9, 1983.

World Health Organization. *The SI for the Health Professions*, 1977.

World Health Organization. *Methods Recommended for Essential Clinical Chemical and Haematological Tests for Intermediate Hospital Laboratories*. Lab, 1986.

Hill, P. *Quality control of biochemical analyses in a clinical laboratory*, 1986. Copies of this excellent small publication are free to laboratory workers in developing countries from Clin-Lab Services Ltd, 46 Farm Road, Edgeware, Middlesex HA8 9LT, United Kingdom. Enclose 3 International Reply Coupons to cover postage.

Reference ranges
For future editions of this manual, the author invites those working in developing countries to comment on the reference ranges quoted in this edition.

28 Tests of Renal Function

28:1 MEASUREMENT OF SERUM OR PLASMA UREA
Diacetyl Monoxime Method[1]

Urea is the main waste product of protein breakdown. It is formed in the liver from carbon dioxide and ammonia, passes into the extracellular fluid, and is excreted almost entirely by the kidneys. The urinary system is described in Chapter 7.

The measurement of urea is an important investigation in diagnosing kidney damage and following its course.

Choice of test method
The diacetyl monoxime method is recommended as a manual colorimetric technique. The stock reagents have good stability at room temperature. Care must be taken however when using the working colour reagent because this is highly corrosive (see later text).

Urea test kits
Manual colorimetric urea test kits based on the diacetyl monoxime method are commercially available, e.g. the bioMérieux *Urée-Kit* (Ref. 61479) priced about £9.00 (1985-1986) for 80 tests. The reagents and test method are different to those described in this subunit. Absorbances can be read in a colorimeter using a green filter (e.g. Ilford No. 604).

An enzyme urea test kit which uses a modification of the Berthelot urease reaction is available from Boehringer. The method requires no protein precipitation stage and incubation can be carried out at room temperature or 37 °C. The kit is called *Urea Color*, Cat. No. 620235 and costs about £26 for 200 tests (1985-1986). Reagents have good stability and a urea standard solution is included.

For the addresses of bioMérieux and Boehringer, see Appendix II.

Most of the test kits do not provide details of calibration. A control serum (not supplied) must be included with each batch of tests. Precautions to prevent water entering the solutions and to protect the developed colour from light as detailed in this subunit, apply when using a diacetyl monoxime urea kit.

Important: For further comments regarding the purchasing and use of clinical chemistry test kits, see 26:1.

Principle of the diacetyl monoxime urea method
Urea reacts with diacetyl monoxime at high temperature in an acid medium in the presence of cadmium ions and thiosemicarbazide. The absorbance of the red colour produced is measured in a colorimeter using a green filter or in a spectrophotometer at 530 nm wavelength.

$$\text{Urea} + \text{diacetyl monoxime} \xrightarrow{100\,°C} \begin{array}{c}\text{Diacetyl-urea}\\\text{compound}\\\textit{Red}\end{array}$$

Calibration
The diacetyl monoxime urea method is calibrated from a solution of urea. This is prepared and diluted to make a series of standards as follows:

Stock urea standard, 125 mmol/l
1. Weigh accurately 0.75 g (750 mg) of pure urea. Transfer the chemical to a 100 ml volumetric flask.

2. Half fill the flask with 1 g/l benzoic acid (Reagent No. 14) and mix to dissolve the urea. Make up to the 100 ml mark with the benzoic acid reagent and mix well.

   The urea concentration in the flask is 125 mmol/l.

3. Transfer the stock urea standard to a storage bottle, label, and store at 2-8 °C. The solution is stable for several months.

Working urea standards 2.5, 5, 10, 15, 20 mmol/l
1. Take five 50 ml volumetric flasks and number them 1 to 5. Pipette accurately into each flask as follows:

Flask	Stock urea, 125 mmol/l
1	1 ml
2	2 ml
3	4 ml
4	6 ml
5	8 ml

2. Make the contents of each flask up to the 50 ml mark with 1 g/l benzoic acid (Reagent No.14) and mix well.

   The concentration of urea in each standard is as follows:

   Flask 1 = 2.5 mmol/l
   2 = 5 mmol/l
   3 = 10 mmol/l
   4 = 15 mmol/l
   5 = 20 mmol/l

3. Transfer each standard solution to a storage bottle, label, and store at 2-8 °C. The working standards are stable for several months.

Preparation of urea calibration graph

1. Take six tubes and label them 'B' (reagent blank) and 1 to 5.

   Pipette 4 ml of freshly prepared urea colour reagent (see *Reagents*) into each tube.

2. Add to each tube as follows:

   Tube
   B .... 20 μl (0.02 ml) distilled water
   1 .... 20 μl standard, 2.5 mmol/l
   2 .... 20 μl standard, 5.0 mmol/l
   3 .... 20 μl standard, 10 mmol/l
   4 .... 20 μl standard, 15 mmol/l
   5 .... 20 μl standard, 20 mmol/l

3. Mix well and continue as described in steps 4 to 6 of the urea assay method.

4. Take a sheet of graph paper and plot the absorbance of each standard (vertical axis) against its concentration in mmol/l (horizontal axis), as described in 25:2. A linear calibration should be obtained.

   The useful working limit (linearity) of the diacetyl monoxime urea method is about 20 mmol/l (120 mg%).

Important: Check the calibrated graph by measuring a control serum as described in the urea method. A new calibration graph should be prepared and checked against controls whenever stock reagents are renewed.

Reagents

— Urea acid reagent   Reagent No. 83
— Diacetyl monoxime, 4 g/l   Reagent No. 28
The above reagents can be stored at room temperature (20-28 °C).

Urea colour reagent
Mix equal volumes of the urea acid reagent and diacetyl monoxime reagent. Allow 4 ml of colour reagent for each tube.

Note: The colour reagent is not stable. Once prepared it can be used for one day only.

Method

Specimen: The method requires 20 μl (0.02 ml) of patient's serum or plasma. For details of urea stability in serum and plasma, see 26:7.

1. Take four or more tubes (depending on the number of tests) and label as follows:

   B   — Reagent blank
   S   — Standard, 10 mmol/l
   C   — Control (see 27:5)
   1,2, etc   — Patients' tests

Note: Whenever resources permit, a full range of standards should be assayed with each batch of tests.

2. Pipette 4 ml of freshly made urea colour reagent into each tube.

   Caution: The colour reagent is highly corrosive, therefore *do not* mouth-pipette.

3. Add to each tube as follows:

   Tube
   B .... 20 μl (0.02 ml) distilled water
   S .... 20 μl standard, 10 mmol/l
   C .... 20 μl control serum
   1,2, etc .... 20 μl patient's serum or plasma

4. Mix well the contents of each tube and incubate at 100 °C for 15 minutes, preferably in a heatblock set at 100 °C or if unavailable in a container of boiling water. Stopper each tube using a *loose* fitting cap or plastic stopper having a small hole through which the steam can escape.

   Note: If using a container of boiling water do not use more water than is necessary to cover the level of fluid in the tubes.

5. Remove the tubes and cool them by placing the tubes in a container of cold water for 5 minutes making sure no water enters the tubes.

   Important: Protect the tubes from direct light because the red compound is sensitive to light. When protected from light, the colour of the solution is stable for up to 1 hour.

6. Read the absorbances of the solutions in a colorimeter using a green filter (e.g. Ilford No. 604) or in a spectrophotometer set at wavelength 530 nm. Zero the instrument with the blank solution in tube B.

7. Calculate the concentration of urea in the control and patients' samples by:

   — Reading the values from the calibration graph providing the reading of the 10 mmol/l standard agrees with the calibration, or if not by

   — Using the following formula:

   $$\text{Urea mmol/l} = \frac{AT}{AS} \times 10$$

   where: AT = Absorbance of test(s) or control
   AS = Absorbance of 10 mmol/l standard

Urea results over 20 mmol/l
Repeat the assay using a 1 in 2 dilution (or more if necessary) of the patient's serum or plasma in distilled water. Multiply the result by the dilution factor.

Summary of Urea Method

For detailed instructions, see text

Pipette into tubes as follows:	BLANK B	STANDARD S	CONTROL C	TEST 1,2, etc
Urea colour reagent (fresh)	4 ml	4 ml	4 ml	4 ml
Distilled water	20 μl	—	—	—
Standard, 10 mmol/l	—	20 μl	—	—
Control serum	—	—	20 μl	—
Patient's serum or plasma	—	—	—	20 μl

Mix well

Incubate at 100 °C for *exactly* 15 minutes

Do not let water enter the tubes

Cool

Protect tubes from light

READ ABSORBANCES

Colorimeter: Green filter, e.g. Ilford No. 604
Spectrophotometer: 530 nm

Zero instrument with blank solution in tube B

Obtain values from the calibration graph if the reading of the 10 mmol/l standard agrees with the calibration. If not, calculate the results as follows:

$$\text{Urea mmol/l} = \frac{\text{Absorbance of test or control}}{\text{Absorbance of 10 mmol/l standard}} \times 10$$

Report patients' results if control value is acceptable

20 μl = 0.02 ml

8. Report the patients' results if the value of the control serum is acceptable.

Quality control

The principles of quality control in clinical chemistry are described in Chapter 27.

For the diacetyl monoxime urea method the following should be attainable:

— OCV, within 3%
— RCV, not exceeding 6%

Approximate urea reference (normal) range

Adults: 3.3-7.7 mmol/l (20-46 mg%)
Infants: 1.3-5.8 mmol/l (8-35 mg%)

To convert from mmol/l to mg%, multiply by 6.
To convert from mg% to mmol/l, divide by 6.

Note: Reference values for serum or plasma urea increase with age. Values are slightly lower in females and also in children.

Interpretation of serum or plasma urea results

Increases

The term uraemia is used to describe the presence of excessive amounts of urea and other nitrogenous waste substances in the blood.

A marked and prolonged increase in urea level is indicative of damaged renal function. Depending on the duration of the damage the term acute or chronic renal failure is used. Many diseases may cause renal failure including primary kidney diseases such as glomerulonephritis (inflammation of the kidney glomeruli), pyelonephritis (inflammation of the pelvis of the kidney), and renal tuberculosis.

Diseases causing obstruction of urine outflow may also lead to kidney failure, e.g. urethral strictures, prostatic enlargement, cancer of the bladder, and urinary schistosomiasis.

Acute renal failure is often due to sudden reduced blood flow to the kidney occurring in haemorrhage, obstetrical and surgical emergencies, malaria, and septicaemia.

Slight increases in urea, (not more than three times the upper limit of the reference range) may occur when there is:

— Dehydration
— Diuretic therapy
— Gastrointestinal blood loss
— Any condition associated with increased protein breakdown such as pneumonia, malaria, meningitis, typhoid, major trauma, and surgical operations.

Decreases

Low urea levels may be found in:

— Pregnancy
— Protein deficiency
— Severe liver disease
— Water overload

REAGENT STRIP TESTS TO MEASURE UREA

The *Urastrat*[2] and *Merckognost Urea*[3] strip tests are suitable for use in emergency situations by health centres and small hospital laboratories that are unable to measure serum or plasma by a colorimetric technique.

Both strip tests are based on the urease reaction, i.e. the release of ammonia following the hydrolysis of urea by the enzyme urease. The ammonia causes a change in colour of the indicator from yellow to blue.

Compared with the *Urastrat* strip test, the *Merckognost Urea* strip test has the advantages that whole blood, serum, or plasma can be used, a wider range of values can be measured, readings are made directly on the test strip (ruler is not required) and can be made at various times, and the strips can be stored at room temperature. *Merckognost* strips, however, are more expensive than *Urastrat* strips.[2, 3]

Full details of how to use the strips are provided by the manufacturers. The storage and control of reagent strip tests are described in 28:7.

Measurement of urea in urine

If required, urinary urea can be measured by the diacetyl monoxime method as described for blood urea. It is however necessary to dilute the urine 1 in 20. The result obtained must then be multiplied by 20 to obtain the concentration of urea in the urine sample.

The amount of urea excreted in a 24 hour urine is approximately 250-600 mmol/l (15-35 g/l).

28:2 MEASUREMENT OF SERUM OR PLASMA CREATININE
Alkaline picrate - Slot Method
(Seaton modified)[4, 5]

Creatinine is a nitrogenous waste product formed from the metabolism of creatine in skeletal muscle. Creatinine diffuses freely throughout the body water. It is filtered from the extracellular fluid by the kidney and excreted in the urine.

Measurement of creatinine, like that of urea, is used as a test of renal function (see *Interpretation of results*).

Choice of test method

The Slot method measures 'true' creatinine and is recommended as a manual colorimetric technique. The Seaton modification uses a single working reagent. There is no protein precipitation stage.

Creatinine test kits

A manual colorimetric creatinine kit based on the alkaline picrate method before and after adding acid (to obtain 'true' creatinine readings) is available from Sigma Chemical Company (see Appendix II for address). The Sigma Creatinine (No. 555-A) Kit costs about £12.00 (1985-1986) for 190 tests. The reagents and technique are different to those described in this subunit.

The Sigma Kit includes standard solutions and details of calibration. Absorbances can be read using a blue-green filter (e.g. Ilford No. 603). The patients' and control values should be read from the calibration graph.

Each batch of patients' tests should include a reagent blank, standard *and* control serum. Results should be reported in μmol/l, not mmol/l or mg/dl as indicated in the test kit. To convert mg% to μmol/l, multiply by 88.5. To convert mmol/l to μmol/l, multiply by 1 000.

Important: For comments regarding the use of clinical chemistry test kits, see 26:1.

Principle of the Slot creatinine method

Creatinine reacts with picric acid in an alkaline medium. The absorbance of the yellow-red colour produced is measured in a colorimeter using a blue-green filter or in a spectrophotometer at 490 nm wavelength.

Unfortunately a number of other compounds similarly react with picric acid giving artificially high results for creatinine if one simply measures the total yellow-red colour produced. A second reading is therefore made after making the solution acid. The colour produced by creatinine is quickly destroyed by acid whereas that given by non-creatinine substances is destroyed more slowly. By subtracting the second reading which is due to non-creatinine substances from the first reading (due to creatinine and non-creatinine substances), the colour produced by the creatinine can be estimated.

Note: The second reading *must* be made within 6 to 10 minutes after the first reading otherwise the acid will completely decolorise the solution.

Creatinine and + Alkaline picric ⟶ Total
non-creatinine   acid reagent   chromogen
substances

                                Yellow-red

Calibration

The Slot creatinine method is calibrated from a solution of creatinine. This is prepared and diluted to make a series of standards as follows:

Stock creatinine standard, 10 mmol/l

1. Weigh accurately 0.113 g of anhydrous creatinine or 0.362 g of creatinine zinc hydrochloride. Transfer the chemical to a 100 ml volumetric flask.

2. Half fill the flask with 100 mmol/l hydrochloric acid (Reagent No. 43) and mix to dissolve the creatinine. Make up to the 100 ml mark with the hydrochloric acid reagent and mix well.

   The creatinine concentration in the flask is 10 mmol/l (10 000 μmol/l).

3. Transfer the stock creatinine standard solution to a storage bottle. Label and store at 2-8 °C. The solution is stable for about 2 months.

Working creatinine standards, 100, 200, 300, 400, 500 μmol/l

1. Take five 100 ml volumetric flasks and number them 1 to 5. Pipette accurately into each flask as follows:

Flask	Stock creatinine, 10 mmol/l
1	1 ml
2	2 ml
3	3 ml
4	4 ml
5	5 ml

2. Make the contents of each flask up to the 100 ml mark with 1 g/l benzoic acid (Reagent No. 14) and mix well.

   The concentration of creatinine in each standard is as follows:

   Flask 1 = 100 μmol/l
          2 = 200 μmol/l
          3 = 300 μmol/l
          4 = 400 μmol/l
          5 = 500 μmol/l

3. Transfer each solution to a storage bottle, label, and store at 2-8 °C. The working standards are stable for about 2 months.

Preparation of creatinine calibration graph

1. Take *two sets* of six tubes and label each set 'B' (reagent blank) and 1 to 5.

   Pipette 2 ml of freshly prepared creatinine working reagent (see *Reagents*) into each tube.

2. Add to each tube as follows:

   Tube
   B .... 0.2 ml (200 μl) acetic acid, 60% v/v
   1 .... 0.2 ml standard, 100 μmol/l
   2 .... 0.2 ml standard, 200 μmol/l
   3 .... 0.2 ml standard, 300 μmol/l
   4 .... 0.2 ml standard, 400 μmol/l
   5 .... 0.2 ml standard, 500 μmol/l

3. Mix well the contents of each pair of tubes and continue as described in steps 4 to 8 of the creatinine method.

4. Take a sheet of graph paper and plot the absorbance of each standard (vertical axis) against its concentration in μmol/l (horizontal axis), as described in 25:2. A linear calibration should be obtained.

The useful working limit (linearity) of the Slot creatinine method is about 500 μmol/l.

Important: Check the calibration graph by measuring a control serum using the creatinine method. A new calibration graph should be prepared and checked against controls whenever stock reagents are renewed.

Reagents
— Sodium dodecyl sulphate,   Reagent No. 69
   40 g/l (sodium lauryl sulphate)
— Phosphate borate buffer,   Reagent No. 54
   pH 12.8
— Picric acid reagent   Reagent No. 59
— Acetic acid, 60% v/v   Reagent No. 3

The above reagents can be stored at room temperature (20-28 °C). Details of their shelf-life can be found under the preparation of each reagent.

Creatinine working reagent
Mix *equal volumes* of the sodium dodecyl sulphate reagent, phosphate borate buffer, and picric acid reagent. Allow 2 ml of working reagent for each tube.
Note: The creatinine working reagent is not stable. Once prepared it can be used for one day only.

Method
Specimen: The method requires 0.4 ml (400 μl) of patient's fresh serum or plasma which must be free from haemolysis (see 26:4).

1. Take *two sets* of four or more test tubes (depending on the number of tests) and label each set as follows:

B   — Reagent blank
S   — Standard, 200 μmol/l
C   — Control (see 27:5)
1,2, etc   — Patients' tests

Two sets of tubes are required in this assay because one set is read after the addition of acid.

Note: Whenever resources permit, a full range of standards should be assayed with each batch of tests.

2. Pipette 2 ml of *freshly* prepared creatinine working reagent into each tube.

3. Add to each tube as follows:
Tube
B .... 0.2 ml (200 μl) distilled water
S .... 0.2 ml standard, 200 μmol/l
C .... 0.2 ml control serum
1,2, etc ...... 0.2 ml patient's serum or plasma

4. Mix well the contents of each pair of tubes and leave at room temperature for 90 minutes.

5. Read the absorbances of one set of solutions in a colorimeter using a blue-green filter (e.g. Ilford No. 603) or in a spectrophotometer set at wavelength 490 nm. Zero the instrument with the blank solution in tube B.

Note: For some colorimeters it may be necessary to use a modified cuvette holder to measure small volumes. No modification is required if using a WPA CO700D colorimeter (see 25:3).

6. Add 50 μl (0.05 ml) of 60% v/v acetic acid reagent to each of the second set of tubes and leave for 6 minutes.

7. Read the absorbances of the second set of solutions. Zero the colorimeter with the acidified blank solution in tube B (second set). Subtract the readings of the second set of tubes from the readings of the first set of tubes. This will give the absorbance of creatinine in the standard, control, and test solutions.

8. Calculate the concentration of creatinine in the control and patients' samples by:

— Reading the values from the calibration graph providing the reading of the 200 μmol/l standard agrees with the calibration, or if not by

— Using the following formula:

$$\text{Creatinine } \mu\text{mol/l} = \frac{AT}{AS} \times 200$$

where AT = Absorbance of test(s) or control
      AS = Absorbance of 200 μmol/l standard

Creatinine results over 500 μmol/l
Repeat the assay using a 1 in 3 dilution of the patient's serum or plasma in distilled water. Multiply the result by 3.

9. Report the patients' results if the value of the control serum is acceptable.

Summary of Creatinine Method

For detailed instructions, see text

Two sets of tubes are required Pipette into each set of tubes as follows:	BLANK B	STANDARD S	CONTROL C	TEST 1,2, etc
Creatinine working reagent (fresh) ...	2 ml	2 ml	2 ml	2 ml
Distilled water	0.2 ml	—	—	—
Standard, 200 μmol/l	—	0.2 ml	—	—
Control serum	—	—	0.2 ml	—
Patient's serum or plasma	—	—	—	0.2 ml

Mix well

Leave at room temperature for 90 minutes

READ ABSORBANCES OF FIRST SET OF TUBES   *Reading 1*

Colorimeter: Blue - Green filter, e.g. Ilford No. 603
Spectrophotometer: 490 nm

Zero instrument with blank solution in tube B (first set of tubes)

Pipette into *second set of tubes:* Acetic acid, 60% v/v	50 μl	50 μl	50 μl	50 μl

Leave *second set of tubes* for 6 minutes

READ ABSORBANCES OF SECOND SET OF TUBES   *Reading 2*

Colorimeter: Blue - green filter e.g. Ilford No. 603
Spectrophotometer: 490 nm

Zero instrument with blank solution in tube B (second set of tubes)

Subtract *Reading 2* from *Reading 1*

Obtain values from calibration graph if the reading of the 200 μmol/l standard agrees with the calibration. If not, calculate the result as follows:

$$\text{Creatinine } \mu\text{mol/l} = \frac{\text{Absorbance of test or control}}{\text{Absorbance of 200 } \mu\text{mol/l standard}} \times 200$$

Report patients' results if control value is acceptable

200 μl = 0.2ml
50 μl = 0.05 ml

Quality control

The principles of quality control in clinical chemistry are described in Chapter 27.

For the Slot creatinine method the following should be attainable:

— OCV, within 4%
— RCV, not exceeding 8%

Approximate creatinine reference (normal) range

Males: 60-130 μmol/l (0.7-1.4 mg%)
Females: 40-110 μmol/l (0.4-1.2 mg%)

To convert μmol/l to mg%, multiply by 0.011.
To convert mg% to μmol/l, divide by 0.011.

Note: Reference values for serum or plasma creatinine are slightly lower in children. Values depend on muscle mass.

Interpretation of serum or plasma creatinine results

Increases

An increase in serum creatinine occurs in renal disease in a similar manner to urea (see 28:1). Creatinine, however, does not increase with age, dehydration, and catabolic states (e.g. fever, sepsis, internal bleeding) to the same extent as urea. Also the rate of creatinine production is little affected by changes in diet such as a low intake of protein (providing this is not prolonged).

The method for measuring creatinine, however, is not as sensitive as the technique used for measuring urea (diacetyl monoxime). Creatinine assays may also be positively interfered with by high ketone levels. This will result in falsely high serum or plasma creatinine concentrations in patients with diabetic ketoacidosis.

Decreases

Diseases associated with muscle wasting reduce the level of creatinine in the blood. In general, however, decreases in concentration are of little significance because serum or plasma creatinine levels are proportional to the muscle mass of an individual.

28:3 TESTING URINE FOR PROTEIN

Most plasma proteins are too large to pass through the glomeruli of the kidney. The small amount of protein which does filter through is normally reabsorbed back into the blood by the kidney tubules. Only trace amounts of protein (less than 0.15 g per 24 h) can therefore be found in normal urine. These amounts are insufficient for detection by routine laboratory tests.

When more than trace amounts of protein are found in urine this is termed proteinuria. The con-

dition is often referred to as albuminuria because when there is glomerular damage most of the protein which passes through the glomerular filter is albumin because this protein molecule is smaller than most of the globulins.

The following methods are used to test for proteinuria:

■ Protein reagent strip test
■ Sulphosalicylic acid test

Note: The heat coagulation test (boiling test) is not recommended because it involves boiling urine specimens which can be dangerous.

Protein Reagent Strip Tests

Urine protein strip tests detect mainly albumin. The test area is impregnated with the indicator tetrabromophenol blue (Ames) or a tetrabromophenolphthalein ethyl ester (Boehringer) and buffered to an acid pH. In the presence of protein there is a change in the colour of the indicator from light yellow to green-blue depending on the amount of protein present.

The strips are very sensitive, detecting as little as 0.1 g/l (10 mg%) of albumin. The reaction is unaffected by turbidity in the urine. Proteins such as globulin, mucoprotein, haemoglobin, and Bence Jones protein give only weak reactions.

Protein testing strips which are available commercially include:

□ *Albustix* (Ames) which measures albumin semiquantitatively:

Scale: Negative, trace, + 0.3 g/l, ++ 1 g/l, +++ 3 g/l, ++++ 20 g/l or more

□ *Albym* (Boehringer) which measures albumin semiquantitatively:

Scale: Negative, about 0.15 g/l, 0.3 g/l, 1 g/l, 5 g/l over 5 g/l.

Note: Albumin test areas can also be found with glucose on *Uristix* (Ames), with glucose and pH on *Combur-Test* (Boehringer), and on many of the multiple strip tests as listed in Chart 28.1 in 28:7.

False reactions

False positive results may be obtained when the urine is contaminated with disinfectants which contain quaternary ammonium compounds, for example cetrimide (cetavlon).

Strongly alkaline urine may also give false positives and overstated results.

Boehringer literature also mentions that false positive results may be obtained during treatment with phenazopyridine or infusion with the plasma expander polyvinylpyrrolidone.

Some strips may also give false positive trace reactions during treatment with chloroquine, quinine, quinidine, and trimethoprim.

Note: The control of reagent strips is described in 28:7.

Sulphosalicylic Acid Test
This test is based on the precipitation of protein by sulphosalicylic acid, especially albumin.

Reagent
— Sulphosalicylic acid, 200 g/l   Reagent No. 80

Method
1. Take two tubes and label one 'C' for comparison and the other 'T' for test.

2. Pour about 2 ml of clear urine into each tube.

   Note: If the urine is cloudy, filter or centrifuge it to obtain a clear sample.

3. Using pH papers or neutral litmus paper, test the reaction of the urine. If neutral or alkaline, add a drop of glacial acetic acid to each tube and mix.

   Caution: Glacial acetic acid is a corrosive and flammable chemical, therefore handle with care away from an open flame.

4. Add 2-3 drops of the sulphosalicylic acid reagent to tube 'T'.

5. Holding both tubes against a dark background, examine for any cloudiness in tube 'T'. Report the appearance in tube 'T' as follows:

   No cloudiness .... Negative
   Slight cloudiness .... +
   Moderate cloudiness .... ++
   Marked cloudiness .... +++
   Cloudiness with precipitate .... ++++

False reactions
False positive reactions may occur if the urine is tested while the patient is receiving tolbutamide (a hypoglycaemic drug), or intensive therapy with penicillin, paraaminosalicylic acid, or sulphonamides. False positive reactions may also occur if the specimen is collected following an intravenous pyelogram (IVP) or an intravenous infusion of the plasma expander polyvinylpyrrolidone.

A high concentration of urates in the urine may cause a false positive result due to precipitation of urate in any acidic urine.

Causes of proteinuria
— Glomerular or tubular urinary disease. Proteinuria accompanies acute glomerulonephritis and is due to increased permeability of the glomerular basement membrane. The degree of proteinuria reflects the severity of the condition and helps in assessing prognosis and response to treatment.

— Pyogenic or tuberculous pyelonephritis.

— Severe lower urinary tract infection.

— Nephrotic syndrome which is a condition characterized by heavy proteinuria and oedema. The oedema is caused by a reduction in the colloid osmotic pressure due to a fall in the level of plasma albumin brought about when the amount of proteinuria rises to 5 or 10 g/l per day (see also end of subunit 30:6).

— Eclampsia when there is moderate to marked proteinuria.

— Urinary schistosomiasis which is usually accompanied by both proteinuria and haematuria.

— Severe febrile illnesses including malaria.

— Occasionally in diabetes. Diabetic nephropathy sometimes causes a nephrotic syndrome.

— Hypertension.

— Accompanying haematuria.

Note: Proteinuria should always be considered to indicate underlying disease until proved otherwise.

Whenever proteinuria is found, the urine should be examined for bacteria, pus cells, red cells, and casts (see 38:11 in Volume II of the Manual).

28:4 DETECTION OF BENCE JONES PROTEIN IN URINE

Bence Jones protein is an abnormal low molecular weight globulin consisting of light chains of immunoglobulins which contain the amino acids found in other proteins except methionine. It may be found in the urine of patients with multiple myeloma which is a malignant disease of the plasma cells, mainly affecting bone.

Tests used to screen for Bence Jones protein are based on demonstrating a protein in the urine which precipitates at 40-60 °C. Bence Jones protein is not well detected by protein reagent strip tests but is precipitated by sulphosalicylic acid.

Heat test to screen for Bence Jones protein
1. Pour about 5 ml of clear freshly collected urine into each of three test tubes.

If the urine is cloudy, centrifuge or filter it to obtain a clear sample.

2. Acidify the urine by adding 1 drop of glacial acetic acid to the first tube, 2 drops to the second tube, and 3 drops to the third tube.

   Note: Precipitation of Bence Jones protein requires the correct degree of acidification.

   Caution: Glacial (concentrated) acetic acid is corrosive and flammable, therefore handle with care away from an open flame.

3. Place the three tubes in a beaker of tap water and insert a 0-100 °C thermometer in one of the tubes.

4. Using a gentle flame slowly heat the beaker of water.

5. When the temperature reaches 40 °C look for cloudiness and precipitation in the tubes. Continue to observe until the temperature reaches 60 °C.

   If a cloudiness appears in one or more of the tubes, continue heating the urine to 100 °C, noting whether the precipitate partially or totally dissolves at 70-100 °C.

Positive test for Bence Jones protein
This is indicated by a cloudiness at 40-60 °C which redissolves over 70 °C. As the urine cools the cloudiness will reappear at about 60 °C.

A false positive test may be obtained if mucin is present.

Note: Other proteins may precipitate at over 70 °C and remain as the urine cools. If other proteins are excreted these may be removed by filtering the hot urine. The specimen should then be allowed to cool and the test repeated.

Important: If Bence Jones protein is suspected, the patient's urine together with a serum sample should be sent to a laboratory able to demonstrate the abnormal protein by protein electrophoresis.

28:5 URINE RELATIVE MASS DENSITY (SPECIFIC GRAVITY)

The relative mass density (d), formerly known as specific gravity (SG), of any liquid is its density compared with distilled water which has a density of 1.000.

By measuring the mass density of urine, information can be obtained regarding the concentrating power of the kidneys.

The following methods are used to test the mass density of urine:

- Urinometer
- Refractometer
- Weighing technique
- Reagent strip test

Specimen: This should be the first urine passed at the beginning of the day with the patient having taken no fluid for 10 hours. The testing of random urine specimens has little clinical value.

Urinometer
This technique uses a specially calibrated hydrometer. The lower the concentration of solutes the further the urinometer will sink in the urine.

A new urinometer must be checked for accuracy by being floated in distilled water. The reading should be 1.000 at the temperature specified on the urinometer. If the reading is not 1.000, subtract the difference in value from each urine reading. For example, if the density of the distilled water is 1.002, subtract 0.002 from each urine reading.

Method
1. Obtain at least 50 ml of urine. Transfer the urine to a cylinder.

   Note: The cylinder and urine must be detergent-free because even a trace of detergent will lower the surface tension of the urine and give an incorrect reading.

2. Immerse the urinometer in the urine and make sure that it floats centrally and does not touch the bottom or sides of the cylinder.

3. Take the reading at the lowest point of the meniscus. This must be done at eye level.

   The scale of the urinometer is calibrated from 1.000-1.060 with each division being equal to 0.001.

Adjustment for temperature
Most urinometers are calibrated for use at 15 °C or 20 °C. For each 3 °C difference, 0.001 must be added if above or subtracted if below the calibration temperature.

Example: If the mass density reading of the urine is 1.022 at 23 °C and the urinometer has been calibrated at 20 °C, the corrected reading is 1.022 + 0.001 = 1.023.

Adjustment for Protein
Subtract 0.001 from the mass density reading for every 4 g protein per litre (0.4 g%) of urine.

Adjustment for Glucose
Subtract 0.001 from the mass density reading for every 15 mmol/l glucose per litre of urine.

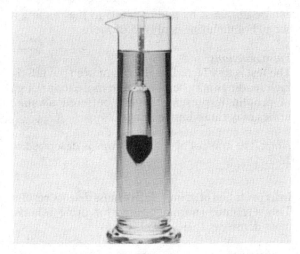

Plate 28.1 Urinometer in a cylinder of urine.

Refractometer

A refractometer measures refractive index. The measurement is based on the number of dissolved particles in the urine. The higher the concentration of particles, the greater the increase in refractive index (refraction). From refractive index measurements a scale of relative mass density (specific gravity) values can be prepared.

Several models of clinical refractometer for measuring urine relative density (specific gravity) are available. The most useful, however, are those instruments that also measure serum total proteins such as the bench model Atago T-2 clinical refractometer[6] shown in Plate 28.2. Urine specific gravity and serum or plasma protein scales of a clinical refractometer are shown in Plate 28.3.

Availability: The Atago T-2 clinical refractometer is included in the Tropical Health Technology Equipment Service to Developing Countries (see Appendix IV, Refractometer).

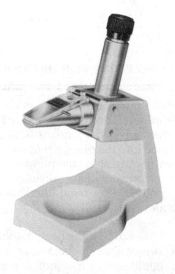

Plate 28.2 Atago T2 clinical refractometer.

Method (based on Atago refractometer T-2)
1. Check that the instrument scale is correctly adjusted by placing a few drops of distilled water on the face of the prism. Gently close the cover plate. With the refractometer facing the light, bring the scale into focus by turning the eyepiece.

   If the boundary line does not coincide with the Wt (water) line, make the necessary adjustment by rotating the scale adjustment knob.

2. To measure urine specific gravity, place one or two drops of urine on the prism surface as shown in Fig. 28.1 and gently close the cover plate.

3. Rotate the eyepiece until the scale becomes clearly visible.

   Observe the point on the urine specific gravity scale where the dark part of the field meets the light area (see Plate 28.3). Read off the urine specific gravity value.

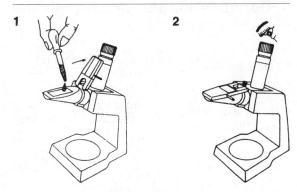

Fig. 28.1 Technique of using Atago refractometer.

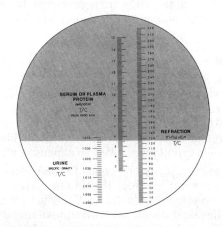

Plate 28.3 Serum protein and urine specific gravity scales of a refractometer.

Important: Although a protein scale is also shown this *must not* be used to measure urine protein. It is calibrated only for measuring *serum total protein* as explained in 30:5.

Weighing Technique

This technique requires the use of an analytical balance capable of weighing to 3 decimal places, i.e. 1 mg sensitivity.

Method

1. Place on each pan of the analytical balance a small beaker containing a few ml of tap water.

2. Using a fine bore Pasteur pipette, transfer water from one beaker to the other until the weight is equal on both sides.

3. Using a dry volumetric pipette, add 10 ml of distilled water to the left hand beaker.

4. Using another dry volumetric pipette, add 10 ml of urine to the right hand beaker.

5. Add milligram weights to the left hand pan, until once again the weight is equal on both sides. Total the number of milligrams used.

6. Calculate the mass density (d) of the urine from the following formula:

$$\text{Urine d} = \frac{10\,000 + \text{Number of milligrams used}}{10\,000}$$

Example
If 270 mg used:

$$\text{Urine d} = \frac{10\,000 + 270}{10\,000}$$

$$= \frac{10\,270}{10\,000}$$

$$= 1.027$$

Note: As described for the urinometer method, adjustments to the value are necessary if the urine contains large amounts of protein or glucose.

Reagent Strip Test

A test area to determine specific gravity in urine can be found on the multiple test strip of Ames called *N-Multistix*. The strip also measures urinary pH, protein, glucose, ketones, bilirubin, blood, nitrite, and urobilinogen. It is an expensive strip.

The reagent test area responds to the concentration of ions in the urine. It contains certain pre-treated polyelectrolytes, the pKa of which changes depending on the ionic concentration of the urine. The indicator bromothymol blue is used to detect the change. Colours range from deep blue-green when the urine is of low ionic concentration, through green to yellow-green when the specimen is of high ionic concentration.

The specific gravity (SG) scale covers the range 1.000 to 1.030 in steps of 0.005. Increased accuracy

can be obtained by adding 0.005 to the reading if the pH of the urine is pH 6.5 or more.

False reactions
The test is unaffected by glucose or urea but falsely high readings may be obtained if more than 0.1 g/l of protein is present. Highly buffered alkaline urines may cause low readings.

Note: The control of reagent strips is described in 28:7.

Interpretation of urine relative mass density results

The reference (normal) range for urine relative mass density is 1.010-1.030.

Low values
A consistently low urine mass density usually indicates poor tubular reabsorption.

Excessive fluid intake, however, will also result in a low mass density. In general, the greater the volume of urine excreted the lower is its density and the lighter its colour.

High values
A high urine mass density may be the result of heavy perspiration, dehydration, or to the presence of substances not normally found in urine such as glucose or protein.

Concentration of urine expressed as osmolality/kg

This is the best way of expressing the concentration of urine because it depends on the number of osmotically active solute particles per unit of solvent whereas mass density depends on the type as well as the number of solute particles. It is however, much simpler to measure the mass density of urine rather than its osmolality. A mass density of 1.002 is equivalent approximately to an osmolality of 100 mosmol/kg and a mass density of 1.025 to about 1000 mosmol/kg.

28:6 TESTING URINE FOR HAEMOGLOBIN

The presence of free haemoglobin in urine is called haemoglobinuria. It occurs with severe intravascular haemolysis when the amount of haemoglobin being released into the plasma is more than can be taken up by haptoglobin (the plasma protein that binds free haemoglobin to prevent it being lost from the body). The renal threshold for free haemoglobin is 1.0-1.4 g/l.

Specimen: Urine containing haemoglobin appears brown or brown-grey in colour and is usually cloudy. It should be tested as soon as possible after it has been passed.

Strip test to detect haemoglobin in urine

The simplest method of detecting haemoglobin in urine is to use a reagent strip test such as the Boehringer strip *Sangur-Test* (also known as *BM-Test Hematurie*). It is a sensitive strip test based on the ability of haemoglobin to catalyze the oxidation of a colour indicator by an organic peroxide to give a blue green complex.

There are separate colour scales for haemoglobin and intact erythrocytes (red cells). An even green colouring of the test area indicates the presence of free haemoglobin or haemolyzed erythrocytes in the urine. Myoglobin gives a similar reaction but myoglobinuria is a rare condition.

A green spotting of the yellow test area indicates the presence of intact erythrocytes in the urine (haematuria).

Differentiation between haemoglobinuria and haematuria is not possible if the urine contains visible amounts of blood.

Note: Test areas for detecting blood in urine in the form of intact red cells and haemoglobin can also be found on several multistrips as listed in 28:7.

False reactions

Low to false negative results are obtained if the urine contains large amounts of ascorbic acid.

False positive reactions can result from the presence of contaminating oxidizing detergents in the urine such as bleach.

Heavy proteinuria (i.e. over 5 g/l protein) may reduce the colour reaction.

Note: The control of reagent strips is described in 28:7.

Causes of haemoglobinuria

Haemoglobinuria occurs with severe intravascular haemolysis. It is associated with:

— Severe falciparum malaria.

— Typhoid fever.

— Glucose-6-phosphate dehydrogenase (G6PD) deficiency following the ingestion of certain drugs.

— *Escherichia coli* septicaemia.

— Incompatible blood transfusion.

— Snake bites that cause acute haemolysis.

— Sickle cell disease crisis with severe haemolysis.

— Severe viral haemorrhagic fever accompanied by intravascular haemolysis

Note: The causes of haematuria and the examination of urine for red cells are described in 38:11 in Volume II of the Manual.

28:7 CONTROL AND SELECTION OF URINE REAGENT STRIP TESTS

A wide range of urine reagent strip test are available. They are rapid and the simpler stable strips are often less expensive than performing chemical tube tests. The reliability of reagent strip tests depends on the correct storage, use and control of the strips.

Correct storage of reagent strips

Read carefully the expiry date and the manufacturer's storage instructions supplied with the strips.

To prevent the deterioration of reagent strips the following are important:

- Protect the strips from moisture and excessive heat and light, but do not refrigerate.

  A desiccant (drying agent) is supplied either in the lid of the container (Boehringer strips) or as a sachet in the container (Ames strips).

- Remove strips only as required. After removing a strip, replace the container top immediately and tightly to prevent moisture from the air entering. This is particularly important when the surrounding humidity is high.

  The reagents in the test areas deteriorate rapidly if they become damp.

Correct use of reagent strips

Manufacturers' instructions must be followed exactly as regards the urine specimen, use of individual strips, timing of reactions, and reading of results.

The following general guidelines apply:

- Collect urine samples in clean, dry, detergent-free containers. The urine should be as fresh as possible and well mixed.

- Before removing a strip, read carefully the manufacturer's instructions on how to test the urine. Become familiar with the test areas and possible reactions.

- Do not use strips that show any discoloration of the test areas.

- Do not contaminate a strip by touching the test areas with the fingers or by laying it down on the bench. Avoid using the strips in the presence of chemical fumes.

- Dip the strip *briefly* in the urine making sure that the test areas are fully immersed. Avoid prolonged contact with the urine because this may result in a dissolving out of the reagents from the test areas.

■ Remove excess urine from the strip by running the edge of the strip along the rim of the urine container.

■ Read carefully the reactions in a good light at exactly the times stated by the manufacturer. Compare the reactions by holding the strip close to the colour chart on the container label, but avoid contaminating the container with urine. If this happens, wipe the label with a cloth moistened with disinfectant.

Quality control of strip tests
Control reference solutions are available from manufacturers for some strips and readers may obtain details of these by writing to Ames Division of Miles Company and Boehringer Mannhein (see Appendix II for addresses).

The performance of most strip tests can also be controlled by checking regularly the strip reactions against those obtained by standard biochemical tests. Control urines of known negative and positive reactions should also be prepared and tested with patients' specimens.

The manufacturers' literature must always be consulted regarding the quality control of different strips and the substances which may interfere with the various reactions.

The problems that have been found in testing urine with reagent strip tests and recommended quality assurance procedures have been described in the paper of Fraser[7]

Selection of urine strip tests
In district laboratories where urines are examined microscopically for bacteria, pus cells (leucocytes), red cells, casts, and parasites, the biochemical testing of urine should include:

Routine
— Protein, to test for proteinuria (see 28:3)
— Glucose, to test for glycosuria (see 31:3)

Either of the following strips is recommended:
☐ *Uristix* (Ames) which detects glucose and measures protein semiquantitatively.
☐ *Combur-Test (BM-Test-3)*, (Boehringer) which detects glucose, measures protein semiquantitatively, and determines pH.

Note: It costs more to use single test strips to screen separately for glucose and protein than using a combined strip with two or three test areas.

Additional when indicated
— Ketones, to test for ketonuria (see 31:4)
— Glucose, quantitative test to assist in the control of diabetes (see 31:3)
— Bilirubin, to investigate jaundice (see 30:3)
— Urobilinogen to investigate jaundice and haemolysis (see 30:4)
— Haemoglobin, to test for haemoglobinuria (see 28:6)

The following strip tests are recommended:
☐ *Ketur Test* (Boehringer) or *Ketostix* (Ames) which detects ketones mainly as acetoacetate (see 31:4).
☐ *Diabur-Test 5000* (Boehringer) which measures urine glucose up to 5 g/l. The value of this strip is discussed in 31:3. It is recommended in preference to *Clinitest*.
☐ *Bilugen-Test* (Boehringer) which detects bilirubin and measures urobilinogen semiquantitatively (see 30:3 and 30:4).
☐ *Sangur-Test* (Boehringer) which detects haemoglobin (see 28:6). It also detects intact red cells but a strip test to test specifically for haematuria is not usually necessary because red cells can be detected microscopically in fresh urine.

Use of half strips
The cost of using strip tests can be significantly reduced by cutting strips in half. A pair of sharp clean scissors must be used to avoid contamination of the test areas. Alternatively, a strip splitter can be used (available from Medistron Ltd, priced about £10 (1985-1986). For address of company, see Appendix II).

Urine strip tests
Further up to date information about the chemical reactions and use of commercially available urine strip tests can be obtained upon request from Ames Division of Miles Laboratories Ltd and Boehringer Mannheim (see Appendix II).

CHART 28.1   BOEHRINGER AND AMES STRIP TESTS FOR URINE TESTING

Reagent strips	Company	Nitrite	pH	Protein	Glucose	Ketones	Urobilinogen	Bilirubin	Blood	Leucocytes	SG
Nitur - Test (BM - Test Nitrite)	B	§									
Albustix	A			§ Qn							
Albym - Test	B			§ Qn							
Glukotest (BM - Test Glucose)	B				§						
Clinistix	A				§						
Diabur - Test 5000 (Chemstrip UG 5000)	B				§ Qn						
Diastix	A				§ Qn						
Ketur - Test (BM - Test Keton, Chemstrip K)	B					§					
Ketostix	A					§					
Ugen - Test (BM - Test Urobilinogene)	B						§ Qn				
Urobilistix	A						§ Qn				
Bilur - Test (BM - Test Bilirubine)	B							§ Sb			
Sangur - Test (Bm - Test Hematurie)	B								§		
Hemastix	A								§		
Uristix	A			§ Qn	§						
Multistix 2	A	§								§	
Keto - Diabur - Test 5000 (Chemstrip UG 5000 K)	B				§ Qn	§					
Gluketur - Test	B				§	§					
Keto - Diastix	A				§ Qn	§					
Bilugen - Test	B						§ Qn	§			
Combur - Test (BM - Test - 3)	B		§ Qn	§ Qn	§						
Ecur - 5 - Test U	B			§ Qn	§	§			§	§	
Hema - Combistix	A		§ Qn	§ Qn	§				§		
Nephur - Test + Leucocytes	B	§	§ Qn	§ Qn	§ Qn				§	§	
N - Combur - Test (Bm - Test - 4)	B	§	§ Qn	§ Qn	§				§		
Combur 5 Test	B	§	§ Qn	§ Qn		§			§		
L - Combur 5 Test (BM - Test - 5L)	B		§ Qn	§ Qn	§	§			§		

Reagent strips	Company	Nitrite	pH	Protein	Glucose	Ketones	Urobilinogen	Bilirubin	Blood	Leucocytes	SG
Labstix	A		§ Qn	§ Qn	§	§			§		
Bili - Labstix SG	A		§ Qn	§ Qn	§	§		§	§		§
Combur 6 Test	B		§ Qn	§ Qn	§	§	§ Qn		§		
Uristix 4	A	§		§ Qn	§					§	
Combur 7 Test (BM - Test - 7)	B		§ Qn	§ Qn	§	§	§ Qn	§	§		
Multistix (2820)	A		§ Qn	§ Qn	§	§	§ Qn	§	§		
Combur 8 Test (Bm - Test - 8)	B	§	§ Qn	§ Qn	§	§	§ Qn	§	§		
N - Multistix SG (2740)	A	§	§ Qn	§ Qn	§	§	§ Qn	§	§		§
Combur - 9 - Test	B	§	§ Qn	§ Qn	§	§	§ Qn	§	§	§	
Multistix 8 SG	A	§	§ Qn	§ Qn	§	§			§	§	§
Multistix 9 SG	A	§	§ Qn	§ Qn	§	§		§	§	§	§

Key: A = Ames Company (see Appendix II)
B = Boehringer Company (see Appendix II)
§ = Substance or reaction tested

Qn = Semi - quantitative result
Sb = Serum bilirubin can also be measured
SG = Specific gravity

Note: Strips which contain more than a few test areas are considerably more expensive than the simpler strips and require more skill to read correctly.

References

1 Wybenga, D. R. Giorgio, Di, Pileggi, J. V. *Clinical Chemistry*, **17**, pp 891-895, 1971.

2 *Urastrat* strips also known as *Urostrat*, are manufactured by General Diagnostics Division of Warner-Lambert Company (see Appendix II). The strips are available in packs of 2 or 10 glass vials, each vial containing 25 strips. When stored at 4 °C and protected from moisture and ammoniacal gases, the strips are stable for about 2 years. An expiry date is printed on each vial. For information about cost and local availability, readers should write to the manufacturer.

3 *Merckognost Urea* strips are manufactured by E. Merck Company (see Appendix II). Each package consists of an aluminium tube containing 60 strips, and a set of reaction vessels. The strips are stable up to the expiry date stated when stored at room temperature, providing the container is kept tightly stoppered. For information about cost and local availability, readers should write to the manufacturer.

4 Slot, C. *Scandinavian Journal of Clinical Laboratory Investigation*, **17**, pp 381-387, 1965.

5 Seaton, B., Ali, A. *Medical laboratory Sciences*, **41**, pp 327-336, 1984.

6 The Atago Clinical Bench Refractometer model T-2 costs about £175 (1985-1986). It measures $150 \times 100 \times 210$ mm and weighs 1.3 Kg. The serum protein scale is from 0 to 12 g/100 ml. The urine specific gravity scale is from 1.000 to 1.050.

7 Fraser, C.G. Urine analysis: current performance and strategies for improvement *British Medical Journal*, **291**, pp 321-323, 1985.

Recommended Reading

Baron, D. N. *A Short Textbook of Chemical Pathology*, Hodder and Stoughton, 4th Edition, 1982. ELBS 1984: £2 ISBN 0 340 27048 9.

Whitby, L. G., Percy-Robb, I. W., and Smith, A. F. *Lecture Notes on Clinical Chemistry*, Blackwell Scientific Publications, Oxford, 3rd Edition, 1984. UK price £9.80. A low cost edition of this book is available from. P G Publishing Private Ltd, Alexandra, PO Box 318, Singapore 9115, Singapore.

29 Function and Measurement of Electrolytes

29:1 FUNCTION OF ELECTROLYTES

Electrolytes are compounds which dissociate in solution to form electrically charged particles, or ions. Positively charged ions are called cations and negatively charged ions are called anions.

In this Chapter, the term electrolytes refers to individual ions.

Electrolytes are important in helping to maintain the stability of the body's internal environment. The electrolytes found in the body's fluids include:

Main cations	Main anions
Sodium (Na^+)	Chloride (Cl^-)
Potassium (K^+)	Bicarbonate (HCO_3^-)
Magnesium (Mg^{++})	Phosphate (HPO_4^{--} $H_2PO_4^-$)
Calcium (Ca^{++})	Sulphate (SO_4^{--})
	Organic acids
	Protein

Sodium, potassium, and bicarbonate are the electrolytes most frequently measured in the laboratory (see 29:2, 29:4).

■ Sodium maintains the correct water balance in body fluids.
■ Sodium and potassium are necessary for heart muscle and other muscle activity.
■ Bicarbonate is important in preserving the acid-base balance in the body.

To maintain electrical neutrality in the body, the proportion of cations to anions must balance.

Electrolytes and water balance

Water constitutes about 60% of the body weight of a healthy adult and about 70% of the weight of a healthy infant.

The total volume of fluid in a healthy adult (weighing approx. 70 kg) is about 42 litres and in an infant (weighing approx. 3 kg) the total fluid volume is just over 2 litres.

Fluid is distributed in the body as:

☐ Intracellular fluid, which is found in the cells of the body.
☐ Extracellular fluid, which is composed of:
— Interstitial fluid, which is found in the spaces between the cells of the body. It is also known as extravascular fluid.
— Plasma, which forms the fluid part of blood and is found in blood vessels (intravascularly).

The intracellular and extracellular fluid areas are separated by selective permeable membranes through which water, electrolyte ions, and small molecules such as glucose, urea, and amino acids diffuse continually to maintain the fluids in equilibrium.

The distribution and concentrations of electrolytes in intracellular and extracellular fluids are as follows:

Intracellular fluid
This constitutes about 28 litres of the body's fluid in an adult and just under 1 litre in an infant. Compared with extracellular fluid, it has a high protein content. It contains the following electrolytes:

Cations: Mainly potassium and magnesium, with lower concentrations of sodium and calcium.

Anions: Mainly protein and phosphate with lower concentrations of chloride, bicarbonate, sulphate, and organic acids.

Extracellular fluid
— Plasma which constitutes about 3.0-3.5 litres in an adult and about 250 ml in an infant. It contains the following electrolytes.

Cations: Mainly sodium, with lower concentrations of potassium, calcium, and magnesium.

Anions: Mainly chloride, with lower concentrations of bicarbonate, inorganic acids, phosphate, and sulphate. Protein is ionized as an anion at pH 7.4.

— Interstitial (extravascular) fluid which constitutes about 11 litres of fluid in an adult and just under 1 litre in an infant. It is made up of lymph, cerebrospinal fluid, pleural fluid, saliva, digestive tract secretions, synovial fluid, amniotic fluid, and aqueous humor.

Through the interstitial fluid, water, electrolytes, oxygen, and food substances pass from the plasma to the cells and waste products are transferred from the cells to the plasma. Interstitial fluid also prevents the cells from being directly affected by any sudden changes in plasma composition.

For the total water content of the body to remain constant the water taken in must equal the water lost from the body as follows:

Body's supply of water	Body's loss of water
Fluids drunk (main supply)	In urine (main loss)
Water in food	In faeces
Water from metabolic activity	In sweat
	In expired air

TOTAL WATER INTAKE	=	TOTAL WATER OUTPUT

Sodium is the main regulator of the osmotic pressure in the body fluids. In health the pressure between the extracellular and intracellular fluids is about equal. When fluid intake is restricted the plasma sodium concentration rises above normal and the extracellular fluid becomes hypertonic. This causes water to pass (by osmosis) from the intracellular fluid to the stronger extracellular fluid until the osmotic pressure balance betwen the two fluids is restored.

Aldosterone, a steroidal hormone produced by the cortex of the adrenal gland, assists in the reabsorption of sodium by the distal kidney tubules. When there is severe salt depletion aldosterone secretion is increased which causes the tubules to reabsorb most or all of the sodium and return it to the extravascular fluid. In this way little or no sodium is lost by being excreted in the urine. Increased kidney tubule reabsorption of sodium increases reabsorption of water. Sodium reabsorption can only take place in exchange for potassium or hydrogen ions. The role of the antidiuretic hormone (ADH) in controlling water balance is explained in 7:2.

Potassium and magnesium, being present in high concentrations inside the cells, are the main osmotic and water balance regulators within the intracellular fluid.

Plasma proteins and capillary blood pressure are important in controlling plasma volume. The higher osmotic pressure of the plasma tends to draw fluid from the tissues into the plasma. This is counter balanced by the hydrostatic (blood) pressure in the capillaries which tends to force fluid out of the plasma into the tissues.

Conditions of fluid inbalance
Losses of body fluid
There are two causes of loss of body fluid:

□ Loss mainly of water alone, i.e. literally dehydration. The dehydrated person becomes thirsty and under normal circumstances drinks to correct the water loss.

Uncorrected dehydration tends to occur therefore in situations in which:

— Persons are unable to obtain sufficient water for themselves, e.g. the unconscious, paralyzed, very young, elderly and feeble, or patients being rapidly ventilated.

— Water is unavailable, e.g. in times of drought or during an emergency at sea.

— There is a deficiency of the antidiuretic hormone (ADH) resulting in excessive urine excretion with inadequate water intake as in diabetes insipidus or severe renal disease.

In water deprivation the fluid loss is shared by the total body fluid. The typical results of laboratory tests in water deprivation are summarized in Table 29.1.

□ Loss of water together with electrolytes is the second and commonest cause of loss of body fluid.

Water containing electrolytes may be lost in the following ways:

— By diarrhoea and vomiting.

— By fluid remaining in the bowel as in paralytic ileus (paralysis of intestinal muscles).

— By excessive sweating as in heat exhaustion.

— By fluid being lost through damaged tissue, e.g. burns.

— By abnormal increased urine excretion due to reduced aldosterone production (e.g. Addisons disease), prolonged use of diuretics, pyelonephritis (salt-losing nephritis), or diabetic ketoacidosis (osmotic diuresis).

In loss of water together with electrolytes, the fluid lost is mainly from the extracellular fluid. More fluid is usually lost from the interstitial fluid than from the plasma because the plasma proteins tend to hold the water in the capillaries. The fluid lost is roughly equivalent to physiological (isotonic) saline which contains 150 mmol/l of sodium and chloride ions and variable amounts of potassium and other dissolved substances. The most important ion lost is sodium because this affects the osmotic pressure of the extracellular fluid.

Note: In diarrhoea and vomiting, unless due to pyloric obstruction, a metabolic acidosis (see later text) can also occur because with the exception of gastric contents, gastrointestinal secretions are alkaline. The potassium lost may cause a significant fall in plasma potassium levels.

If the fluid loss is not corrected, the plasma volume may also become depleted. Adequate blood circulation depends on the correct volume of plasma being maintained. A severe loss of water and salt from the body can therefore lead to a state of shock with low blood pressure, muscular weakness and wrinkled skin.

Note: The results of laboratory tests in losses of body fluid are summarized in Table 29.1.

Table 29.1 Laboratory Test Results in Losses of Body Fluid

LOSS OF WATER ALONE

Laboratory findings after about 36-48 h without water (12-24 h in infants):

Blood tests
- Increased sodium and chloride
- Increased total protein
- Increased urea
- Raised packed cell volume (haematocrit)
- Increased haemoglobin

Urine tests
- Raised relative mass density (specific gravity)
- Increased sodium and chloride
- Ketones detected (late stages)
- Protein detected (late stages)
- Red cells and casts may be found (late stages)

LOSS OF WATER WITH ELECTROLYTES

Laboratory findings in moderate to severe water and salt depletion:

Blood tests
- Normal or reduced sodium and chloride
- Increased urea (late stages)
- Raised packed cell volume
- Increased haemoglobin

Urine tests
- Reduced relative mass density
- Absent or reduced sodium and chloride

Note: In the management of patients with salt and water depletion a simple test for urine chloride (see 29:3) may be of value when facilities are not available for measuring serum or plasma electrolytes.

Oedema

In this condition of fluid imbalance, abnormally large amounts of interstitial fluid accumulate in the tissue spaces of the body. Gross oedema can lead to salt and water depletion.

The main causes of oedema are as follows:

— Low concentration of plasma proteins resulting in insufficient osmotic pressure to draw water from the tissues back into the plasma. Reduced plasma protein levels occur in protein calorie malnutrition, conditions of famine, diseases of the liver which cause reduced protein production, or when there is a leak of plasma proteins through damaged capillaries as in burns, anoxia, infections, or allergic reactions.

— Blocked or damaged lymphatic vessels preventing the removal of protein from interstitial fluid, e.g. lymphatic filariasis.

— Sodium retention in the extracellular fluid caused by secondary excess of aldosterone, e.g. in heart failure when stimulation of secretion of the hormone is increased.

— Increase in capillary blood pressure resulting in little or no transfer of water from the tissues back into the plasma, e.g. in congestive heart failure, venous thrombosis, and occasionally in pregnancy due to increased pressure on leg veins.

Electrolytes and acid-base balance

For the healthy functioning of the body's cells the reaction (pH) of the extracellular fluid must be kept within the narrow limits of pH 7.37-7.45. This corresponds to a hydrogen ion concentration of 36-44 nmol/l.

During normal metabolic activity, acids are continually being formed. Unless these acids are neutralized immediately and eventually excreted they can seriously affect the acid-base balance in the body. Such acids include carbonic acid, sulphuric acid, acetoacetic acid and phosphoric acids.

Carbonic acid (H_2CO_3) influences acid-base balance the most because it is produced in large amounts from the aerobic metabolism of organic compounds in the tissues.

The balance between acid and base ions is held constant by:

☐ Buffering systems operating in the cells and fluids. The most important is the bicarbonate system which operates in the plasma. The main acid-base regulating reaction is as follows:

$$H^+ \quad + \quad HCO_3^- \quad \rightleftharpoons \quad H_2CO_3$$
Acidic ion   Bicarbonate ion   Carbonic acid

The bicarbonate content of the buffer is controlled by the kidneys.

In the cells the reduced haemoglobin-oxyhaemoglobin and protein buffer systems are important. When the haemoglobin molecule becomes deoxygenated it takes up hydrogen ions from the carbonic acid. When it becomes oxygenated the hydrogen ions are dissociated and join with the bicarbonate to form carbonic acid.

The dihydrogen phosphate-monohydrogen phosphate system has a buffering effect inside the cells and also in the extracellular fluids, especially urine.

☐ The regulating action of the lungs.
To maintain a pH of between 7.37-7.45 the proportion of bicarbonate to carbonic acid in the body fluids must be 20 to 1. The formation of carbonic acid in the cells, its breakdown to bicarbonate, and final removal by the lungs as carbon dioxide are explained in 6:2.

If the plasma carbon dioxide is too high, the respiratory centre is stimulated to increase respiration and excrete more carbon dioxide until the correct pH of the blood is restored. If the carbon dioxide concentration is too low, respiration is depressed so that less carbonic acid in the form of carbon dioxide leaves the lungs which then increases the pH of the blood.

☐ Reabsorption mechanisms of the kidney tubules. The renal tubules contain the enzyme carbonic anhydrase which catalyzes the combination of carbon dioxide and water to form carbonic acid. The acid dissociates into hydrogen ions and bicarbonate ions. The hydrogen ions are secreted into the urine in return for sodium ions and the bicarbonate together with the sodium passes into the plasma to restore the bicarbonate level.

The kidneys excrete hydrogen ions mainly in the form of dibasic phosphate. Sulphate, acetoacetate, and other anions from buffered acids are also excreted and possibly ammonium ions.

Disturbances of acid-base balance

Disorders of acid-base balance are due to increases or decreases in the concentration of bicarbonate or carbonic acid in the blood caused by:

— Introduction into or production in the body of excessive amounts of acidic or base ions that cannot be neutralized by the normal acid-base regulating mechanisms.

— Disorders of pulmonary or renal function.

Acid-base disturbances can be of metabolic or respiratory origin. They are described as metabolic if involving a change in bicarbonate concentration and as respiratory if related to a change in carbon dioxide in solution.†

† Carbon dioxide in solution is directly proportional to the partial pressure (P) of carbon dioxide (PCO_2) in the lungs and arterial blood.

Depending on whether the pH of the intracellular fluid falls below pH 7.37 or rises above pH 7.45, metabolic and respiratory acid-base disturbances are described as acidosis (acidaemia) or alkalosis (alkalaemia):

☐ Metabolic acidosis (bicarbonate deficit)
☐ Metabolic alkalosis (bicarbonate excess)
☐ Respiratory acidosis (carbonic acid excess)
☐ Respiratory alkalosis (carbonic acid deficit)

Alkalosis occurs less frequently than acidosis.

Metabolic acidosis

This is caused either by a reduction of bicarbonate, e.g. following severe diarrhoea, or by an excess of acids in the extracellular fluid, e.g. in diabetic or starvation ketosis when there is an excess of acetoacetic acid.

The overproduction of acid radicles is the commonest cause of metabolic acidosis. Renal failure

where the body cannot excrete acid is another common cause.

Respiratory acidosis

This is due to an increase in carbon dioxide (CO_2) caused by a failure of the lungs to expel it. Ventilatory failure may occur in chronic bronchitis, severe pneumonia, chest injury, damage to respiratory muscle, or following drug overdose.

Metabolic alkalosis

This may be caused either by an increase in bicarbonate or by a deficiency of acids. An excess of bicarbonate is usually due to taking large amounts of bicarbonate salts to relieve gastric hyperacidity. The urine becomes alkaline and bicarbonate ions will be excreted in the urine until the pH of the plasma returns to its correct value. Hydrochloric acid may be lost by severe or prolonged vomiting due to pyloric obstruction.

Potassium depletion may also cause metabolic alkalosis because this encourages the secretion of hydrogen ions by the renal tubules in exchange for sodium.

Respiratory alkalosis

This occurs whenever there is a depletion of carbonic acid due to voluntary hyperventilation or occasionally in association with liver failure, encephalitis, meningitis, or salicylate overdose.

Note: Laboratory tests to investigate acid-base disorders include the measurement of blood pH, carbon dioxide as PCO_2† and bicarbonate (from heparinized anaerobically collected arterial blood). A blood gas analyzer equipped with special electrodes is used to measure the pH and PCO_2 and from these two measurements the bicarbonate can be calculated.‡

† PCO_2 is the partial pressure (P) of carbon dioxide (CO_2) in the gas phase in equilibrium with dissolved CO_2. It is measured in kPa (SI units) or mm Hg (non-SI units).

‡ Plasma bicarbonate ion concentration refers to the amount of bicarbonate (HCO_3^-) in plasma. What is called the standard bicarbonate concentration is the amount of bicarbonate in plasma after the blood has been fully oxygenated and equilibrated in the laboratory to a PCO_2 of 5.3 kPa (40 mm Hg) at 37 °C before separation of the plasma. Both measurements are expressed in mmol/l.

A further measurement that is sometimes made is base excess. This is the amount of strong acid that would be required to titrate 1 litre of fully oxygenated blood to a H^+ of 40 nmol/l (pH 7.4) at 37 °C where the PCO_2 is 5.3 kPa.

In district laboratories unable to analyze blood gases, a titrimetric technique can be used to measure bicarbonate as described in 29:4.

The results of laboratory tests in acid-base disorders are summarized in Table 29.2.

Measuring partial pressure of oxygen (PO₂)

In the investigation of respiratory disorders, especially in conditions of anoxia, measurement of arterial PO_2 with PCO_2 is of value. Measurement of PO_2 also requires the use of a blood gas analyzer.

Table 29.2 Results of Laboratory Tests in Conditions of Acidosis and Alkalosis (before compensation)

	Blood pH	PCO₂	Plasma bicarbonate
Reference range	Arterial 7.37-7.45 Venous 7.32-7.39	35-46 mm Hg (4.5-6.0 kPa)	23-31 mmol/l
Metabolic acidosis	Low ↓	Normal or low	Low ↓↓
Respiratory acidosis	Low ↓	Raised ↑	Raised ↑
Metabolic alkalosis	Raised ↑	Normal or high	Raised ↑↑
Respiratory alkalosis	Raised ↑	Low ↓	Low ↓

29:2 MEASUREMENT OF SODIUM AND POTASSIUM IN SERUM OR PLASMA

The importance of the electrolytes sodium and potassium is explained in 29:1.

Techniques for measuring sodium and potassium

The following techniques are available for measuring sodium and potassium in serum or plasma:

- Flame emission spectrometry using a flame photometer (more correctly termed flame emission spectrometer) which measures the concentration of sodium and potassium in mmol/l.

- Ion selective electrode (ISE) using an ISE analyzer which measures (senses) the activity of sodium and potassium ions and converts the activity measurements to mmol/l.

- Dry reagent (solid phase) technology using sodium and potassium slides or strips and a reflectance meter which measures the concentration of sodium and potassium in mmol/l.

Choice of technique

Up until recently, flame emission spectrometry using a flame photometer was judged to be the only reliable technique for measuring sodium and potassium in body fluids. Few district hospital laboratories in a developing country are able to afford to buy a flame photometer or to maintain a regular gas supply which is needed to operate the system.

An ISE analyzer has the advantage that no gas supply is needed but the analyzer is expensive to buy and the running and maintenance costs are extremely high for a district hospital laboratory (see later text).

Use of sodium and potassium reagent slides or strips and a reflectance meter is the simplest of the systems and it is possible that this technique may make it possible in the future for district hospital laboratories to measure electrolytes. The systems, however, are only just becoming available. Clinical evaluations of the various systems are underway and as yet (1986) there is no information regarding the performance of the systems in tropical and developing countries.

FLAME EMISSION SPECTROMETRY

Principle

Using compressed air, diluted serum or plasma is sprayed as a fine mist of droplets (nebulised) into a non-luminous gas flame which becomes coloured by the characteristic emission of the sodium or potassium metallic ions in the sample. Light of a wavelength corresponding to the metal being measured is selected by a light filter or prism system and allowed to fall on a photosensitive detector system. The amount of light emitted depends on the concentration of metallic ions present.

Many expensive flame photometers are used with an internal lithium standard. The sample is diluted in a diluent which contains a known and constant amount of lithium. The energy emitted in the flame by sodium or potassium is compared with the output from the lithium, enabling the sodium or potassium concentration in mmol/l to be calculated.

Components of a flame photometer

The basic components of a flame photometer are as follows:

Nebuliser (atomizer)

In this, the sample is mixed with air and sprayed to the burner at a constant and reproducible rate. An air compressor is used to provide a stream of air to draw in and nebulise the sample.

Mixing chamber with baffles

In the mixing chamber the atomized sample and fuel are mixed. The baffles deflect any large droplets to waste allowing only the small droplets to reach the flame.

Burner

This converts the metallic ions to uncharged atoms and excites them to emit light. To maintain a steady blue flame both the gas and air pressures have to be carefully controlled.

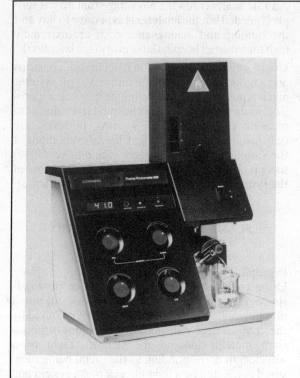

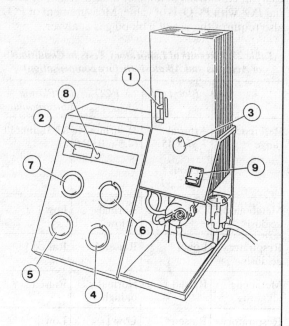

Plate 29.1 Corning model 410 flame photometer. *Courtesy of Corning.*
Components 1 Filter selector 2 Digital display 3 Inspection flap 4 Fuel adjustment control
5 Blank control 6 Coarse sensitivity control 7 Fine sensitivity control 8 Decimal push button
9 Power switch

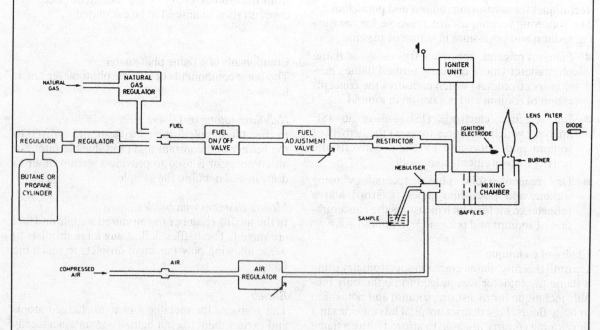

Fig. 29.1 Working principle of a flame photometer.

Lens and filter system
A lens focuses the light emitted from the flame and a narrow band filter selects the wavelength of the metal being measured.

Photosensitive detector system
A diode is used to convert the emitted light into an electric current which is measured. In newer types of flame photometers, sodium and potassium results are displayed directly in mmol/l.

Note: The basic structure of a flame photometer is shown in Fig. 29.1 and Plate 29.1.

The operating structures and maintenance of a flame photometer vary from one manufacturer to another. It is essential to follow exactly the manufacturer's operating and maintenance instructions.

Types of flame photometer
Instruments such as the Radiometer FLM 3 flame photometer, Gilford Microflame Photometer and Corning Model 480 flame photometer are equipped with an internal lithium standard. Such instruments simultaneously measure sodium and potassium and provide digital readouts of the concentration units. Instruments with an internal standard are very expensive.

Other flame photometers such as the Corning Model 410 medical flame photometer measure sodium and potassium by comparing the light emitted from the sample with that from standard solutions. Separate dilutions are required for measuring each electrolyte. The Corning Model 410 flame photometer is shown in Plate 29.1. It can be fitted with a lineariser module (recommended) which gives direct concentration readouts for sodium and potassium. Corning also make available an air compressor (No. 856) for use with the Model 410 which has been specially designed for operation in conditions of high temperature and humidity. A dilutor is also available.

Cost and availability of Corning Model 410C flame photometer
The 410C flame photometer complete with filters, standards solutions, lineariser module, and instruction manual costs about £845 (1986).

An air compressor and fuel regulator are *essential* to operate the flame photometer. The No. 586 air compressor (for tropical climates) costs about £283.50 (1986). Fuel regulators are available for use with propane, butane, or natural gas, priced about £26. The Corning 805 Dilutor complete with connections and manual costs about £395 (1986).

Quality control
The following are important when measuring sodium and potassium using a flame photometer:

☐ Collect the specimen correctly. The blood must not be collected from an arm receiving an electrolyte or dextrose intravenous infusion. Haemolysis of the specimen must be avoided (see 26:4) and the plasma or serum must be separated from the cells within 2½ hours. A suitable anticoagulant is lithium heparin. An anticoagulant which contains sodium or potassium must not be used. If preferred, *fresh* serum can be used.

☐ Dilute the serum or plasma with care. Good quality calibrated pipettes or a sensitive dilutor must be used to measure the very small amount of sample used in the test. A diluent recommended by the manufacturer of the instrument should be used. This must be free from bacteria or moulds. A suitable preservative to prevent the growth of moulds is formalin (1-2 drops per litre of diluent). Commercially prepared diluents contain preservatives.

Note: Small strands of fibrin, bacteria, or moulds can cause inaccuracies by interrupting or blocking the flow of sample through the nebuliser.

☐ Prepare standards accurately or preferably use those supplied by the manufacturer. The standards should be stored in plastic (polypropylene) containers to prevent sodium contamination which can occur if glass bottles are used.

☐ Use chemically clean containers to prevent contamination of samples. Do not use the thumb to cover containers during mixing because perspiration from the thumb contains a high concentration of electrolytes.

☐ Use a stable well-maintained flame photometer. The components of a flame photometer must be cleaned regularly and maintained as instructed by the manufacturer. The nebuliser needs to be well rinsed after use.

☐ Make sure that the gas supply is of the correct pressure and of the type recommended for use with the flame photometer.

☐ Use an air supply that is clean, free from water, and at the correct pressure. If condensation in the air supply tubing (due to conditions of high temperature and humidity) is a problem, an air compressor with a water separator should be used or a compressor designed for use in humid climates such as the Corning air compressor No. 856 (see previous text).

☐ Include adequate control samples with each batch of tests. The principles of quality control in clinical chemistry are described in Chapter 27.

When measuring sodium and potassium using a flame photometer, the following should be attainable:

Sodium:	— OCV, of around 1%
	— RCV, not exceeding 2%
Potassium:	— OCV, of around 1.5%
	— RCV, not exceeding 3%

ISE TECHNIQUE

Principle

The principle of measuring sodium and potassium using ion selective electrodes (ISEs) is similar to that used for measuring pH except sodium and potassium ion selective electrodes are used instead of a hydrogen selective electrode.

An ion selective electrode consists of a detector electrode and an electrically conductive membrane which separates the sample solution of unknown activity from a solution of fixed ion activity which fills the electrode. A difference in ionic composition of the two solutions causes an electrical potential difference to develop across the membrane. Changes in potential across the selective membrane are measured with respect to a reference electrode, the potential of which is constant. The change in potential difference between the reference electrode and the ion selective electrode for the sample is compared with the potential difference for a calibration solution of known composition.

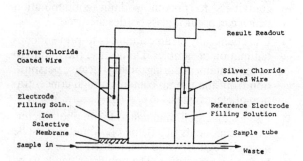

Fig. 29.2   Diagram to show the parts of an ion selective electrode analyser.
Courtesy of Dr S. C. H. Smith.

Components of an ISE analyzer

Structurally an ISE analyzer is based on an electrochemical cell. Its basic components are as follows:

Detector electrode and ion selective membrane
Sodium ISE: This is made of a special glass which is selective for sodium, i.e. only sodium ions are free to move to any extent.

Potassium ISE: This is usually constructed from polyvinyl chloride (PVC) in which the antibiotic valinomycin is immobilized. The valinomycin selectively transports potassium ions across the membrane.

Reference electrode
This is usually a calomel (Hg/Hg_2Cl_2) or silver chloride ($Ag/AgCl$) electrode. The electrical potential of the reference electrode must remain constant for long periods.

Voltmeter
This measures the potentials developed. Sodium and potassium results are displayed digitally.

Electrolyte solution
The circuit of the electrochemical cell is completed by an electrolyte solution. A silver coated wire enables the electric cell to be completed with the reference electrode.

Types of ISE analyzer

There are two types of ISE analyzer:

— ISE analyzers that carry out measurements on diluted samples, e.g. Beckman Electrolyte II, and ISE's found in some multichannel analyzers such as the Hitachi 705 or Technicon RA 1000.

— ISE analyzers that carry out measurements on undiluted samples. Examples of this type of analyzer include the 'stat' Orion 1020, Corning 614, Kone Microlyte, Nova 1, and Radiometer KNA 1. When using this direct type of ISE analyzer anticoagulated whole blood can be used. Samples do not require centrifuging or dilution and therefore results can be obtained quickly. A direct ISE analyzer is shown in Plate 29.2.

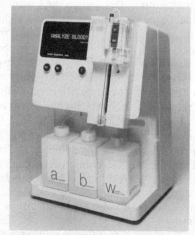

Plate 29.2 ISE analyzer. *Courtesy of Orion.*

Cost and availability of Orion 1020 ISE analyzer
Model 1020 Na/K analyzer costs about US $5000. This price includes battery/charger unit (can be operated from a battery for 45 minutes), 2 bottles of standards, 1 bottle reference electrode filling solution, 1 bottle daily wash solution, electrodes (×1 each Na, K, and reference), 2 reference membrane assemblies, 1 fluid bath module, and essential waste bottle and tubing.

Electrodes require replacement every 6-12 months. Na and K electrodes cost US $50-55 and reference electrode US $150. Sample probe replacement (every year) costs US $55 and reference membrane assembly (every 2-3 m) costs US $.65.

The standard and reference filling solutions cost US $120 (×4 standard A, ×1 standard B, ×1 reference filling solution). Electrode rinsing and daily wash solutions cost US $15/

125 ml. A box of 6 controls (3.5 ml /vial) costs US $30. Tubing requires replacement every few months and this costs US $55 per kit.

Note: Prices quoted are International prices (1985-1986). Further details of local agents etc can be obtained from Orion Research Inc. (see Appendix II).

ISE measurement of electrolytes

ISE analyzers measure (sense) the electrochemical *activity* of ions whereas flame photometers measure the *concentration* of ions. Activity values are lower than concentration values, e.g. at a sodium concentration of 140 mmol/l in normal plasma the measured sodium activity would be about 105. To avoid confusion, most ISE analyzer manufacturers adjust the activity measurements of their instruments to give readings that are compatible with the concentration results given by flame photometers. The necessary adjustment is made by using specially formulated calibration solutions (produced by the manufacturers) and therefore these solutions *cannot* be interchanged between instruments.

Samples containing high concentrations of lipid or protein

By flame photometry a falsely low sodium concentration is obtained (pseudohyponatraemia) because of the space taken up by the lipid and protein whereas a correct result is obtained when using a *direct* ISE analyzer because the activity of the ion in the plasma water is measured.

Cost of analyzing sodium and potassium by ISE

While ISE analyzers do not require flammable gases, air compressors, or large quantities of distilled water for their operation, compared with flame photometers ISE analyzers can be very expensive to operate and maintain.

Unlike flame photometers, ISE analyzers incur running costs even when they are not being used because the electrodes must be kept washed at regular intervals with fresh conditioning solutions. Electrodes usually require replacing every 6-12 months (even if only a few determinations are performed).

Most direct ISE analyzers cost £3000-£4500 (1985-1986). Estimations of running costs will depend on the number of electrolyte determinations performed.[1] For small workloads, e.g. around 10 samples per day, an ISE analyzer can be seven times more expensive to operate than a flame photometer. For larger workloads, e.g. 100 tests per day, the running costs may be only three times more expensive. Comparison of ISE running costs against using electrolyte dry reagent slides or strips and a reflectance meter are not yet available but the latter systems should be less expensive.

Quality control

Regular maintenance of an ISE analyzer on a daily basis is *essential* to ensure reliable performance. This includes cleaning the fluid transport system, conditioning the electrodes, changing the membranes that cover the electrode tips, and performing calibration routines to assess electrode condition. Electrodes require replacing usually every 6-12 months due to loss of sensitivity and selectivity.

Full details of quality control procedures, daily maintenance and replacement of electrodes and other parts of an ISE analyzer will be found in the manufacturer's instruction manual. These must be followed exactly. Special control solutions are required. These are often aqueous control solutions which are not ideal. Some commercially available control sera for use with ISE analyzers do not give satisfactory results.

Important: If considering purchasing an ISE analyzer, obtain full details from the manufacturer of costs (including prices of the required solutions, replacement electrodes and other parts), availability of spares and consumables, maintenance, and control procedures. Make sure a demonstration of operation and maintenance can be provided.

ISE Working Group

At the time of this Manual going to press (1986), a European Working Group is studying the introduction of commercial ISE analyzers into clinical practice (for calcium as well as sodium and potassium). Further information about ISE analyzers can be obtained by writing to the European Group. Letters should be addressed to Dr A H J Mass, Dept of Cardiology, University Hospital, Catharijnesingel 101, Utrecht, Netherlands or to Mr P M G Broughton, Wolfson Research Laboratories, Queen Elizabeth Medical Centre, Birmingham B15 2TH, UK.

ELECTROLYTE DRY REAGENT SLIDES OR STRIPS

As mentioned under *Choice of technique* at the beginning of this subunit, the use of stable dry reagent slides and strips and a reflectance meter (measures reflected light) is a recently developed technology for measuring sodium and potassium.

The three systems that are in use or are being developed for measuring electrolytes are as follows:

- *Kodak Ektachem DT60* analyzer, manufactured by Eastman Kodak Company.
- *Seralyzer* system, manufactured by Ames Division Miles Laboratories Ltd.
- *Reflotron* system, manufactured by Boehringer Mannheim.

   All three systems can be used for measuring a wide range of substances in blood (see 26:1). For up to date information, availability and cost of equipment, test slides or strips and controls and the *results of clinical evaluations*, readers should write to Eastman Kodak, Ames Division Miles Laboratories and Boehringer Mannheim (for addresses, see Appendix II).

Approximate reference (normal) ranges for sodium and potassium

Sodium:

134-146 mmol/l (134-146 mEq/l)

Potassium:

Adults: 3.6-5.0 mmol/l (3.6-5.0 mEq/l)
Newborns: 4.0-5.9 mmol/l (4.0-5.9 mEq/l)
Values are highest immediately after birth.

Interpretation of sodium results

Increases

An elevated sodium level is known as hypernatraemia. It is nearly always due to dehydration with the rise in sodium (also chloride and urea) being due to a concentrating effect.

A high sodium level must be reported as soon as possible. Severe hypernatraemia (sodium level that has reached 155 mmol/l) is a serious finding which requires immediate correction to prevent coma and death.

Decreases

A low sodium level is known as hyponatraemia. It is a commoner finding than hypernatraemia. A greatly reduced level (as low as 125 mmol/l) indicates a dangerous condition and must be reported as soon as possible.

A low sodium level may accompany any severe illness including viral and bacterial infections, malaria, heart attacks, heart failure, strokes, and tumours of the brain and lung. Other causes of hyponatraemia include:

— Surgery or severe accident.
— Side effect of some drugs.
— When loss of salt and water is replaced by water only.
— Inadequate salt intake.
— Loss of sodium in the urine as in salt-losing nephritis.
— Hypoadrenalism (Addison's disease). In tropical countries hypoadrenalism can be caused by tuberculosis of the adrenal glands.

Interpretation of potassium results

Increases

A raised potassium level is known as hyperkalaemia. Levels above 6.5 mmol/l are particularly dangerous and must be reported *immediately* because fatal disorders of heart rhythm can occur suddenly.

An important cause of hyperkalaemia is renal failure. Other causes include adrenal insufficiency and excessive potassium chloride treatment with diuretics to compensate for potassium losses.

Falsely high potassium result: This can occur if a blood sample is haemolyzed due to poor venepuncture technique, a sample is left for a long time

(e.g. overnight) without the plasma or serum being removed or if whole blood is refrigerated before it is centrifuged. Red cells contain a high concentration of potassium.

Decreases

A low potassium level is called hypokalaemia. Causes include:

— Inadequate intake of potassium in the diet.
— Therapy with certain drugs such as diuretics, laxatives, corticosteroids.
— Cushing's syndrome.
— Conditions associated with prolonged diarrhoea or loss of other gut fluids.

Misleading sodium and potassium results due to an electrolyte or dextrose infusion

Misleading sodium and potassium values may be obtained if blood is collected from an arm receiving an intravenous electrolyte or dextrose infusion. This should be suspected if a grossly abnormal result is obtained from a post-surgical patient especially if the test has not been requested urgently. If an electrolyte infusion is the cause, a chloride result will give the best clue to this type of error since the chloride will be artificially high due to the infusion of physiological saline which contains 150 mmol/l chloride.

29:3 SEMIQUANTITATIVE ESTIMATION OF CHLORIDE IN URINE

When unable to measure plasma electrolytes, a simple test to estimate chloride in urine may be of value in the management of patients with salt and water depletion. Loss of water together with dissolved salts results in the conservation of sodium and chloride by the kidneys and therefore a lower concentration of sodium chloride in the urine.

Depending on the amount of sodium chloride excreted in the urine a patient can be classified as a mild, moderate, or severe case of salt and water depletion.

Principle of test

When acidified silver nitrate is added to urine, silver chloride is the only salt which is precipitated. The degree of precipitation (cloudiness) is therefore a measure of the chloride concentration in the urine.

Reagents

— Acidified silver nitrate   Reagent No. 7

— Standard solutions containing 150, 75, 50, 30, 7.5, 3.0 mmol/l sodium chloride

Preparation of sodium chloride standards 150, 75, 50, 30, 7.5, 3.0 mmol/l
1. Take six large tubes and label them 150, 75, 50, 30, 7.5, and 3.0.

2. Pipette into each tube as follows:

Tube	Distilled water	Physiological saline
150	—	10.0 ml
75	5.0 ml	5.0 ml
50	6.7 ml	3.3 ml
30	8.0 ml	2.0 ml
7.5	9.5 ml	0.5 ml
3.0	9.8 ml	0.2 ml

3. Stopper each tube and mix well.

4. Take six small tubes (2 to 5 ml capacity) and label them 150, 75, 50, 30, 7.5, and 3.0 mmol/l.

    Transfer 1 ml from each of the larger tubes to the set of small tubes.

5. Add 1 ml of acidified silver nitrate reagent to each of the small tubes, stopper and mix.

    Caution: Do not mouth-pipette the reagent because it is corrosive. Handle it with care because although colourless it will stain skin, clothes, bench surfaces, etc, and the brown colour is difficult to remove.

    Note: The small standard tubes can be kept for 3 or 4 days providing they are kept tightly stoppered and in a cool place.

Method of estimating urinary chloride
1. Pipette 1 ml of clear urine into a test tube of the same size as the small standard tubes.

    If the urine is cloudy, filter or centrifuge it to obtain a clear sample for testing.

2. Add 1 ml of acidified silver nitrate reagent to the urine and mix.

    Caution: Do not mouth-pipette the reagent because it is corrosive. Handle it with care because although colourless it will stain skin, clothes, bench surfaces, etc, and the brown colour is difficult to remove.

3. Examine the urine for a cloudiness. Estimate the approximate concentration of chloride in the urine by matching the cloudiness with the standards. Matching is best carried out against a dark background.

4. Report the approximate chloride concentration in the urine in mmol/l.

Note: If the urine remains clear after adding the reagent report the test as 'no chloride detected'.

Interpretation of results
The sodium chloride content in urine from a patient with moderate to severe salt and water depletion will be less than 10 mmol/l (or less than 20 mmol/l per 24 h). The salt deficiency will not be corrected until the amount of sodium chloride being excreted reaches 65 mmol/l or more.

Fantus test
This is not recommended as a test for estimating urinary chloride because the titration end point is unreliable when the chloride content is low.

29:4 MEASUREMENT OF SERUM OR PLASMA BICARBONATE
Titrimetric Method[2]

As explained in 29:1, bicarbonate is important in regulating acid-base balance in the body.

Principle of titrimetric method
A known amount of strong hydrochloric acid is added to a fresh sample of serum or plasma. The carbon dioxide formed is expelled by shaking the sample. The hydrogen ions that remain are titrated against sodium hydroxide using the indicator phenol red.

Reagents
— Sodium chloride, 10 g/l carbon   Reagent No. 67
   dioxide-free
— Hydrochloric acid, 10 mmol/l   Reagent No. 45
   carbon dioxide-free
— Sodium hydroxide, 10 mmol/l   Reagent No. 75
   carbon dioxide-free
— Bicarbonate standard,   Reagent No. 16
   25 mmol/l
— Phenol red indicator   Reagent No. 52
— Antifoaming agent, i.e. isoamyl alcohol or *Triton X100*

The 10 mmol/l hydrochloric acid and sodium hydroxide solutions require preparation weekly.

The phenol red indicator is stable indefinitely when stored in a tightly-capped plastic bottle.

Method

Specimen: The test requires 0.2 ml (200 μl) of patient's *fresh* plasma or serum. The sample must be free from haemolysis (see 26:4) and analyzed as soon as possible after collection. The test is performed in duplicate.

1. Add an antifoaming agent (*Triton X100* or isoamyl alcohol) to the plasma or serum sample by touching the end of a thin glass rod into the agent and then rotating the rod in the plasma or serum.

2. Prepare a comparison solution against which the end-point colour of the test and standard solution can be matched:

   — Pipette 6.0 ml of the carbon dioxide-free 10 g/l sodium chloride solution into a small conical (Erlenmeyer) flask or if unavailable into a small beaker.
   — Add 0.1 ml (100 μl) of fresh test plasma or serum and mix.
   — Add 0.1 ml of phenol red indicator, stopper the flask and mix gently. The colour of the diluted sample will turn pink.

3. Take four small conical flasks or small beakers (same size as used for the comparison solution) and label as follows:

   T1, T2   — Test (performed in duplicate)
   S1, S2   — Standard (performed in duplicate)

4. Pipette into each flask or beaker as follows:

	S1	S2	T1	T2
Sodium chloride, 10 g/l	4 ml		4 ml	
Bicarbonate standard, 25 mmol/l	0.1 ml		—	
Patient's fresh serum or plasma	—		0.1 ml	
Hydrochloric acid, 10 mmol/l	1 ml		1 ml	

5. Swirl each flask rapidly to expel the carbon dioxide which forms from the reaction of the bicarbonate with the hydrochloric acid. Leave each flask for at least 1 minute before titrating.

6. Add 0.1 ml (100 μl) of phenol red indicator to each flask and mix.

7. Fill a microburette with 10 mmol/l sodium hydroxide solution (carbon dioxide-free, see *Reagents*).

8. Titrate the contents of each flask or beaker with the 10 mmol/l sodium hydroxide until a pink colour which matches the colour in the comparison flask (or beaker) is reached and persists for about 15 seconds. This is the end point of the reaction.

Note: Near the end-point the colour tends to turn and then fade after each drop of sodium hydroxide is added.

9. Note how much sodium hydroxide has been added. Calculate the bicarbonate concentration in the standard and patient's sample as follows:

   Serum bicarbonate in mmol/l = A $\times$ 100

   where: A = 1.00 − Volume of sodium hydroxide used

Bicarbonate standard value
This should be within the range 24-26 mmol/l. The reason for including a bicarbonate standard is to check that the concentrations of the 10 mmol/l hydrochloric acid and 10 mmol/l sodium hydroxide solutions are correct.

Quality control

The principles of quality control in clinical chemistry are described in Chapter 27. For the estimation of plasma bicarbonate by the titrimetric method the following should be attainable:

— OCV, of around 10%
— RCV, not exceeding 20%

Approximate bicarbonate reference (normal) range

23-31 mmol/l (23-31 mEq/l)

No calculation is required to convert from mmol/l to mEq/l because 1 mEq is numerically the same as 1 mmol for monovalent ions.

Note: The titrimetric bicarbonate technique measures the bicarbonate concentration rather than the total carbon dioxide content of the sample which would be about 1-3 mmol/l higher for normal persons.

Interpretation of results

Bicarbonate levels may be affected by a variety of respiratory and metabolic disturbances which affect acid-base balance.

Increases
Raised bicarbonate levels are due either to a fai-

Summary of Bicarbonate Method

For detailed instructions, see text

Preparation of Comparison Solution
Pipette into a small conical flask or beaker as follows:

Sodium chloride, 10 g/l	6.0 ml
Patient's fresh serum or plasma	0.1 ml
(treated with antifoaming agent)	
Phenol red indicator	0.1 ml

Mix well

Measurement of bicarbonate Pipette into small flasks or beaker as follows:	STANDARD S1 S2	TEST T1 T2
Sodium chloride, 10 g/l	4 ml	4 ml
Bicarbonate standard, 25 mmol/l	0.1 ml	—
Patient's fresh serum or plasma .... (treated with antifoaming agent)	—	0.1 ml
Hydrochloric acid, 10 mmol/l	1 ml	1 ml

Swirl each flask or beaker to expel carbon dioxide

Leave for 1 minute

Add 0.1 ml of phenol red indicator to each flask and mix

Titrate with sodium hydroxide, 10 mmol/l solution until the colour matches the comparison flask

Serum bicarbonate mmol/l = A × 100

where: A = 1.00 – Volume of sodium hydroxide used

Average results of duplicate tests

Standard value should be 24-26 mmol/l

0.1 ml = 100 μl

lure of the lungs to excrete carbon dioxide efficiently (respiratory acidosis) when the levels are raised to compensate for the increased pCO_2 or to excessive amounts of circulating bicarbonate (metabolic alkalosis).

Decreases
Decreased bicarbonate levels can be caused either by increased utilization of bicarbonate (metabolic acidosis) or very occasionally by loss of carbon dioxide due to hyperventilation (respiratory alkalosis).

Note: The terms respiratory acidosis and alkalosis and metabolic acidosis and alkalosis are explained at the end of subunit 29:1.

References

1   Broughton, P. M. G., and Woodford, F. P. *Journal of Clinical Pathology*, **36**, p 1028, 1983.

2   Hodes, M. E. *Standard Methods of Clinical Chemistry*, **1**, pp 19-22, 1953.

Recommended Reading

Baron, D. N. *A Short Textbook of Chemical Pathology*, Hodder and Stoughton, 4th Edition, 1982. ELBS edition 1984 available at £2.

Whitby, L. G., Percy-Robb, I. W., Smith, A. F. *Lecture Notes on Clinical Chemistry*, Blackwell Scientific, 3rd Edition, 1984.

Walmsley, R. N., and White, G. H. *A Guide to Diagnostic Clinical Chemistry*, Blackwell, 1983.

Acknowledgement

The author wishes to acknowledge the assistance of Dr S C H Smith, Senior Biochemist, Dept of Clinical Chemistry, Birmingham Maternity Hospital, for contributing artwork and text describing ISE analyzers and their use in measuring sodium and potassium.

30

Tests to Investigate Liver, Pancreatic, and Gastrointestinal Diseases

30:1 INVESTIGATION OF LIVER DISEASES

The liver is a complex organ which forms part of the reticuloendothelial system, converts toxic substances to harmless compounds, produces bile, and is involved in the metabolism of bilirubin, proteins, carbohydrates, lipids, hormones, and vitamins (see 8:4).

In tropical countries diseases of the liver are common and often severe.

Common causes of liver disease in tropical countries

□ Hepatitis due to hepatitis viruses and less frequently to other viruses (e.g. yellow fever virus, Marburg and Ebola viruses, Epstein-Barr virus, cytomegalovirus), bacteria such as *Leptospira interrogans*, parasites including *Toxoplasma gondii*, and certain drugs and toxins.

□ Cirrhosis caused by alcohol and dietary toxins. The ingestion of alkaloid toxins in 'bush teas' is a cause of veno-occlusive disease (narrowing of central and sublobular hepatic veins) in the West Indies, parts of Africa and the Middle East. An excess of hepatic copper is linked to infantile cirrhosis in India.

□ Hepatoma, especially in areas where there is a high incidence of viral hepatitis.

□ Parasitic diseases, especially visceral leishmaniasis, hepatic amoebiasis, hepatosplenic schistosomiasis, hepatic hydatid disease, repeated infection with malaria parasites, and severe infections with *Opisthorchis* and *Fasciola* species.

Tests used to investigate liver disorders

In district laboratories the following tests are most frequently used to investigate the causes of liver disease and jaundice, to assess the extent of liver damage, and to monitor a patient's progress:

- Serum or plasma total bilirubin
- Serum or plasma alkaline phosphatase
- Serum or plasma aspartate aminotransferase
- Serum or plasma albumin
- Urine bilirubin and urobilinogen

Note: Other tests may also be required, e.g. serum protein electrophoresis and measurement of serum alpha-feto protein. For such investigations,

specimens will need to be sent to the Regional Laboratory for analysis (see 26:7).

Tests used to investigate liver disorders should be requested specifically. It is a waste of valuable resources to perform *routinely* a full range of 'liver function tests' on every patient requiring investigation when some patients may not require such comprehensive testing.

Jaundice

Liver disorders are often associated with jaundice (icterus). Visible jaundice occurs when the concentration of bilirubin in the plasma rises to more than twice its normal limit, i.e. about 34 μmol/l (2 mg%). The whites of the eyes appear yellow and the skin and body fluids also become pigmented.

Types of bilirubin

Bilirubin is a product of red cell breakdown (see 8:4). The term unconjugated or indirect bilirubin refers to bilirubin before it is conjugated (joined to glucuronic acid) in the liver. It circulates in the plasma bound to albumin and is water-insoluble. It cannot be filtered out by the kidney glomeruli and is therefore not found in urine.

Conjugated or direct bilirubin refers to bilirubin which has been conjugated in the liver to form water-soluble mono- and diglucuronides of bilirubin. In certain forms of jaundice (not haemolytic) it can be found in urine.

Haemolytic jaundice

In haemolytic (prehepatic) jaundice, more bilirubin is produced than the liver can metabolize, e.g. in severe haemolysis (breakdown of red cells). The excess bilirubin which builds up in the plasma is mostly of the unconjugated type and is therefore not found in the urine.

Hepatocellular jaundice

In hepatocellular (hepatic) jaundice, there is a build up of bilirubin in the plasma because it is not transported, conjugated, or excreted by the liver cells because they are damaged, e.g. in viral hepatitis. The excess bilirubin is usually of both the unconjugated and conjugated types with bilirubin being found in the urine.

Obstructive jaundice

In obstructive (posthepatic) jaundice, bilirubin builds up in the plasma because its flow is obstructed in the small bile channels or in the main bile duct.This can be caused by gall stones or a tumour obstructing or closing the biliary tract. The excess bilirubin is mostly of the conjugated type and is therefore found in the urine. The term cholestasis is used to describe a failure of bile flow.

Chart 30.1 Common Findings in Tests used to Investigate Jaundice

Tests	Haemolytic Jaundice	Hepatocellular Jaundice	Obstructive Jaundice
SERUM OR PLASMA			
Bilirubin	Slight to moderately raised	Slight to moderately raised	Moderate to markedly raised
Alkaline phosphatase	Normal	Slight to moderately raised	Moderate to markedly raised
Aspartate aminotransferase	Normal to slightly raised	Moderate to markedly raised	Slight to moderately raised
Albumin	Normal	Reduced if disease is prolonged	Normal or reduced
URINE			
Bilirubin	Negative	Positive	Positive (strongly)
Urobilinogen	Increased	Normal or slightly increased	Normal or absent

Note: In differentiating hepatocellular disease from obstructive jaundice, serum or plasma alkaline phosphatase and aspartate aminotransferase tests are of particular value. Alkaline phosphatase levels are lower and aspartate aminotransferase levels are usually much higher in hepatocellular disease than in obstructive jaundice.

In viral hepatitis, aspartate aminotransferase levels are markedly raised.

Note: Jaundiced patients often have both hepatocellular and obstructive features. It is usual to find some obstruction when there is damage to liver cells and following obstruction there is usually some liver cell damage.

30:2 MEASUREMENT OF SERUM OR PLASMA TOTAL BILIRUBIN
Modification of Jendrassik and Grof Method[1]

The metabolism of bilirubin is described and illustrated in 8:9.

Choice of test method
A method based on that developed by Jendrassik and Grof is recommended as a manual colorimetric method for measuring serum or plasma bilirubin.

Compared with some other methods (e.g. Malloy and Evelyn, Lathe and Ruthven, Watson and Powell), the Jendrassik and Grof method can be performed with greater precision and is more rapid, sensitive and specific. Methods which use methanol are not recommended.[2] In the method described only the measurement of total bilirubin is described. Differentiation between haemolytic jaundice (unconjugated bilirubinaemia) and obstructive jaundice (conjugated bilirubinaemia) can be made by testing the urine for bilirubin (see 30:3) or by haematological tests.

Bilirubin test kits
Sigma Chemical Company produce a manual colorimetric bilirubin test kit (Ref. 605-D) based on the Jendrassik and Grof method. The technique is rapid and there is minimal interference from haemolysis.

The Sigma kit is priced about £14 for a maximum of 100 tests (1985-1986). It includes a protein-based bilirubin standard of approx. 166 μmol/l (10 mg%) which is reconstituted with 3 ml of water. Details of calibration are given and all the reagents are supplied. Each kit contains 10 vials of diazo reagent in lyophilized form. When prepared each 10 ml vial of *working* diazo reagent is sufficient for 20 tests and has a shelf life of 5 days at 0-5 °C.

Note: For further comments regarding the purchasing and use of clinical chemistry kits, see 26:1.

Principle of the Jendrassik and Grof total bilirubin method
Sulphanilic acid is diazotized by the nitrous acid produced from the reaction between sodium nitrite and hydrochloric acid.

Bilirubin reacts with the diazotized sulphanilic acid (diazo reagent) to form azobilirubin. Caffeine is an accelerator and gives a rapid and complete conversion to azobilirubin. The pink acid azobilirubin is converted to blue azobilirubin by an alkaline tartrate reagent and the absorbance of the blue-green solution is read in a colorimeter using an orange filter or in a spectrophotometer at wavelength 600 nm. Measurement of the azobilirubin in an alkaline medium removes turbidity and increases specificity. There is very little interference by other pigments at 600 nm wavelength.

Bilirubin + caffeine/ + diazo $\longrightarrow$ Acid
        benzoate   reagent   azobilirubin

Acid azobilirubin + alkaline $\longrightarrow$ Alkaline
                   tartrate   azobilirubin
                                      Blue-green

Calibration

The bilirubin assay is most easily calibrated from a serum of high bilirubin concentration. The Nyegaard *Seronorm Bilirubin Paediatric* serum (value around 340 μmol/l) is recommended because it is of animal origin (no risk of containing hepatitis viruses) and has good stability. For the address of Nyegaard and Co, see Appendix II.

In its lyophilized form, *Seronorm Bilirubin Paediatric* has a shelf-life of at least 3 years when stored in the dark at 2-8 °C. After reconstitution (with distilled water) it is stable for 4 days in the dark at 2-8 °C. When stored frozen (in amounts ready for use) at −20 °C or below, the serum can be kept for several weeks. There is a 3% decrease in value per week at −20 °C. It costs about £17 for 6 × 3 ml (1985-1986).

Other bilirubin reference sera

If unable to obtain *Seronorm Bilirubin Paediatric*, a reference serum of high bilirubin content (about 350 μmol/l) can also be obtained from Laboratories biotrol or Boehringer Mannheim (for addresses see Appendix II).

The biotrol product is called *C.A.M-Trol Bilirubine High level* (ref. A02333). It is of bovine origin, costs about £19 for 5 × 2 ml (1985-1986) and in lyophilized form is stable for 2 years in the dark at 2-8 °C and a few hours when reconstituted.

The Boehringer product is called *Precibil* (ref. 158046). It is a *human-based* product, costs about £12 for 4 × 2 ml (1985-1986) and is stable in lyophilized form for about 2 years in the dark at 2-8 °C and 2 days at 2-8 °C when reconstituted.

Bilirubin standards
1. Reconstitute the *Seronorm Bilirubin Paediatric* serum (or other reference serum) exactly as instructed by the manufacturer.

    Important: Bilirubin is unstable. It is rapidly destroyed by ultraviolet light, therefore protect the serum from daylight and fluorescent light.

2. Prepare five standards by taking five small containers and numbering them 1 to 5. Pipette

accurately into each as follows:

Container	Reference serum	Physiological saline
1	0.1 ml	0.9 ml
2	0.2 ml	0.8 ml
3	0.5 ml	0.5 ml
4	0.8 ml	0.2 ml
5	Neat serum	—

Mix well the contents in each container.

Important: Protect the bilirubin from direct light by wrapping black paper or aluminium foil around each container.

3. Calculate the concentration of bilirubin in each standard by multiplying the concentration of bilirubin in the serum (as given by the manufacturer) by the following factors:

    Standard, 1: multiply by 0.1
              2:        „   0.2
              3:        „   0.5
              4:        „   0.8
              5:        „   1.0 (neat serum)

    Example
    If the reference serum contains 340 μmol/l bilirubin, the concentration in each of the standards would be 34 μmol/l, 68 μmol/l, 170 μmol/l, 272 μmol/l, and 340 μmol/l.

Note: The manufacturer's calibration instructions which accompany the serum can also be followed but these usually recommend the use of four instead of five standards.

Preparation of bilirubin calibration graph
1. Take ten tubes and label them 1 to 5 and B1 to B5 (each standard requires its own blank (B) solution as in the test method).

2. Pipette 1 ml of caffeine-benzoate reagent (see *Reagents*) into each tube.

    Caution: Caffeine is a harmful chemical, therefore handle with care and *do not* mouth-pipette.

3. Add to each tube as follows:

    Tube
    1 and 1B ..... 0.1 ml (100 μl) standard No. 1
    2 and 2B .... 0.1 ml standard No. 2
    3 and 3B .... 0.1 ml standard No. 3
    4 and 4B .... 0.1 ml standard No. 4
    5 and 5B .... 0.1 ml standard No. 5

4. Add 0.5 ml of diazo reagent (see *Reagents*) to tubes 1, 2, 3, 4, 5 and mix well.

Summary of Bilirubin Method

For detailed instructions, see text

Pipette into tubes as follows:	STANDARD S	STANDARD BLANK SB	CONTROL C	CONTROL BLANK CB	TESTS 1,2, etc	TEST BLANKS 1B, 2B, etc
Caffeine - benzoate reagent ..	1 ml	1 ml	1 ml	1 ml	1 ml	1 ml
Standard serum	0.1 ml	0.1 ml	—	—	—	—
Control serum	—	—	0.1 ml	0.1 ml	—	—
Patient's serum or plasma .	—	—	—	—	0.1 ml	0.1 ml
Diazo reagent	0.5 ml	—	0.5 ml	—	0.5 ml	—
Sulphanilic acid, 5 g/l	—	0.5 ml	—	0.5 ml	—	0.5 ml

Mix well

Leave at room temperature for   5 minutes

Alkaline tartrate reagent ..	1 ml	1 ml	1 ml	1 ml	1 ml	1 ml

Mix well

READ ABSORBANCES

Colorimeter: Orange filter, e.g. Ilford No. 607
Spectrophotometer: 600 nm

Zero the instrument with distilled water

Read the blanks first

Subtract blank readings

Obtain values from the calibration graph if the result of the standard agrees with the calibration. If not, calculate the results as follows:

Total bilirubin μmol/l $= \dfrac{\text{Absorbance of test or control}}{\text{Absorbance of standard}} \times$ Concentration of standard

Report patients' results if control value is acceptable

0.1 ml = 100 μl
0.5 ml = 500 μl

5. Add 0.5 ml of sulphanilic acid, 5 g/l reagent (see *Reagents*) to tubes 1B, 2B, 3B,4B, 5B and mix well.

6. Leave for 5 minutes at room temperature (20-28 °C).

   Note: A variety of waiting times are recommended for the Jendrassik and Grof method. Using caffeine-benzoate, 99.5% of the colour is developed within 30 seconds.[2]

7. Continue as described in steps 7 to 8 of the total bilirubin method.

8. Take a sheet of graph paper and plot the absorbance of each standard (vertical axis) against its concentration in μmol/l (horizontal axis) as described in 25:2.

   The useful working limit (linearity) of the Jendrassik and Grof method is about 350 μmol/l.

Important: Check the calibration graph by measuring a control serum as described in the total bilirubin method. A new calibration graph should be prepared and checked against controls whenever stock reagents are renewed.

Reagents
— Sulphanilic acid, 5 g/l	Reagent No. 79
— Sodium nitrite, 5 g/l	Reagent No. 76
— Caffeine-benzoate reagent	Reagent No. 23
— Alkaline tartrate reagent	Reagent No. 10

All the reagents except the sodium nitrite reagent are stable at room temperature (20-28 °C) for about 6 months. The sodium nitrite reagent must be stored at 2-8 °C. It is stable for at least 1 month when kept tightly stoppered.

Diazo reagent

Mix: 20.0 ml sulphanilic acid, 5 g/l reagent
     0.5 ml sodium nitrite , 5 g/l reagent

When kept tightly stoppered at 2-8 °C, the diazo reagent is stable for up to 72 hours.

Method
Specimen: The method requires 0.2 ml (200 μl) of patient's serum or plasma from EDTA or heparin anticoagulated blood. The specimen should be as fresh as possible (not more than 24 hours old).

Samples from infants: Icteric plasma from infants can be diluted 1 in 2 (0.1 ml plasma and 0.1 ml physiological saline) or if highly icteric 1 in 4 (0.05 ml plasma and 0.15 ml physiological saline). Multiply the result by two or by four according to which dilution is used.

Important: Protect the specimen from daylight and fluorescent light because bilirubin is *rapidly* destroyed by ultraviolet light.

1. Take six or more tubes (depending on the number of tests) and label as follows:
   S ....Standard
   SB ....Standard blank
   C ....Control serum (see 27:5)
   CB ....Control blank
   1,2, etc ....Patients' tests
   1B, 2B, etc ....Patients' blanks

2. Pipette 1 ml of caffeine-benzoate reagent into each tube.

3. Add to each tube as follows:
   Tube
   S, SB ....0.1 ml standard serum
                         (170-340 μmol/l)
   C, CB ....0.1 ml control serum
   1, 1B, 2, 2B, etc ...0.1 ml patient's serum or
                         plasma
   Mix well.

4. Add 0.5 ml of diazo reagent to tubes S, C, 1, 2, etc and mix well.

5. Add 0.5 ml of sulphanilic acid, 5 g/l reagent to tubes SB, CB, 1B, 2B, etc and mix well.

6. Leave at room temperature (20-28 °C) for 5 minutes.

7. Add 1 ml of alkaline tartrate reagent to each tube and mix well.

   Note: With the addition of this reagent any turbidity in the solutions will clear.

8. Read immediately the absorbances of the solutions (blanks first) in a colorimeter using an orange filter (e.g. Ilford No. 607) or in a spectrophotometer set at wavelength 600 nm. Zero the instrument with distilled water.

   Subtract the blank readings from the standard, control and patients' samples i.e. subtract reading SB from S, CB from reading C, B1 from 1, etc.

   Note: for some colorimeters it may be necessary to use a modified cuvette holder to read the small volumes. No modification is required if using a WPA CO700D Colorimeter (see 25:3).

9. Calculate the concentration of total bilirubin in the control and patients' samples by:

   — Reading the values from the calibration graph providing the reading of the standard agrees with the calibration, or if not by

— Using the following formula:

Concentration of total bilirubin in μmol/l =

$$\frac{AT}{AS} \times \text{concentration of standard}$$

where: AT = Absorbance of test(s) or control
       AS = Absorbance of standard

Bilirubin values greater than 350 μmol/l (20 mg%)
Repeat the assay after diluting the serum or plasma 1 in 4 in physiological saline. Multiply the result by four.

10. Report the patients' results if the value of the control serum is acceptable.

Quality control
The principles of quality control in clinical chemistry are described in Chapter 27.

For the Jendrassik and Grof total bilirubin method the following should be attainable.

— OCV of around 6%
— RCV not exceeding 12%

Approximate total bilirubin reference (normal) range
Adults: 3-21 μmol/l (0.2-1.3 mg%)
Newborns: 8-67 μmol/l (0.5-4.0 mg%)*
* Highest values in the first 3-5 days of life.

To convert μmol/l to mg%, multiply by 0.06.
To convert mg% to μmol/l, multiply by 17.

Interpretation of serum or plasma bilirubin results
A rise in the level of bilirubin in the blood is called hyperbilirubinaemia. The main causes are as follows:

☐ Overproduction of bilirubin caused by an excessive breakdown of red cells. The bilirubin is of the unconjugated type (see 30:1). In tropical countries haemolysis is due mainly to:

— Severe falciparum malaria
— Sickle cell disease haemolytic crisis
— Haemolysis associated with glucose-6-phosphate dehydrogenase deficiency and hereditary spherocytosis.
— Antigen antibody reactions as in haemolytic disease of the newborn, autoimmune haemolytic anaemias, or following an incompatible blood transfusion.

— Toxins from bacteria, snake venoms, drugs, or herbs.

☐ Liver cell damage in which there is usually an increase in both conjugated and unconjugated bilirubin (see 30:1). The commonest causes are:

— Hepatitis caused by hepatitis viruses and other viruses.
— Malaria
— Leptospirosis
— Relapsing fever
— Brucellosis
— Typhoid
— Chemicals, plant toxins and drugs

☐ Metabolic disturbances in the liver involving defective conjugation, transport and, or, excretion of bilirubin. Examples include:

— type of neonatal jaundice, often referred to as 'physiological jaundice' in which the conjugation system of an infant is insufficiently developed at birth (see also later text).
— rare inherited disorders of conjugation such as Gilbert's and Crigler-Najjar syndromes.

☐ Partial or complete stopping of the flow of bile through bile channels with a build up of conjugated bilirubin in the blood. Cholestasis can be due to:

— Obstruction of the extra-hepatic biliary ducts by gallstones, tumours (especially hepatomas and carcinoma of the pancreas), cholangitis (inflammation of the biliary ducts), or by helminths such as *Opisthorchis* or *Fasciola* species. Occasionally heavy *Ascaris* infections, especially in children, may result in blockage of the common bile duct.
— Pressure on the small bile ducts as may occur in hepatitis or as a side effect of drugs.

Note: Mild to moderate hyperbilirubinaemia may also be found in association with any serious condition such as a terminal illness, or following major trauma, surgery, or blood transfusion.

Neonatal jaundice
As previously described, a type of neonatal jaundice known as 'physiological' jaundice may develop in a newborn baby if the conjugation mechanism of the infant is not fully developed. The jaundice begins to appear on the second day after birth and is of longer duration in premature infants.

Other common causes of neonatal jaundice in tropical countries are as follows:

— Glucose-6-phosphate dehydrogenase deficiency, especially in Papua New Guinea, Malaysia, Singapore and other parts of South-East Asia. The jaundice develops soon after birth.

— Infections, particularly septicaemia, congenital syphilis, toxoplasmosis, and viral infections. The jaundice usually develops 3-4 days after birth.

— ABO haemolytic disease of the newborn in which jaundice occurs usually within 24 hours of birth.

In neonatal jaundice the level of unconjugated bilirubin is important. Levels in excess of 340 μmol/l (20 mg%) in the normal child may result in the unconjugated bilirubin being deposited in the basal ganglion of the brain, a condition known as kernicterus. This may cause permanent damage to the brain cells of the infant. It is therefore important to measure the serum or plasma bilirubin at regular intervals. Even at bilirubin levels much lower than 340 μmol/l the premature child is especially at risk as is the child with acidosis or low serum or plasma albumin levels because the levels of 'free' bilirubin not bound to albumin are much higher and it is this type of bilirubin that causes kernicterus.

30:3 TESTING URINE FOR BILIRUBIN

Bilirubin is not normally detected in the urine. When it is found, the condition is referred to as bilirubinuria.

Urine containing 8.4 μmol/l (0.5 mg%) or more of bilirubin has a characteristic yellow-brown colour (hepatocellular jaundice) or a yellow-green appearance (obstructive jaundice).

The following methods are used to test for bilirubinuria:

■ Fouchet's tube test
■ *Ictotest*
■ Bilirubin strip tests

Specimen: Freshly passed urine is required. It should be protected from daylight and fluorescent light because bilirubin is rapidly oxidized by ultraviolet light to biliverdin which is not detected by the reagents used in the tube, tablet, or strip tests.

Fouchet's Tube Test
This test is recommended for detecting bilirubin in urine because it is sensitive, inexpensive and easy to perform.

Barium chloride is used to precipitate the sulphates in the urine. Any bilirubin present becomes attached to the precipitated barium sulphate. When Fouchet's reagent is added to the precipitate, the iron III (ferric) chloride oxidizes the bilirubin to green-blue biliverdin.

Reagents
— Barium chloride, 0.48 mol/l   Reagent No. 12
  (10% w/v)
— Fouchet's reagent   Reagent No. 40

Method
1. Dispense about 5 ml of fresh urine into a tube or small bottle.

   A 5 ml (5 cc) syringe can be used to dispense the specimen. It is not necessary to use a calibrated pipette.

   Note: If the urine is alkaline, acidify it by adding one or two drops of glacial (concentrated) acetic acid.

2. Add 2.5 ml of barium chloride reagent and mix well.

   A syringe or graduated 3 ml plastic bulb pipette (see 2:4) can be used to add the reagent.

3. Filter or centrifuge to obtain a precipitate.

4. Add 1 drop of Fouchet's reagent to the precipitate on the filter paper (after unfolding the paper) or to the sediment in the tube (after discarding the supernatant urine).

Results
Bilirubin present ... Immediate blue-green colour
                     around the drop of Fouchet's reagent.

Bilirubin absent .... No blue-green colour.

Note: Any pink mauve colour which develops is due to salicylates in the urine.

Ictotest
Ictotest (Ames) is a tablet reagent test. It is based on the joining of bilirubin to a stable diazonium solid salt to produce blue-purple azobilirubin. The reaction is specific for bilirubin. When the tablet is moistened, carbon dioxide escapes which leads to a mixing of the chemical components.

Details of use, reaction, and storage of *Ictotest* tablets are supplied by the manufacturer. It is particularly important that the storage instructions are followed *exactly* because even the slightest moisture from the air will cause deterioration of the reagents. Only tablets which appear *completely dry* (white) should be used.

Ictotest is less sensitive than Fouchet's test but more sensitive than most of the bilirubin strip tests. It detects as little as 1.7 μmol/l (0.1 mg%) of bilirubin in the urine.

False reactions

False negative results may be given if the urine contains high levels of ascorbic acid.

Difficulty in reading reactions may occur if the urine contains beetroot dye. Beetroot dye can be recognized however by its acid-base reactions. If the urine is made alkaline the dye becomes colourless and if made acid the colour returns.

Bilirubin Strip Tests

Strip tests to detect bilirubinuria include:

☐ *Bilugen-Test* (Boehringer) which is a double test strip. It detects bilirubin in urine and also tests for raised levels of urine urobilinogen.

The bilirubin reaction is based on the coupling of bilirubin with 2,6-dichlorobenzene-diazonium tetrafluoroborate in an acid medium to give a reddish-violet azo dye. For the reaction of the urobilinogen test area, see 30:4.

The practical sensitivity of *Bilugen-Test* for bilirubin is 9 μmol/l (0.5 mg%).

☐ *Bilur-Test* (Boehringer, also known as *BM-Test-Bilirubine*). This is a double strip test. It detects bilirubin in urine and tests for significant rises of bilirubin in serum.

The sensitivity of the urine bilirubin test area is similar to *Bilugen-Test*. The serum bilirubin scale has a practical sensitivity of 14 μmol/l (0.8 mg%) with a top value (+++) that corresponds to 58 μmol/l (3.5 mg%) or more of serum total bilirubin.

Note: Bilirubin test areas are also included on many of the multiple strip tests manufactured by both Boehringer and Ames companies.

False reactions

False negative reactions may occur if the urine contains large amounts of ascorbic acid. Sensitivity of the urine bilirubin test is also reduced by nitrite which may be present with some bacterial urinary infections.

False positive reactions may be produced by drugs that colour the urine red or turn red in an acid environment, e.g. phenazopyridine.

Note: The control of reagent strips is described in 28:7.

Causes of bilirubinuria

Bilirubin can be found in the urine whenever there is an increase of conjugated bilirubin in the blood. Bilirubinuria occurs therefore in obstructive jaundice when there is an increase of conjugated bilirubin in the blood and also in hepatocellular jaundice

when the blood usually contains both conjugated and unconjugated bilirubin.

Bilirubin is not found in the urine in haemolytic jaundice or in other conditions in which the excess bilirubin in the blood is of the unconjugated type.

In the early stages of viral hepatitis, bilirubinuria together with raised aminotransferase levels can be found before a patient becomes clinically jaundiced.

30:4 TESTING URINE FOR UROBILINOGEN

As explained in 8:9 it is normal to find small amounts of urobilinogen in the urine derived from that which is reabsorbed from the intestine. The concentration of urobilinogen in the urine is therefore dependent on the amount of bilirubin being produced and entering the intestine and on the ability of the liver to excrete the urobilinogen coming to it from the intestine.

Urine is often tested for increases in urobilinogen when investigating haemolysis or liver disorders in which liver function is impaired.

The following methods are used to test for increased urobilinogen in urine:

■ Ehrlich's test
■ Urobilinogen strip tests

Specimen: Freshly passed urine is required because urobilinogen which is colourless is rapidly oxidized to the orange pigment urobilin which is not detected by Ehrlich's test or by the urobilinogen strip tests.

Note: If a delay in testing urine is unavoidable a technique must be used which detects urobilin in urine such as the Schlesinger test. Details of this test can be found in textbooks of clinical biochemistry.

Ehrlich's Test (Watson's modification)

Urobilinogen reacts with *p*-dimethylaminobenzaldehyde to form a red condensation product. The intensity of colour produced corresponds to the concentration of urobilinogen present. Bilirubin interferes with the reaction and therefore if present it must first be removed by reacting the urine with barium chloride.

Reagents

— Hydrochloric acid, 50% v/v   Reagent No. 44
— Ehrlich's reagent   Reagent No. 32
— Chloroform or amyl alcohol

Method

1. Take two small tubes and label one 'T' (test) and the other 'C' (comparison).

2. Dispense 5 ml of *fresh* urine into each tube. A 5 ml (5 cc) syringe can be used to dispense the specimen. It is not necessary to use a calibrated pipette.

   Note: If the urine contains bilirubin, mix equal volumes of the specimen with 0.48 mol/l barium chloride (Reagent No. 12). Centrifuge or filter to obtain a clear supernatant or filtrate to test for urobilinogen.

3. Add 0.5 ml of Ehrlich's reagent to tube 'T' and mix.

   Add 0.5 ml of 50% v/v hydrochloric acid to tube 'C' and mix.

   A graduated plastic bulb pipette (see 2:4) can be used to dispense the reagent.

4. Leave both tubes at room temperature (20-28 °C) for 5 minutes.

5. *Looking down through the tubes*, examine for a definite red colour in tube 'T' as compared with tube 'C'.

   If present, check that the red colour is due to urobilinogen and not to porphobilinogen:
   — Add 1-2 ml of chloroform or amyl alcohol. Mix well and allow to settle.
   — Look for a red colour in the chloroform or amyl alcohol layer, indicating the presence of urobilinogen. If the red colour is not in this layer it is due to porphobilinogen.*

   * Porphobilinogen is excreted in the urine of patients with acute idiopathic porphyria, a rare inherited disease that affects nerves and muscles.

Results
Increased urobilinogen … Red colour in tube 'T'
Normal urobilinogen …. Pink colour in tube 'T'
No urobilinogen ……… Similar colours in tubes 'T' and 'C'

False reactions
A false negative reaction may occur if the urine contains nitrite as in some bacterial urinary infections. The nitrite will oxidize the urobilinogen to urobilin which is not detected by Ehrlich's reagent. A negative reaction may also occur if a patient is receiving intensive antimicrobial therapy. The antimicrobials will reduce the number of bacteria in the intestine and so prevent urobilinogen being formed.

Besides porphobilinogen, other substances which react with Ehrlich's reagent include the metabolite indican and drugs such as *p*-aminosalicylic acid and sulphonamides.

Note: Heating the test solution, as is sometimes recommended, does not intensify the reaction.

The increase in colour produced by heat is due to the presence of indole derivatives.

Urobilinogen Strip Tests
The urobilinogen strip tests manufactured by Boehringer are specific for urobilinogen and not affected by the substances that interfere in the Ehrlich's test. A pink-red azo dye is formed by 4-methoxybenzene-diazonium tetrafluoroborate when it combines with urobilinogen.

The reaction of the Ames urobilinogen strip tests is a modification of the Ehrlich's test and is therefore not specific for urobilinogen (see *False reactions*). In this strip test, *p*-dimethylaminobenzaldehyde reacts with urobilinogen to produce a brown-orange colour.

The strip tests give semiquantitative results. They detect normal and increased amounts of urobilinogen. They cannot be used to demonstrate the absence of urine urobilinogen.

Urobilinogen strip tests include:

☐ *Ugen-Test* (Boehringer, also known as *BM-Test-Urobilinogene*). This is a single test strip which is specific for urobilinogen.

   Scale: Normal, 17, 70, 149, 200 μmol/l.

   No change in colour or colours lighter than that shown for 17 μmol/l (1 mg%) indicate a normal result.

☐ *Bilugen-Test* (Boehringer) which is a double test strip. It measures urine urobilinogen semiquantitatively and also detects urine bilirubin.

   The urobilinogen reaction and scale for *Bilugen-Test* are the same as that described for *Ugen-Test*.

☐ *Urobilistix* (Ames) which is a single strip test. As previously explained it is not specific for urobilinogen.

   Scale: 1.6, 16, 33, 66, 131, 197 μmol/l. Reactions up to 16 μmol/l indicate a normal result.

False reactions
The strips manufactured by both Boehringer and Ames do not react with porphobilinogen within the time specified for the urobilinogen reaction. With phenazopyridine (found in some disinfectants), a rapid red colour is formed due to the acidity of the buffers impregnating both strips.

Ames urobilinogen strip tests may give false positive reactions if the urine contains indole, skatole, indican, breakdown products of chlorophyl, PAS metabolites, and sulphonamide amines. Nitrite may inhibit the reaction and give a false negative result.

Boehringer urobilinogen strips may give a false negative result in the presence of formaldehyde concentrations of over 200 mg / 100 ml urine.

Note: The control of reagent strips is described in 28:7.

Interpretation of urine urobilinogen results
Increases
— Haemolytic disease when the amount of bilirubin being produced is increased leading to greater amounts of urobilinogen being formed.
— Paralytic ileus or enterocolitis when there is an increase in the production of urobilinogen in the intestine.
— Hepatocellular damage or hepatic congestion, resulting in less of the absorbed urobilinogen being excreted by the liver. The urobilinogen then passes into the general circulation leading to more being excreted by the kidneys.
— Cirrhosis of the liver.

Decreases
— Obstruction of bile ducts preventing the flow of bilirubin to the intestine for conversion to urobilinogen.
— Hepatocellular damage preventing the conjugation and excretion of bilirubin for conversion to urobilinogen.
— Absence or reduction of the normal intestinal bacterial flora (necessary to convert conjugated bilirubin to urobilinogen), leading to little or no urobilinogen being produced. This may occur in neonates or following intensive antimicrobial therapy.

Note: In viral hepatitis, urine urobilinogen is at first increased but as liver cell damage increases the small biliary ducts become obstructed leading to a reduction or even an absence of urobilinogen in the urine. In the recovery stages, urine urobilinogen again increases due to the bilirubin, now in excess, being able to pass through the biliary ducts into the intestine.

30:5 MEASUREMENT OF SERUM OR PLASMA TOTAL PROTEIN
Biuret Method[3]

The main plasma protein fractions are globulins, albumin, and fibrinogen. The important role of plasma proteins in the control of water balance in the body is described in 29:1. Plasma proteins also have important nutritive, transporting, protective, buffering, and enzymatic functions. Many blood coagulation factors are also proteins.

Difference between serum and plasma: Serum is obtained from clotted blood. It contains globulins and albumin but no fibrinogen. The fibrinogen is converted to insoluble fibrin as the blood clots.

Choice of test method
The Biuret method is recommended as a manual colorimetric technique for measuring serum or plasma total protein.

Serum total protein can also be measured refractometrically using a refractometer such as the Atago T-2 model (see later text). Only a small drop of sample is required and no reagents are needed. Studies comparing the Biuret method and the refractometric technique indicate that the two methods are interchangeable for clinical purposes.[4] It would appear that the refractometric method is no more affected by lipaemia and high glucose and urea values than the Biuret method and definitely less affected by haemolysis and raised bilirubin levels.

Total protein test kits
Several Biuret manual colorimetric total protein test kits are commercially available. The bioMérieux *Protéines-Kit* includes sufficient bovine albumin 100 g/l standard to calibrate both the total protein and albumin tests. The kit costs about £13 (1985-1986) for 400 tests (as performed by the micro method described in this subunit).

Although the bioMérieux kit is convenient and among the lower priced of the commercially produced kits, not many laboratories will be able to afford to use it on a regular basis. The reagents for the manual non-kit method are however easy to make and can be prepared much more economically in the laboratory.

Important: For further comments regarding the purchasing and use of clinical chemistry tests kits, see 26:1.

Principle of Biuret method
Protein molecules are composed of amino acids arranged in long chains called peptide chains. The links which join the amino acids together are known as peptide bonds.

In the Biuret reaction the cupric ions in the reagent join with the peptide bonds of the protein molecules in an alkaline solution to form a blue-violet coloured complex. The absorbance of the colour produced is measured in a colorimeter using a yellow-green filter or in a spectrophotometer at 540 nm wavelength.

The use of blank solutions is recommended to avoid errors due to turbidity.

Note: The Biuret method can also be used for measuring total protein in transudates and exudates. It is not however suitable for measuring protein in urine or cerebrospinal fluid. Testing for protein in urine is described in 28:3 and in cerebrospinal fluid in 31:6.

$$\text{Proteins} + \underset{\text{Alkaline pH}}{\text{Copper ions}} \longrightarrow \underset{\underset{\textit{Blue-violet}}{\text{complex}}}{\text{Protein-copper}}$$

Calibration
Standards to calibrate the Biuret total protein method (and also the albumin method, see 30:6) are most easily prepared from a bovine albumin 100 g/l solution. Such a solution is available from bioMérieux called *Proteitrol* (No. 62441), and costs about £10 (1985-1986) for 25 ml. If unable to obtain the bioMérieux product, a 100 g/l protein standard is also available from Sigma Company called *Albumin Stock Standard* (No. 905-10) and costs about £16 (1985-1986) for 28 ml. For the addresses of bioMérieux and Sigma companies, see Appendix II.

Alternatively, an expired bottle of human serum albumin (from pharmacy or blood transfusion laboratory) can be used. This should be reconstituted as instructed on the bottle and stored at 2-8 °C. If a sterile needle and syringe are used to withdraw the amount required, the serum can be kept for several months. The concentration of albumin will be stated on the bottle label. Five standards should be prepared.

Working total protein standards 20, 40, 60, 80, 100 g/l (prepared from 100 g/l albumin standard)
1. Take five small containers (about 5 ml capacity) and number them 1 to 5. Pipette accurately into each as follows:

Container	Albumin 100 g/l	Protein Diluent Reagent No. 60
1	0.4 ml	1.6 ml
2	0.8 ml	1.2 ml
3	1.2 ml	0.8 ml
4	1.6 ml	0.4 ml
5	2.0 ml	—

2. Mix well the contents in each container.

The concentration of albumin in each of the standards is as follows:

Container 1 = 20 g/l
2 = 40 g/l
3 = 60 g/l
4 = 80 g/l
5 = 100 g/l

3. Label and store at 2-8 °C. The standard solutions are stable for several months.

Preparation of the protein calibration graph
1. Take six tubes and label them 'B' (reagent blank) and 1 to 5.

2. Pipette 2.5 ml of Biuret reagent (see *Reagents*) into each tube.

3. Add to each tube as follows:
Tube
B .... 50 μl (0.05 ml) distilled water
1 .... 50 μl standard, 20 g/l
2 .... 50 μl standard, 40 g/l
3 .... 50 μl standard, 60 g/l
4 .... 50 μl standard, 80 g/l
5 .... 50 μl standard, 100 g/l
Mix well.

4. Continue as described in steps 5 and 6 of the total protein method.

5. Take a sheet of graph paper and plot the absorbance of each standard (vertical axis) against its concentration in g/l (horizontal axis), as described in 25:2. A linear calibration should be obtained.

The useful working limit (linearity) of the Biuret total protein method is about 100 g/l (10 g%).

Important: Check the calibration graph by measuring a control serum as described in the total protein method. A new calibration graph should be prepared and checked against controls whenever stock reagents are renewed.

Reagents
— Biuret reagent   Reagent No. 18
— Biuret blank reagent   Reagent No. 17

The above reagents when stored in tightly stoppered bottles are stable indefinitely at room temperature (20-28 °C).

Method
Specimen: The method requires 0.1 ml (100 μl) of patient's serum or plasma. The blood must be collected with the minimum of venous stasis and precautions should be taken to avoid haemolysis (see 26:4).

1.Take six or more tubes (depending on the number of tests) and label as follows:

B   — Reagent blank
S   — Standard, 60 g/l
            (see *Calibration*)
C   — Control serum (see 27:5)
CB   — Control serum blank
1, 2, etc   — Patients' tests
1B, 2B, etc   — Patients' test blanks

Summary of Total Protein Method

For detailed instructions, see text

Pipette into tubes as follows:	STANDARD BLANK B	STANDARD S	CONTROL C	CONTROL BLANK CB	TESTS 1,2, etc	TEST BLANKS 1B, 2B, etc
Biuret reagent	2.5 ml	2.5 ml	2.5 ml	—	2.5 ml	—
Biuret blank reagent	—	—	—	2.5 ml	—	2.5 ml
Distilled water	50 μl	—	—	—	—	—
Standard 60 g/l	—	50 μl	—	—	—	—
Control serum	—	—	50 μl	50 μl	—	—
Patient's serum or plasma	—	—	—	—	50 μl	50 μl

Mix well

Leave at 37 °C for 10 minutes or at room temperature for 30 minutes

READ ABSORBANCES

Colorimeter: Yellow - green filter, e.g. Ilford No. 605
Spectrophotometer: 540 nm

Zero the instrument with blank solution in tube B

Read the control and test blanks first

Subtract blank readings

Obtain values from the calibration graph if the result of the 60 g/l standard agrees with the calibration. If not, calculate the results as follows:

$$\text{Total protein g/l} = \frac{\text{Absorbance of test or control}}{\text{Absorbance of 60 g/l standard}} \times 60$$

Report patients' results if control value is acceptable

50 μl = 0.05 ml

Note: Whenever resources permit, a range of standards should be assayed with each batch of tests.

2. Pipette 2.5 ml of Biuret reagent into tubes B, S, C, 1, 2, etc.

3. Pipette 2.5 ml of Biuret blank reagent into tubes CB, 1B, 2B, etc.

4. Add to each tube as follows:

   Tube
   B .... 50 μl distilled water
   S .... 50 μl standard, 60 g/l
   C, CB .... 50 μl control serum
   1, 1B, 2, 2B, etc .... 50 μl patient's serum
   or plasma

   Mix well.

5. Leave at 37 °C for 10 minutes or at room temperature (20-28 °C) for 30 minutes.

   The same temperature must be used in the test method as used to prepare the calibration graph.

6. Read the absorbances of the solutions (blanks first) in a colorimeter using a yellow-green filter, e.g. Ilford No. 605 or in a spectrophotometer set at 540 nm. Zero the instrument with the blank solution in tube B.

   Subtract the blank readings from the control and patients' samples, i.e. subtract CB from C, 1B from 1, 2B from 2, etc.

   Note: For some colorimeters it may be necessary to use a modified cuvette holder to read the small volumes. No modification is required if using a WPA CO700D Colorimeter (see 25:3).

7. Calculate the concentration of total protein in the control and patients' samples by:

   — Reading the values from the calibration graph providing the reading of the 60 g/l standard agrees with the calibration, or if not by
   — Using the following formula:

   $$\text{Total protein g/l} = \frac{AT}{AS} \times 60$$

   where AT = Absorbance of test(s) or control
   AS = Absorbance of 60 g/l standard

8. Report the patients' results if the value of the control serum is acceptable.

Quality control
The principles of quality control in clinical chemistry are described in Chapter 27.
For the Biuret total protein method the following

should be attainable:
— OCV, around 2%
— RCV, not exceeding 4%

Approximate total protein reference (normal) range
60-81 g/l (6.0-8.1 g%)

To convert from g/l to g%, divide by 10.
To convert from g% to g/l, multiply by 10.

Note: Values are lower when lying down (by 10%).

USE OF A REFRACTOMETER
An indirect way of estimating serum or plasma total protein in health centres and small hospital laboratories unable to measure total protein colorimetrically is to use a refractometer with a built-in scale for serum proteins.

A simple to operate clinical refractometer calibrated for serum or plasma proteins is the Atago bench T-2 refractometer. The instrument requires only a small drop of serum or plasma. It is shown in Plate 28.2 and Plate 28.3 in 28:5 (also used to measure urine specific gravity).

As explained in 28:5, the instrument measures the refractive index of a specimen. Assuming that the substances in serum other than protein, do not vary greatly in their concentration, the protein content of the serum or plasma can be calculated using a conversion factor. The protein scale of the refractometer is based on using such a conversion factor. The operation of the instrument is similar to that described in 28:5 for testing urine. The scale giving serum or plasma total protein concentration is used to read off the results.

The accuracy of the instrument can be checked as directed in the manufacturer's instruction booklet. Most commercially available control sera cannot be used to check the instrument because the refractometer scale of protein values is based on the concentration of solutes as found in normal unaltered serum.

Note: A refractometer cannot be used to measure protein in urine or cerebrospinal fluid.

Interpretation of serum or plasma total protein results
Increases
A rise in serum or plasma total protein is not common. When it occurs it is usually due to:

— Haemoconcentration, following shock, severe vomiting, or diarrhoea.
— Increased globulin production associated with chronic infections such as tuberculosis, kala-azar, and tropical splenomegaly.

— The presence of abnormal globulins, as in multiple myeloma, macroglobulinaemia, or lymphoma.
— Collagen vascular diseases and some forms of liver disease.

Falsely raised value: This may be obtained if the specimen contains dextran from an intravenous infusion.

Decreases
A decrease in the total protein level is more common and may be caused by:

— Low protein intake as in the severe form of protein energy malnutrition known as kwashiorkor.
— Malabsorption as in chronic pancreatitis, coeliac disease, and sprue.
— Loss of protein from the body in urine as in the nephrotic syndrome. Protein can also be lost from the skin following severe burns or from the bowel as in ulcerative colitis and other forms of protein-losing gastroenteropathy.
— Liver disease associated with a reduction in protein synthesis, although the total protein may be within the reference range because the albumin levels fall and the globulin levels rise at the same time.
— An increase in the body's need for protein. e.g. following surgery or serious tissue damage when protein is required for energy and repair. High protein demands lead to hypoalbuminaemia (low albumin levels).

30:6 MEASUREMENT OF SERUM OR PLASMA ALBUMIN[5, 6]

Albumin is synthesized entirely in the liver and is present in the plasma in greater concentration than globulins. It diffuses easily through damaged membranes and is more readily filtered out by the kidneys than most globulins because its molecules are smaller.

Serum or plasma albumin levels are mainly measured to investigate liver diseases, protein energy malnutrition, disorders of water balance, nephrotic syndrome, and protein-losing gastrointestinal diseases.

Choice of test method
The bromocresol green (BCG) binding method is recommended as a manual colorimetric technique for measuring serum or plasma albumin.

Albumin test kits
Manual colorimetric test kits that measure albumin by the bromocresol green binding method are available commercially but most are expensive. The Sigma kit No. 630 is priced about £13.80 for 100 tests (1985-1986). For the address of Sigma chemical company, see Appendix II.

Principle of the BCG albumin method
Bromocresol green is an indicator which is yellow between pH 3.5-4.2. When it binds to albumin the colour of the indicator changes from yellow to blue-green. The absorbance of the colour produced is measured in a colorimeter using an orange filter or in a spectrophotometer at 632 nm wavelength. Turbidity in the solutions is avoided by the addition of Brij-35.

$$\text{Albumin} + \text{BCG pH 4.2} \longrightarrow \text{Albumin-BCG complex}$$
$$\textit{Blue-Green}$$

Calibration
The bromocresol green method for albumin can be calibrated from the same 100 g/l standard solution of albumin as used for calibrating the total protein method (see 30:5).

Albumin standards 10, 20, 30, 40, 50 g/l
1. Take five small containers (5 ml capacity) and number them 1 to 5. Pipette accurately into each as follows:

Container	Albumin 100 g/l	Protein Diluent Reagent No. 60
1	0.2	1.8
2*	0.4	1.6
3	0.6	1.4
4*	0.8	1.2
5	1.0	1.0

* These two standards which correspond to 20 g/l and 40 g/l need not be pipetted if they have already been prepared for calibrating the total protein method.

2. Mix well the contents in each container.
The concentration of albumin in each of the standards is as follows:

Container 1 = 10 g/l
2 = 20 g/l
3 = 30 g/l
4 = 40 g/l
5 = 50 g/l

3. Label and store at 2-8 °C. The standard solutions are stable for several months.

Preparation of the albumin calibration graph

1. Take six tubes and label them 'B' (reagent blank) and 1 to 5.

2. Pipette 4 ml of BCG reagent (see *Reagents*) into each tube.

   Note: Allow the BCG reagent to come to room temperature before use.

3. Add to each tube as follows:

   Tube
   B .... 20 μl (0.02 ml) distilled water
   1 .... 20 μl standard, 10 g/l
   2 .... 20 μl standard, 20 g/l
   3 .... 20 μl standard, 30 g/l
   4 .... 20 μl standard, 40 g/l
   5 .... 20 μl standard, 50 g/l

4. Mix well but avoid frothing of the reagent. If air bubbles are present the absorbance readings will be incorrect.

5. Continue as described in steps 5 and 6 of the test method.

6. Take a sheet of graph paper and plot the absorbance of each standard solution (vertical axis) against its concentration in g/l (horizontal axis), as described in 25:2.

   The useful working limit (linearity) of the bromocresol green method for albumin is about 50 g/l (5 g%).

   Important: Check the calibration graph by measuring a control serum as described in the albumin method. A new calibration graph should be prepared and checked against controls whenever stock reagents are renewed.

Reagent
— Bromocresol green (BCG)   Reagent No. 19
  reagent

   When stored at 2-8 °C the BCG reagent is stable for several months. It should be allowed to warm to room temperature (20-28 °C) before use.

Method
Specimen: The method requires 20 μl (0.02 ml) of patient's serum or plasma. The blood must be collected with the minimum of venous stasis and haemolysis should be avoided (see 26:4).

1. Take four or more tubes (depending on the number of tests) and label as follows:

B   — Reagent blank
S   — Standard, 30 g/l (see *Calibration*)
C   — Control (see 27:5)
1, 2, etc   — Patients' tests

2. Pipette 4 ml of BCG reagent (warmed to room temperature) into each tube.

3. Add to each tube as follows:

   Tube
   B .... 20 μl (0.02 ml) distilled water
   S .... 20 μl standard, 30 g/l
   C .... 20 μl control serum
   1, 2, etc ...... 20 μl patient's serum or plasma

   Note: If a patient's sample appears turbid, prepare a serum blank by mixing 20 μl of patient's serum or plasma in 4 ml of succinate buffer (Reagent No. 78).

4. Mix *well* but avoid frothing of the solutions. If air bubbles are present the absorbance readings will be incorrect.

5. Read *immediately* the absorbances of the solutions in a colorimeter using an orange filter (e.g. Ilford No. 607) or in a spectrophotometer set at 632 nm. Zero the instrument with the reagent blank solution in tube B.

   Note: If using a serum blank, read its absorbance after zeroing the instrument with distilled water. Subtract this reading from the reading of the patient's BCG sample (read against the reagent blank solution).

6. Calculate the concentration of albumin in the control and patients' samples by:

   — Reading the values from the calibration graph providing the reading of the 30 g/l standard agrees with the calibration, or if not by

   — Using the following formula:

   $$\text{Albumin g/l} = \frac{\text{AT}}{\text{AS}} \times 30$$

   where: AT = Absorbance of test(s) or control
           AS = Absorbance of 30 g/l standard

7. Report the patients' results if the value of the control serum is acceptable.

Quality control
The principles of quality control in clinical chemistry are described in Chapter 27.

For the bromocresol green albumin method the

Summary of Albumin Method

Pipette into tubes as follows:	BLANK B	STANDARD S	CONTROL C	TEST 1,2, etc
Bromocresol green (BCG) reagent ...	4 ml	4 ml	4 ml	4 ml
Distilled water	20 μl	—	—	—
Standard, 30 g/l	—	20 μl	—	—
Control serum	—	—	20 μl	—
Patient's serum or plasma	—	—	—	20 μl

Mix *well* but avoid frothing

READ ABSORBANCES IMMEDIATELY

Colorimeter: Orange filter, e.g. Ilford No. 607
Spectrophotometer: 632 nm

Zero instrument with blank solution in tube B

Obtain values from the calibration graph if the result of the 30 g/l standard agrees with the calibration. If not, calculate the results as follows:

$$\text{Albumin g/l} = \frac{\text{Absorbance of test or control}}{\text{Absorbance of 30 g/l standard}} \times 30$$

Report patients' results if control value is acceptable

$20 \ \mu l = 0.02 \ ml$

following should be attainable:
— OCV, around 3%
— RCV, not exceeding 6%

Approximate albumin reference (normal) range
30-45 g/l

To convert from g/l to g%, divide by 10.
To convert from g% to g/l, multiply by 10.

Note: Albumin levels are lower in infants and when individuals are lying down (by 10%).

Interpretation of serum or plasma albumin results
Increases
Serum or plasma albumin levels are rarely raised, except artefactually by prolonged venous stasis.

Decreases
Many of the causes of low total protein levels (see 30:5) are the result of hypoalbuminaemia, especially the nephrotic syndrome. The pathogenesis and management of nephrotic syndrome have been described in the paper of Cohen.[14] Several parasitic infections cause a reduction in the synthesis of albumin.

Note: The BCG method is not very accurate at low levels of serum albumin, giving results with positive bias when the albumin is less than 20g/l. This is probably unimportant in clinical practice.

30:7 MEASUREMENT OF SERUM OR PLASMA ASPARTATE AMINOTRANSFERASE ACTIVITY
Reitman-Frankel Kit Method[7, 8]

The enzymes, aspartate aminotransferase (AST), previously known as glutamate oxaloacetate transaminase (GOT), and alanine aminotransferase (ALT), formerly known as glutamate pyruvate transaminase (GPT), are concerned with amino acid metabolism.

Large amounts of AST are present in the liver, kidneys, cardiac muscle, and skeletal muscle. Small amounts of the enzyme are present in the brain, pancreas, and lungs. ALT is found principally in the liver with only small amounts being present in other organs. When there is liver cell damage the serum or plasma levels of both enzymes are raised.

Note: Although ALT is often regarded as being more specific for detecting liver cell damage, the difference in the raised levels of the two enzymes is small and does not justify measuring both AST and ALT. Most laboratories do not measure ALT

except under special circumstances. The determination of serum or plasma AST is preferred to that of ALT because aspartate aminotransferase enzyme activity is also a useful indicator of myocardial damage (see *Interpretation of AST results*).

Choice of test method
The Reitman-Frankel AST method is suitable because it can be performed as a manual colorimetric end-point technique. The reagents are however complex to prepare and therefore the use of ready-made reagents (substrate and colour reagent) purchased separately or in kit form is recommended.

The bioMérieux *Transaminases-Kit GOT/AST* is an economically priced kit† which uses reagents that are stable for several years at 2-8 °C. Individual reagents can also be purchased separately. A pyruvate (standard) solution is provided in the kit. The only reagent not included in the kit is the 0.4 mol/l sodium hydroxide solution but this can be easily prepared in the laboratory.

† **BioMérieux Transaminases-Kit GOT/AST (Ref. 61691)**
The kit costs about £8.50 (1986) for approx. 200 tests using *half* volumes of reagents as described in this subunit. When stored at 2-8 °C the reagents are stable for several years. For the address of bioMérieux, see Appendix II.

Note: If unable to obtain the bioMérieux kit, a manual colorimetric kit based on the Reitman-Frankel method is also available from Biotrol Company. It is called *TGO Colorimetric* (Ref. A 02516) and priced about £11 (1986) for 120 tests (using half volumes of reagents). The expiry dates of the reagents are not as long as those in the bioMérieux kit and the reagents cannot be bought separately.

Principle of Reitman-Frankel AST method
AST is incubated at 37 °C for exactly 60 minutes in a pH 7.5 buffered substrate containing aspartate and α-ketoglutarate. AST catalyzes the transfer of the amino group from aspartate to ketoglutarate, forming oxaloacetate and glutamate.

The oxaloacetate reacts with 2,4-dinitrophenylhydrazine (DNPH) to form 2,4-dinitrophenylhydrazone which in an alkaline medium gives a red-brown colour. The absorbance of the colour produced is measured in a colorimeter using a green filter or in a spectrophotometer at 505 nm wavelength.

$$\text{Aspartate} + \alpha\text{-keto-glutarate} \underset{\substack{\text{pH 7.5} \\ \text{60 mins}}}{\overset{\substack{\text{AST} \\ 37\,°C}}{\rightleftharpoons}} \text{Glutamate} + \text{Oxalo-acetate}$$

$$\text{DNPH} \xrightarrow{\text{Alkaline pH}}$$

Red - Brown

Calibration of bioMérieux AST Kit

The Reitman-Frankel AST kit method is calibrated from a pyruvate standard solution (bioMérieux product R4). It is supplied in the kit (61691) but can also be bought separately (bioMérieux Ref. 61741, costing about £4 for 9 ml).

The method of calibration is as follows:

1. Take six tubes and label them 'B' (blank) and 1 to 5. Pipette accurately into each as follows:

Tube	Reagent 1†	Reagent 4‡
B	0.50 ml	—
1	0.45 ml	0.05 ml
2	0.40 ml	0.10 ml
3	0.35 ml	0.15 ml
4	0.30 ml	0.20 ml
5	0.25 ml	0.25 ml

† Buffered AST (GOT) substrate
‡ Pyruvate solution

2. Add 0.1 ml (100 μl) of distilled water to each tube and mix well.

3. Add 0.5 ml of *Reagent 3* (colour reagent) to each tube and mix well.

4. Leave for 20 minutes at room temperature (20-28 °C).

5. Add 5 ml of 0.4 mol/l sodium hydroxide solution (see *Reagents*) to each tube and mix well.

6. Leave for 5 minutes at room temperature.

7. Read the absorbances of the pyruvate standard solutions in a colorimeter using a green filter (e.g. Ilford No. 604) or in a spectrophotometer set at wavelength 505 nm. Zero the instrument with the reagent blank solution in tube B.

8. Take a sheet of graph paper and plot the absorbance of each standard (vertical axis) against its equivalent AST (GOT) activity (horizontal axis). Use international units per litre (U/l).

AST U/l in each standard are as follows:

    Tube 1 = 11 U/l
             2 = 26 U/l
             3 = 46 U/l
             4 = 72 U/l
             5 = 103 U/l

Note: A non-linear (curved line) graph will be obtained (see 25:2).

Important: Check the calibration graph by measuring a control serum as described in the AST kit method. A new calibration graph requires preparation and checking against controls every 2 months or whenever new reagents are used.

Reagents (bioMérieux Kit 61691)

— *Reagent 1*, AST (GOT) pH 7.5 phosphate buffered substrate containing 200 mmol/l aspartate and 2 mmol/l α-ketoglutarate

— *Reagent 3*, colour reagent containing 1 mmol/l 2,4-dinitrophenylhydrazine (DNPH)

— *Reagent 4*, pyruvate standard

— Sodium hydroxide, 0.4 mol/l   Reagent No. 71 (0.4N)

Note: bioMérieux *Reagent No. 2* is not required for measuring AST.

When stored at 2-8 °C the AST substrate and colour reagent are stable for several years. The colour reagent should be protected from light. The sodium hydroxide reagent can be stored at room temperature (20-28 °C). It is stable indefinitely.

Method

Specimen: The method requires 0.1 ml (100 μl) of patient's fresh serum or plasma which must be free from haemolysis (see 26:4). For details of blood collection and the stability of AST activity in serum and plasma, see 26:7. If the serum or plasma is lipaemic this should be reported.

Use of half volumes: To reduce costs, the volumes of samples and reagents used in this method are half those stated in the bioMérieux kit procedure.

1. Take four or more tubes (depending on the number of tests) and label as follows:

    B   — Reagent blank
    S   — Standard (pyruvate)
    C   — Control serum (see 27:5)
    1, 2, etc   — Patients' tests

2. Pipette 0.5 ml of *Reagent 1* (substrate) into the control and patients' tubes (C, 1, 2, etc). Transfer these tubes to a heat-block or water bath set at 37 °C.

After 5 minutes add to the tubes as follows:

C .... 0.1 ml (100 μl) control serum
1, 2, etc .... 0.1 ml patient's serum

Mix and incubate at 37 °C for exactly 60 minutes. Start timing after adding serum to the first tube.

Summary of AST Method
Using Reagents from bioMérieux Kit 61691

Pipette into tubes as follows:	BLANK B	STANDARD S	CONTROL C	TESTS 1,2, etc
Reagent 1 (substrate)	—	—	0.5 ml	0.5 ml
Warm the substrate in tubes C, and tests 1,2, etc at 37 °C for 5 minutes				
Control serum	—	—	0.1 ml	—
Patient's serum	—	—	—	0.1 ml
Incubate tubes C, and tests 1,2, etc at 37 °C for exactly 60 minutes				
Just before 60 minutes is due pipette: Distilled water	0.1 ml	0.1 ml	—	—
Reagent 1 (substrate)	0.5 ml	0.3 ml	—	—
Reagent 4 (pyruvate)	—	0.2 ml	—	—
At *exactly* 60 minutes, pipette as follows: Reagent 3 (Colour reagent)	0.5 ml	0.5 ml	0.5 ml	0.5 ml
Mix well				
Leave at room temperature for 20 minutes				
Sodium hydroxide, 0.4 mol/l	5 ml	5 ml	5 ml	5 ml
Mix well				
Leave at room temperature for 5 minutes				
READ ABSORBANCES *Colorimeter:* Green filter, e.g. Ilford No. 604 *Spectrophotometer:* 505 nm Zero instrument with blank solution in tube B				
Obtain values in U/l from the calibration graph				
Report patients' results if control value is acceptable				

0.1 ml = 100 μl
0.2 ml = 200 μl
0.3 ml = 300 μl
0.5 ml = 500 μl

3. Just before 60 minutes is due, pipette into the blank and standard tubes as follows:

    B .... 0.1 ml distilled water
                0.5 ml *Reagent 1*

    S .... 0.1 ml distilled water
                0.3 ml *Reagent 1*
                0.2 ml *Reagent 4*

4. At *exactly* 60 minutes, remove tubes C, 1, 2, etc from the heat-block or water bath and place them in the rack with tubes B and S.

5. Add *immediately* 0.5 ml of *Reagent 3* to each tube and mix well. Leave at room temperature (20-28 °C) for 20 minutes.

6. Add 5 ml of 0.4 mol/l sodium hydroxide reagent to each tube and mix well. Leave at room temperature for 5 minutes.

7. Read the absorbances of the standard, control, and patients' samples in a colorimeter using a green filter (e.g Ilford No. 604) or in a spectrophotometer set at wavelength 505 nm. Zero the instrument with the reagent blank solution in tube B.

    The colours of the solutions are stable for up to 1 hour.

8. Read off the AST activity in U/l in the control and patients' sample from the calibration graph, making sure that the reading of the standard which corresponds to AST 72 U/l agrees with the calibration curve.

    AST results over 103 U/l:
    Repeat the assay using a 10 minute incubation time (instead of 60 minutes). Multiply the result by six.

9. Report the patients' results if the value of the control serum is acceptable.

Quality control
The principles of quality control in clinical chemistry are described in Chapter 27.

For the Reitman-Frankel method of measuring AST activity the following should be attainable:

— OCV, around 8%
— RCV, should not exceed 16%

Approximate AST reference (normal) range
Up to 42 U/l (tested at 37 °C)
Note: Other methods give much lower reference

values, particularly UV colorimetric methods in which incubation is carried out at 25 °C.

Interpretation of serum or plasma AST results
Liver disease
Very high AST activities usually accompany liver disease especially when there is hepatocellular damage, e.g. in hepatitis. In general, the higher the AST activity the greater the degree of liver damage. In viral hepatitis, the serum or plasma AST is often raised before the patient appears jaundiced and remains elevated for as long as the virus remains active.

Obstructive liver disease is usually accompanied by only a small or moderate AST rise especially in the early stages.

Myocardial infarction
An important cause of elevated serum AST is myocardial infarction i.e. destruction of an area of heart muscle because its blood supply has been cut off due to a blood clot in a coronary artery.

The enzyme level rises soon after the coronary vessel becomes blocked, reaches its highest value 12 to 24 hours after the infarct and returns to normal usually within 48 hours. In general, the more extensive the infarct, the higher the AST peak level.

Other causes of raised AST levels
Because AST is widely distributed in body tissues many other diseases involving cellular injury may be accompanied by increases in AST levels, e.g. severe bacterial infections, malaria, pneumonia, infectious mononucleosis, pulmonary infarcts, and tumours.

AST activity is also increased in some muscle disorders and following surgery, injury, or blood transfusion.

AST activity is artefactually increased when haemolysis is present or if the blood has been stored unseparated.

30:8 MEASUREMENT OF SERUM OR PLASMA ALKALINE PHOSPHATASE ACTIVITY
Nitrophenyl Phosphate Kit Method (Bessey, Lowry and Brock)[9, 10]

Alkaline phosphatase enzymes have maximum activity in the pH range 9.6-10.0. Their exact biochemical role in the tissues is not known but because they are often found attached to cell membranes they are thought to be concerned with the transport of phosphate across cell membranes.

Alkaline phosphatase enzymes are found in many tissues, particularly in liver and bone and also in the small intestine, kidneys, and placental tissue. Their activity in serum or plasma is usually measured to investigate diseases of the liver or bone, especially tumours, abscesses, hydatid cyst, and biliary obstruction. To establish whether a raised serum or plasma alkaline phosphatase activity is of bone or liver origin further tests are required such as the measurement of 5-nucleotidase or gamma-glutamyl transferase. These enzymes are also raised when increased levels of alkaline phosphatase are of hepatic origin. Alternatively, alkaline phosphatase isoenzymes may be measured. For further testing and information the Regional Clinical Chemistry Laboratory should be contacted.

Choice of test method

A suitable manual colorimetric technique is the Bessey Lowry and Brock method which uses 4-nitrophenylphosphate (NPP) as substrate. The use of ready-made reagents and standards purchased separately or in kit form is recommended because the reagents are complex to prepare in district laboratories.

The Merck *Merckotest Alkaline Phosphatase* kit is based on the Bessey Lowry and Brock method. It is economically priced and provides all the reagents required including the 4-nitrophenyl standard solution.

Merckotest Alkaline Phosphatase Kit, (Ref. 3304)
The kit costs about £12.00 (1985-1986) for approx. 200 tests using *half* volumes of reagents as described in this sub-unit. The buffer and 4-nitrophenyl solution are stable for 1 year when stored at 2-8 °C. The substrate is supplied in tablet form (20 tablets/kit). Each tablet is added to 10 ml of buffer and this buffer-substrate solution is stable for 4 weeks at 2-8 °C. For the address of Merck Company, see Appendix II.

Note: If unable to obtain the Merck kit a similar alkaline phosphatase kit is available from Boehringer (Ref. 123889). It is priced about £11.00 (1985-1986) for approx. 200 tests using half volumes of reagents but the kit does *not* include the sodium hydroxide reagent or the standard solution. The standard solution is however available free of charge upon request. The stability of the buffer substrate solution is given as only 1 week at 2-8 °C.

Principle of Bessey Lowry and Brock alkaline phosphatase method

Alkaline phosphatase is incubated at 37 °C for exactly 30 minutes in a pH 10.5 buffered substrate which contains 4-nitrophenylphosphate (NPP). The enzyme hydrolyzes the substrate liberating 4-nitrophenol and inorganic phosphate.

Following the addition of sodium hydroxide (NaOH) the reaction is stopped and the absorbance of the yellow colour produced is measured in a colorimeter using a deep violet filter or in a spectrophotometer at 400 nm wavelength.

$$\text{NPP} \xrightarrow[\substack{37\,°C \\ 30\ mins}]{\substack{\text{Alk. phosphatase}}} \text{Phosphate} + \text{4-nitrophenol}$$

pH 10.5 $\text{NaOH} \rightarrow$

Yellow anion

Calibration of Merck Phosphatase Kit

The kit is calibrated using a 4-nitrophenol standard solution. This is supplied in the *Merckotest alkaline phosphatase kit* (3304) as a concentrate which requires diluting before use as instructed.

The method of calibration is as follows:

1. Dilute the standard solution (bottle ④) as instructed.

2. Take six tubes and label them 'B' (blank) and 1 to 5. Pipette accurately into each tube as follows:

Tube	Diluted standard	NaOH 0.02 mol/l
B	—	5.0
1	0.5	4.5
2	1.0	4.0
3	1.5	3.5
4	3.0	2.0
5	5.0	—

Mix well the solutions in tubes 1 to 4.

3. Read the absorbances of the standards in a colorimeter using a deep violet filter (e.g. Ilford No. 600) or in a spectrophotometer set at 400 nm wavelength. Zero the instrument with the sodium hydroxide solution in tube B.

4. Take a sheet of graph paper and plot the absorbance of each standard (vertical axis) against its equivalent alkaline phosphatase activity in international units per litre (U/l).

The U/l of alkaline phosphatase activity in each standard is as follows:

Tube 1 = 10 U/l
       2 = 20 U/l
       3 = 30 U/l
       4 = 60 U/l
       5 = 100 U/l

Important: Check the calibration graph by measuring a control serum as described in the alkaline

Summary of Alkaline Phosphatase Kit Method
Using Reagents from Merck Kit 3304

Pipette into tubes as follows	STANDARD S	CONTROL C	CONTROL BLANK CB	TESTS 1, etc	TEST BLANKS 1B, etc
Solution ② (substrate) ...	—	0.5 ml	0.5 ml	0.5 ml	0.5 ml
Warm at 37 °C for 5 minutes					
Control serum	—	50 μl	—	—	—
Patient's serum	—	—	—	50 μl	—
Mix well					
Incubate tubes C, and tests 1, etc at 37°C for *exactly* 30 minutes					
Solution ③ (NaOH, 0.02 mol/l)	3.5 ml	5 ml	5 ml	5 ml	5 ml
Mix well					
Control serum	—	—	50 μl	—	—
Patient's serum	—	—	—	—	50 μl
Standard solution (diluted)	1.5 ml	—	—	—	—
Mix well					
READ ABSORBANCES					
Colorimeter: Deep violet filter, e.g. Ilford No. 600 *Spectrophotometer:* 400 nm Zero the instrument with distilled water.					
Subtract blank readings					
Obtain values in U/l from the calibration graph					
Report patients' results if control value is acceptable					

$50 \ \mu l = 0.05 \ ml$

phosphatase kit method. A new calibration graph should be prepared and checked against the controls whenever new stock reagents are used.

Reagents (Merck Kit 3304)

— *Solution* ①, 50 mmol/l glycine-sodium hydroxide buffer at pH 10.5. It also contains 0.5 mmol/l magnesium chloride.

Prepare by making the contents of bottle ① up to 200 ml with distilled water. Mix well and store at 2-8 °C. The buffer is stable for 1 year.

— *Solution* ②, 4-nitrophenyl phosphate substrate. Each tablet contains 5.5 mmol/l 4-nitrophenyl phosphate.

Prepare by dissolving 1 substrate tablet from bottle ② in 10 ml of the buffer solution ①. Store at 2-8 °C. The solution is stable for 4 weeks.

— *Solution* ③, sodium hydroxide 0.02 mol/l.

Prepare by making 5 ml of concentrate from bottle ③ up to 1 litre with distilled water. Mix well and store at room temperature or 2-8 °C.

Method

The method requires 100 μl (0.1 ml) of fresh patient's serum or plasma which must be free from haemolysis (see 26:4). For details of the stability of alkaline phosphatase in serum and plasma, see 26:7.

1. Take 5 or more tubes (depending on the number of tests) and label as follows:

   S   — Standard (4-nitrophenol)
   C   — Control serum (see 27:5)
   CB   — Control blank
   1, etc   — Patients' sera
   1B, etc   — Patients' blanks

2. Pipette 0.5 ml of *solution* ② into tubes C, CB, and patients' 1, 1B, etc. Transfer these tubes to a 37 °C heat-block or water bath to warm the substrate.

3. After 5 minutes add to the control and patients' sample tubes *only* (i.e. C, 1, etc) as follows:

   C   ....50 μl (0.05 ml) of control serum
   1, etc   ......50 μl (0.05 ml) of patient's serum

   Mix and incubate at 37 °C for *exactly* 30 minutes.

4. After 30 minutes add *solution* ③ to the tubes as follows:

   S   .... 3.5 ml *solution* ③, mix well
   C, CB, 1, 1B, etc ...5 ml *solution* ③, mix well

5. Add to the standard, control blank and patients' blank tubes as follows:

S   .... 1.5 ml standard solution,† mix well
CB   ...... 50 μl control serum, mix well
1B, etc ..50 μl patient's serum, mix well

† Use the *diluted* standard solution as used for calibrating the assay (see step 1 of *Calibration of assay*).

6. Read the absorbances of the standard, control, and patients' samples and their blanks in a colorimeter using a deep violet filter (e.g. Ilford No. 600) or in a spectrophotometer set at 400 nm wavelength. Zero the instrument with distilled water.

   Subtract the readings of the blanks from the control and patients' samples, i.e. subtract reading CB from C, 1B from B, etc.

7. Read off the alkaline phosphatase activity in the control and patients' samples in U/l from the previously prepared calibration curve making sure that the reading of the standard solution, which is equivalent to 30 U/l, agrees with the calibration graph.

   Values greater than 100 U/l
   If a patient's result is greater than 100 U/l, repeat the assay after diluting the serum 1 in 5 with physiological saline. Multiply the result by five.

8. Report the patient's results if the value of the control serum is acceptable.

Quality control

The principles of quality control in clinical chemistry are described in Chapter 27.

For the Bessey, Lowry and Brock serum or plasma alkaline phosphatase method the following should be attainable.

— OCV, around 10%
— RCV, should not exceed 20%

Approximate serum or plasma alkaline phosphatase reference (normal) range

Adults: 20-90 U/l

Children: Up to 350 U/l (1-12 y)

Highest values are found in rapidly growing children. Levels up to 500 U/l may be found during puberty because of rapid bone growth during this period.

Interpretation of alkaline phosphatase results

Interpretation of serum or plasma alkaline phosphatase levels is often difficult because of the various tissue sources of the enzyme. Results must be evaluated together with other clinical and biochemical findings.

Levels of one to one and a half times the upper reference range limit are not always significant. Such levels may be found in the elderly in the absence of obvious disease. Younger people may at times show mild rises which return to normal later.

When definite persistent increases in alkaline phosphatase of more than twice the upper reference range occur, then a definite cause must be sought. The reasons for such increases include:

— Obstructive jaundice, in which there is a marked increase in the level of the enzyme.

— Hepatocellular disease in which there is a slight to moderate rise.

— Hepatoma, secondary carcinoma, amoebic abscess, and hydatid cyst, in which a marked increase in alkaline phosphatase may occur with normal levels of serum or plasma aspartate aminotransferase and serum or plasma bilirubin.

— Many bone diseases including osteomalacia and rickets, and also renal rickets, healing fractures, bone tumours, Paget's disease, and hyperparathyroidism

Note: Physiological increases in serum or plasma alkaline phosphatase occur in puberty and pregnancy.

30:9　TESTS TO INVESTIGATE PANCREATIC AND GASTROINTESTINAL FUNCTIONS

In district hospital laboratories, the investigation of pancreatic and gastrointestinal disorders is usually limited to the following tests:

■ Measurement of serum or plasma amylase: to assist in the diagnosis of acute pancreatitis (see 30:10).

■ Semi-quantitative estimation of trypsin in duodenal juice or faeces: to investigate cystic fibrosis and chronic pancreatitis (see 30:11).

■ Detection of occult blood in faeces: to investigate gastrointestinal bleeding (see 30:12).

■ Examination of faeces for increased fat content: to investigate conditions causing steatorrhoea (see 30:13).

■ Testing of faecal specimens for lactose and pH: to assist in the diagnosis of lactase deficiency (see 30:14).

Testing of gastric juice for free hydrochloric acid
Although the measurement of free hydrochloric acid in gastric juice is frequently requested to investigate peptic ulceration, the test has little value. Radiological and visual studies are the main means of diagnosing peptic ulceration.

Investigation of achlorhydria
Sometimes it is useful to know whether achlorhydria (lack of gastric acid) is present, for example when the pain has returned after a vagotomy operation for a duodenal ulcer, or to investigate malabsorption (particularly of iron), pernicious anaemia, or carcinoma of the stomach.

In such cases it is usually sufficient to collect a sample of gastric juice after the patient has fasted overnight and measure the pH of the juice using a pH meter or narrow-range pH papers.

30:10　MEASUREMENT OF SERUM OR PLASMA AMYLASE
Caraway Method[11, 12]

Amylase is an enzyme which is present in large amounts in the cells of the pancreas. The secretion of the enzyme and its role in the digestive process and carbohydrate metabolism are described in Chapter 8.

Acute inflammation of the pancreas (pancreatitis) causes the release of amylase into the circulation. Measurement of serum or plasma amylase is usually requested to assist in the differentiation of acute pancreatitis from other acute abdominal disorders.

Choice of test method
The Caraway amylase method described is a simple rapid manual colorimetric technique which uses a small amount of specimen and a starch substrate that can be easily prepared in the laboratory.

If available, a commercial test kit which uses a dye marked starch substrate such as the *Phadebas Amylase Test* is recommended (see following text).

Amylase Test Kits
A test kit which uses a dye labelled substrate and therefore measures the amount of starch hydrolyzed by amylase (e.g. *Phadebas Amylase Test*) is preferred to a kit in which the amount of starch which remains after hydrolysis is measured using an iodine solution.

The *Phadebas Amylase Test* kit uses a blue dyed polysaccharide substrate in tablet form. Amylase activity is proportional to the amount of polysaccharide hydrolyzed in 15 minutes at 37 °C as shown by the depth of blue colour produced. The reaction is stopped by sodium hydroxide and after filtering or centrifuging to remove the unhydrolyzed solid substrate, the absorbance of the blue solution is measured in a colorimeter using an orange filter or in a spectrophotometer at 620 nm. Results in U/l are read from a calibration chart provided.

The *Phadebas Amylase Test* is manufactured by Pharmacia Diagnostics (see Appendix II). It costs about £16.00 (1985-1986) for 50 tablets which have a shelf-life from manufacture of 3 years when stored at 2-8 °C. The 0.5 mol/l sodium hydroxide solution which is required is not provided but can be easily prepared in the laboratory. Control sera which give values for the *Phadebas Amylase Test* are listed at the end of 27:5.

Note: A *Phadebas isoamylase test* which measures amylase of pancreatic origin is also available from Pharmacia but this is a more complex and longer technique and costs almost three times as much as *Phadebas Amylase Test*.

Principle of the Caraway amylase method

Amylase is incubated at 37 °C for exactly 7½ minutes in a pH 7.0 phosphate buffered starch substrate. The enzyme hydrolyzes the starch to maltose and other fragments.

The amount of starch which remains unhydrolyzed at the end of the incubation period is shown by the addition of an iodine solution. The iodine reacts with the unhydrolyzed starch to give a violet blue-black colour, the absorbance of which is measured in a colorimeter using a red filter or in a spectrophotometer at 660 nm wavelength.

Enzyme activity is measured by the difference in absorbance of the starch-iodine complex of the sample against that of a reagent blank in which there is no hydrolysis. The result is expressed in international units per litre (U/l).

Amylase units

A Caraway unit of amylase is defined as the amount of amylase per 100 ml of serum or plasma that hydrolyzes 5 mg of starch in 15 minutes at 37 °C to the point at which it no longer gives a blue colour with iodine.

The factor of 1480 which is used to calculate amylase activity in U/l at the end of the test method is derived from:

$$\frac{100}{0.02} \times \frac{0.4}{5} \times \frac{15}{7.5} \times 1.85$$

where:
Amount of serum or plasma used in the test is 0.02 ml.
Amount of starch used = 0.4 mg.
Incubation time = 7.5 minutes.
The figure 1.85 is the arbitrary factor used to convert Caraway units/100 ml to U/l.

$$\text{Starch} \xrightarrow[\text{pH 7.0} \quad 37\,°C]{\text{Amylase}} \text{Maltose and other fragments}$$

Unhydrolyzed + Iodine ⟶ Starch-iodine complex
starch   *Violet blue-black*

Difference in absorbance
of starch-iodine complex
against reagent blank
gives amylase activity

Reagents
— Starch substrate, pH 7.0   Reagent No. 77
— Stock iodine solution   Reagent No. 47

The buffered starch substrate can be stored at room temperature (20-28 °C) and is stable for about 1 year. The stock iodine reagent when stored at 2-8 °C in a brown bottle is stable for about 2 months.

Working iodine reagent
Prepare by mixing 1 ml of stock iodine solution with 9 ml of distilled water.

Method
Specimen: The method requires 20 µl (0.02 ml) of patient's *fresh* serum or heparinized plasma that is free from haemolysis.

Note: Plasma from oxalated, EDTA, or citrated anticoagulated blood must not be used.

1. Take three graduated tubes (or tubes pre-marked to hold 10 ml) and label as follows:

   C   — Control serum (see 27:5)
   T   — Patient's test
   B   — Reagent blank

2. Pipette 1 ml of *well-mixed* starch substrate into each tube.

3. Place tubes C and T in a heat block or water bath set at 37 °C for 3 minutes to warm the substrate.

4. Without removing the tubes from the heat block or water bath add:

   C .... 20 µl (0.02 ml) control serum
   T .... 20 µl   patient's test serum

   Mix and incubate at 37 °C for *exactly* 7½ minutes.

   Important: Avoid contaminating the samples with saliva from the mouth (do not mouth-pipette) or perspiration from the thumb or fingers. Both saliva and perspiration contain amylase.

Summary of Amylase Method

Pipette in graduated tubes (or tubes premarked to hold 10 ml) as follows:	CONTROL C	TEST T	BLANK B
Starch substrate, *well-mixed*	1 ml	1 ml	1 ml

Warm tubes C and T at 37 °C for 3 minutes

Control serum	20 µl	—	—
Patient's serum	—	20 µl	—

Mix well

Incubate tubes C and T at 37 °C for *exactly* 7½ mins

Working iodine reagent	1 ml	1 ml	1 ml

Mix well

Make volume in each tube up to 10 ml with distilled water and *mix well*

READ ABSORBANCES

Colorimeter: Red filter, e.g. Ilford No. 608
Spectrophotometer: 660 nm

Zero instrument with distilled water

Calculate results as follows:

$$\text{Amylase U/l} = \frac{\text{Absorbance of blank} - \text{Absorbance of test or control}}{\text{Absorbance of blank}} \times 1480$$

Report patients' results if control is acceptable

20 µl = 0.02 ml

5. After exactly 7½ minutes, remove tubes C and T from the water bath. *Immediately* add 1 ml of working iodine reagent to tube C and T.

   Pipette 1 ml of working iodine reagent into tube B.

   Note: If the substrate is colourless after adding the working iodine reagent to the patient's test sample this means that the amylase level is very high. Dilute the patient's serum or plasma 1 in 6 with physiological saline (i.e. 20 μl patient's sample mixed with 0.1 ml saline) and repeat the test using 20 μl of the diluted sample. The final result must be multiplied by six.

6. Make the volume in each tube up to the 10 ml mark with distilled water and mix well.

7. Read immediately the absorbances of the test, control and reagent blank in a colorimeter using a red filter (e.g. Ilford No. 608) or in a spectrophotometer set at 660 nm. Zero the instrument with distilled water.

8. Calculate the amylase activity in U/l in the control and patient's samples from the following formula:

$$\text{Amylase U/l} = \frac{AB - AT}{AB} \times 1480^*$$

   where:
   AB = Absorbance of reagent blank
   AT = Absorbance of control or test
   * For an explanation of this factor, see *Principle of test*

   Results over 735 U/l
   Dilute the patient's serum or plasma 1 in 6 with physiological saline (20 μl and 0.1 ml saline) and repeat the assay using 20 μl of the diluted sample. Multiply the result by six.

9. Report the patient's result if the value of the control serum is acceptable.

Quality control
The principles of quality control in clinical chemistry are described in Chapter 27.

For the Caraway amylase method the following should be attainable:

— OCV, of around 6%
— RCV, not exceeding 12%

Approximate amylase reference (normal) range
70-340 U/l

To convert Caraway units /100 ml to international units /litre (U/l), multiply by 1.85. This is an arbitrary factor.

Interpretation of amylase results
Acute pancreatitis
Very high concentrations of serum or plasma amylase (over 1850 U/l) are virtually diagnostic of acute pancreatitis or acute episodes of chronic relapsing pancreatitis. When chronic pancreatitis has reached the stage of scarring and calcification, the serum amylase level is usually normal.

With acute pancreatitis, the rise in serum or plasma amylase is often very brief with the enzyme reaching its highest level within 12-24 hours and returning to normal within 48-72 hours.

Slight to moderate increases of serum amylase must be interpreted carefully. They are not diagnostic of acute pancreatitis unless the blood has been collected too late to catch the peak level.

Other laboratory findings
In acute pancreatitis the white cell count is raised. A serious condition is indicated if the serum or plasma albumin and calcium and blood haematocrit levels fall and the serum or plasma bilirubin and urea levels rise.

Other conditions giving raised amylase values
Serum or plasma amylase levels of approximately 740-1500 U/l may be due to:

— Renal failure
— Salivary gland obstruction or inflammation as with mumps
— Diabetic ketoacidosis
— Opiate drugs
— Alcoholism
— Hypothermia
— Almost any acute abdominal emergency, and also cholecystitis, perforated peptic ulcer, or appendicitis.

Falsely raised amylase level
Falsely elevated amylase levels may result if the serum is markedly turbid.

Measurement of Amylase in Urine
Urinary amylase (sometimes referred to as diastase) is raised in acute pancreatitis and in other conditions where serum or plasma amylase activity is increased. The measurement of urinary amylase can be helpful because unlike serum or plasma amylase, the urinary level remains elevated for 4-6 days after an attack of acute pancreatitis.

Urinary amylase is measured in the same way as serum or plasma amylase. The reference range for urine amylase is up to 300 U/l per hour.

30:11 SEMIQUANTITATIVE ESTIMATION OF TRYPSIN IN FAECES
X-ray Film Method[13]

Trypsin is an enzyme that is produced and secreted as trypsinogen by the pancreas. It is the main proteolytic enzyme in pancreatic juice, catalyzing the hydrolysis of proteins to small polypeptides (see Chapter 8).

The estimation of trypsin is requested to investigate pancreatic exocrine deficiency as in cystic fibrosis or chronic pancreatitis.

Choice of test method
A simple inexpensive gelatin test which gives a semiquantitative estimation of trypsin is described. It uses only a single reagent and a piece of unused (unexposed) X-ray film.

Principle of gelatin trypsin test
Dilutions of fresh duodenal juice or fresh emulsified faeces are made in 10 g/l sodium carbonate solution. Each dilution is placed on an area of unused (unexposed) X-ray film. The gelatin coating of the film acts as a protein substrate for the enzyme.

Following incubation at 37 °C for 30 minutes, the proteolytic activity of the enzyme is noted. The trypsin level is reported as the highest dilution of duodenal juice or faeces that gives complete digestion of the gelatin as shown by a clearing of the film.

Note: The test is less reliable if faeces are used because bacterial trypsin is normally present in faeces. Whenever possible the test should be performed using duodenal juice.

Reagent
— Sodium carbonate, 10 g/l   Reagent No. 66
  (1% w/v)

  The reagent is stable for several months at room temperature.

Method
1. Obtain a piece of unused X-ray film and cut out a square measuring 60 mm × 60 mm.

2. Using a grease pencil on the emulsion side, mark off the piece of film into 9 squares of equal size (i.e. each square measuring 20 × 20 mm).

   Mark the squares (in the right hand corner) 8, 16, 32, 64, 128, 256, 512, 1024, and C (control).

3. Place the marked film, emulsion side up, in the bottom of a petri dish (90 mm diameter) on a piece of damp filter paper.

4. Prepare dilutions from 1 in 8 to 1 in 1024 of the duodenal juice or emulsified fresh faeces as follows:

   — Take eight small tubes and number them 1 to 8.

   — Pipette 3.5 ml of the sodium carbonate reagent into tube 1 and 2.0 ml into the remaining tubes 2-8.

   — Add 0.5 ml of duodenal juice or emulsified faeces to tube 1, and mix.

   — Transfer 2 ml of the mixed suspension from tube 1 to tube 2, and mix. Repeat the procedure up to and including tube 8, discarding the final 2 ml.

5. Using a small bore plastic bulb pipette (see 2:4), place one small drop from each dilution onto its appropriate square of film, starting with the 1 in 1024 dilution (square 1024).

6. Pipette 1 drop of the sodium carbonate reagent onto the control (C) square.

7. Cover the petri dish and place it in a 37 °C incubator for 30 minutes.

8. At the end of 30 minutes, transfer the petri dish to a refrigerator for 5 minutes to allow the gelatin to harden.

9. Remove the piece of film from the petri dish and allow a gentle stream of water to flow over the surface of the film to wash off the dilutions and digested gelatin.

10. Examine the squares for digestion of the gelatin as shown by a clearing of the film.

11. Report the trypsin activity as the highest dilution that gives complete digestion (clearing) of the gelatin.

Control
The control square should show no proteolytic activity although the appearance of the gelatin may appear slightly altered.

Interpretation of results
Normal levels of trypsin
This is shown by digestion of the gelatin up to a dilution of at least 1 in 64 of faeces or 1 in 512 of duodenal juice.

Deficiency of trypsin
This is shown by no digestion of the gelatin or not beyond a dilution of 1 in 8 of faeces or 1 in 32 of duodenal juice.

30:12 TESTING FAECES FOR OCCULT BLOOD

Bleeding into the gastrointestinal tract may be rapid with the vomiting of blood (haematemesis) or the passage of blood through the rectum (melaena). When the bleeding is chronic with only small amounts of blood being passed in the faeces, the blood (or its breakdown products) is not recognized in the faeces and is referred to as occult (hidden) blood.

Requests for occult blood testing are usually made to investigate the cause of iron deficiency anaemia or to assist in the diagnosis of peptic ulceration or cancer of the gastrointestinal tract.

Choice of test

Chemical tests to detect occult blood are based on the principle that haemoglobin and its derivatives react in a similar way to peroxidase enzymes, i.e. they catalyze the transfer of an oxygen atom from a peroxide such as hydrogen peroxide to a chromogen such as benzidine, *o*-tolidine, guaiacum, 2,6-dichlorophenolindophenol or aminophenazone. Oxidation of the chromogen is shown by the production of a blue, blue-green, or pink colour.

Benzidine and o-tolidine tests
Tests which use benzidine or *o*-tolidine are not recommended because both these chemicals are known to have carcinogenic properties.

Occult blood tests differ in their sensitivity. Highly sensitive tests can be misleading because they detect trace amounts of blood which can be found in normal faeces or they give false positive reactions when faeces contains dietary substances which have peroxidase-like activity. Tests of low sensitivity can also be misleading because they may fail to detect small amounts of blood which are pathological. There is no chemical test for occult blood which is completely free from false positive and false negative reactions. Occult blood tests are essentially screening tests and their results must be interpreted with care.

The aminophenazone occult blood test is a suitable test for district laboratories. The reagents can be easily prepared in the laboratory.

Occult blood test kits
Generally available test kits include:

■ *Okokit* tablet test, available from Hughes and Hughes

Ltd. It uses guaiacum and is an intermediate to low sensitivity test with a 2 year shelf-life from manufacture.

■ *Hemoccult* slide and tape tests, available from Smith Kline Diagnostics. They use guaiacum and are of intermediate to low sensitivity tests with a 2 year shelf-life from manufacture.

■ *Quick-Cult* slide and tape tests, available from Laboratory Diagnostics Company Inc. They use guaiacum and are of intermediate to low sensitivity tests with a 3 year shelf-life from manufacture.

■ *Peroheme 40* paper test, available from BDH Diagnostics. This uses 2,6-dichlorophenolindophenol as the chromogen and is a more sensitive test than the other products mentioned above. It has a 1 year shelf-life from manufacture.

Note: For further information about the above mentioned kits, including prices and local availability readers should contact each manufacturer (addresses can be found in Appendix II).

Principle of the aminophenazone test

Haemoglobin and its derivatives catalyze the transfer of oxygen from hydrogen peroxide to aminophenazone. Oxidation of the aminophenazone produces a blue colour.

Reagents

— Acetic acid, 10% v/v   Reagent No. 2
— Alcohol, 95% v/v   Reagent No. 9
— Hydrogen peroxide (H_2O_2)   Reagent No. 46
  10 vols solution*

   * A 10 vols (volume) hydrogen peroxide solution means that 1 volume will give 10 volumes of oxygen at NTP on complete degradation. If the solution available is 100 vols, dilute 1 in 10 with distilled water to obtain a 10 vols solution. Store in a tightly stoppered dark bottle away from light and heat.

Working Aminophenazone reagent
The amounts given are sufficient for 1 test with positive and negative controls. Prepare fresh as follows:

Alcohol, 95% v/v .... 15 ml
Acetic acid, 10% v/v .... 1 ml
4-Aminophenazone* (4-aminoantipyrine) .. 0.4 g

* Accurate weighing is not necessary. For easy preparation, mark a small tube to hold 0.4 g of the chemical. Between use keep the marked tube attached to the bottle of chemical with an elastic band.

Dissolve the aminophenazone in the alcohol solution and *immediately before use* add the acetic acid. Mix well.

Method

1. Dispense about 7 ml of distilled water into a wide bore test tube.

   A 10 ml syringe may be used to dispense the water.

2. Add a sample of faeces about 10-15 mm in diameter (taken from various parts of the specimen). Using a glass or plastic rod, emulsify the faeces in the water.

3. Allow the faecal particles to settle or centrifuge the emulsified specimen.

4. Take three *completely clean* tubes and label them:

   T   — Patient's test
   Neg   — Negative control
   Pos   — Positive control

5. Add to into each tube as follows:
   Tube

   T ......5 ml supernatant fluid from emulsified faeces
   Neg ...5 ml distilled water
   Pos ... 5 ml distilled water in which 50 μl (0.05 ml) of whole blood has been mixed

   A 5 ml syringe may be used to dispense the faecal supernatant fluid and distilled water.

6. Layer 5 ml of working aminophenazone reagent on top of the fluid in each tube (i.e. pipette down the side of each tube). Do *not* mix.

   A 5 ml syringe may be used to dispense the reagent.

7. Add 10 drops of the 10 vols hydrogen peroxide solution. Do *not* mix. Allow to stand for 1 minute.

8. Look for the appearance of a blue colour where the aminophenazone reagent meets the sample or control solutions.

   Report the results as follows:

No colour change	Negative
Pale blue	Positive +
Dark blue	Positive ++
Blue-black	Positive +++

Negative control: This should show no colour change
Positive control: This should show a positive reaction.

False reactions

A false positive reaction may occur if the faeces contains peroxidase-like substances particularly meat (myoglobin), fish, or green vegetables. To avoid this it is best if the patient does not eat these foods for at least 1 day before the test specimen is obtained.

A false negative reaction may be obtained if the faeces contains a high concentration of ascorbic acid.

Note: If the test is negative but there is high clinical suspicion, a further two specimens should be tested to detect bleeding which may be intermittent.

Interpretation of results

The commonest causes of positive occult blood tests in tropical and other developing countries are hookworm infection, peptic ulcer, and bleeding from oesophageal varices due to cirrhosis of the liver.

Other causes include carcinoma in the gastrointestinal tract, erosive gastritis due to alcohol or drugs, or swallowed blood from recurrent nosebleeds.

30:13 EXAMINATION OF FAECES FOR EXCESS FAT

Most dietary fat is absorbed in the small intestine with very little being excreted in the faeces. Normal fat absorption requires the presence of bile salts, pancreatic and intestinal lipase, and a normal intestinal mucosa.

Steatorrhoea

Disorders of fat absorption cause excessive amounts of fat to be excreted in the faeces. The condition is referred to as steatorrhoea.

In tropical countries, steatorrhoea is associated with post-infective tropical malabsorption (tropical sprue), giardiasis, strongyloidiasis, capillariasis, chronic pancreatitis, and less commonly to pancreatic or biliary obstruction.

Microscopical examination of faeces for fat

Fatty stools are pale in colour, bulky, float on water, and are often frothy with an offensive odour.

Excess fat in faeces may occur as:

■ Neutral fat globules

- Fatty acid crystals
- Soapy flakes

Method
1. Make a thin preparation of the faeces in physiological saline on a slide. Cover with a cover glass (avoid trapping air bubbles).

2. Examine the preparation for excess neutral fat globules, fatty acid crystals, and soapy fats using the 10× and 40× objectives with the condenser iris closed sufficiently to give good contrast.

   Constant focusing is necessary because fat does not sediment but tends to float in the preparation.

Neutral fat globules
These are easily recognized because they are highly refractile, colourless, and variable in size and shape with an oily look. They can be stained orange-red with a concentrated alcoholic solution of Sudan III or a saturated solution of oil red 0 in isopropanol (the stain can be run under one end of the cover glass).

If a drop of ethanol or ether is added, the fat globules will dissolve. Patients taking liquid paraffin excrete droplets of oil which are identical in appearances to the fat globules present in steatorrhoea.

Fatty acids
Fatty acids usually appear as groups of needle-like colourless crystals. They do not stain with Sudan III or oil red 0, but melt easily if *gentle* heat is applied to the preparation. Fatty acid crystals dissolve in ethanol and ether.

Soapy fats
Soaps also form masses of needle-like colourless crystals. They can be distinguished from fatty acid crystals because they do not melt with heat and they do not dissolve in ethanol or ether unless first treated with acetic acid. Soapy fats occur as flakes (soapy plaques).

Interpretation of microscopical findings
The presence of excess neutral fat globules in the faeces of a person taking a normal diet suggests lipase deficiency due to pancreatic disease. Neutral fat is the unsplit form of fat which is found in food before it is digested.

The presence of excess fatty acids and soapy fats (split fats that have not been absorbed) in faeces suggests malabsorption.

Measurement of faecal fat
The results of faecal fat tests are often unsatisfactory due to errors of collection, effects of constipation and diet, and to unsuitable test methods.

Few district hospital laboratories are equipped to perform faecal fat estimations. The laboratory methods available for determining faecal fats involve considerable health risks to those involved in the collection of faeces and the performance of the estimation.

Because of the unreliability of results and the unsafe nature of the procedure, many clinical chemistry laboratories no longer measure faecal fats.

30:14 INVESTIGATION OF LACTASE DEFICIENCY

Lactase is an enzyme which converts lactose to glucose and galactose. If lactase is deficient, lactose is not digested or absorbed but ferments to lactic acid with the production of gas. This causes abdominal pain and diarrhoea which may be persistent and severe especially in young children.

When there is lactase deficiency faecal specimens usually contain lactose and have a low pH due to the presence of lactic acid.

Lactase deficiency is indicated if a faecal specimen:

- Contains ++ or more of sugar (lactose)
- Has a pH of 6.0 or below

Testing for lactose in faeces
The simplest method of detecting lactose in a fluid faecal specimen is to use Benedict's reagent or *Clinitest.*

If using Benedict's reagent, the specimen is tested in the same way as described for urine in 31:3

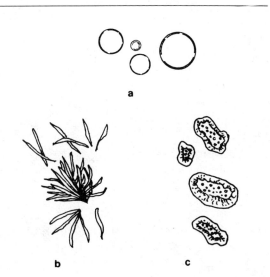

Fig. 30.1 *a* **Neutral fat globules.** *b* **Fatty acids** *c* **Soapy plaques.**

except that 8 drops of freshly passed fluid faecal specimen are used instead of urine.

If using *Clinitest*, add 5 drops of freshly passed fluid specimen to 10 drops of clean water. After boiling has stopped mix the contents of the tube and note the colour of the fluid. A yellow-brown colour indicates the presence of ++ sugar (lactose).

Testing of pH of faeces
The pH of a faecal fluid specimen can be tested using a pH meter or narrow range pH papers.

low cost edition of this book is available from P. G. Publishing Private Ltd, Alexandra, PO Box 318, Singapore 9115, Singapore.

References

1   American Association for Clinical Chemistry Inc. *Selected Methods for the Small Clinical Chemistry Laboratory*. Ed. Willard, R., and Meites, F and S., 1982.

2   Doumas, B. T., *et al*. Standardization in bilirubin assays: Evaluation of selected methods and stability of bilirubin solutions. *Clinical Chemistry*, 19, **9**, pp 984-993, 1973.

3   Doumas, B. T. *Clinical Chemistry*, **21**, pp 1159-1166, 1975.

4   Studies comparing the biuret colorimetric method and refractometric technique for estimating serum total protein are available upon request from the American Optical Company, (for address, see Appendix II).

5   Spencer, K., and Price, C. P. *Annals of Clinical Biochemistry*, **14**, pp 105-115, 1977.

6   Doumas, B. T., Watson, W. A., and Biggs, H. G. *Clinica Chimica Acta* 31, p 87, 1971.

7   Reitman, S., and Frankel, S. *American Journal of Clinical Pathology*, **28**, pp 56-63, 1957.

8   bioMérieux *Clinical Chemistry Catalogue*, p 125, 1984.

9   Bessey, O. A., Lowry, O. H., and Brock, M. J. *Journal of Biological Chemistry*, **164**, p 321, 1946.

10 Merck, *Directions for Use, Clinical Chemistry, Diagnostica Merck*, 1982/83.

11 Caraway, W. T. *American Journal of Clinical Pathology*, **32**, pp 97-99, 1959.

12 Martinek, R. G. *Clinica Chimica Acta*, **9**, pp 590-592, 1964.

13 Gordon, I. G., Levin, B., and Whitehead, T. P. *British Medical Journal*, **1**, p 463, 1952.

14 Cohen, J. D., Nephrotic syndrome, *Medicine Digest*, **12**, (10), pp 4-10, 1986.

Recommended Reading
Baron, D. N. *A Short Textbook of Chemical Pathology*, Hodder and Stoughton, 4th Edition, 1982. ELBS 1984: £2 ISBN 0 340 27048 9.

Whitby, L. G., Percy-Robb, I. W., and Smith, A. F. *Lecture Notes on Clinical Chemistry*, Blackwell Scientific Publications, 3rd Edition, 1984, UK price £9.80. A

31

Measurement of Blood Glucose and Calcium
Urinary Sugar and Ketones
Cerebrospinal Fluid Tests

31:1 MEASUREMENT OF PLASMA GLUCOSE
Glucose Oxidase Method (GOD-PAP)[1, 2, 3]

The body's need for glucose and the role of insulin and other factors in regulating blood glucose levels are described in 8:2.

Plasma glucose is measured mainly in the diagnosis and management of diabetes mellitus. Good control of blood glucose levels in diabetics helps to prevent or delay the development of complications which may lead to blindness, kidney failure, coronary thrombosis, and gangrene of the lower limbs.

Blood glucose measurements must be carried out on the day and *at the time requested*. Collection times are usually related to food intake, insulin treatment, or both. The time the blood is collected must be written on the specimen container and on the patient's request form.

Provision must be made for urgent glucose measurement requests which may be necessary outside the normal working hours of the laboratory. Both severe hyperglycaemia (high glucose levels) and hypoglycaemia (low glucose levels) can result in loss of consciousness (coma) and therefore require urgent investigation.

Terms used to describe the collection of blood glucose specimens
Fasting specimen
This refers to blood collected after a period of no food intake. For adults the fasting time is usually 10 to 16 hours. For children the fasting time is 6 hours unless a longer time is indicated, e.g. when investigating hypoglycaemia. The drinking of plain water does not break the fast.

Post-prandial specimen
This describes blood collected after a meal has been taken. The sample is usually taken as a 2 h post-prandial specimen.

Random specimen
This refers to a blood sample collected at any time, regardless of food intake.

Note: The collection of blood for glucose tolerance tests is described in 31:2.

Choice of test method
In the first edition of this manual an *o*-toluidine glucose method was recommended in preference to a glucose oxidase method for reasons of cost, reagent stability, and simplicity of technique. Caution was expressed regarding the handling of the highly corrosive and toxic *o*-toluidine reagent.

With the further development of glucose oxidase techniques, reagents have become more stable and methods easier to perform. There is also now very little difference in cost between glucose oxidase and *o*-toluidine manual colorimetric methods. For these reasons and also because the working *o*-toluidine reagent is so irritating and corrosive, a glucose oxidase method is recommended and described in this edition of the manual. There is also some evidence that *o*-toluidine may be a carcinogen.

A further advantage of the glucose oxidase method is that the reaction is carried out at 37 °C not at 100 °C like the *o*-toluidine method.

Note: Copper and ferricyanide blood glucose reduction methods are not recommended because they are not sufficiently selective for glucose.

Glucose test kits
Several manual colorimetric glucose oxidase kits are available commercially. Most, however, do not include a protein precipitation stage. The total volume for measuring in many of the kits is only 1.01 ml which means that both sample and reagent volumes will probably need to be doubled (an important consideration when evaluating the cost of using a kit). Details of calibration are not included in the instructions which accompany most glucose oxidase kits.

Important: For further comments regarding the purchasing and use of clinical chemistry test kits, see 26:1.

Principle of glucose oxidase-peroxidase method
Glucose oxidase (GOD) catalyzes the oxidation of glucose to give hydrogen peroxide (H_2O_2) and gluconic acid. In the presence of the enzyme peroxidase (POD), the hydrogen peroxide is broken down and the oxygen released reacts with 4-aminophenazone (4-aminoantipyrine) and phenol to give a pink colour.

The absorbance of the colour produced is measured in a colorimeter using a green filter or in a spectrophotometer at 515 nm.

$$Glucose + oxygen \xrightarrow{GOD} Gluconic\ acid + H_2O_2$$

$$H_2O_2 + aminophenazone + phenol \xrightarrow{POD} Coloured\ complex$$
Pink

Note: A protein precipitation stage is required because the phenol is contained in the protein precipitant reagent. It also helps to achieve more reliable results by removing certain substances (particularly urate) which may be present in samples in sufficient concentration to interfere in the final stage of the reaction.[6]

To reduce costs, the glucose oxidase method described in this subunit uses smaller volumes of patients' and control samples and reagents than described in other publications.

Calibration

The glucose oxidase method is calibrated from a solution of glucose. This is prepared and diluted to make a series of standards as follows:

Stock glucose standard, 100 mmol/l
1. Weigh accurately 1.8 g of dry anhydrous glucose (analytical reagent grade).

   Note: To ensure that the glucose is dry, heat it in an open container in an oven at 60-80 °C for about 4 hours. Remove and close the container immediately. When cool, weigh the glucose.

2. Transfer the glucose to a 100 ml volumetric flask. Half fill the flask with 1 g/l benzoic acid (Reagent No. 14) and mix until the glucose is fully dissolved. Make up to the 100 ml mark with the benzoic acid reagent and mix well.

   The glucose concentration in the flask is 100 mmol/l.

3. Transfer to a storage bottle and label. When stored at 2-8 °C the stock standard is stable for about 6 months. If stored frozen in tightly stoppered containers the stock standard is stable for at least 1 year.

Working glucose standards 2.5, 5, 10, 20, 25 mmol/l
1. Take five 100 ml volumetric flasks and number them 1 to 5. Pipette accurately into each flask as follows:

Flask	Stock glucose, 100 mmol/l
1	2.5 ml
2	5.0 ml
3	10.0 ml
4	20.0 ml
5	25.0 ml

2. Make the contents of each flask up to the 100 ml mark with 1 g/l benzoic acid (Reagent No. 14) and mix well.

The concentration of glucose in each standard is as follows:

Flask	1 = 2.5 mmol/l
	2 = 5.0 mmol/l
	3 = 10.0 mmol/l
	4 = 20.0 mmol/l
	5 = 25.0 mmol/l

3. Transfer each solution to a storage bottle and label. Store at room temperature (20-28 °C). The working standards are stable for about 2 months.

Preparation of glucose calibration graph
1. Take six tubes and label them 'B' (reagent blank) and 1 to 5. Pipette 1.5 ml of protein precipitant reagent into each tube.

2. Add to each tube as follows:

Tube	
B	50 µl (0.05 ml) distilled water
1	50 µl standard, 2.5 mmol/l
2	50 µl standard, 5 mmol/l
3	50 µl standard, 10 mmol/l
4	50 µl standard, 20 mmol/l
5	50 µl standard, 25 mmol/l

3. Continue as described in steps 5 to 7 of the glucose method.

4. Take a sheet of graph paper and plot the absorbance of each standard (vertical axis) against its concentration in mmol/l (horizontal axis) as described in 25:2. A linear calibation should be obtained.

The useful working limit (linearity) of the glucose oxidase method is about 25 mmol/l.

Important: Check the calibration graph by measuring a control serum as described in the urea method. A new calibration graph should be prepared and checked against controls whenever stock reagents are renewed.

Reagents
— Protein precipitant reagent   Reagent No. 61
— Colour reagent   Reagent No. 26

The protein precipitant reagent can be stored at room temperature (20-28 °C). It is stable indefinitely. The colour reagent requires storage at 2-8 °C. When refrigerated it has a shelf-life of about 3 months.

Method

Specimen: The method requires 50 μl (0.05 ml) of patient's plasma from a fluoride-oxalate specimen. Details of blood collection and the stability of glucose in plasma can be found in 26:7.

Note: Serum can also be used providing the assay is carried out within 30 minutes of collecting the blood (without fluoride preservative the glucose is broken down by glycolysis). The use of capillary or venous whole blood should be avoided because the concentration of glucose in red cells is not constant.

The glucose oxidase method described in this subunit can also be used for measuring glucose in cerebrospinal fluid (see step 3.).

1. Take four or more tubes (depending on the number of tests) and label as follows:

    B   — Reagent blank
    S   — Standard, 10.0 mmol/l
    C   — Control (see 27:5)
    1, 2, etc   — Patients' tests

    Note: Whenever resources permit, a range of standards should be assayed with each batch of tests.

2. Pipette 1.5 ml of protein precipitant reagent into each tube.

3. Add to each tube as follows:

    Tube
    B .... 50 μl (0.05 ml) distilled water
    S .... 50 μl standard, 10 mmol/l
    C .... 50 μl control serum
    1, 2, etc .... 50 μl patient's plasma
    Mix well.

    Important: If a glucose request is urgent because a patient is thought to be in a hypoglycaemic (low glucose) coma, to avoid any possible delay set up an additional tube containing 100 μl of plasma (divide the result by two).

    Measurement of glucose in cerebrospinal fluid (c.s.f.):
    Use 0.2 ml (200 μl) of c.s.f. and divide the result by four (a fasting lumbar c.s.f. glucose is normally 40-80% of the blood glucose).

4. Centrifuge the control and patients' samples (tubes C, 1, 2, etc) for 3-5 minutes at medium to high speed to obtain clear supernatant fluids.

5. Transfer 0.5 ml from the blank, standard, control, and patients' samples to a second set of tubes (labelled as in step 1).

6. Add 1.5 ml of colour reagent to each tube and *mix well*.

Incubate at 37 °C in a heat-block or water bath for 10 minutes. Shake occasionally to ensure adequate aeration of the samples.

7. Read the absorbances of the solutions in a colorimeter using a green filter (e.g. Ilford No. 604) or in a spectrophotometer set at wavelength 515 nm. Zero the instrument with the blank solution in tube B.

    Note: For some colorimeters it may be necessary to use a modified cuvette holder to measure small volumes. No modification is required if using a WPA model CO700D Colorimeter (see 25:3).

8. Calculate the concentration of glucose in the control and patients' samples by:

    — Reading the values from the calibration graph providing the result of the 10 mmol/l standard agrees with the calibration or if not by

    — Using the following formula:

    $$\text{Glucose mmol/l} = \frac{AT}{AS} \times 10.0$$

    where : AT = Absorbance of test(s) or control
                AS = Absorbance of 10 mmol/l standard

    Glucose results below 2.2 mmol/l
    Repeat the assay using 0.1 ml (100 μl) of patient's plasma.
    Multiply the result by two.

    Glucose results over 25.0 mmol/l
    Repeat the assay after diluting the plasma 1 in 2, i.e. mix 50 μl plasma with 50 μl distilled water and use 50 μl of this diluted sample in the test.

9. Report the patients' results if the value of the control serum is acceptable.

Quality control

The principles of quality control in clinical chemistry are described in Chapter 27.

For the glucose oxidase method the following should be attainable:

— OCV, of around 3%
— RCV, not exceeding 6%

Approximate glucose reference (normal) range
Adults
— Fasting (plasma) 3.6-6.4 mmol/l (see *Note*)
— Random (plasma) 3.3-7.4 mmol/l (see *Note*)
Children
— Fasting (plasma) 2.4-5.3 mmol/l (see *Note*)
     Newborn values are slightly lower, i.e. 1.1-4.4 mmol/l

Summary of Glucose Method

For detailed instructions, see text

Pipette into tubes as follows:	BLANK B	STANDARD S	CONTROL C	TESTS 1,2, etc
Protein precipitant reagent	1.5 ml	1.5 ml	1.5 ml	1.5 ml
Distilled water	50 μl	—	—	—
Standard, 10.0 mmol/l	—	50 μl	—	—
Control serum	—	—	50 μl	—
Patient's plasma	—	—	—	50 μl

Mix well

Centrifuge tubes C, and tests 1, 2, etc to obtain clear supernatant fluids

Take a second set of tubes and label B, S, C, 1, 2, etc

Transfer from first to second set of tubes	0.5 ml	0.5 ml	0.5 ml	0.5 ml
Add colour reagent to second set of tubes	1.5 ml	1.5 ml	1.5 ml	1.5 ml

Mix well

Incubate at 37 °C for 10 minutes. Shake occasionally.

READ ABSORBANCES

Colorimeter: Green filter, e.g. Ilford No. 604
Spectrophotometer: 515 nm

Zero instrument with blank solution in tube B

Obtain values from the calibration graph if the result of 10 mmol/l standard agrees with calibration. If not, calculate the results as follows:

$$\text{Glucose mmol/l} = \frac{\text{Absorbance of test or control}}{\text{Absorbance of 10.0 mmol/l standard}} \times 10$$

Report patients' results if control value is acceptable

50 μl = 0.05 ml

To convert from mmol/l to mg%, multiply by 18.
To convert from mg% to mmol/l, divide by 18.

Note: In current practice, reference ranges have little real use. Plasma glucose results are now compared to definitive numerical criteria as detailed below (see *Interpretation of results*).

Venous plasma values are about 15% higher than whole blood values (except in anaemia).

There is little difference between values obtained from venous plasma and capillary plasma when the glucose concentration is normal. When the glucose is raised however, the value obtained from capillary plasma will be slightly higher than that from venous plasma.

Interpretation of blood glucose results
Increases

A raised blood glucose level is called hyperglycaemia. When definite it is diagnostic of diabetes mellitus. In an adult with symptoms, a random venous plasma glucose of 11.1 mmol/l or more on two occasions or a fasting value of 7.8 mmol/l or more on two occasions is diagnostic. Random values below 7.8 mmol/l and fasting values below 6.4 mmol/l exclude a diagnosis of diabetes mellitus.

Diabetes in tropical and developing countries

Diabetes is widespread throughout the world. It is known to affect more than 30 million people with a sharp rise in prevalence having been reported from those developing countries in which the disease has been studied. Untreated diabetes is an important cause of premature death, prolonged illhealth, and disability. Diabetic persons are also at risk of acute infections of the skin (e.g. boils, carbuncles), candidiasis, and pulmonary tuberculosis.

A description of the main clinical forms of diabetes can be found in 8:2. Many of the genetic, immunological, and environmental factors that cause or lead to diabetes are not fully understood and sufficient information from most developing countries is not yet available. With reference to Africa, it appears that the bulk of African diabetics belong to the non-insulin dependent [Type 2] group and that the typical insulin dependent [Type 1] diabetes is rare. Genetic and immunological factors play a smaller role in causing diabetes in Africans. Environmental factors such as malnutrition, alcohol, and widespread infections (mainly viral) are clearly more important.[4]

One form of diabetes, referred to as the J (Jamaica) type, has been observed in the West Indies and also in Africa, Indonesia, India, Pakistan, Malaysia, Fiji, and Papua New Guinea. It affects mainly children and non-obese young adults. It is characterized by a resistance to ketosis even though the diabetes is of a severe form that requires high doses of insulin. Nearly all patients have a history of severe malnutrition in childhood.

Another form of diabetes which is also common in tropical countries especially in Brazil, South India, Indonesia, Nigeria, and Zaire is associated with pancreatitis in which the pancreas becomes fibrosed and calcified. It has been reported as having an onset in youth but is found in all age groups. There is often a history of severe malnutrition in childhood and in some populations it appears to be linked to a build up of cyanide in the body from eating cassava where this is the main food consumed.

In its 1980 *Diabetes Report*,[5] WHO recommends the establishment of special centres in developing countries to integrate the care of diabetics and to promote improved diagnosis and research into diabetes. Further information regarding health services and the management of diabetes can also be found in this *Report.*

A mild hyperglycaemia may accompany pancreatic disease or pituitary and adrenal disorders. Steroid therapy may also cause hyperglycaemia due to reduced carbohydrate metabolism.

Transient hyperglycaemia often occurs following severe stress, e.g. after surgery, injury, shock, infections, or severe burns.

Decreases

A low blood glucose level is called hypoglycaemia. Persistent occurrences of hypoglycaemia with glucose levels less than 2.2 mmol/l accompanied by symptoms such as fainting, fits, sweating, hunger, pallor, confusion, or violence, should be investigated.

Causes of hypoglycaemia include kwashiorkor, severe liver disease, alcoholic excess, insulin secreting tumours, Addison's disease, and certain drugs. Commonly, however, markedly reduced blood glucose levels occur following the overtreatment of diabetes.

Neonatal hypoglycaemia: Newborn infants may suffer hypoglycaemia when blood glucose levels fall below 1.1 mmol/l. Infants particularly at risk are underweight poorly nourished babies, twins, premature infants, and babies born of diabetic mothers. It is important to detect hypoglycaemia of the newborn because without treatment brain damage may occur.

False glucose values

A falsely high glucose level will result if a blood sample is collected from an arm receiving a glucose (dextrose) intravenous (i.v.) infusion.

A falsely low value may be obtain if the plasma is markedly icteric.

REAGENT STRIP TESTS TO MEASURE
BLOOD GLUCOSE

The semiquantitative measurement of blood glucose by a reagent strip method that covers the range 1-44 mmol/l (20-800 mg%) is suitable for use in emergency situations by health centres and small hospital laboratories unable to measure blood glucose by a colorimetric technique.

Two strips are currently available (1986) to estimate blood glucose over the range 1-44 mmol/l:

☐ *Visidex II* (replaced *Visidex I*), manufactured by Ames Division Miles Laboratories (see Appendix II).

☐ *Haemo-Glukotest 20-800R* (also known as *BM-Test-Glycemie 20-800R*, and *Chemstrip G*), manufactured by Boehringer Mannheim (see Appendix II).

Both strips use glucose oxidase methods. Full instructions are supplied with the products and these must be followed exactly. There are two separate test areas on each strip which make it possible to assay glucose in the range 1 to 44 mmol/l. Test results are stable for several days as detailed in the manufacturers' information sheets.

Cost of blood glucose strips

In some countries *Visidex II* is less expensive than *Haemo-Glukotest 20-800R*. Details of availability and local prices can be obtained by writing to Ames and Boehringer companies (see Appendix II). Foil packed strips are considerably more expensive than strips sold in containers. Costs can however be reduced by cutting (vertically) the strips in half using sharp scissors. There appears to be no loss of accuracy when using half strips[10].

Quality control and storage of blood glucose strips

Control glucose solutions are available for testing *Visidex II* and *Haemo-Glukotest 20-800R*. Full details are available from Ames and Boehringer companies.

Both *Visidex II* and *Haemo-Glukotest 20-800R* strips can be stored at room temperature (below 30 °C).They must be kept tightly stoppered in their containers, protected from humidity and bright light.

Visidex II has an expiry date of 6 months from the time the container is opened. *Haemo-Glukotest 20-800R* has greater stability with an expiry date of 2 years from when the container is opened. Both *Visidex II* and *Haemo-Glukotest 20-800R* are packaged in containers which hold 50 strips.

Note: Evaluations of *Visidex II* and *Haemo-Glukotest 20-800R* have been published.[8, 9, 10]

Blood glucose meters for reading strip tests

While a meter such as the Boehringer *Reflolux* (battery/mains) provides a more accurate reading of *Haemo-Glukotest 20-800R* strips (*Visidex II* cannot be read using a meter), in most cases a visually read strip will give acceptable accuracy for the diagnosis and management of diabetic patients.[11]

Most meters are expensive and should not be purchased unless servicing facilities are available and those operating the meters are trained carefully in their use and control.

GLYCOSYLATED HAEMOGLOBIN[12]

Red cells normally contain some haemoglobin A in glycosylated form i.e. attached to a glucose residue. Glycosylated haemoglobin A is referred to as Hb A_1. The main glycosylated fraction is Hb A_{1c} and its concentration in the blood is proportional to the average blood glucose level that existed over the previous 2-3 months. The glucose remains complexed to the haemoglobin molecule for the lifetime of the red cell and therefore the concentration of glycosylated haemoglobin circulating in red cells is a guide to the average blood glucose level over a period of the previous 8-12 weeks (lifespan of red cells).

Measurement of glycosylated haemoglobin can sometimes help in assessing the control of diabetic patients, particularly non-insulin dependent diabetics whose blood glucose levels do not change markedly. The test is of less value in diabetics where blood glucose levels range from high to low. This is because when averaged the glucose level may be 'normal'.

Microchromatographic and ion-exchange resin colorimetric methods for measuring glycosylated haemoglobin are available but expensive.† Reference ranges for Hb A_1 are usually 5-9% of the total haemoglobin but each laboratory should work out its own range. The expected values for uncontrolled diabetics when using the *Glycohemoglobin Hb A_1 test* kit are quoted as greater than 8.5%.

† Glycohemoglobin Hb A_1 test kit

This is a rapid ion-exchange resin colorimetric test manufactured by Human GmbH (for address, see Appendix II). It costs about £26 for 20 tests (1985-1986). Whole blood is lyzed and mixed with a cation-exchange resin. A resin separator is used to remove the resin from the supernatant fluid which contains the glycohaemoglobin. The percentage of glycohaemoglobin is determined by measuring the absorbances of the glycohaemoglobin fraction and total haemoglobin fraction (from lyzed blood) at 415 nm, calculating the ratio of the absorbances and comparing this ratio with that of the standard preparation provided.

31:2 GLUCOSE TOLERANCE TESTS

A glucose tolerance test (GTT) measures the ability of the body to tolerate, or cope with, a standard dose of glucose. The degree of tolerance to the glucose, as shown by changes in the blood levels, is mainly dependent on the rate of glucose absorption and on the insulin response. As the glucose is absorbed, the level of glucose in the blood rises and the normal response is for insulin to be released from the pancreas to lower the glucose level. Tolerance is reduced when insulin is insufficient or absent.

Glucose tolerance tests are usually requested to investigate glycosuria or when a random or fasting blood glucose is suggestive but not diagnostic of diabetes. It happens only rarely however that the result of a fasting or random blood glucose is difficult to interpret and a GTT is necessary.

Note: Glucose tolerance tests are used far too frequently in most clinical practices and should be discouraged unless absolutely necessary. If glycosuria is found, measurement of fasting glucose should be performed *before* the patient is subjected to a GTT.[17]

Preparation of the patient
— Before the test the patient should be on a diet containing not less than 150 g of carbohydrate per day for at least 3 days. If the GTT is performed following starvation or a diet low in carbohydrate, glucose tolerance will be reduced which will make the results of the test difficult to interpret.

— Ideally the test should be performed in the morning. The patient should be instructed not to eat, drink (except plain water), or smoke for 10-16 hours before the test.

For infants the fasting time from food is as follows:

Infants less than 4 months:	4 hour fast
Infants aged 4-6 months:	6 hour fast
Infants aged 6-24 months:	8 hour fast

— Patients should be reassured if anxious. Outpatients should be allowed to rest for about 20 minutes before starting the test especially if they have had to walk a considerable distance to reach the hospital. Excessive exercise, excitement, or fear may reduce glucose tolerance.

— During the test the patient should, if possible, be sitting up. If lying down the patient should be positioned on the right side to ensure rapid emptying of the stomach.

— Ideally the patient should have no other disease at the time a glucose tolerance test is performed.

Method of performing a glucose tolerance test
1. Prepare a GTT chart for the patient on which to record collection times and test results. A layout of such a chart is shown at the end of this method.

2. Collect a fasting venous blood sample into a bottle or tube containing fluoride-oxalate (Reagent No. 37). Label the container 'fasting blood'.

3. Give the patient 75 g of glucose (D-glucose monohydrate) in 250-350 ml water, to be drunk in 5 to 15 minutes.[5] To reduce nausea a few drops of lemon juice may be added to the water.

Note: For children, the recommended glucose dose is 1.75 g per kilogram body weight to a maximum of 75 g.

4. Make a note of the time and enter on the GTT chart the times at which the blood samples are to be collected, i.e. 1 hour and 2 hours after the glucose water has been drunk.

Collection times
Formerly blood samples were collected at 30 minute intervals but studies have shown that it is the fasting and 2 hour post glucose samples that are of major diagnostic value.[5] The 1 hour post glucose sample is of value to support a clinical diagnosis of diabetes especially when symptoms of the disease are absent.

5. Instruct the patient to rest quietly and not to eat, drink, exercise, smoke, or leave the hospital during the test. Inform the patient when the test will be completed.

Important: If the patient should feel faint, very nauseated or begin to perspire excessively, call a medical officer.

6. Collect each blood sample at the correct time, labelling each container with the collection time.

7. Measure the glucose concentration in each of the three blood specimens using the method described in 31:1.

8. Enter the patient's results on the GTT chart if the value of the control serum is acceptable.

Example of GTT Chart Layout

Collection times	*Plasma Glucose Results*
Fasting	..........mmol/l
1 hour*	..........mmol/l
2 hours*	..........mmol/l

*After drinking the glucose water

Interpretation of GTT venous plasma glucose results
The following diagnostic criteria (WHO) are for venous plasma glucose results:

Healthy	Fasting	< 6.4 mmol/l
	2 hour specimen	< 7.8 mmol/l
	Intermediate specimen	< 11.1 mmol/l
Diabetic	Fasting	≥ 7.8 mmol/l
	2 hour specimen	≥ 11.1 mmol/l
Impaired glucose tolerance	Fasting	< 7.8 mmol/l
	2 hour specimen	7.9-11.0 mmol/l
	Intermediate specimen	≥ 11.1 mmol/l

Notes

□ For asymptomatic patients, two abnormal values of greater than 11.1 mmol/l are needed to make a diagnosis of diabetes mellitus.

□ Generally, young children show an increase in glucose tolerance and elderly persons show a tendency towards a reduction in tolerance.

□ With malabsorption, there is very little rise in the blood glucose value after glucose intake (flat GTT showing increased tolerance but this is of very limited value as a diagnostic test since young healthy adults have a flat curve).

31:3 TESTING URINE FOR GLUCOSE

Almost all the glucose which passes from the blood into the glomerular filtrate is normally reabsorbed back into the circulation by the kidney tubules. Usually less than 0.8 mmol/l (15 mg%) is excreted in the urine. The term glycosuria refers to the presence of more than the usual amount of glucose in the urine.

Renal threshold for glucose
The highest level that the blood glucose reaches before glycosuria occurs is referred to as the renal threshold for glucose. In health it is about 9-10 mmol/l (160-180 mg%) which represents the normal maximum reabsorptive capacity of the kidney tubules.

Requests for tests to detect glycosuria are usually made to screen for diabetes. The semiquantitative estimation of glucose in a series of urine specimens from a known diabetic can provide information on the degree of blood glucose control.

The following methods are used to test for glycosuria:

■ Glucose reagent strip test
■ *Clinitest*
■ Benedict's tube test

Glucose Reagent Strip Test
A reagent strip test is recommended in preference to *Clinitest* or Benedict's test for detecting glycosuria because it is specific for glucose and also a safer test to perform.

Several urine glucose strip tests are commercially available. They are all based on a glucose oxidase reaction. Glucose is oxidized to gluconolactone by the enzyme glucose oxidase (specific for glucose) with the release of hydrogen peroxide. A chromogen is then oxidized by the hydrogen peroxide and a peroxidase enzyme is used to convert the chromogen from a reduced colourless state to a coloured oxidized state.

$$\text{Glucose} + \underset{\text{(From the air)}}{\text{Oxygen}} \xrightarrow{\text{Glucose oxidase}} \underset{\text{acid}}{\text{Gluconic}} + \underset{\text{peroxide}}{\text{Hydrogen}}$$

$$\underset{\text{peroxide}}{\text{Hydrogen}} + \text{Chromogen} \xrightarrow{\text{Peroxidase}} \underset{\text{COLOURED}}{\text{Chromogen oxidized}}$$

The various glucose reagent strips differ from one another chemically as regards the type of chromogen and buffer system used. There are also differences in the stability and sensitivity of the different strips and the degree of interference from substances other than glucose which may be present in the urine. The manufacturers' literature must therefore be read carefully.

Strip tests are available for both detecting and measuring glucose semiquantitatively in urine. Strips that measure glucose in urine are recommended.

Strips to detect glucose in urine
These include:

□ *Clinistix* (Ames) which will detect about 5.5 mmol/l (0.5%) or more of glucose.

□ *Glukotest* (Boehringer, also known as *BM-Test-Glucose*) will detect 2.2 mmol/l (0.2%) or more of glucose.

Note: Glucose detecting test areas can also be found with ketones on the test strips *Keto-Diastix* (Ames) and *Gluketur-Test* (Boehringer) and on several other test strips as listed in Chart 28.I in 28:7.

Strips to measure glucose semiquantitatively
These include:

□ *Diastix* (Ames) which detects 5.5 mmol/l of glucose and measures it semiquantitatively up to 111 mmol/l (2%).

  Scale: Negative, 5.5, 14, 28, 55, 111 mmol/l or more.

□ *Diabur-Test 5000* (Boehringer) which detects 5.5 mmol/l of glucose and measures it semiquantitatively up to 280 mmol/l (5%).

  Scale: Negative, 5.5, 14, 28, 56, 111, 167, 280 mmol/l.

Important: *Diabur-Test 5000* enables a glucose specific strip test to be used to measure glucose in urine instead of Benedict's test or *Clinitest* which are not specific for glucose and also dangerous because they involve boiling urine with caustic chemicals.

Note: Glucose semiquantitative test areas can also be found with ketones on *Keto-Diastix* (Ames) with glucose values up to 111 mmol/l and *Keto-Diabur-Test 5000* (Boehringer) with values up to 280 mmol/l, and on several other test strips (ranges up to 56 mmol/l and 111 mmol/l) as listed in Chart 28.I in 28:7.

When testing the urine of diabetics for glucose and ketones, it is usually less costly to use a combined strip than two separate single test strips.

False reactions

A number of urinary or contaminating substances may give false negative or false positive glucose strip test results. The most commonly occurring of these interfering substances are as follows:

— Oxygen receptors in the urine, i.e. substances which (when present in moderate to large amounts) can be oxidized by the hydrogen peroxide in preference to the chromogen. This can lead to a loss in sensitivity of the strip. Such substances include ascorbic acid and certain drug metabolites.

  Similarly, moderate to large amounts of acetoacetate in urine as can be found in specimens from out-of-control diabetics, may interfere and give misleading results with some strips.

— Catalase, when present in high concentration in the urine (as in severe *E. coli* infections) can destroy hydrogen peroxide and so cause a false negative result.

— Disinfectants such as bleach which oxidize the chromogen directly and therefore cause a false positive reaction.

Note: The control of reagent strips is described in 28:7.

Clinitest

Clinitest (Ames) is a modification of the Benedict's tube test in tablet form.

Clinitest tablet contains copper sulphate, sodium carbonate, sodium hydroxide, and citric acid. As the diluted urine acts upon the tablet, the citric acid is neutralized by sodium carbonate and by sodium hydroxide with the production of intense heat and the release of carbon dioxide. The heat produced brings the mixture to the boil and the copper ions are reduced by the glucose.

The reaction is not specific for glucose. Substances which reduce copper ions in the *Clinitest* are similar to those listed for Benedict's test (see later text). Because the reaction is not specific for glucose, it is possible for a urine to give a positive *Clinitest* but a negative reagent strip test (glucose-specific).

It is also possible when testing a urine to obtain a positive strip test and a negative *Clinitest*. This is because *Clinitest* is unable to detect less than 13.8 mmol/l (250 mg%) of glucose in the urine whereas the strip tests are more sensitive, detecting as little as 5.5 mmol/l (100 mg%) or less of glucose.

Note: Wherever possible the use of *Clinitest* should be avoided. A strip test such as *Diabur-Test 5000* should be used because it is not only specific for glucose but also a safer method of measuring glucose in urine (see previous text).

Benedict's Tube Test

Whenever possible this test should be replaced by a safe glucose-specific strip test such as *Diabur-Test 5000*. Benedict's test is described for those laboratories unable to obtain urine strip tests.

Reagents
— Benedict's reagent   Reagent No. 13
— Glucose control solution*

  * Prepare by dissolving 1 gram of glucose in 100 ml of 1 g/l benzoic acid (see Reagent No. 14). The solution is stable for several months at room temperature (20-28 °C).

Method
1. Take three or more tubes (depending on the number of tests), and label as follows:

   POS   — Positive control
   NEG   — Negative control
   1, 2, etc,   — Patients' tests

2. Deliver 2 ml of Benedict's reagent into each tube.

   A plastic 2 ml or 2.5 ml syringe or graduated plastic bulb pipette (see Appendix IV, Syringe, Plastic bulb pipette) can be used to dispense the reagent. It is not necessary to use a calibrated pipette.

3. Add to each tube as follows:
   Tube
   POS   ....0.2 ml glucose control solution
   NEG   ....0.2 ml of distilled water
   1, 2, etc ....0.2 ml of fresh urine

   A plastic 1 ml graduated syringe (see Appendix IV, Syringe) can be used to dispense the 0.2 ml of glucose, water, and urine.

4. Mix the contents of each tube.

5. Place the tubes in a heat-block set at 100 °C or if unavailable in a container of boiling water for *exactly* 5 minutes.

6. Remove the tubes and examine the solution in each tube for a precipitate and change of colour.

Report the sugar concentration as follows:

Appearance of Solution	Sugar Concentration
Blue, clear or cloudy	Nil
Green, no precipitate	Trace
Green, with precipitate	+ (Approx. 0.5%)
Brown and cloudy	++ (Approx. 1.0%)
Orange and cloudy	+++ (Approx. 1.5%)
Red and cloudy	++++ (2.0% or more)

Note: The negative control (tube NEG) should show no change of colour. The positive control (tube POS) should show a ++ reaction (1.0%) of reducing substance.

Substances which may also reduce Benedict's reagent
These include other sugars which may occasionally be present in urine such as galactose, lactose, fructose, and pentose.

False positive reactions may also be obtained if certain drugs are present, e.g. salicylates, penicillin, streptomycin, isoniazid, and *p*-aminosalicylic acid.

Chemicals present in urine which may reduce Benedict's reagent include creatinine, urate, and ascorbic acid.

Causes of glycosuria
— A rise in the concentration of blood glucose with the kidney tubules being unable to reabsorb the increased amount of glucose in the glomerular filtrate.

Raised renal threshold for glucose
If the blood glucose level is high but the filtration rate is slow or the flow of blood to the kidneys is reduced as in heart failure, sodium depletion, or shock, there will be a rise in the renal threshold for glucose. Glucose will not appear in the urine until the blood glucose is well over 10 mmol/l (180 mg%). With diabetes mellitus the renal threshold for glucose is often raised, especially in elderly diabetics, those with cardiac failure, or those in diabetic coma with shock.

— A reduced rate of reabsorption of glucose by the kidney tubules as occurs in serious tubular damage or an inherited defect of tubular absorption causing a lowering of the glucose renal threshold. Glucose appears in the urine when the blood glucose level is well below 10 mmol/l (180 mg%). This is often referred to as renal glycosuria.

Fanconi syndrome
When glucose, amino acids, phosphate, and other substances are excreted due to impaired reabsorption this is termed the Fanconi syndrome.

— An increase in the rate of glomerular filtration as may sometimes occur during pregnancy.

Important: The blood glucose level should be measured (see 31:1) whenever glucose is found in the urine and the patient is not a known diabetic or receiving glucose intravenously.

31:4 TESTING URINE FOR KETONES

Acetoacetate, *beta*-hydroxybutyrate and acetone are collectively referred to as ketone bodies or simply ketones. The excretion of more than a trace of these substances in the urine is called ketonuria.

Formation of ketones
As explained in 8:2, the metabolism of glucose normally provides the body with its energy requirements. If, however, the intake of glucose is insufficient as in starvation, or glucose metabolism is defective due to a lack of insulin as occurs in untreated or uncontrolled diabetes, the body obtains its energy by breaking down fats. It is this increase in fat metabolism which leads to a build up of ketones in the body. An accumulation of ketones in the body is called ketosis.

Ketones are toxic to the brain and if present in sufficiently high concentration in the blood they can contribute to the coma found in diabetic ketoacidosis. They are strong acids and may overcome the buffering systems in the blood and so cause ketoacidosis. With coma due to ketoacidosis, ketonuria is always present.

Urine ketone tests detect acetoacetate and acetone. *Beta*-hydroxybutyrate is not detected.

The following methods are used to test for ketonuria:
- Ketone reagent strip test
- *Acetest*
- Nitroprusside tube or tile test

The reactions of these tests are similar. Acetoacetate and acetone react with sodium nitroprusside* in an alkaline medium to give a violet dye complex. The strips are more sensitive to acetoacetate than acetone.

* The accepted international name for sodium nitroprusside is sodium pentacyanonitrosylferrate.

Ketone Reagent Strip Test
The urine must be tested soon after it is passed before the acetoacetate is carboxylated to acetone.

Several ketone strip tests are available commercially. They include:

□ *Ketostix* (Ames) which will detect 0.5-1.0 mmol/l of acetoacetate. It is less sensitive to acetone.

Scale: Negative, + (small), ++ (moderate), +++ (large)

□ *Ketur-Test* (Boehringer, also known as *BM-Test-Keton* and *Chemstrip K*), which has a similar sensitivity to *Ketostix*, detecting 0.5 mmol/l of acetoacetate and 7-12 mmol/l of acetone.

Scale: Negative, + (0.5-4 mmol/l), ++ (4-10 mmol/l), +++ (more than 10 mmol/l)

Note: Similar ketone test areas can also be found with glucose on *Keto-Diastix* (Ames), *Gluketur-Test* (Boehringer), and *Keto-Diabur-Test 5000* (Boehringer). The latter strip is particularly useful because it measures urine glucose from 5.5 mmol/l to 280 mmol/l (i.e. up to 5%). Ketone test areas are also included on most of the multiple strip tests. These are listed in Chart 28.I in 28:7.

False reactions
Ames' literature mentions that some high specific gravity / low pH urine samples may give trace positive reactions. False positive reactions (trace or less) may also occur with highly pigmented urine especially specimens that contain large amounts of L-dopa metabolites.

Boehringer literature advises that phenylketones give an orange-red colour reaction which is easy to distinguish from the mauve-purple reaction due to ketones.

Note: The control of reagent strips is described in 28:7.

Acetest
Acetest (Ames) is also based on a nitroprusside reaction but is more sensitive than the strip tests in detecting ketones, especially acetone. It will detect 0.012 mmol/l acetoacetate and 4.3 mmol/l acetone.

Acetest has about the same stability as the ketone strip tests. It is however packaged in bottles of 100 tablets. The same storage conditions that apply to strip tests also apply to the storage of *Acetest* tablets. They must be kept tightly stoppered in their container with the desiccant supplied. If the tablets appear moist and dark coloured, this indicates reagent deterioration, and they must *not* be used.

False reactions
These are the same as those given by Ames for their ketone strip tests.

Nitroprusside Tube or Tile Test
The nitroprusside tube or tile test is a sensitive technique for detecting ketones in urine. Fresh urine is reacted with a dry reagent containing sodium nitroprusside, ammonium sulphate, and sodium carbonate. In an alkaline medium, sodium nitroprusside reacts with acetoacetate and acetone to give a mauve-purple colour.

Reagent
— Nitroprusside dry reagent   Reagent No. 51

Method
1. Transfer about 0.5-1.0 g of nitroprusside reagent to the bottom of a small test tube or to a well of a white porcelain tile.

2. Add 1 drop of fresh urine, sufficient to moisten the reagent.

3. For 1 minute observe the moistened reagent for the development of a mauve-purple colour.

   Note: If using a tube, any change in colour can be seen more easily if the tube is held against a white piece of paper.

4. Report the test as follows:
   No colour change ..... Ketones not detected
   Slight purple colour .... + Ketones
   Moderate purple .... ++ Ketones
   Dark purple .... +++ Ketones

False reactions
Weak false positive reactions may occur if the urine contains L-dopa or large amounts of phenyl-pyruvic acid (found in the rare disorder phenylketonuria).

Causes of ketonuria
— Untreated diabetes. The finding of ketonuria in a diabetic being treated usually indicates an out-of-control state.

— Conditions of starvation when fat metabolism is increased.

— Eating a diet that is very low in carbohydrates.

— Severe dehydration following prolonged vomiting or diarrhoea.

— Glycogen storage disease.

Testing of Serum or Plasma for Ketones
The testing of serum or plasma for ketones can assist in the investigation of hyperglycaemic patients. The same tests that are used to detect ketones in urine can be used to test for ketones in serum or plasma. Results can be interpreted as follows:

Negative or weakly positive serum/plasma ketones in hyperglycaemic patient
Indicates hyperglycaemia with no ketoacidosis (hyperosmolar non-ketotic coma).

Strongly positive serum/plasma ketones (ketonuria also present) in hyperglycaemic patient
Indicates hyperglycaemia with ketoacidosis.

31:5 MEASUREMENT OF SERUM TOTAL CALCIUM
Cresolphthalein Complexone Method[16]

The measurement of serum calcium is usually requested to investigate bone diseases and malabsorption.

Plasma calcium
Calcium is present in plasma in three forms:

□ Free ionized calcium which makes up 50-65% of plasma calcium.

□ Calcium bound to protein (mainly albumin) which forms 30-45% of the plasma calcium.

□ Calcium complexed to other molecules such as citrate, bicarbonate, and phosphate. This form makes up the remaining 5-10% of the total plasma calcium.

Most calcium assays (including the cresolphthalein complexone method) measure total calcium although it is only the free ionic calcium which is biologically active.

Choice of test method
In the first edition of this manual a methylthymol blue calcium method was described. This method is now no longer recommended because it has relatively poor precision. An improved method which uses cresolphthalein complexone (CPC) is described.

Calcium test kits
Very few CPC manual colorimetric test kits are available. Most kits use a methylthymol blue technique.

Principle of CPC method
Cresolphthalein complexone (CPC) forms a violet coloured complex with calcium. The absorbance of the colour produced is measured in a colorimeter using a yellow filter or in a spectrophotometer at 575 nm wavelength. Interference from magnesium is reduced by including 8-hydroxyquinoline in the working CPC reagent. The ethanediol in the reagent suppresses the ionisation of the o-cresolphthalein complexone and helps to give a clear solution.

Specimens which appear slight to moderately icteric or haemolyzed may be assayed. A correction, however, should be made when a patient's serum or plasma albumin level is low (see end of test method).

Calcium + CPC ⟶ Calcium CPC complex
Violet

Calibration
The CPC calcium method is calibrated (to check for linearity) from a calcium solution. This is diluted to make a series of standards as follows:

Stock calcium standard, 10 mmol/l
The 10 mmol/l calcium stock standard is best purchased as a ready-made solution from BDH Chemicals Ltd (No. 221884B, approx. £5 for 500 ml, 1985-1986 price) or other manufacturer.

If unable to purchase the ready-made solution, a 10 mmol/l calcium stock standard solution can be prepared as follows:

1. Weigh accurately 100 mg of *dried* calcium carbonate (analytical reagent grade).

   To ensure that the calcium carbonate is dry, heat it in an open container in an oven at 80-100 °C for about 4 hours. Remove and close the container immediately. When cool, weigh the chemical.

2. Transfer the weighed calcium carbonate to a 100 ml volumetric flask. Add about 10 ml of distilled water followed by 0.7 ml of concentrated hydrochloric acid. Mix until the chemical is fully dissolved.

   Caution: Concentrated hydrochloric acid is corrosive, therefore handle with care. *Do not* mouth-pipette.

3. Make up to the 100 ml mark with distilled water and mix well.

Transfer the stock 10 mmol/l calcium standard to a *completely clean* plastic storage bottle. Label and store at room temperature (20-28 °C). The stock standard is stable for about 1 year.

Working calcium standards 1.00, 1.50, 2.00, 2.50, 3.00 mmol/l
1. Take five *completely clean* plastic bottles of about 20 ml capacity and number them 1 to 5. Pipette accurately into each as follows:

Bottle	Stock Calcium 10 mmol/l	Distilled water
1	1.0 ml	9.0 ml
2	1.5 ml	8.5 ml
3	2.0 ml	8.0 ml
4	2.5 ml	7.5 ml
5	3.0 ml	7.0 ml

2. Mix well the contents in each bottle.

The concentration of calcium in each standard is as follows:

Bottle 1 = 1.00 mmol/l
         2 = 1.50 mmol/l
         3 = 2.00 mmol/l
         4 = 2.50 mmol/l
         5 = 3.00 mmol/l

3. Label each bottle and store at room temperature (20-28 °C). The working standard solutions are stable for several weeks.

Preparation of calcium calibration graph
1. Take six tubes (preferably plastic) and label 'B' (reagent blank) and 1 to 5.

   Pipette 5 ml of working CPC reagent (see *Reagents*) into each tube.

2. Add to each tube as follows:
   Tube
   B .... 50 μl (0.05 ml) distilled water
   1 .... 50 μl standard, 1.00 mmol/l
   2 .... 50 μl standard, 1.50 mmol/l
   3 .... 50 μl standard, 2.00 mmol/l
   4 .... 50 μl standard, 2.50 mmol/l
   5 .... 50 μl standard, 3.00 mmol/l

   Mix well.

3. Using completely clean cuvettes, read the absorbances of the standard solutions in a colorimeter using a yellow filter (e.g. Ilford No. 606) or in a spectrophotometer set at 575 nm. Zero the instrument with the blank solution in tube B.

4. Take a sheet of graph paper and plot the absorbance of each standard solution (vertical axis) against its concentration in mmol/l (horizontal axis) as described in 25:2. A linear calibration should be obtained.

   The useful working limit (linearity) of the CPC calcium method is about 3.00 mmol/l.

Important: The calibration graph requires checking against controls whenever new stock CPC reagent is prepared. The calibration graph should not be used for obtaining patients' results.

Reagents
— CPC stock reagent   Reagent No. 27

Working CPC reagent
This should be prepared weekly. Prepare by dissolving *completely* 0.1 g (100 mg) of 8-hydroxyquinoline* in 100 ml of stock CPC reagent (the chemical dissolves slowly).

* Available from BDH Chemicals and other manufacturers.

The working CPC reagent is stable for 1 week when stored at 2-8 °C. It should have an absorbance of about 0.2 when measured at 575 nm against distilled water. If over 0.2, this indicates a dirty container or cuvette or the deterioration or contamination of the stock CPC reagent which must then be renewed.

Method
Specimen: The method requires 0.1 ml (100 μl) of patient's serum. Plasma should not be used. The specimen should be a fasting one and collected with the minimum of venous stasis (see 26:4). Prolonged stasis can increase the calcium concentration by up to 0.25 mmol/l. The patient should not be receiving EDTA therapy.

For details of the stability of calcium in whole blood and serum, see 26:7.

1. Take *two sets* of four or more tubes (depending on the number of tests) and label as follows:
   B   — Reagent blank
   S   — Standard, 2.00 mmol/l
   C   — Control
   1, 2, etc   — Patients' tests

   Important: Two sets of tubes are required because calcium assays must be performed in duplicate and the absorbances of the two tests must not differ more than ± 0.02. The slightest calcium contamination from tubes or pipettes will give incorrect results. Glassware used in calcium assays should be acid-washed (in 5% v/v hydrochloric acid) to remove all traces of calcium, well rinsed in tap water, followed by deionized or distilled water, and allowed to dry. It is advisable to keep a set of acid-washed tubes, pipettes, and cuvettes for use only in calcium assays.

2. Pipette 5 ml of working CPC reagent into each tube.

   Caution: The working CPC reagent is harmful, therefore handle with care and *do not* mouth-pipette.

3. Pipette into each set of tubes as follows:
   Tube
   B   .... 50 μl (0.05 ml) distilled water
   S   .... 50 μl standard, 2.00 mmol/l
   C   .... 50 μl control serum (see 27:5)
   1, 2, etc .... 50 μl patient's serum

   Mix *well* for several seconds.

4. Using completely clean cuvettes, read the absorbances of the solutions in a colorimeter using a yellow filter (e.g. Ilford No. 606) or in a spectrophotometer set at 575 nm. Zero the

Summary of Calcium Method

For detailed instructions, see text

Two sets of tubes are required Pipette into each set of tubes as follows:	BLANK B	STANDARD S	CONTROL C	TESTS 1,2, etc
Working CPC reagent	5 ml	5 ml	5 ml	5 ml
Distilled water	50 μl	—	—	—
Standard, 2.00 mmol/l	—	50 μl	—	—
Control serum	—	—	50 μl	—
Patient's serum	—	—	—	50 μl

Important: Use *completely clean* tubes and pipettes

Mix well for several seconds

READ ABSORBANCES

Colorimeter: Yellow filter, e.g. Ilford No. 606
Spectrophotometer: 575 nm

Zero instrument with blank solution in tube B

Use *completely clean* cuvettes

Calculate results in mmol/l as follows:

$$\text{Calcium mmol/l} = \frac{\text{Absorbance of test or control}}{\text{Absorbance of 2.00 mmol/l standard}} \times 2.00$$

Average results of duplicate tests

Report patients' results if control value is acceptable

50 μl = 0.05 ml

instrument with the blank solution in tube B.

5. Calculate the concentration of calcium in the control and patients' samples from the following formula:

$$\text{Calcium mmol/l} = \frac{AT}{AS} \times 2.00$$

where AT = Absorbance of test or control
AS = Absorbance of 2.00 standard

Calcium results greater than 3.00 mmol/l
Dilute the serum 1 in 2 with distilled water and repeat the assay. Multiply the result by two.

6. Report the patients' results if the value of the control serum is acceptable.

Correction of calcium result when a patient's serum or plasma albumin is low
When a patient's serum or plasma albumin level is below 40 g/l, the calcium result should be corrected using the following formula:

Corrected calcium mmol/l =

$$\frac{40 - \text{albumin g/l}}{40} + \text{Calcium result in mmol/l}$$

Example: Patient's calcium result is 1.85 mmol/l
Patient's albumin level is 25 g/l

$$\text{Corrected calcium mmol/l} = \frac{40 - 25}{40} + 1.85$$

$$= 2.23 \text{ mmol/l}$$

Report both the patient's uncorrected and corrected calcium results.

Note: The above correction can also be applied when a high level of albumin, e.g. due to dehydration, is present.

Quality control
The principles of quality control in clinical chemistry are described in Chapter 27. For the CPC calcium method, the following should be attainable:

— OCV, of around 2%
— RCV, not exceeding 4%

Approximate total calcium reference (normal range)
Adults: 2.25-2.60 mmol/l (9.0-10.4 mg%)
Newborns: 1.85-3.45 mmol/l (7.4-13.8 mg%)

To convert from mmol/l to mg%, multiply by 4.
To convert from mg% to mmol/l, divide by 4.

Note: Calcium values are lower when lying down. Values are also influenced by diet.

Interpretation of serum total calcium results
Increases
A rise in the level of blood calcium is known as hypercalcaemia. The main causes are as follows:

— Malignancies and bony metastatic deposits.
— Primary hyperparathyroidism (increased functioning of the parathyroid glands).
— Excessive intake of calcium or vitamin D, or both.
— Sarcoidosis (a granulomatous disease commonly affecting the skin, lymphatic glands, or the bones of the hand) causing increased sensitivity to vitamin D.
— Myelomatosis.
— Conditions leading to bone wastage especially poliomyelitis and childhood fractures.

Note: A falsely high calcium level will result if there is excessive venous stasis when a blood sample is collected (see 26:4) because this will cause an increase in plasma proteins leading to a rise in the level of protein-bound calcium.

Decreases
A lowering of the blood calcium level is referred to as hypocalcaemia. It can cause muscular spasm especially of the hands and feet when it is called tetany. Conditions in which hypocalcaemia occurs include:

— Deficient intake or absorption of calcium.
— Vitamin D deficiency due to poor diet or malabsorption. Inadequate vitamin D results in osteomalacia in which there is an excessive loss of calcium and phosphorus from bone, leading to bone softening. When osteomalacia affects growing bones this is referred to as rickets.
— Steatorrhoea with faulty absorption of vitamin D, calcium, and phosphates.
— Hypoparathyroidism (decreased functioning of the parathyroid glands).
— Acute pancreatitis with calcium being bound by the liberated fatty acids.
— Neonatal hypocalcaemia, usually due (a few days after birth) to cow's milk feeding which leads to an increase in serum inorganic phosphate.
— Hypoalbuminaemia causing a reduction of plasma-bound calcium and therefore of serum total calcium. Correction for this is described at the end of the test method.

31:6 BIOCHEMICAL TESTING OF CEREBROSPINAL FLUID

The biochemical testing of cerebrospinal fluid (c.s.f.) is performed to assist in the diagnosis of meningitis and other disorders of the central nervous system. It usually includes:

■ Measurement of glucose
■ Measurement of total protein

Other c.s.f. investigations
The testing of c.s.f. for pathogens and cells is described and illustrated in 38:12 in Volume II of the Manual.

Specimen: It is usual to collect two samples of c.s.f. in sterile containers. Sample No. 1 (about 1 ml) is used for culture and sample No. 2 (2-3 ml) is used for microscopy, cell count, and biochemical testing.

Sample No. 2 is used for the measurement of glucose and protein because there is less chance of it containing blood if the lumbar puncture is traumatic. If blood is present in the c.s.f. it is unsuitable for cell counting and the measurement of glucose and protein.

MEASUREMENT OF CSF GLUCOSE

Glucose in c.s.f. can be measured as follows:

☐ Colorimetrically using a glucose oxidase method.
☐ Semiquantitatively using Benedict's reagent if a colorimeter is not available.

> *Important*: c.s.f. glucose must be measured as soon as possible (within 20 minutes) after it has been withdrawn otherwise a false low result will be obtained due to glycolysis. If a delay is unavoidable, sample No. 2 must be collected into fluoride-oxalate preservative (Reagent No. 37). This will prevent glycolysis. The fluoride-oxalate will not interfere with the measurement of protein.

Glucose oxidase method for measuring c.s.f. glucose
This is the same method as described for measuring serum or plasma glucose in 31:1 except four times the amount of c.s.f. (fresh or fluoride-oxalate c.s.f. is used (i.e. 0.2 ml) and the result is divided by four. More c.s.f. is used because the concentration of glucose in c.s.f. is much less than that found in serum or plasma and markedly reduced levels occur in meningitis.

Benedict's semiquantitative c.s.f. glucose method
Benedict's method for measuring c.s.f. glucose

requires 1 ml of *fresh* or fluoride-oxalated c.s.f. (usually the supernatant fluid from centrifuged No. 2 sample).

Reagent
— Benedict's reagent*   Reagent No. 13
* This is the same reagent as used for urine testing.

Method
1. Take five tubes and label them 1, 2, 3, 4, and C (Control). Pipette into each tube as follows:

Tube	1	2	3	4	C
ml of Benedict's reagent	2.0	2.0	2.0	2.0	2.0
ml of c.s.f.	0.1	0.2	0.3	0.4	—

Caution: Do not mouth-pipette the reagent or c.s.f. A 2 ml syringe or graduated plastic bulb pipette (see 2:4) can be used to deliver the reagent, and a pipette with pipette-filler or an automatic pipetter can be used to dispense the c.s.f.

2. Mix the contents of each tube and place all five tubes in a container of *boiling* water for 5 minutes.

3. Remove the tubes and compare the colour of the solutions in tubes 1 to 4 with that in the control tube. Make a note of the tubes in which reduction (R) has occurred. Reduction of the reagent is indicated by a change in colour from blue (as seen in the control tube) to blue-brown.

4. Interpret and report the results as follows:

	Reactions				c.s.f. Glucose	
Tube	1	2	3	4	mmol/l	mg%
	—	—	—	—	0 - 1.1	0 - 20
	—	—	—	R	1.2 - 1.7	21 - 30
	—	—	R	R	1.8 - 2.2	31 - 40
	—	R	R	R	2.3 - 2.8	41 - 50
	R	R	R	R	> 2.8	> 50

Key
R = Reduction reaction (Blue-brown solution)
— = No reduction (blue-solution, like control)
> = Greater than

Use of *Dextrostix* for estimating c.s.f. glucose
A reagent strip test for measuring blood glucose such as

Dextrostix should not be used for estimating glucose in c.s.f. because the blue colours produced do not correspond to the colour scale produced for blood glucose.

Interpretation of c.s.f. glucose results

Usually the concentration of glucose in c.s.f. is a half to two thirds of that found in serum or plasma i.e. 2.5-4.0 mmol/l (45-72 mg%).

Decreases

Low c.s.f. glucose levels are found in most forms of meningitis, particularly pyogenic meningitis when glucose may even be absent. In viral meningitis however, the c.s.f. glucose is often normal.

Increases

A raised c.s.f. glucose is found when there is a raised blood glucose and sometimes with encephalitis or following damage to cerebral capillaries.

MEASUREMENT OF CSF PROTEIN

Total protein in c.s.f. can be measured as follows:

☐ Colorimetrically using a trichloroacetic acid method.
☐ Visual comparative semiquantitative method when a colorimeter is not available.

Pandy's test

This is a simple technique that is sometimes used to screen for increases in c.s.f. globulin when it is not possible to measure c.s.f. total protein.

Colorimetric trichloroacetic acid total protein method

Required

— Trichloroacetic acid, 50 g/l (5% w/v) Reagent No. 81
— Protein standards prepared from a protein solution or serum of known protein concentration.

Preparation of protein standards using a serum of known protein concentration

— Dilute the serum 1 in 10 by mixing 1 ml of serum with 9 ml of physiological saline. Calculate the protein value of the diluted serum by dividing its original value by 10.

Example: If the protein value of the serum is 78 g/l (7.8 g%), the protein value after dilution will be 7.8 g/l (780 mg%).

— Take five tubes and number them 1 to 5. Pipette into each tube as follows:

Tube No:	1	2	3	4	5
ml of saline:	1.9	1.8	1.7	1.6	1.5
ml of diluted serum:	0.1	0.2	0.3	0.4	0.5

Mix well the contents of each tube.

— Calculate the concentration of protein in each of the five standards as follows:

No. 1:	Divide value of *diluted* serum	by 20
2:		by 10
3:		by 6.6
4:		by 5.0
5:		by 4.0

Preparation of a calibration graph

1. Take five tubes and label them 1 to 5.

   Pipette 2.4 ml of 50 g/l trichloroacetic acid into each tube.

   Caution: The trichloroacetic acid solution is corrosive and has an irritating vapour, *do not* mouth-pipette.

2. Add 0.8 ml of standard solution to each tube (standard No. 1 to tube No. 1 etc.). Mix the contents of each tube and leave for 5 minutes.

3. Remix each standard solution taking care not to introduce air bubbles. Read the absorbance of each in a colorimeter using a blue filter (e.g. Ilford No. 602) or in a spectrophotometer at wavelength 450 nm. Zero the instrument with distilled water.

4. Take a sheet of graph paper and plot the absorbance of each standard (vertical axis) against its concentration in g/l (horizontal axis). Draw a straight line passing through zero and the points plotted.

Method

The method requires 0.8 ml of c.s.f. (usually the supernatant fluid from No. 2 sample). Fluoride-oxalate c.s.f. can also be used.

1. Pipette 2.4 ml of 50 g/l trichloroacetic acid solution into a tube.

2. Add 0.8 ml of c.s.f. Mix and leave for 5 minutes.

   Note: If after adding the c.s.f. a heavy precipitate forms, set up the test again using a 1 in 5 dilution of the c.s.f. (0.2 ml c.s.f. mixed with 0.8 ml of physiological saline gives a 1 in 5 dilution; use 0.8 ml of the diluted fluid).

   Blank solution: If the c.s.f. is coloured yellow or red, prepare a blank solution by adding 0.8 ml of c.s.f. to 2.4 ml of physiological saline.

3. Remix the contents of the tube, taking care not to introduce air bubbles. Read the absorbance of the precipitated protein in a colorimeter using a blue filter (e.g. Ilford No. 602) or in a spectrophotometer set at wavelength 450 nm. Zero the instrument with distilled water or with a blank solution.

4. Read off the concentration of c.s.f. protein in grams per litre (g/l) from the previously prepared calibration graph.

   Note: If the concentration is over 1.5 g/l (150 mg%), repeat the test using a 1 in 5 dilution of the c.s.f. (see previous text). The calibration graph should be linear for values up to 1.5 g/l.

Visual comparative method for measuring protein
Required
— Trichloroacetic acid, 50 g/l   Reagent No. 81 (5% w/v)
— Protein standards containing 0.44 g/l (44 mg%), 0.88 g/l (88 mg%), and 1.10 g/l (110 mg%) protein

Preparation of protein standard solutions
The standards may be easily prepared from a 22% albumin solution (as used in blood transfusion work), as follows:

— Take three screw-cap bottles of 50 ml capacity and label them 0.44 g/l, 0.88 g/l, and 1.10 g/l.

Pipette into each bottle as follows:

Bottle	22% Albumin Solution*
0.44 g/l	0.1 ml
0.88 g/l	0.2 ml
1.10 g/l	0.25 ml

* If only a 30% albumin solution is available, make a 22% solution by mixing 1.6 ml of distilled water with 4.4 ml of the 30% solution.

— Add 50 ml of distilled water (sterile if possible) to each bottle, stopper, and mix well.

Store the solutions at 2-8 °C. Renew every month or before if they become contaminated.

Method
The method requires 0.5 ml of c.s.f. (usually the supernatant fluid from No. 2 sample).

1. Take four tubes and label them 1, 2, 3, and P (Patient).

2. Pipette into each tube as follows:

Tube:	1	2	3	P
ml trichloroacetic acid, 50 g/l:	1.5	1.5	1.5	1.5
ml 0.44 g/l standard:	0.5	—	—	—
ml 0.88 g/l standard:	—	0.5	—	—
ml 1.10 g/l standard:	—	—	0.5	—
ml c.s.f.:	—	—	—	0.5

Caution: *Do not* mouth-pipette the trichloroacetic acid or c.s.f. Use a pipette with pipette-filler, a plastic bulb pipette, or a dispenser.

3. Mix the contents of each tube, and leave for 5 minutes.

4. Remix the solutions in each tube, and make an estimate of the approximate amount of protein in the c.s.f. by comparing the cloudiness in the patient's tube (P) with that in each of the three standard tubes.

   Report the approximate protein concentration in grams per litre (g/l).

   Note: It is easier to match the turbidity in the patient's tube with that in the standard tubes if a printed card is held behind the tubes.

Values greater than 1.10 g/l (110 mg%)
If the turbidity in the patient's tube is greater than 1.10 g/l, repeat the test after diluting the c.s.f. 1 in 5 in physiological saline (0.1 ml of c.s.f. added to 0.4 ml of saline will give a 1 in 5 dilution). Multiply the result by 5.

Pandy's globulin test
This screening test detects rises in c.s.f. globulin. It is only of value when it is not possible to perform a total protein estimation.

Required
— Phenol, saturated solution   Reagent No. 53

Method
Specimen: The test requires one drop of c.s.f. or supernatant c.s.f. sample.

1. Pipette about 1 ml of saturated phenol solution into a small tube.

   Caution: Phenol is a highly corrosive and harmful chemical, therefore *do not* mouth-pipette. Use a graduated plastic bulb pipette or a pipette with pipette-filler.

2. Using a plastic bulb pipette (see 2:4), and holding the tube at eye level against a dark background, add 1 large drop of c.s.f. (supernatant fluid from centrifuged No. 2 sample). Do *not* mix.

3. Look for an immediate cloudiness around the drop of c.s.f., indicating the presence of excess globulin. Report the test as:

   Pandy's test positive .... Immediate cloudiness
   Pandy's test negative .... No cloudiness

   Note: After a few minutes the cloudiness may disappear.

Interpretation of c.s.f. protein results

The c.s.f. total protein is normally 0.15-0.40 g/l (15-40 mg%). The range for ventricular fluid is slightly lower. Values up to 1.0 g/l (100 mg%) are normal for newborn infants. Only traces of globulin are found in normal c.s.f. (insufficient to give a positive Pandy's test).

An increase in total protein and a positive Pandy's test occurs in all forms of meningitis, in amoebic and trypanosomiasis meningoencephalitis, cerebral malaria, brain tumours, cerebral injury, spinal cord compression, poliomyelitis, the Guillain-Barré syndrome (often the only abnormality), and polyneuritis. Increases in c.s.f. protein also occur in diseases which cause changes in plasma proteins such as multiple myeloma.

When the total protein exceeds 2.0 g/l (200 mg%), the fibrinogen level is usually increased sufficiently to cause the c.s.f. to clot. This may occur in severe pyogenic meningitis, spinal block, or following haemorrhage.

Note: c.s.f. biochemical and microbiological findings in meningitis and other diseases of the central nervous system are summarized on pages 169-170 in Volume II of the Manual.

References

1 Trinder, P. *Annals of Clinical Biochemistry*, **6**, p 24, 1969.

2 Barham, D. and Trinder, P. *Analyst*, **97**, pp 142-145, 1972.

3 Richardson, T. *Annals of Clinical Biochemistry*, **14**, pp 223-226, 1977.

4 Oli, J. M. Diabetes mellitus in Africans. *Journal of the Royal College of Physicians of London*, **17**, 4, pp 224-227, 1983.

5 World Health Organization. *WHO Expert Committee on Diabetes Mellitus*, Technical Report Series, **646**, 1980.

6 World Health Organization. *Evaluation of Performance of Diagnostic Reagent sets used in Health Laboratories with Limited Resources: Appendix A. Glucose*. LAB/83.2. Copies can be obtained from WHO, 1211-Geneva, 27 Switzerland.

7 Jones, G. R., *et al*. *British Medical Journal*, 281:1358 (letter), 1980.

8 Spruce, B. A., Worth, R. C., and Ward, J. D. A comparative study of *Visidex II* and *BM Glycaemie 20-800* blood glucose test strips. *Diabetologia*, **27**, 334A, 1984.

9 Betteridge, D. J., *et al*. Assessment of *Visidex II*, a new blood glucose monitoring system. *Practical Diabetes*, Vol. I, **1**, Sept., 1984.

10 Nankervis, A. T., *et al*. Appraisal of a new rapid enzyme strip. *Medical Journal of Australia*, **2**, pp 677-8, 1980.

11 Alberti, K. G. M. M., Skrabalo, Z. Standardization of biochemical methods in the diagnosis and management of diabetes with particular reference to developing countries. *IDF Bulletin*, January, 1982.

12 Gill, G. V. Diabetes - some recent advances. *Medicine Digest*, 8, **12**, pp 5-14, 1982.

13 National Diabetes Data Group (NDDG). Classification and diagnosis of diabetes mellitus and other categories of glucose intolerance. *Diabetes*, **28**, p 1039, 1979.

14 Caraway, W. T. *Standard Methods of Clinical Chemistry*, **4**, pp 239-247, 1963.

15 Zurkowski, P. *Clinical Chemistry*, **10**, pp 451-453, 1964.

16 Clark, W. L., Baginski, E. S., Marie, S. S., and Zak, B. *Microchemical Journal*, **20**, pp 22-32, 1975.

17 Fraser C. G. Personal Communication, 1986.

Recommended Reading

World Health Organization, *WHO Expert Committee on Diabetes Mellitus*, Technical Report Series, **646**, 1980.

Baron, D. N. *A Short Textbook of Chemical Pathology*, Hodder and Stoughton, 4th Edition, 1982. ELBS: 1984 £2 ISBN 0 340 27048 9.

Whitby, L. G., Percy-Robb, I. W., and Smith, A. F. *Lecture Notes on Clinical Chemistry*, Blackwell Scientific Publications, Oxford, 3rd Edition, 1984. UK price £9.80. A low cost edition of this book is available from, P G Publishing Private Ltd, Alexandra, PO Box 318, Singapore 9115, Singapore.

APPENDIX I

PREPARATION OF REAGENTS

PREPARATION AND STORAGE OF REAGENTS

This appendix includes details of how to prepare and store the reagents used in the techniques described in this Manual. In addition to the details given under individual reagents, the following also apply:

- Weigh as accurately as possible chemicals that are to be used to make buffers, volumetric solutions, and standard solutions.

  Note: The technique of preparing accurate solutions is described fully in 24:8.

- Always label clearly all reagents. Include the full name of a reagent and where appropriate, its concentration and date of preparation.

- If a reagent is *Harmful*, *Toxic*, *Corrosive*, or *Flammable*, indicate this on the bottle label.

  Note: Hazard safety symbols are illustrated and described under 'The Safe Use of Chemicals and Reagents' in 2:5.

- Store reagents in completely clean bottles that have *leak-proof* screw-caps or stoppers. Use brown bottles for storing light sensitive reagents.

- Protect all reagents from sunlight and excessive heat. Store light sensitive reagents and stock solutions of stains in the dark and unstable reagents at 2-8 °C (as indicated under individual reagents).

  Note: The phrase 'room temperature' as used in this Appendix, refers to 20-28 °C.

- Filter stains as required, into stain dispensing containers.

For further details regarding the preparation of reagents, dilution of solutions, use of SI units, and the safe storage and use of chemicals in the laboratory, including how to pipette safely, readers are referred to 24:5 - 24:8 and 2:4 - 2:5.

Distilled water

For all the reagents described in this Appendix, deionized water can be used instead of distilled water. For most stains and reagents not used in clinical chemistry tests, boiled filtered water or water filtered through a *Sterasyl* candle filter (see 3:7) can be used if distilled or deionized water is not available.

Useful Tables

1 g	= 1 000 mg	1 litre	= 1 000 ml
1 g	= 1 000 000 µg	1 ml	= 1 000 µl
0.1 g	= 100 mg	1 mol	= 1 000 mmol
0.01 g	= 10 mg	1 mol	= 1 000 000 µmol
1 000 µg	= 1 mg	1 mmol	= 1 000 µmol

Acetic acid, 3% v/v   No. 1
To make 100 ml:

Acetic acid, glacial .... 3 ml
Distilled water .... 97 ml

1. Fill a 100 ml cylinder to the 97 ml mark with water.
2. Add 3 ml of glacial acetic acid, i.e. to the 100 ml mark.

   Caution: Glacial acetic acid is corrosive and flammable. It is also irritating to the eyes, therefore handle it with great care, away from any open flame, and in a well ventilated room. Do *not* mouth- pipette the acid.

3. Transfer to a clean leak-proof bottle, and mix well.
4. Label the bottle and store at room temperature. The reagent is stable indefinitely.

Acetic acid, 10% v/v   No. 2
To make 100 ml:

Acetic acid, glacial .... 10 ml
Distilled water .... 90 ml

1. Fill a 100 ml cylinder to the 90 ml mark with water.
2. Add 10 ml of glacial acetic acid, i.e. to the 100 ml mark.

   Caution: See text under Reagent No. 1.

3. Transfer to a clean leak-proof bottle, and mix well.
4. Label the bottle and store at room temperature. The reagent is stable indefinitely.

Acetic acid, 60% v/v   No. 3
To make 100 ml:

Acetic acid, glacial .... 60 ml
Distilled water .... 40 ml

1. Fill a 100 ml cylinder to 40 ml mark with water.
2. Add 60 ml of glacial acetic acid, i.e. to the 100 ml mark.

   Caution: See text under Reagent No. 1

3. Transfer to a clean leak-proof bottle, and mix well.
4. Label the bottle, and mark it *Corrosive* and *Harmful*. Store the reagent at room temperature in a safe place. It is stable indefinitely.

Acid alcohol, 0.5% v/v   No. 4
This is a 0.5% v/v hydrochloric acid solution in 70% v/v alcohol.
To make about 500 ml:

Ethanol or methanol, absolute .... 350 ml
Water .... 150 ml
Hydrochloric acid, concentrated .... 2.5 ml

1. Fill a 500 ml cylinder to the 150 ml mark with water.
2. Add 350 ml of absolute ethanol or methanol,* i.e. to the 500 ml mark.

   * Technical grade is adequate.

   Caution: Ethanol and methanol are highly flammable, therefore use well away from an open flame.
3. Add 2.5 ml of concentrated hydrochloric acid.

   Caution: Concentrated hydrochloric acid is a corrosive chemical with an injurious vapour, therefore handle it with great care in a well ventilated room. Do *not* mouth-pipette.
4. Transfer to a clean leak-proof bottle and mix well.
5. Label the bottle and mark it *Flammable*. Store at room temperature in a safe place. The reagent is stable indefinitely.

Acid pepsin solution   No. 5
To make about 100 ml:

Pepsin .... 0.5 g
Hydrochloric acid, concentrated .... 0.7 ml
Distilled water .... 100 ml

1. Weigh the pepsin and transfer it to a clean leak-proof bottle of 100 ml capacity.
2. Measure 100 ml of water and add about half of it to the bottle. Dissolve the pepsin in the water. Add the remainder of the water.
3. Add 0.7 ml of concentrated hydrochloric acid and mix well.

   Caution: Concentrated hydrochloric acid is a corrosive chemical with an injurious vapour, therefore handle it with great care in a well ventilated room. Do *not* mouth-pipette.
4. Label the bottle and store at 2-8 °C. The reagent is stable for several months.

Acidified ethanol solution   No. 6
To make about 100 ml:

Acetic acid, glacial .... 0.45 ml
Ethanol, absolute .... 90 ml
Distilled water .... 10 ml

1. Using a 100 ml cylinder, measure 90 ml of absolute ethanol.

   Caution: Absolute ethanol is highly flammable, therefore use it well away from an open flame.
2. Add 10 ml of water, i.e to the 100 ml mark.
3. Add 0.45 ml of glacial acetic acid.

   Caution: See note under Reagent No. 1.
4. Transfer to a clean leak-proof bottle, and mix well.
5. Label the bottle and mark it *Flammable*. Store at room temperature in a safe place. The reagent is stable indefinitely.

Acidified silver nitrate   No. 7
To make 500 ml:

Silver nitrate .... 14.5 g
Nitric acid, 7.7 mol/l (50% v/v)* .... to 500 ml

*Prepare by mixing 250 ml of concentrated nitric acid with 250 ml of distilled water. Add the acid to the water.

Caution: Concentrated nitric acid is a highly corrosive chemical, therefore handle it with care.

1. Weigh the silver nitrate and transfer it to a 500 ml volumetric flask.

   Caution: Silver nitrate is an oxidizing and corrosive chemical, therefore handle it with care.
2. Half fill the flask with the nitric acid solution (7.7 mol/l), and mix until the silver nitrate is completely dissolved.
3. Make up to the 500 ml mark with the nitric acid solution (7.7 mol/l), and mix well.

   Caution: Make sure the flask is tightly stoppered. Although the solution appears colourless, silver nitrate will stain skin, clothing, the laboratory bench, etc. The brown stain is very difficult to remove.
4. Transfer to a dark glass bottle.
5. Label the bottle and mark it *Corrosive*.
6. Store at room temperature out of direct sunlight. The reagent is stable for several months.

Acridine orange, stock solution   No. 8
To make 100 ml:

Acridine orange .... 0.1 g
Distilled water .... 100 ml

1. Weigh the acridine orange and transfer it to a dark, clean, leak-proof bottle of 100 ml capacity.
2. Measure 100 ml of water and add about half of it to the bottle. Mix until the acridine orange is fully dissolved. Add the remainder of the water and mix well.
3. Label the bottle and store it at room temperature. The solution is stable for several weeks.

Working acridine orange solution
Prepare as described in 13:11.

Alcohol, 95% v/v   **No. 9**
To make 100 ml:

Ethanol, absolute .... 95 ml
Distilled water .... 5 ml

1. Using a 100 ml cylinder, measure 95 ml of absolute ethanol.

    Caution: Absolute ethanol is highly flammable, therefore use it well away from an open flame.

2. Add 5 ml of water, i.e. to the 100 ml mark.

3. Transfer to a clean leak-proof bottle and mix well.

4. Label the bottle and mark it *Flammable*. Store at room temperature in a safe place. The reagent is stable indefinitely.

Alkaline tartrate reagent   **No. 10**
To make 100 ml:

Potassium sodium tartrate .... 35.0 g
Sodium hydroxide .... 7.5 g
Distilled water .... to 100 ml

1. Weigh the potassium sodium tartrate and sodium hydroxide and transfer to a 100 ml volumetric flask.

    Caution: Sodium hydroxide is a corrosive deliquescent chemical, therefore handle it with care and make sure the stock bottle of chemical is tightly stoppered after use.

2. About half fill the flask with water and mix until the chemicals are fully dissolved.

3. Make up to the 100 ml mark with water and mix well.

4. Transfer to a clean leak-proof bottle. Label the bottle and mark it *Corrosive*. Store at room temperature. The reagent is stable for at least 6 months.

Alkaline water   **No. 11**
To make about 100 ml:

Sodium bicarbonate .... 2 g
(sodium hydrogen carbonate)
Water .... 100 ml

1. Weigh the sodium bicarbonate and transfer it to a clean leak-proof bottle.

2. Measure the water, add to the chemical, and mix until the sodium bicarbonate is fully dissolved.

3. Label the bottle, and store it at room temperature. The reagent should be discarded if it shows signs of contamination.

Barium chloride, 0.48 mol/l (10% w/v)   **No. 12**
To make 500 ml:

Barium chloride .... 50 g
Distilled water .... to 500 ml

1. Weigh the barium chloride and transfer it to a 500 ml volumetric flask.

    Caution: Barium chloride is a poisonous chemical which is injurious to health when inhaled or swallowed.

2. Half fill the flask with water and mix to dissolve the chemical.

3. Make up to the 500 ml mark with water and mix well.

4. Transfer to a clean leak-proof bottle. Label the bottle and mark it *Toxic*. Store at room temperature. The reagent is stable for several months.

Benedict's reagent (qualitative)   **No. 13**
Purchase ready-made, or prepare as follows:
To make 500 ml:

Copper II sulphate, 5-hydrate* .... 8.6 g
*Use analytical grade
Sodium carbonate, anhydrous .... 50.0 g
tri-Sodium citrate .... 86.4 g
Distilled water .... to 500 ml

1. Weigh the copper sulphate, and transfer it to a clean beaker. Measure about 75 ml of water, add to the beaker, and stir to dissolve the chemical.

2. Weigh the sodium carbonate and sodium citrate. Transfer these to a 500 ml volumetric flask.

3. Half fill the flask with water and mix to dissolve the chemicals (placing the flask in a container of hot water for a few minutes will help to dissolve the chemicals. Allow to cool).

4. Add the copper sulphate solution to the volumetric flask, a little at a time, mixing after each addition. Rinse out the beaker with distilled water to make sure all the copper sulphate is transferred to the flask.

5. Make up to the 500 ml mark with water, and mix well.

6. Transfer to a clean leak-proof plastic bottle. Label the bottle. Store at room temperature. When kept tightly stoppered the reagent is stable indefinitely.

Benzoic acid, 1 g/l (0.1% w/v)   **No. 14**
To make 1 litre:

Benzoic acid .... 1 g
Distilled water .... to 1 litre

1. Heat about 500 ml of distilled water to 50-70 °C.

2. Weigh the benzoic acid, and transfer it to a 1 litre volumetric flask.

3. Half fill the flask with the hot water, and mix to dissolve the chemical. Allow to cool.

4. When cool, make up to the 1 litre mark with water and mix well.

5. Transfer to a clean leak-proof bottle. Label the bottle. Store at room temperature. The solution is stable indefinitely.

Beyer's stock solution   No. 15
To make about 107 ml:

Copper II chloride dihydrate .... 0.7 g
(CuCl$_2$.2H$_2$O)
Acetic acid, glacial .... 7 ml
Formalin solution, 20% v/v* .... 100 ml

*Prepare by mixing 20 ml of concentrated formaldehyde solution (37-40% v/v) with 80 ml of distilled or filtered water.

Caution: Formaldehyde solution is a toxic chemical with an irritating and harmful vapour, therefore handle it with care in a well ventilated room.

1. Weigh the copper II chloride and transfer it to a clean leak-proof bottle.

2. Measure the formalin solution and acetic acid, and add to the bottle. Mix until the copper II chloride is completely dissolved.

   Caution: Glacial acetic acid is corrosive and flammable. It is also irritating to the eyes, therefore handle it with care away from any open flame and in a well ventilated room. Do *not* mouth-pipette.

3. Label the bottle and mark it *Corrosive* and *Toxic*. Store at room temperature in a safe place. The reagent is stable indefinitely.

   Working Beyer's solution
   Dilute the stock solution 1 in 10 in distilled or filtered water, e.g. mix 2 ml of stock solution with 18 ml of water.

Bicarbonate standard, 25 mmol/l   No. 16
To make 100 ml:

Sodium bicarbonate* .... 0.21 g
(Sodium hydrogen carbonate)

*Use analytical grade *dry* sodium bicarbonate

Distilled water, ... to 100 ml
carbon dioxide-free*

*Prepare by boiling distilled water for several minutes to expel the carbon dioxide. Bottle the boiled water while it is still warm and store in a tightly stoppered bottle. Use when it has cooled to room temperature.

1. Weigh *accurately* the sodium bicarbonate and transfer it to a 100 ml volumetric flask.

2. Make up to the 100 ml mark with the carbon dioxide-free water and mix until the chemical is completely dissolved.

3. Transfer to a clean leak-proof bottle and stopper tightly. Label the bottle and store at 2-8 °C. Prepare fresh standard every week.

Biuret blank reagent   No. 17
To make 1 litre:

Potassium sodium tartrate .... 9 g
Potassium iodide .... 5 g
Sodium hydroxide, ... 100 ml
6 mol/l (Reagent No. 74)
Distilled water .... to 1 litre

1. Weigh the potassium sodium tartrate and potassium iodide, and transfer these to a 1 litre volumetric flask.

2. About half fill the flask with water and mix until the chemicals are completely dissolved.

3. Add 100 ml of 6 mol/l sodium hydroxide, and mix.

4. Make up to the 1 litre mark with distilled water and mix well.

5. Transfer to a clean leak-proof bottle and label. Store at room temperature. The reagent is stable indefinitely.

Biuret reagent   No. 18
To make 1 litre:

Copper II sulphate, 5-hydrate* .... 3 g
* Analytical grade is required
Potassium sodium tartrate .... 9 g
Potassium iodide .... 5 g
Sodium hydroxide, ... 100 ml
6 mol/l (Reagent No. 74)
Distilled water .... to 1 litre

1. Weigh the copper II sulphate and transfer it to a 1 litre volumetric flask. About half fill the flask with water and mix until the chemical is fully dissolved.

2. Weigh the potassium sodium tartrate and potassium iodide and transfer these to the flask. Mix until they are completely dissolved.

3. Add 100 ml of 6 mol/l sodium hydroxide and mix well.

4. Transfer to a clean leak-proof bottle and label. Store at room temperature. The reagent is stable indefinitely.

Bromocresol green (BCG) reagent   No. 19
To make 1 litre:

Succinic acid	5.6 g
Sodium hydroxide	1.0 g
Sodium azide	0.1 g
Stock BCG, 10 mmol/l†	8.0 ml
Brij-35 solution, 250 g/l‡	2.5 ml
Distilled water	to 1 litre

† Purchase from BDH Chemicals Ltd (code No. 22116 2U, priced in 1986 about £3.50 for 250 ml).

‡ Prepare by dissolving 25 g of solid Brij-35 (obtainable from BDH Chemicals Ltd, code No. 56003 4B priced in 1986 about £7.20 for 500 g) in about 20 ml of warm distilled water. When dissolved, make up to 100 ml with distilled water and mix gently.

1. Half fill a 1 litre volumetric flask with distilled water.

2. Weigh the succinic acid and sodium azide and dissolve in the water.

3. Weigh the sodium hydroxide and add to the flask. Mix until dissolved.

4. Measure *accurately* the stock BCG solution, add to the flask, and mix.

5. Add the Brij-35 solution and make up to about 950 ml with distilled water. Mix gently but avoid frothing.

6. Check the pH of the reagent. It should be pH 4.2 ± 0.05 at room temperature.

   Important: If the pH is not correct, it must be adjusted by adding (drop by drop) 10 g/l (1% w/v) sodium hydroxide if below pH 4.2, or 50 g/l (5% w/v) succinic acid if over pH 4.2.

7. Make up to the 1 litre mark with distilled water and mix.

8. Transfer to a dark brown bottle and label. Store at 2-8 °C. The reagent is stable for several months.

Buffered saline, pH 7.0-7.1   No. 20
This can be prepared by adding 0.4-0.7 ml of 10 g/l *di*-sodium hydrogen phosphate* to every 500 ml of physiological saline (Reagent No. 58). Check the pH using narrow range pH papers or a pH meter.

* Prepare by dissolving 1 g *di*-sodium hydrogen phosphate in 100 ml distilled water.

Buffered water, pH 7.1-7.2   No. 21
This is best prepared from stock phosphate buffer solutions A and B as follows:

Stock phosphate solution A

Sodium dihydrogen phosphate, 1-hydrate ($NaH_2PO_4.H_2O$)	27.6 g
Distilled water	to 1 litre

1. Weigh accurately the chemical and transfer it to a 1 litre volumetric flask.

2. Half fill the flask with water, and mix to dissolve the chemical. Make up to the 1 litre mark with distilled water, and mix well. Transfer to a clean, leak-proof bottle.

3. Label the bottle 'Stock phosphate solution A'. Store in a cool place or preferably at 2-8 °C. The solution is stable for several months.

Stock phosphate solution B

di-Sodium hydrogen phosphate, anhydrous (Na_2HPO_4)	28.39 g
Distilled water	to 1 litre

Prepare as described above for solution A. Label the bottle 'Stock phosphate solution B'. Store in a cool place or preferably at 2-8 °C. The solution is stable for several months.

To make 1 litre buffered water, pH 7.2:

Stock phosphate solution A	140 ml
Stock phosphate solution B	360 ml
Distilled water	500 ml

1. Measure accurately the stock phosphate solutions and water, transfer to a clean leak-proof bottle, and mix well. Check the pH using narrow range pH papers or a pH meter.

   Alternatively, measure the stock phosphate solutions, transfer to a litre volumetric flask, and make up to the mark with water. Transfer to a clean leak-proof bottle, and mix well. Check the pH using narrow range pH papers or a pH meter.

2. Label the bottle and store it at room temperature. The buffer is stable for several months.

Burrow's stain   No. 22
To make 100 ml:

Thionin	0.02 g
Ethanol, absolute (absolute alcohol)	3 ml
Acetic acid, glacial	3 ml
Distilled water	94 ml

1. Weigh the thionin* and transfer it to a leak-proof bottle of 100 ml capacity.

   * If an accurate balance is not available to weigh the 0.02 g (20 mg) of thionin, transfer a small amount of the powdered stain to a small tube and dip the end of a wet (water-wetted) swab stick (or unburnt end of a match stick) in the powder. This will give approximately 20 mg.

2. Measure the ethanol and acetic acid and add these to the bottle. Mix until the thionin is completely dissolved.

   Caution: Ethanol is highly flammable and glacial acetic acid is corrosive, flammable, and has an irritating vapour, therefore handle these chemicals with care, well away from any open flame, in a well ventilated room. Do *not* mouth-pipette.

3. Add the water and mix well.

4. Label the bottle and store preferably at 2-8 °C. Renew every 3 months.

Caffeine-benzoate reagent No. 23
To make 500 ml:

Sodium acetate, trihydrate .... 46.5 g
Sodium benzoate .... 28.0 g
di-Sodium EDTA* .... 0.5 g
(* ethylenediamine tetra-acetic acid, *di*sodium salt)
Caffeine .... 19.0 g
Distilled water .... to 500 ml

1. Weigh the sodium acetate, sodium benzoate, and *di*-sodium EDTA, and transfer these to a 500 ml volumetric flask.

2. About half fill the flask with water and mix to dissolve completely the chemicals.

3. Add the caffeine and mix to dissolve.

4. Make up to the 500 ml mark with water and mix well.

5. Filter the reagent into a clean leak-proof bottle. Label the bottle and store it at room temperature. The reagent is stable for at least 6 months.

Carbol fuchsin No. 24
This is the same as the carbol fuchsin stain used in the Ziehl-Neelsen technique described in 34:6 in Volume II of the Manual (Reagent No. 19). For completeness, the preparation of the stain is also described in this Volume.

To make about 1115 ml:

Basic fuchsin .... 10 g
Ethanol or methanol, absolute* .... 100 ml
Phenol .... 50 g
Distilled water .... 1 litre

* Technical grade is adequate.

1. Weigh the basic fuchsin on a piece of clean paper (preweighed), and transfer the powder to a bottle of at least 1.5 litre capacity.

2. Measure the ethanol (ethyl alcohol) or methanol (methyl alcohol), and add to the bottle. Mix at intervals until the basic fuchsin is fully dissolved.

   Caution: Methanol and ethanol are highly flammable, therefore use well away from an open flame.

3. With great care, weigh the phenol in a beaker. Measure the water, and add some of it to the beaker to dissolve the phenol. Transfer to the bottle of stain, and mix well.

   Caution: Phenol is a highly corrosive, toxic, and hygroscopic chemical, therefore handle it with *great care*. To avoid spilling phenol on the balance pan, remove the beaker when adding or subtracting the chemical.

4. Add the remainder of the water, and mix well.

5. Label, and store at room temperature. The stain is stable indefinitely.

For use: Filter a small amount of the stain into a dropper bottle or other suitable stain dispensing container.

Citric acid-Tween solution No. 25
To make 1 litre:

Citric acid .... 12.91 g
di-Sodium hydrogen phosphate, ... 27.61 g
hydrated ($Na_2HPO_4.12H_2O$)
Tween 80 .... 50 ml
Merthiolate .... 0.1 g
Distilled water .... to 1 litre

1. Weigh the citric acid and *di*-sodium hydrogen phosphate and transfer these to a 1 litre volumetric flask.

2. Half fill the flask with warm water and mix until the chemicals are completely dissolved.

3. Add 50 ml of Tween 80 and make up to the 1 litre mark with water.

4. Transfer to a clean leak-proof bottle. Add 0.1 g merthiolate (preservative) and mix gently but well.

5. Label the bottle and store at room temperature. The solution is stable for several months.

Colour reagent for glucose assay No. 26
To make 230 ml:

4-Aminophenazone, 5 g/l† .... 16 ml
Fermcozyme 952 DM‡ .... 4 ml
Phosphate buffer (Reagent No. 55) .... 60 ml
Distilled water .... 150 ml

† Prepare by dissolving 0.5 g of 4-aminophenazone* (4-aminoantipyrine) in 100 ml of distilled water.

* Obtainable from Koch-Light Ltd, BDH Chemicals Ltd, other chemical manufacturer.

‡ Obtainable direct from Fermco Laboratories or from Hughes and Hughes or other agent. For the addresses of these companies, see Appendix II.

Fermcozyme 952 DM contains 1250 U/ml of glucose oxidase and 1 mg/ml of peroxidase. It is available in 50 ml bottles, priced about £12.00 for 50 ml (1986). It is a stable product with a shelf-life from manufacture in excess of 2 years. It requires storage at 2-8 °C.

1. Measure the aminophenazone, *Fermcozyme*, phosphate buffer, and water, and transfer these to a dark coloured, clean, leak-proof bottle. Mix well.

2. Label the bottle and store at 2-8 °C. When refrigerated the colour reagent is stable for about 3 months.

CPC stock reagent   No. 27
To make 500 ml:

Ethanediol* .... 38 ml
2-Amino-2-methyl-l-propanol* .... 13 ml
o-Cresolphthalein complexone .... 0.015 g
(*CPC*)*

* Available from BDH Chemicals Ltd and other manufacturers. The *o*-cresolphthalein complexone can be purchased from BDH Chemicals in 1 g amounts (No. 200272L),
priced about £5.00 (1986).

1. Half fill a 500 ml volumetric flask with distilled water.

2. Measure the ethanediol and 2-amino-2-methyl-l-propanol, add these to the flask, and mix.

3. Weigh accurately the *o*-cresolphthalein complexone (CPC) and add to the flask. Mix until the CPC is completely dissolved.

4. Make up to the 500 ml mark with distilled water and mix well.

5. Transfer the reagent to a *completely clean* dark coloured leak-proof bottle, and label. Store at 2-8 °C. The stock CPC reagent is stable for 3-4 weeks.

Working CPC reagent
Prepare as described in 31:5.

Diacetyl monoxime, 4 g/l   No. 28
To make 500 ml:

Diacetyl monoxime .... 2 g
Distilled water .... to 500 ml

1. Weigh the diacetyl monoxime and transfer it to a 500 ml volumetric flask.

2. Half fill the flask with water and mix until the chemical is completely dissolved.

3. Make up to the 500 ml mark with water and mix well.

4. Transfer to a clean leak-proof bottle and label. Store preferably at 2-8 °C. The reagent is stable for at least 6 months.

Dill-Glazko eosin   No. 29
To make 101 ml:

Eosin (yellowish) powder .... 0.05 g
Chloroform .... 100 ml
Hydrochloric acid, 1 mol/l (1 N) .... 1 ml

1. Weigh the eosin on a piece of clean paper, (pre-weighed) and transfer to a clean, leak-proof, brown bottle.

2. Measure the chloroform, and add to the bottle.

   Caution: Chloroform is a volatile and danger-ous substance, which is injurious to health when inhaled. Use with care, avoiding contact with eyes and skin.

3. Measure the hydrochloric acid 1 mol/l solution, and add to the bottle.

4. Stopper the bottle, and mix for 2-3 minutes.

5. Allow the reagent to settle.

6. Remove the upper layer of the reagent, and discard.

7. Label the bottle and mark it *Harmful*.

   Store at room temperature away from direct sunlight, with the top of the bottle tightly stop-pered. The reagent is stable for several months.

Delafield haematoxylin   No. 30
It is recommended that this stain be bought ready-made from Paramount Reagents, (see Appendix II) or other supplier.

When purchased ready made from Paramount Reagents, Delafield haematoxylin costs approx. £1.80 for 100 ml or £4.50 for 500 ml (1986).

For those laboratories wishing to make their own stain the following formula can be used:

Haematoxylin .... 4.0 g
Ammonium alum .... 8.0 g
Potassium permanganate .... 0.2 g
Ethanol, absolute .... 125 ml
Distilled water .... 400 ml

1. Weigh the haematoxylin and transfer it to a clean bottle or flask.

2. Measure the absolute ethanol and add it to the haematoxylin. Stopper the flask or bottle and stand it in a container of hot water to help the haematoxylin to dissolve. Do not heat over an open flame (ethanol is highly flammable). Mix well and when cool, filter.

3. Weigh the ammonium alum and transfer to a bottle or flask. Add 400 ml of hot water (40-50 °C) to help the ammonium alum to dissolve. When dissolved, add the solution to the filtered haematoxylin solution and mix well.

4. Dissolve the potassium permanganate in about 10 ml of distilled water and add this to the stain (this will 'ripen' the stain, i.e. enable it to be used immediately). Mix well.

5. Label the bottle and store it at room tempera-ture. The stain is stable for several months.

Dobell's iodine   No. 31
To make about 200 ml:

Iodine .... 4 g
Potassium iodide .... 8 g
Distilled water .... 200 ml

1. Weigh the potassium iodide, and transfer it to a clean leak-proof brown bottle of 250 ml capac-ity.

2. Measure 200 ml of water and add to the bottle.

Mix well until the chemical is completely dissolved.

3. Weigh the iodine and add it to the potassium iodide solution. Mix well to dissolve the iodine.

    Caution: Iodine is injurious to health if inhaled or allowed to come into contact with the eyes.

    Note: Iodine will not dissolve in water. It is important, therefore, to add the potassium iodide to the water first, followed by the iodine.

4. Label the bottle and mark it *Harmful*. Store at room temperature away from direct sunlight. The solution is stable for several months.

For use: Transfer about 10 ml of the iodine solution to a small brown dropper bottle or insert a dropping pipette through the cap of a small brown bottle.

Note: If Lugol's iodine is available, a suitable solution for staining protozoal cysts can be made by diluting Lugol's iodine 1 in 2 with 25% v/v acetic acid, i.e. mix 10 ml of Lugol's iodine with 10 ml of 25% v/v acetic acid. This solution gives good staining of nuclei without overstaining.

Erhlich's reagent   No. 32
To make about 200 ml:

4-Dimethylaminobenzaldehyde .... 4 g
Hydrochloric acid, concentrated .... 40 ml
Distilled water .... 160 ml

1. Weigh the 4-dimethylaminobenzaldehyde, and transfer it to a clean, leak-proof brown bottle.

2. Measure the water and add to the chemical. Mix to dissolve.

3. Add the concentrated hydrochloric acid, and mix well.

    Caution: Concentrated hydrochloric acid is a corrosive chemical with an injurious vapour, therefore handle it with great care in a well ventilated room.

4. Label the bottle and mark it *Corrosive*. Store at room temperature. The reagent is stable for several weeks if protected from daylight.

Eosin stain, 5 g/l (0.5% w/v)   No. 33
To make about 100 ml:

Eosin powder .... 0.5 g
Distilled water .... 100 ml

1. Weigh the eosin on a clean piece of paper (pre-weighed), and transfer the powder to a clean, leak-proof, brown bottle of 100 ml capacity.

2. Add 100 ml of water, and mix to dissolve the stain.

3. Label the bottle, and store it at room temperature. The stain is stable indefinitely.

For use: Transfer a small amount of the stain to a bottle with a cap into which a dropper can be inserted.

Ethanol iodine solution   No. 34
To make about 100 ml:

Ethanol, 70% v/v* .... 100 ml
Iodine crystals . As needed to give brown colour

* Prepare by mixing 30 ml of distilled water with 70 ml of absolute ethanol (ethyl alcohol).

1. Dissolve sufficient iodine in the 70% ethanol to give a medium brown colour.

    Note: The colour should not be too dark otherwise the iodine will interfere with the trichrome staining. Neither should the colour be too light because the mercuric chloride left in the preparation will not be removed adequately.

2. Protect the reagent from direct sunlight. Label the container and mark it *Flammable*.

Field's stain A   No. 35
To make 500 ml:

Field's stain A powder* .... 6 g
Distilled water (hot) .... 500 ml

* Obtain from Paramount Reagents, BDH Chemicals Ltd, or other reliable supplier.

1. Weigh the powder on a piece of clean paper (pre-weighed), and transfer it to a large Pyrex beaker or high density polyethylene reagent bottle (see 3:2).

2. Measure the water and heat to boiling.

3. Add the hot water to the stain and mix to dissolve the powder.

4. When cool, filter the stain into a clean bottle.

5. Label the bottle and store it at room temperature. The stain is stable indefinitely.

Field's stain B   No. 36
To make 500 ml:

Field's stain powder B* .... 5 g
Distilled water (hot) .... 500 ml

*Obtain from Paramount Reagents, BDH Chemicals Ltd, or other reliable supplier.

Prepare as described for Field's stain A (Reagent No. 35). Label the bottle and store at room temperature. The stain is stable indefinitely.

Fluoride-oxalate reagent   No. 37
To make 100 ml:

Sodium fluoride .... 1 g
Potassium oxalate .... 3 g
Distilled or deionised water .... to 100 ml

1. Weigh the sodium fluoride and potassium oxalate and transfer these to a 100 ml volumetric flask.

2. Half fill the flask with water and mix until the

chemicals are completely dissolved. Make up to the 100 ml mark with water and mix well.

3. Transfer to a clean leak-proof bottle, and label. Store at room temperature. The reagent is stable for several months.

Preparation of containers
Dispense 0.1 ml of reagent into small containers and allow the water content to evaporate (cover the containers with a thin cloth). When dry, stopper the containers.

For use: The amount of fluoride-oxalate in each tube is sufficient to preserve 1 ml of blood. After adding the blood, mix gently. The fluoride prevents glycolysis and the oxalate prevents clotting of the blood. Fluoride-oxalated blood or c.s.f. can also be used in protein and urea tests.

Formol detergent solution   No. 38
To make 500 ml:

Formaldehyde, concentrated solution ..... 10 ml
Detergent solution* .... 10 ml
Clean water .... 480 ml

* This can be *Lipsol, Fairy Liquid, Decon, Teepol*, or other washing-up detergent.

1. Measure the water and transfer to a storage bottle.

2. Measure the detergent solution and add to the water.

   Note: If using the *Faecal formol detergent schisto kit* (Appendix IV, see FDK.010), 10 ml can be measured using one of the labelled sedimentation containers.

3. Measure the formaldehyde solution* and add to the water. Mix well.

   See **Note** above.

   Caution: Concentrated formaldehyde solution is a toxic chemical with a vapour that is irritating to the eyes and mucous membranes, therefore handle it with great care in a well ventilated room.

4. Label the bottle and store at room temperature. The solution is stable indefinitely.

Formol saline, 10% v/v   No. 39
To make 500 ml:

Physiological saline .... 450 ml
(Reagent No. 58)
Formaldehyde solution, concentrated ..... 50 ml

1. Measure the physiological saline and transfer it to a clean leak-proof bottle.

2. Measure the formaldehyde solution and add to the saline. Mix well.

   Caution: Concentrated formaldehyde solution is a toxic chemical with a vapour that is irritating to the eyes and mucous membranes, there-

fore handle it with great care in a well ventilated room.

3. Label the bottle and store at room temperature in a safe place. The reagent is stable indefinitely.

Fouchet's reagent   No. 40
To make 100 ml:

Trichloroacetic acid (TCA) .... 25 g
Iron III chloride (ferric chloride), ... 10 ml
100 g/l (10% w/v)*
Distilled water .... to 100 ml

* Prepare by dissolving 10 g of the chemical in 100 ml of distilled water.

1. Rapidly weigh the TCA in a beaker. Add 30-40 ml of distilled water, and stir to dissolve the chemical.

   Caution: TCA is a strongly corrosive and deliquescent chemical, therefore avoid contact with the eyes and skin and make sure the stock bottle of chemical is tightly stoppered after use.

2. Using a funnel, transfer the dissolved acid to a 100 ml volumetric flask.

3. Add 10 ml of the iron III chloride solution, and mix. Make up to the 100 ml mark with distilled water, and mix well.

4. Transfer the reagent to a small brown bottle (one in which a dropper can be inserted).

5. Label the bottle, and mark it *Corrosive*. Store at room temperature. The reagent is stable for several months.

Giemsa stain   No. 41
Purchase ready-made or prepare using the following formula.

To make about 500 ml:

Giemsa powder .... 3.8 g
Glycerol (glycerine) .... 250 ml
Methanol (methyl alcohol), ... 250 ml

Correction: In Volume II, the text under methanol (Reagent No. 35) should   read 'Technical Grade is not suitable'.

1. Weigh the Giemsa on a piece of clean paper (preweighed), and transfer to a *dry* brown bottle of 500 ml capacity which contains a few glass beads.

   Note: Giemsa stain will be spoilt if water enters the stock solution during its preparation or storage.

2. Using a *dry* cylinder, measure the methanol, and add to the stain. Mix well.

   Caution: Methanol is toxic and highly flammable, therefore handle it with care and use well away from an open flame.

3. Using the same cylinder, measure the glycerol,

and add to the stain. Mix well.

4. Place the bottle of stain in a water bath at 50-60 °C, or if not available at 37 °C, for up to 2 hours to help the stain to dissolve. Mix well at intervals.

5. Label the bottle, and mark it *Flammable and Toxic*. Store at room temperature in the dark. If kept well-stoppered, the stain is stable for several months.

For use: Filter a small amount of the stain into a dry stain dispensing container.

Glycerol jelly   No. 42
To make about 310 ml:

Gelatin .... 15 g
Glycerol (glycerine) .... 50 ml
Distilled water .... 250 ml

1. Measure the water and heat to boiling.

2. Weigh the gelatin and add to the hot water. Stir until the gelatin is completely dissolved.

3. Measure the glycerol and mix with the gelatin water.

4. Dispense in 10-20 ml amounts in screw-cap bottles, and allow to gel. Label each bottle and store at 2-8 °C.

For use: Liquefy a container of glycerol jelly by placing it in hot water (about 50 °C). Mix with the faecal sediment as described in 13:9.

Hydrochloric acid, 100 mmol/l   No. 43
(0.1 mol/l)
To make 500 ml:

Hydrochloric acid, concentrated .... 4.5 ml
Distilled water .... to 500 ml

1. Half fill a 500 ml volumetric flask with water.

2. Measure 4.5 ml of concentrated hydrochloric acid and add this to the water.

   Caution: Concentrated hydrochloric acid is a corrosive chemical with an injurious vapour, therefore handle it with great care in a well ventilated rooom. Do *not* mouth-pipette.

3. Make up to the 500 ml mark with water and mix well.

4. Transfer to a clean leak-proof bottle and label. Store at room temperature. The reagent is stable indefinitely.

Hydrochloric acid, 50% v/v   No. 44
To make 100 ml:

Hydrochloric acid, concentrated .... 50 ml
Distilled water .... 50 ml

1. Using a cylinder, measure 50 ml of water and transfer to a leak-proof screw cap bottle.

2. Measure 50 ml of concentrated hydrochloric acid and add to the water. Cap the bottle and mix well.

   Caution: See Reagent No. 43.

3. Label the bottle and mark it *Corrosive*. Store at room temperature in a safe place. The reagent is stable indefinitely.

Hydrochloric acid, 10 mmol/l   No. 45
carbon dioxide-free (for bicarbonate assays)
To make 100 ml:

Hydrochloric acid, 100 mmol/l* .... 10 ml

*Purchase as an accurate 100 mmol/l (0.1 mol/l) volumetric solution or prepare from a 1 mol/l volumetric solution.

Sodium chloride, 10 g/l .... to 100 ml
carbon dioxide-free (see Reagent No. 67).

1. Pipette *accurately* 10 ml of 100 mmol/l hydrochloric acid into a 100 ml volumetric flask.

2. Make up to the 100 ml mark with the carbon dioxide-free sodium chloride solution and mix. Renew daily.

Hydrogen peroxide, 10 vols solution   No. 46
To make 100 ml:

Hydrogen peroxide, 30% w/v* .... 10 ml
Distilled water .... 90 ml

* A 30% w/v hydrogen peroxide solution is available from BDH Chemicals and other suppliers of chemicals. It contains 100 volumes.

1. Measure 90 ml of water and transfer to a clean, leak-proof brown bottle.

2. Measure 10 ml of 30% w/v hydrogen peroxide and add to the water. Cap the bottle and mix well.

   Caution: Hydrogen peroxide is a corrosive and oxidizing chemical, therefore handle it with care. Always store it in a cool dark place, preferably at 2-8 °C because exposure to warmth and light causes oxygen to be evolved with a build up of pressure, which may lead to an explosion.

3. Label the bottle and mark it *Corrosive* and *Oxidizing*. Store in a cool dark place, preferably at 2-8 °C.

Iodine, stock solution, 50 mmol/l   No. 47
To make 1 litre:

Potassium iodate .... 3.57 g
Potassium iodide .... 45.00 g
Hydrochloric acid, concentrated .... 9.0 ml
Distilled water .... to 1 litre

1. Weigh the potassium iodate and potassium iodide, and transfer these to a 1 litre volumetric flask.

2. Add about 800 ml of water and mix until the chemicals are completely dissolved.

3. Measure the concentrated hydrochloric acid and *slowly*, with mixing, add this to the flask.

   Caution: Concentrated hydrochloric acid is a corrosive chemical with an injurious vapour, therefore handle it with care and use in a well ventilated room. Do *not* mouth-pipette.

4. Make up to the 1 litre mark with water and mix.

5. Transfer to a clean, leak-proof brown bottle and label. Store at room temperature away from sunlight. The reagent is stable for about 1 year.

Working iodine solution
Prepare as described in 30:10.

Lactophenol solution   No. 48
To make about 110 ml:

Phenol .... 25 g
Lactic acid .... 25 ml
Glycerol .... 50 ml
Distilled water .... 25 ml

1. Rapidly weigh the phenol in a preweighed beaker.

2. Measure the water and add to the phenol. Mix to dissolve the phenol. Transfer to a clean, leak-proof, brown bottle.

   Caution: Phenol is a highly corrosive, toxic, and hygroscopic chemical, therefore handle it with great care. To avoid damaging the balance pan, remove the beaker when adding or subtracting the chemical. Make sure the stock bottle of phenol is tightly stoppered after use.

3. Measure the lactic acid and glycerol and add to the bottle. Cap the bottle and mix well.

4. Label the bottle and mark it *Toxic* and *Corrosive*. Store at room temperature in a safe place. The reagent is stable for many months.

Methylene blue-saline, 0.1% w/v   No. 49
To make 100 ml:

Physiological saline (Reagent No. 58) .... 100 ml
Methylene blue .... 0.1 g

1. Weigh the methylene blue and transfer it to a clean leak-proof bottle.

2. Measure the saline and add to the dye. Mix until the methylene blue is completely dissolved.

3. Label the bottle and store it at room temperature. Discard the stain if it becomes contaminated.

For use: Filter a small amount of the stain into a dropper bottle.

Nigrosin stain   No. 50
To make about 120 ml:

Acetic acid, glacial .... 10 ml
Methanol, absolute .... 50 ml
Nigrosin, saturated aqueous solution* .... 10 ml
Distilled water .... 50 ml

*Prepare by dissolving sufficient *water-soluble* nigrosin in about 12 ml of warm distilled water until no more can be dissolved. Filter 10 ml.

1. Measure the water and transfer it to a clean, leak-proof, brown bottle.

2. Measure the acetic acid and methanol and add these to the water.

   Caution: Glacial acetic acid is a corrosive and flammable chemical with an irritating vapour and methanol is highly flammable. Handle, therefore, these chemicals with care, well away from any open flame and in a well ventilated room.

3. Add the nigrosin stain and mix well. Label the bottle and store it at room temperature. The reagent is stable for many months and can be reused.

Nitroprusside dry reagent   No. 51
To make about 153 g:

Ammonium sulphate .... 100 g
Sodium carbonate, anhydrous .... 50 g
Sodium nitroprusside* .... 3 g

* The accepted international name for sodium nitroprusside is pentacyanonitrosyl ferrate.

1. Weigh the sodium nitroprusside, and transfer it to a clean, wide-necked, plastic screw-cap container.

   Caution: Sodium nitroprusside is a poisonous chemical, therefore handle it with care.

2. Using a pestle or the end of a clean test tube (made of thick glass), grind the crystals to a powder.

3. Weigh the sodium carbonate and ammonium sulphate, and transfer these to the container.

4. Cap the container and mix the powders by shaking.

5. Label the container and mark it *Toxic*. Store at room temperature. The reagent is stable for several months.

PBS, pH 7.2, see Reagent No. 57

Phenol red indicator   No. 52
To make 100 ml:

Phenol red powder .... 0.1 g
Sodium hydroxide, 50 mmol/l* .... 5.7 ml

*Prepare by mixing 5 ml of 100 mmol/l sodium hydroxide (purchase as ready-made 100 mmol/l volumetric solution) with 5 ml of carbon dioxide-free distilled water (see following text).

Distilled water, ... to 100 ml
carbon dioxide-free*

*Prepare by boiling distilled water for several minutes to expel the dissolved carbon dioxide. While still warm, transfer the boiled water to a clean, leak-proof bottle and stopper tightly. Use when the water has cooled to room temperature.

1. Weigh the phenol red in a small preweighed plastic bottle. Add 5.7 ml of 50 mmol/l sodium hydroxide and mix until the powder is completely dissolved.

2. Using a funnel, transfer the dissolved dye to a 100 ml volumetric flask. Use a little of the carbon dioxide-free distilled water to rinse out the bottle to make sure all the phenol red is transferred to the flask.

3. Make up to the 100 ml mark with carbon dioxide-free water.

4. Transfer the reagent to a plastic bottle, cap tightly, and mix well.

5. Label the bottle and store at room temperature. The solution is stable indefinitely.

Phenol, saturated solution No. 53
To make about 30 ml:

Phenol crystals .... 2 g
Distilled water .... 30 ml

1. Weigh the phenol in a beaker (preweighed). Add the water, and stir to dissolve the chemical. Transfer to a clean, leak-proof bottle and mix well.

   Caution: Phenol is a highly corrosive, toxic, and hygroscopic chemical, therefore handle it with great care. To avoid damaging the balance pan, always remove the beaker when adding or subtracting the chemical. Make sure the stock bottle of phenol is tightly stoppered after use.

2. Label the bottle, and mark it *Corrosive*. Store at room temperature in a safe place. The reagent is stable indefinitely.

Phosphate borate buffer, pH 12.8 No. 54
To make 500 ml:

tri-Sodium orthophosphate .... 9.5 g
di-Sodium tetraborate .... 9.5 g
Distilled water .... to 500 ml

1. Weigh the sodium orthophosphate and sodium tetraborate, and transfer these to a 500 ml volumetric flask.

2. Half fill the flask with water and mix to dissolve the chemicals.

3. Measure the pH and adjust to pH 12.8 by adding 1 mol/l sodium hydroxide (Reagent No. 72). About 110 ml will be required.

4. Make up to the 500 ml mark with water and mix well.

5. Transfer to a clean leak-proof bottle, and label. Store at room temperature. The reagent is stable indefinitely.

Phosphate buffer for glucose colour reagent No. 55
To make 500 ml:

di-Sodium hydrogen orthophosphate .... 10 g
anhydrous (Na_2HPO_4)
Potassium dihydrogen orthophosphate ...... 10 g
(KH_2PO_4)
Sodium azide .... 2 g
Distilled water .... to 500 ml

1. Weigh the chemicals and transfer these to a 500 ml volumetric flask.

2. Half fill the flask with water and mix to dissolve the chemicals. Make up to the 500 ml mark with water and mix well.

3. Transfer the reagent to a clean leak-proof bottle (preferably plastic), and label. Store at room temperature. The reagent is stable for several months.

Phosphate buffered saline, pH 7.0 No. 56
To make about 200 ml:

Stock phosphate solution A* .... 39 ml
Stock phosphate solution B* .... 61 ml
Distilled water .... 100 ml
Sodium chloride .... 1.7 g

*See Reagent No. 21.

1. Mix the phosphate solutions with the water. Add the sodium chloride and mix to dissolve.

2. Check the pH using narrow range pH papers or a pH meter. Store the reagent in a cool place or preferably at 2-8 °C. The reagent is stable for several weeks. Renew if it becomes contaminated.

Phosphate buffered saline, pH 7.2 No. 57
To make about 200 ml:

Stock phosphate solution A* .... 28 ml
Stock phosphate solution B* .... 72 ml
Distilled water .... 100 ml
Sodium chloride .... 1.7 g

*See Reagent No. 21.

1. Mix the phosphate solutions with the water. Add the sodium chloride, and mix well to dissolve.

2. Check the pH using narrow range pH papers or a pH meter. Store the reagent in a cool place or

preferably at 2-8 °C. The reagent is stable for several weeks. Renew if it becomes contaminated.

Physiological saline, 8.5 g/l   No. 58
(0.85% w/v)
To make 1 litre:

Sodium chloride .... 8.5 g
Distilled water .... to 1 litre

1. Weigh the sodium chloride, and transfer it to a clean leak-proof bottle premarked to hold 1 litre.
2. Add distilled water to the 1 litre mark, and mix until the salt is fully dissolved.
3. Label the bottle, and store it at room temperature. The reagent is stable for several months. Discard if it becomes contaminated.

Picric acid reagent (13 g/l)   No. 59
This reagent is a saturated solution of picric acid, i.e it contains 13 g of the chemical per litre. It is best purchased in this form (BDH No. 22035) because picric acid is not available as a dry chemical for weighing like other chemicals. It is always supplied containing about 50% water (*dry* picric acid is explosive).

If saturated picric acid cannot be obtained, a saturated solution can be prepared from picric acid containing 50% water as follows:

1. Weigh about 11 g of the well mixed moist picric acid in a beaker.
2. Add the chemical to 500 ml of distilled water and mix at intervals for several hours to produce a saturated solution.
3. Transfer to a clean, leak-proof brown bottle. Label the bottle and mark it *Harmful*. Store at room temperature. The reagent is stable indefinitely.

Protein diluent   No. 60
To make 1 litre:

Sodium chloride .... 9 g
Sodium azide .... 1 g
Distilled water .... to 1 litre

1. Weigh the sodium chloride and sodium azide, and transfer these to a 1 litre volumetric flask or leak-proof bottle pre-marked to hold 1 litre.
2. Half fill the flask or bottle with water and mix until the chemicals are completely dissolved.
3. Make up to the 1 litre mark with water and mix well.
4. Label the bottle and store at room temperature. The reagent is stable indefinitely.

Protein precipitant reagent   No. 61
To make 500 ml:

Sodium tungstate, dihydrate .... 5 g
di-Sodium hydrogen phosphate, ... 5 g
anhydrous (Na_2HPO_4)
Sodium chloride .... 4.5 g
Phenol .... 0.5 g
Hydrochloric acid, 1 mol/l* .... 62 ml
Distilled water .... to 500 ml

*Prepare by diluting concentrated hydrochloric acid 1 in 10, i.e half fill a 100 ml volumetric flask with distilled water, add 9 ml of concentrated hydrochloric acid (do *not* mouth-pipette), make up to the 100 ml mark with distilled water, and mix well.

1. Weigh the sodium tungstate, di-sodium hydrogen phosphate, and sodium chloride, and transfer these to a 500 ml volumetric flask.
2. Half fill the flask with distilled water and mix until the chemicals are completely dissolved.
3. Add 62 ml of 1 mol/l hydrochloric acid solution and mix.
4. Weigh the phenol and add to the flask. Mix to dissolve.

   Caution: Phenol is a highly corrosive and hygroscopic chemical, therefore take great care when weighing the chemical and transferring it to the flask. After use, make sure the stock bottle of phenol is tightly stoppered.
5. Make up to the 500 ml mark with distilled water and mix well.
6. Transfer the reagent to a clean leak-proof bottle and label. Store at room temperature. The reagent is stable indefinitely.

Saline, see Reagent No. 58

SAF (sodium acetate, acetic acid,   No. 62
formaldehyde) fixative
To make about 995 ml:

Sodium acetate .... 15 g
Acetic acid, glacial .... 20 ml
Formaldehyde, concentrated solution ..... 40 ml
Water (need not be distilled) .... 925 ml

1. Measure the water and transfer about half of it to a clean leak-proof bottle.
2. Weigh the sodium acetate and add this to the bottle. Mix to dissolve the chemical.
3. Measure the acetic acid and add to the bottle. Mix.

   Caution: Glacial acetic acid is corrosive and flammable. It is also irritating to the eyes, therefore handle it with great care, away from any open flame, and in a well ventilated room.
4. Measure the formaldehyde solution and add to

the bottle. Mix.

Caution: Concentrated formaldehyde solution is a toxic chemical with a vapour that is irritating to the eyes and mucous membranes, therefore handle it with great care in a well ventilated room.

5. Add the remainder of the water and mix well.

6. Label the bottle and mark it *Toxic* and *Corrosive*. Store at room temperature in a safe place. The reagent is stable indefinitely.

Saponin solution   No. 63
See Reagent No. 64

Saponin-saline solution   No. 64
This is a 1% w/v solution of saponin in physiological saline.

To make about 500 ml:

Saponin (white, pure grade) .... 5 g
Physiological saline (Reagent No. 58) .... 500 ml

1. Weigh the saponin and transfer this to a clean leak-proof bottle.

   Caution: Saponin powder is a harmful chemical, therefore handle it with great care and avoid inhaling the powder.

2. Measure the saline and add about half of it to the bottle. Mix gently (by swirling) to dissolve the chemical (standing the bottle in hot water will help the saponin to dissolve).

3. Add the remainder of the saline and mix gently but well (avoid excess frothing).

4. Label the bottle and store it preferably at 2-8 °C. The reagent is stable for several months.

For use: Transfer a small amount to a dropper bottle.

Schaudinn's fixative   No. 65
To make approximately 750 (stock solution):

Mercury (II) chloride .... 35 g
(mercuric chloride)
Ethanol, 95% v/v .... about 250 ml
Distilled water .... 500 ml
Acetic acid, glacial .... See *For use*

1. Weigh the mercury II chloride, and transfer to a heat resistant flask or bottle.

   Caution: Mercury (II) chloride is a poisonous chemical, therefore handle it with care.

2. Measure the water, add to the flask, and mix.

3. Place the flask in a container of boiling water to dissolve the mercury (II) chloride.

4. When the chemical is completely dissolved, allow the saturated solution to cool to room temperature (the excess chemical will crystallize out).

5. Pour the clear supernatant fluid into a measuring cylinder, and note the volume.

6. Add 95% v/v ethanol in the proportion of one part of alcohol to two parts of the mercury (II) chloride solution.

   Caution: Ethanol (ethyl alcohol) is highly flammable, therefore use it well away from an open flame.

7. Transfer the reagent to a clean, leak-proof bottle and mix. Label the bottle '*Stock Schaudinn's Reagent*' and mark it *Toxic*. Store at room temperature in a safe place. The reagent is stable indefinitely.

For use:
Immediately before required, add 5 ml of glacial acetic acid to 95 ml of *Stock Schaudinn's Reagent*.

Caution: Glacial acetic acid is corrosive and flammable. It is also irritating to the eyes, therefore handle it with great care, away from any open flame, and in a well ventilated room. Do *not* mouth-pipette the acid.

Sodium carbonate   No. 66
To make 250 ml:

Sodium carbonate, hydrated .... 2.5 g
Distilled water .... to 250 ml

1. Weigh the sodium carbonate, and transfer to a 250 ml volumetric flask.

2. Half fill the flask with water and mix to dissolve the chemical.

3. Make up to the 250 ml mark with water and mix well.

4. Transfer the solution to a clean, leak-proof bottle. Label the bottle and store at room temperature. The reagent is stable for several months.

Sodium chloride, 10 g/l   No. 67
carbon dioxide-free
To make 500 ml:

Sodium chloride .... 5 g
Distilled water, ... to 500 ml
carbon dioxide-free*

* For preparation, see Reagent No. 45.

1. Weigh the sodium chloride and transfer to a 500 ml volumetric flask.

2. Half fill the flask with carbon dioxide-free water and mix to dissolve the chemical.

3. Make up to the 500 ml mark with the carbon dioxide-free water. Transfer to a clean leak-proof bottle, cap tightly, and mix.

4. Label the bottle and store at room temperature. Renew weekly.

Sodium citrate anticoagulant   No. 68
To make about 100 ml:

tri-Sodium citrate .... 3.8 g
Distilled water .... 100 ml

1. Weigh the sodium citrate and transfer it to a clean leak-proof bottle.

2. Add 100 ml of water and mix to dissolve the chemical.

3. Label the bottle and store preferably at 2-8 °C. Renew every 6 weeks.

Sodium dodecyl sulphate, 40 g/l   No. 69
To make 500 ml:

Sodium dodecyl sulphate .... 20 g
Distilled water .... to 500 ml

1. Weigh the sodium dodecyl sulphate and transfer it to a 500 ml volumetric flask.

   Caution: Sodium dodecyl sulphate is a harmful chemical, therefore handle it with care.

2. Half fill the flask with water and mix until the chemical is completely dissolved.

3. Make up to the 500 ml mark with water and mix.

4. Transfer to a clean leak-proof bottle. Label and mark the bottle *Harmful*. Store at room temperature in a safe place. The reagent is stable indefinitely but should be discarded if it becomes turbid.

Sodium hydroxide, 3% w/v   No. 70
To make about 100 ml:

Sodium hydroxide .... 3 g
Distilled water .... 100 ml

1. Weigh the sodium hydroxide and transfer it to a clean leak-proof bottle.

   Caution: See Reagent No. 72.

2. Measure the water and add to the bottle (preferably plastic). Mix until the chemical is completely dissolved.

3. Label the bottle and mark it *Corrosive*. Store at room temperature. The reagent is stable indefinitely.

Sodium hydroxide, 0.4 mol/l (0.4N)   No. 71
To make 1 litre:

Sodium hydroxide .... 16 g
Distilled water .... to 1 litre

1. Weigh the sodium hydroxide and transfer it to a 1 litre volumetric flask.

   Caution: See Reagent No. 72.

2. Half fill the flask with distilled water and mix until the chemical is fully dissolved.

3. Make up to the 1 litre mark with distilled water and mix well.

4. Transfer to a clean *leak-proof* bottle (preferably plastic). Label the bottle and mark it *Corrosive*. Store at room temperature. The reagent is stable indefinitely.

Note: A 0.4 mol/l solution of sodium hydroxide can also be prepared from a 1 mol/l volumetric solution of sodium hydroxide (dilute 400 ml of 1 mol/l sodium hydroxide to 1 litre with distilled water).

Sodium hydroxide 1 mol/l (4% w/v)   No. 72
Purchase ready-made as a 1 mol/l volumetric solution or prepare as follows:

To make 1 litre:

Sodium hydroxide .... 40.01 g
Distilled water .... to 1 litre

1. Weigh the sodium hydroxide, and transfer it to a 1 litre volumetric flask.

   Caution: Sodium hydroxide is a corrosive deliquescent chemical, therefore handle it with care, and make sure the stock bottle of chemical is tightly stoppered after use.

2. Half fill the flask with water, and mix to dissolve the chemical. Make up to the 1 litre mark with water, and mix well.

3. Transfer to a clean leak-proof bottle (preferably plastic). Label the bottle, and mark it *Corrosive*. Store at room temperature. The reagent is stable indefinitely.

Sodium hydroxide, 10 g/l   No. 73
To make 100 ml:

Sodium hydroxide .... 1 g
Distilled water .... to 100 ml

1. Weigh the sodium hydroxide and transfer it to a 100 ml volumetric flask.

   Caution: See Reagent No. 72.

2. Half fill the flask with water and mix to dissolve the chemical.

3. Make up to the 100 ml mark with water and mix.

4. Transfer to a clean leak-proof bottle (preferably plastic). Label the bottle and store at room temperature. The reagent is stable indefinitely.

Sodium hydroxide, 6 mol/l   No. 74
To make 500 ml:

Sodium hydroxide .... 120 g
Distilled water .... to 500 ml

1. Rapidly weigh the sodium hydroxide in a large beaker.

   Caution: See Reagent No. 72.

2. Add about 150 ml of water and mix to dissolve the chemical.

3. Transfer to a 500 ml flask, rinsing out the beaker with water to make sure all the dissolved chemical is transferred to the flask.

4. Make up to the 500 ml mark with water and mix well.

5. Transfer to a clean leak-proof bottle (preferably plastic). Label the bottle and mark it *Corrosive*. Store at room temperature. The reagent is stable indefinitely.

Sodium hydroxide, 10 mmol/l (0.01 mol/l) carbon dioxide-free (for bicarbonate assays)　　No. 75

To make 100 ml:

Sodium hydroxide, 100 mmol/l* .... 10 ml
Sodium chloride, 10 g/l .... to 100 ml
carbon dioxide-free (see Reagent No. 67).

*Purchase as a ready-made 100 mmol/l (0.1 mol/l) volumetric solution or prepare from a 1 mol/l (1000 mmol/l) volumetric solution.

1. Half fill a 100 ml volumetric flask with the carbon dioxide-free sodium chloride solution.

2. Measure the 100 mmol/l sodium hydroxide solution (do *not* mouth-pipette), add to the flask, and mix.

3. Make up to the 100 ml mark with the carbon dioxide-free sodium chloride solution, and mix. Renew daily.

Sodium nitrite, 5 g/l (0.5% w/v)　　No. 76
To make 100 ml:

Sodium nitrite .... 0.5 g
Distilled water .... to 100 ml

1. Weigh the sodium nitrite and transfer it to a 100 ml volumetric flask.

2. Half fill the flask with water and mix until the chemical is completely dissolved.

3. Make up to the 100 ml mark with water and mix well.

4. Transfer to a clean leak-proof bottle and label. Store at 2-8 °C. Renew monthly.

Starch substrate, pH 7.0　　No. 77
To make 1 litre:

di-Sodium hydrogen phosphate, ... 26.60 g
anhydrous (Na_2HPO_4)
Sodium chloride .... 1.75 g
Benzoic acid .... 8.60 g
Soluble starch .... 0.40 g
Distilled water .... to 1 litre

1. Weigh the *di*-sodium hydrogen phosphate, sodium chloride, and benzoic acid. Transfer

these chemicals to a heat resistant beaker or flask.

2. Add about 500 ml of water and mix. Place the beaker or flask in a container of water and heat to boiling. Mix at intervals to dissolve the chemicals.

3. Weigh the starch and dissolve it in about 10 ml of cold distilled water.

4. With *mixing*, stir in the starch suspension to the hot solution in the beaker. Continue mixing until the solution reaches 100 °C. Allow to boil for 1 minute.

5. Cool to room temperature. Transfer to a 1 litre volumetric flask and make up to the 1 litre mark with water. Mix well.

6. Transfer to a clean leak-proof bottle and label. Store at room temperature. The reagent is stable for about 1 year.

Note: Before use, mix the reagent well.

Succinate buffer, pH 4.2　　No. 78
To make 1 litre:

Succinic acid .... 5.6 g
Sodium hydroxide .... 1.0 g
Sodium azide .... 0.1 g
Distilled water .... to 1 litre

1. Weigh the chemicals and transfer them to a 1 litre volumetric flask.

2. Half fill the flask with distilled water and mix until the chemicals are completely dissolved.

3. Make up to the 1 litre mark with distilled water and mix well.

4. Check that the pH of the buffer is pH 4.2 ± 0.05 at room temperature. If the pH is not 4.2, adjust it using 10 g/l (1% w/v) sodium hydroxide or 50 g/l (5% w/v) succinic acid (add drop by drop).

5. Transfer to a clean leak-proof bottle and label. Store at 2-8 °C. The buffer is stable for several months.

Sulphanilic acid, 5 g/l　　No. 79
To make 500 ml:

Sulphanilic acid .... 2.5 g
Hydrochloric acid, concentrated .... 7.5 ml
Distilled water .... to 500 ml

1. Weigh the sulphanilic acid and transfer to a 500 ml volumetric flask.

   Caution: Sulphanilic acid is a harmful chemical, therefore handle it with care.

2. Half fill the flask with water.

3. Measure the hydrochloric acid and add to the flask.

   Caution: See Reagent No. 43.

4. Mix until the sulphanilic acid is completely dissolved. Make up to the 500 ml mark with water and mix well.

5. Transfer to a clean leak-proof bottle. Label the bottle and mark it *Harmful*. Store at room temperature. The reagent is stable for about 6 months.

Sulphosalicylic acid, 200 g/l   No. 80
(20% w/v)
To make 250 ml:

Sulphosalicylic acid .... 50 g
Distilled water .... to 250 ml

1. Weigh the acid, and transfer it to a 250 ml volumetric flask (or bottle premarked to hold 250 ml).

2. Half fill the flask with water and mix to dissolve the acid.

3. Make up to the 250 ml mark with water and mix well. Transfer to a clean leak-proof bottle. Label the bottle, and store at room temperature. The reagent is stable for several months.

Trichloroacetic acid, 50 g/l   No. 81
(5% w/v)
To make 100 ml:

Trichloroacetic acid (TCA) .... 5 g
Distilled water .... to 100 ml

1. Weigh the TCA in a beaker (preweighed). Add about 30 ml of the water, and stir to dissolve the TCA.

   Caution: TCA is a strongly corrosive and deliquescent chemical with an irritating vapour, therefore handle it with care in a well ventilated room. Make sure the stock bottle of the chemical is tightly stoppered after use.

2. Transfer to a 100 ml volumetric flask. Make up to the mark with distilled water, and mix well.

3. Transfer to a clean leak-proof bottle. Label, and mark it *Corrosive*. Store at room temperature. The reagent is stable indefinitely.

Trichrome stain   No. 82
To make about 102 ml:

Chromotrope 2R .... 0.60 g
Light green SF .... 0.15 g
Fast green FCF .... 0.15 g
Phosphotungstic acid .... 0.70 g
Acetic acid, glacial .... 1 ml
Distilled water .... 100 ml

1. Weigh the dry ingredients and transfer them to a clean leak-proof bottle.

2. Measure the acetic acid (do *not* mouth-pipette) and add to the bottle.
   Caution: See Reagent 1.

3. After about 30 minutes, measure the water and add to the bottle.

4. Cap the bottle and mix until the stains and phosphotungstic acid are completely dissolved.

For use: Transfer the stain to a staining jar (Coplin type is suitable) and use as described in 13:10. The stain can be reused several times.

Urea acid reagent   No. 83
To make 500 ml:

Thiosemicarbazide .... 0.05 g
Cadmium sulphate .... 1.60 g
Sulphuric acid, concentrated .... 44.0 ml
ortho-Phosphoric acid .... 66.0 ml
Urea working standard, 2.5 mmol.l* ..... 1.5 ml
Distilled water .... to 500 ml

*See 28:1.

1. About half fill a 500 ml volumetric flask with water.

2. Measure the sulphuric acid and *slowly*, with mixing, add it to the water. Considerable heat will be evolved.

   Important: The acid *must* be added to the water. Concentrated sulphuric acid is a highly corrosive and deliquescent chemical, therefore handle it with *great care*.

3. Measure the phosphoric acid and slowly with mixing, add it to the flask.

   Caution: Concentrated phosphoric acid is a *highly corrosive* acid, therefore handle it with great care.

4. Allow the solution to cool to room temperature.

5. Measure the thiosemicarbazide and cadmium sulphate and add these to the solution. Mix to dissolve (make sure the stopper of the flask is tight fitting).

6. Measure the urea standard solution, and add it to the flask.

7. Make up to 500 ml mark with water and mix.

8. With care, transfer the reagent to a clean, dark, leak-proof bottle, Label, and mark the bottle *Corrosive* and *Toxic*. Store at room temperature. The reagent is stable for at least 6 months.

Zinc sulphate solution, 33% w/v   No. 84
To make approximately 500 ml:

Zinc sulphate .... 165 g
Distilled water .... 500 ml

1. Weigh the zinc sulphate and transfer it to a clean leak-proof bottle of 1 litre capacity.

2. Measure the water and add it to the chemical.

3. Stopper the bottle, and mix well.

4. Stand the bottle in a container of hot water to dissolve the zinc sulphate. Mix until the chemical is completely dissolved.

5. Allow the solution to cool to room temperature.

6. Using a hydrometer, check the relative density of the solution. If the density is not within 1.180-1.200, add more chemical or water to bring the solution within the correct density range.

7. Label the bottle and store at room temperature. When stored with the bottle top tightly stoppered, the solution is stable for several weeks. The relative density should be checked periodically.

APPENDIX II

ADDRESSES OF MANUFACTURERS

AND OTHER

USEFUL ADDRESSES

ALPHA LABORATORIES LTD
169 Oldfield Lane
Greenford, England UB6 8PW

AMERICAN OPTICAL COMPANY
(Scientific Instrument Division)
Box 123, Buffalo
NY 14240, USA

AMES DIVISION MILES LABORATORIES LTD
PO Box 37, Stoke Court,
Stoke Poges, Slough,
Bucks, England SL2 4LY

ARNOLD R HORWELL LTD
73 Maygrove Road
West Hampstead
London, England NW6 2BP

ATAGO COMPANY LTD
32–10 Honcho Itabashi-ka
Tokyo 173, Japan

AZLON PRODUCTS LTD
172 Brownhill Road
London, England SE6 2DL

BAIRD AND TATLOCK LTD
PO Box 1, Romford
Essex, England RM1 1HA

BDH CHEMICALS LTD
Poole
England BH12 4NN

J BIBBY SCIENCE PRODUCTS LTD
Stone, Staffordshire,
England ST15 0SA

BIOMÉRIEUX INTERNATIONAL DEPARTMENT
Marcy l'Etoile
69260 Charbonnieres-les-Bains
France

BOEHRINGER MANNHEIM GmbH
D-6800 Mannheim 31
Germany

BOSCH COMPANY
7455 Jungingen
Hohenzollern, Germany

BUFFALO MEDICAL SPECIALTIES MFG INC
PO Box 17247, 14205 Myerlake Circle,
Clearwater, FL 3350, USA

CAMLAB LTD
Nuffield Road, Cambridge
Cambridgeshire, England CB4 1TH

CLANDON SCIENTIFIC LTD
Lysons Avenue, Ash Vale,
Aldershot, Hampshire
England GU12 5QR

COMPUR ELECTRONIC GmbH
D-8000 Munchen
Western Germany

CORNING LABORATORY DIVISION LTD
Stone, Staffordshire
England ST15 0BG

CORDIS LABORATORIES INCORPORATED
PO Box 370428
Miami, Florida 33137, USA

CORNING MEDICAL LTD
Halstead, Essex
England CO9 2DX

DELPHI INDUSTRIES LTD
27 Ben Lomond Crescent
Pakuranga, Auckland
New Zealand

DIFCO LABORATORIES
PO Box 1058A
Detroit, MI 48232, USA

DYNATECH LABORATORIES LIMITED
Daux Road, Billingshurst
Sussex, England RH14 9SJ

EASTMAN KODAK CO
343 State Street, Rochester
NY 14650, USA

FAIREY INDUSTRIAL CERAMICS LTD
Stone, Staffordshire
England ST15 0PU

FERMCO LABORATORIES
PO Box, 5110
Chicago, USA

FUJIZOKI PHARMACEUTICAL CO LTD
6–7 Shimoochiai 4-chome
Shinjuku-ku Tokyo 161, Japan

GALLENKAMP, FISONS plc
Scientific Equipment Division
Belton Road West
Loughborough, Leicestershire
England LE11 0TR

GENERAL DIAGNOSTICS
Division of Warner-Lambert Company
Morris Plains
New Jersey 07950, USA

GQF MANUFACTURING COMPANY
PO Box 1552
Savannah, Ga 31402, USA

HAMLO
(Aid to medical laboratories
in developing countries)
Wilhelminapark 52
3581 NM Utrecht
The Netherlands

HAWKSLEY AND SONS LTD
12 Peter Road, Lancing
West Sussex, England BN15 8TH

HETTICH ZENTRIFUGEN
Postfach 4255
D-7200 Tuttlingen, Germany

HOECHST COMPANY
Hoechst Aktiengesellschaft
Postfach 80 03 20
6230 Frankfurt (M) 80, Germany

HOOK AND TUCKER INSTRUMENTS LTD
Vulcan Way, New Addington
Croydon, England CR0 9UG

HUGHES AND HUGHES LTD
Elms Industrial Estate
Church Road, Harold Wood,
Romford, Essex, England RM3 0HR

HUMAN GmbH
Im Maisel 14
D-6204 Taunusstein 4 (Neuhof)
Germany

INSTITUT PASTEUR
3 bd Raymond Poincaré
BP 3-92430
Marnes-la-Coquette, France

ISMUNIT ISTITUTO IMMUNOLOGICO ITALIANO
00040 Pomezia (Roma)
Via Castagnetta, Italy

KARTELL PLASTICS LTD
Via delle industrie
PO Box 18
20082 Noviglio (Milano), Italy

LABORATOIRES BIOTROL
1 rue de Foins
75140 Paris, France

LABORATORY DIAGNOSTICS COMPANY LTD
Morganville,
NJ 07751, USA

LIC LTD
129 Groveley Road
Sunbury on Thames
Middlesex, England TW16 7JZ

LIP (EQUIPMENT AND SERVICES) LTD
111 Dockfield Road
Shipley, West Yorkshire
England BD17 7AS

E LLOYD AND CO
Churchworks, Byron Hill Road
Harrow-on-the-Hill
Middlesex, England HA2 0HY

LUCKHAM LTD
Labro Works, Victoria Gardens
Burgess Hill, Sussex
England RH15 9QN

MANESTY MACHINES LTD
Evans Road, Speke
Liverpool, England L24 9LQ

MEDIN STAAL
2015 13J, Haarlem
Zijlweg 154, Netherlands

MEDISTRON LTD
6 Lawson-Hunt Industrial Park
Broadbridge Heath, Horsham
West Sussex, England RH12 3JR

W MEMMERT COMPANY
Fabrik fur Laboratoriumsgerate
854 Schwabach
Postfach 1520, Germany

E MERCK
D-6100 Darmstadt,
Germany

MIDDLEMASS FABRICATORS LTD
Honeysome Industrial Estate
Honeysome Road, Chatteris
Cambs, England PE16 6FA

NYEGARD COMPANY
Post Box 4220, Torshov
Oslo 4, Norway

OHAUS SCALE CORPORATION
29 Hanover Road, Florham Park
New Jersey 07932, USA

ORION RESEARCH INCORPORATED
840 Memorial Drive
Cambridge, MA 02139, USA

PARAMOUNT REAGENTS LTD
Mast House, Derby Road,
Bootle, Merseyside
England L20 1EA

PATH/PACT
4 Nickerson Street
Seattle, Washington 98109-1699, USA

PHARMACIA LTD
AB Fortia, Box 604
S-75125, Uppsala, Sweden

RUDOLPH BRAND GmbH
Laborgerate und Vakuumtechnik
Postfach 310
D-6980 Wertheim, West Germany

SCIENTIFIC INDUSTRIES INTERNATIONAL INC LTD
PO Box 26, Loughborough
Leicestershire, England LE11 1DB

SHANDON SOUTHERN PRODUCTS LTD
Chadwick Road, Astmoor
Runcorn, Cheshire
England WA7 1PR

SIGMA CHEMICAL CO LTD
Fancy Road, Poole
England BH17 7TG

SMITH KLINE RIT
Biological Division
Rue de l'Institut 89
1330 Rixensart, Belgium

STERILIN LTD
Sterilin House, Clockhouse Lane
Feltham, Middlesex, England TW14 8QS

STUART SCIENTIFIC CO LTD
Holmthorpe Avenue
Holmethorpe Industrial Estate
Redhill, Surrey, England RH1 2NJ

SWS FILTRATION LTD
Great Chesterford, Saffron Walden
Essex, England CB10 1PL

TEACHING AIDS AT LOW COST
PO Box 49, St Albans
Herts, England AL1 4AX

TROPICAL HEALTH TECHNOLOGY
14 Bevills Close, Doddington
March, Cambridgeshire
England PE15 0TT

TRUMETER COMPANY LTD
Milltown St, Radcliffe,
Manchester, England M26 9NX

WALDEN PRECISION APPARATUS LTD
The Old Station, Linton
Cambridge, England CB1 6NW

WELLCOME DIAGNOSTICS
Temple Hill, Dartford
England DA1 5AH

WELLCOME REAGENTS LTD
Beckenham, Kent
England BR3 3BS

HISTOPATHOLOGICAL SERVICES TO DEVELOPING COUNTRIES

For hospitals and health centres that have no access to reliable and regular histopathological services, use can be made of overseas institutions that maintain an interest in tropical pathology. Material is sent by airmail post, and the reports returned by airmail. One such service is provided in London, and further advice can be obtained from:

Dr Sebastian Lucas
Dept of Histopathology
School of Medicine, UCL
University St
London WC1E 6JJ
United Kingdom

APPENDIX III

USEFUL TABLES

SI Units (see also 1:5)

Prefix	Symbol	Function
femto	f	10^{-15}
pico	p	10^{-12}
nano	n	10^{-9}
micro	μ	10^{-6}
milli	m	10^{-3}
* ⎡ centi	c	10^{-2} ⎤
⎢ deci	d	10^{-1} ⎥
⎣ deca	da	10^{1} ⎦
hecto	h	10^{2}
kilo	k	10^{3}
mega	M	10^{6}
giga	G	10^{9}
tera	T	10^{12}

*Use not recommended

Length

1 dm	= 10^{-1} m (0.1 m)
1 cm	= 10^{-2} m (0.01 m)
1 mm	= 10^{-3} m (0.001 m)
*1 μm	= 10^{-6} m (0.000 001 m)
1 nm	= 10^{-9} m (0.000 000 001 m)
1 km	= 1000 m (10^{3} m)
1 m	= 10 dm
1 m	= 100 cm
1 m	= 1000 mm
1 m	= 1 000 000 μm
1 m	= 1 000 000 000 nm
1 cm	= 10 mm
1 cm	= 10 000 μm
1 mm	= 1000 μm
1 m	= 3.281 feet
1 km	= 0.62137 mile
1 inch	= 2.54 cm

Mass

1 kg	= 10^{3} g (1000 g)
1 mg	= 10^{-3} g (0.001 g)
1 μg	= 10^{-6} g (0.000 001 g)
1 ng	= 10^{-9} g (0.000 000 001 g)
1 pg	= 10^{-12} g (0.000 000 000 001 g)
1 kg	= 1000 g
1 g	= 1000 mg
1 g	= 1 000 000 μg
1 g	= 1 000 000 000 ng
1 g	= 1 000 000 000 000 pg
1 mg	= 0.001 g
1 mg	= 1000 μg
1 kg	= 2.205 lb

Volume

1 dl	= 10^{-1} l (0.1 l)
1 cl	= 10^{-2} l (0.01 l)
1 ml	= 10^{-3} l (0.001 l)
1 μl	= 10^{-6} l (0.000 001 l or 1 mm³)
1 nl	= 10^{-9} l (0.000 000 001 l)
1 pl	= 10^{-12} l (0.000 000 000 001 l)
1 l	= 10 dl
1 l	= 1000 ml
1 l	= 1 000 000 μl
1 l	= 1 000 000 000 nl
1 dl	= 100 cm³, formerly 100 ml
1 ml	= 1000 μl
1 pint	= 0.568 l
1 l	= 1.760 pints
1 l	= 0.22 gallons

Amount of substance

1 mmol	= 10^{-3} mol (0.001 mol)
1 μmol	= 10^{-6} mol (0.000 001 mol)
1 nmol	= 10^{-9} mol (0.000 000 001 mol)
1 mol	= 1000 mmol
1 mol	= 1 000 000 μmol
1 mol	= 1 000 000 000 nmol
1 mmol	= 1000 μmol
1 mmol	= 1 000 000 nmol
1 μmol	= 1000 nmol

Temperature conversion

To convert °C to °F:
multiply by 9, divide by 5, and add 32.

To convert °F to °C:
subtract 32, multiply by 5, and divide by 9.

0 °C	= 32 °F
10 °C	= 52 °F
20 °C	= 68 °F
30 °C	= 86 °F
36.9 °C	= 98.4 °F
40 °C	= 104 °F
50 °C	= 122 °F
100 °C	= 212 °F

Pressure

Approx. conversion: $\dfrac{\text{mm Hg} \times 2}{15} = \text{kPa}$

lb/sq inch x 6.895 = kPa

ATOMIC MASSES AND VALENCIES OF SOME ELEMENTS

Element	Symbol	Relative Atomic Mass	Valence
Aluminium	Al	26.9815	3
Antimony	Sb	121.75	3, 5
Barium	Ba	137.34	2
Cadmium	Cd	112.40	2
Calcium	Ca	40.08	2
Carbon	C	12.011	2, 4
Chlorine	Cl	35.453	1, 3, 5, 7
Chromium	Cr	51.996	2, 3, 6
Cobalt	Co	58.9332	2, 3
Copper	Cu	63.546	1, 2
Fluorine	F	19.9984	1
Gold	Au	196.8665	1, 3
Hydrogen	H	1.0079	1
Iodine	I	126.9045	1, 3, 5, 7
Iron	Fe	55.847	2, 3, 6
Lead	Pb	207.2	2, 4
Lithium	Li	6.941	1
Magnesium	Mg	24.305	2
Manganese	Mn	54.9380	2, 3, 4, 6, 7
Mercury	Hg	200.59	1, 2
Molybdenum	Mo	95.94	2, 3, 4, 5, 6
Nickel	Ni	58.7	2, 3
Nitrogen	N	14.0067	3, 5
Oxygen	O	15.9994	2
Phosphorus	P	30.9738	3, 5
Platinum	Pt	195.09	2, 4
Potassium	K	39.098	1
Selenium	Se	78.96	2, 4, 6
Silicon	Si	28.086	4
Silver	Ag	107.868	1
Sodium	Na	22.9898	1
Sulphur	S	32.06	2, 4, 6
Tin	Sn	118.69	2, 4
Tungsten	W	183.85	2, 4, 5, 6
Zinc	Zn	65.38	2

Note: The atomic weights quoted are the 1973 values* based on carbon 12.
*IUPAC. *Atomic weights of the elements,* 1973.

MOLE PER LITRE SOLUTIONS OF SOME CONCENTRATED ACIDS

Acetic acid, glacial, 99.6% w/w:	Approx. 17.50 mol/l
Hydrochloric acid, 1.16, 32% w/w:	Approx. 10.20 mol/l
Hydrochloric acid, 1.18, 36% w/w:	Approx. 11.65 mol/l
Nitric acid, 1.42, 70% w/w:	Approx. 15.80 mol/l
Sulphuric acid, 1.84, 97% w/w:	Approx. 18.00 mol/l

To make approx. 1 mol/l solutions from concentrated acids

Concentrated acids	ml diluted to 1 litre
Acetic acid, (glacial), 99.6% w/w	57 ml
Hydrochloric acid, 32% w/w	98 ml
Hydrochloric acid, 36% w/w	86 ml
Nitric acid, 70%, w/w	63 ml
Sulphuric acid, 97% w/w	56 ml

RELATIVE MOLECULAR MASSES OF SOME SUBSTANCES

Substance	Symbol	Relative Molecular Mass (taken to two decimal places)
Acetic acid	CH_3COOH	60.08
Ammonium carbonate	$(NH_4)_2CO_3$	96.09
Ammonium chloride	NH_4Cl	53.50
Ammonium molybdate	$(NH_4)_2MoO_4$	196.03
Ammonium nitrate	NH_4NO_3	80.05
Ammonium oxalate	$(NH_4)_2C_2O_2 \cdot H_2O$	142.12
Barium chloride	$BaCl_2$	208.27
Barium hydroxide	$Ba(OH)_2 \cdot 8H_2O$	315.51
Boric acid (boracic acid)	H_3BO_3	61.84
Calcium chloride	$CaCl_2$	110.98
CopperII sulphate (cupric)	$CuSO_4$	159.61
	$CuSO_4 \cdot 5H_2O$	249.69
Hydrochloric acid	HCl	36.47
Iron III chloride	$FeCl_3$	162.22
(Ferric chloride)	$FeCl_3 \cdot 6H_2O$	270.32
Lead nitrate	$Pb(NO_3)_2$	331.23
Lithium carbonate	Li_2CO_3	73.89
Magnesium chloride	$MgCl_2 \cdot 6H_2O$	203.33
Mercury II chloride	$HgCl_2$	271.52
(Mercuric chloride)		
Molybdic acid	H_2MoO_4	161.97
	$H_2MoO_4 \cdot H_2O$	179.98
Nitric acid	HNO_3	63.02
Phosphoric acid	H_3PO_4	98.00
Potassium carbonate	K_2CO_3	138.20
	$K_2CO_3 \cdot 1\frac{1}{2}H_2O$	165.24
Potassium chloride	KCl	74.55
Potassium cyanide	KCN	65.11
Potassium dichromate	$K_2Cr_2O_7$	294.21
Potassium ferricyanide	$K_3Fe(CN)_6$	329.25
Potassium ferrocyanide	$K_4Fe(CN)_6 \cdot 3H_2O$	422.39
Potassium hydrogen phosphate	K_2HPO_4	174.18
Potassium dihydrogen phosphate	KH_2PO_4	136.09
Potassium hydroxide	KOH	56.10
Potassium hypochlorite	$KClO$	90.55
Potassium iodate	KIO_3	214.02
Potassium iodide	KI	166.02
Potassium nitrate	KNO_3	101.10
Potassium nitrite	KNO_2	85.10
Potassium oxalate	$K_2C_2O_4 \cdot H_2O$	184.23
Potassium permanganate	$KMnO_4$	158.03
Potassium phosphate	K_3PO_4	212.27
Potassium sulphate	K_2SO_4	174.26
Potassium tartrate	$K_2C_4H_4O_6 \cdot \frac{1}{2}H_2O$	235.27
Potassium thiocyanate	$KSCN$	97.18
Silver nitrate	$AgNO_3$	169.89
Sodium azide	NaN_3	65.02
Sodium barbital (Sodium diethyl barbiturate)	$NaC_8H_{11}N_2O_3$	206.18
Sodium benzoate	$NaC_7H_5O_2$	144.11
Sodium carbonate	Na_2CO_3	106.00
	$Na_2CO_3 \cdot H_2O$	124.02
Sodium chlorate	$NaClO_4$	106.45
Sodium chloride	$NaCl$	58.45

Substance	Symbol	Relative Molecular Mass (taken to two decimal places)
Sodium chromate	Na_2CrO_4	162.00
Sodium citrate	$Na_3C_6H_5O_7 \cdot 2H_2O$	294.12
Sodium cyanide	$NaCN$	49.02
Sodium dithionite	$Na_2S_2O_4 \cdot 2H_2O$	210.16
Sodium ferricyanide	$Na_3Fe(CN)_6 \cdot H_2O$	298.97
Sodium ferrocyanide	$Na_4Fe(CN)_6 \cdot 10H_2O$	484.11
Sodium fluoride	NaF	42.00
Sodium bicarbonate	$NaHCO_3$	84.02
Sodium hydroxide	$NaOH$	40.01
Sodium metabisulphite	$Na_2S_2O_5$	190.13
Sodium molybdate	$Na_2MoO_4 \cdot 2H_2O$	241.98
Sodium nitrate	$NaNO_3$	85.01
Sodium nitrite	$NaNO_2$	69.01
Sodium nitroprusside	$Na_2(NO)Fe(CN)_5 \cdot 2H_2O$	297.97
Sodium oxalate	$Na_2C_2O_4$	134.01
Sodium perchlorate	$NaClO_4 \cdot H_2O$	140.47
Sodium phosphate	$Na_3PO_4 \cdot 12H_2O$	380.16
Sodium sulphate	Na_2SO_4	142.06
Glauber's salt	$Na_2SO_4 \cdot 10H_2O$	322.22
Sodium sulphite	Na_2SO_3	126.06
Sodium thiosulphate	$Na_2S_2O_3 \cdot 5H_2O$	248.21
Sodium tungstate	$Na_2WO_4 \cdot 2H_2O$	329.95
Sulphuric acid	H_2SO_4	98.08
Zinc acetate	$Zn(C_2H_3O_2)_2 \cdot 2H_2O$	219.50
Zinc chloride	$ZnCl_2$	136.29

SQUARE ROOTS OF 0.1 TO 4.00

	0.00	0.01	0.02	0.03	0.04	0.05	0.06	0.07	0.08	0.09
0.1	0.32	0.33	0.35	0.36	0.37	0.39	0.40	0.41	0.42	0.44
0.2	0.45	0.46	0.47	0.48	0.49	0.50	0.51	0.52	0.53	0.54
0.3	0.55	0.56	0.57	0.57	0.58	0.59	0.60	0.61	0.62	0.62
0.4	0.63	0.64	0.65	0.66	0.66	0.67	0.68	0.69	0.69	0.70
0.5	0.71	0.71	0.72	0.73	0.73	0.74	0.75	0.76	0.76	0.77
0.6	0.77	0.78	0.79	0.79	0.80	0.81	0.81	0.82	0.82	0.83
0.7	0.84	0.84	0.85	0.85	0.86	0.87	0.87	0.88	0.88	0.89
0.8	0.89	0.90	0.91	0.91	0.92	0.92	0.93	0.93	0.94	0.94
0.9	0.95	0.95	0.96	0.96	0.97	0.97	0.98	0.98	0.99	0.995

	0.00	0.01	0.02	0.03	0.04	0.05	0.06	0.07	0.08	0.09
1.0	1.00	1.01	1.01	1.02	1.02	1.03	1.03	1.03	1.04	1.04
1.1	1.05	1.05	1.06	1.06	1.07	1.07	1.08	1.08	1.09	1.09
1.2	1.10	1.10	1.11	1.11	1.11	1.12	1.12	1.13	1.13	1.14
1.3	1.14	1.15	1.15	1.15	1.16	1.16	1.17	1.17	1.18	1.18
1.4	1.18	1.19	1.19	1.20	1.20	1.20	1.21	1.21	1.22	1.22
1.5	1.23	1.23	1.23	1.24	1.24	1.25	1.25	1.25	1.26	1.26
1.6	1.27	1.27	1.27	1.28	1.28	1.29	1.29	1.29	1.30	1.30
1.7	1.30	1.31	1.31	1.32	1.32	1.32	1.33	1.33	1.33	1.34
1.8	1.34	1.35	1.35	1.35	1.36	1.36	1.36	1.37	1.37	1.38
1.9	1.38	1.38	1.39	1.39	1.39	1.40	1.40	1.40	1.41	1.41
2.0	1.41	1.42	1.42	1.43	1.43	1.43	1.44	1.44	1.44	1.45
2.1	1.45	1.45	1.46	1.46	1.46	1.47	1.47	1.47	1.48	1.48
2.2	1.48	1.49	1.49	1.49	1.50	1.50	1.50	1.51	1.51	1.51
2.3	1.52	1.52	1.52	1.53	1.53	1.53	1.54	1.54	1.54	1.55
2.4	1.55	1.55	1.56	1.56	1.56	1.57	1.57	1.57	1.58	1.58
2.5	1.58	1.58	1.59	1.59	1.59	1.60	1.60	1.60	1.61	1.61
2.6	1.61	1.62	1.62	1.62	1.63	1.63	1.63	1.63	1.64	1.64
2.7	1.64	1.65	1.65	1.65	1.66	1.66	1.66	1.67	1.67	1.67
2.8	1.67	1.68	1.68	1.68	1.69	1.69	1.69	1.69	1.70	1.70
2.9	1.70	1.71	1.71	1.71	1.72	1.72	1.72	1.72	1.73	1.73
3.0	1.73	1.74	1.74	1.74	1.75	1.75	1.75	1.75	1.76	1.76
3.1	1.76	1.76	1.77	1.77	1.77	1.78	1.78	1.78	1.78	1.79
3.2	1.79	1.79	1.79	1.80	1.80	1.80	1.81	1.81	1.81	1.81
3.3	1.82	1.82	1.82	1.83	1.83	1.83	1.83	1.84	1.84	1.84
3.4	1.84	1.85	1.85	1.85	1.86	1.86	1.86	1.86	1.87	1.87
3.5	1.87	1.88	1.88	1.88	1.88	1.88	1.89	1.89	1.89	1.90
3.6	1.90	1.90	1.90	1.91	1.91	1.91	1.91	1.92	1.92	1.92
3.7	1.92	1.93	1.93	1.93	1.93	1.94	1.94	1.94	1.94	1.95
3.8	1.95	1.95	1.95	1.96	1.96	1.96	1.97	1.97	1.97	1.97
3.9	1.98	1.98	1.98	1.98	1.99	1.99	1.99	1.99	2.00	2.00
4.0	2.00	2.00	2.01	2.01	2.01	2.01	2.02	2.02	2.02	2.02

APPENDIX IV

TROPICAL HEALTH TECHNOLOGY

EQUIPMENT SERVICE

TO DEVELOPING COUNTRIES

TROPICAL HEALTH TECHNOLOGY
LABORATORY EQUIPMENT SERVICE
to
DEVELOPING COUNTRIES

This Appendix lists those products which are available at low cost to medical workers in developing countries from the non-profit organization Tropical Health Technology. The Service is mainly to assist district hospital laboratories and community-based laboratories in rural areas.

Descriptions of the products, prices, and ordering information can be found in the *Supplement* which developing country readers will find in the back cover of the Manual.

Note: The *Supplement* will also be sent to readers of the Manual in other countries if such persons are planning to work in developing countries and may wish to use the Service. Requests for the **Laboratory Equipment Service to Developing Countries Supplement** should be addressed to Tropical Health Technology, 14 Bevills Close, Doddington, March, Cambridgeshire PE15 0TT, United Kingdom. Please enclose a self-addressed envelope (size, not less than 270 x 190 mm).

Nomogram for calculating relative centrifugal force (RCF)

To calculate RCF value at any point along the tube or flask measure the radius in mm from the centre of the centrifuge spindle to the particular point. Draw a line from this radius value on the right-hand column to the appropriate centrifuge speed on the left-hand column. The RCF value is the point where the line crosses the centre column.

The nomogram is based om the formula:
RCF $= 11.18 \times 10^{-7} \times RN^2$
R = Radius in mm from centrifuge spindle to point in tube.
N = Speed of spindle in rpm.

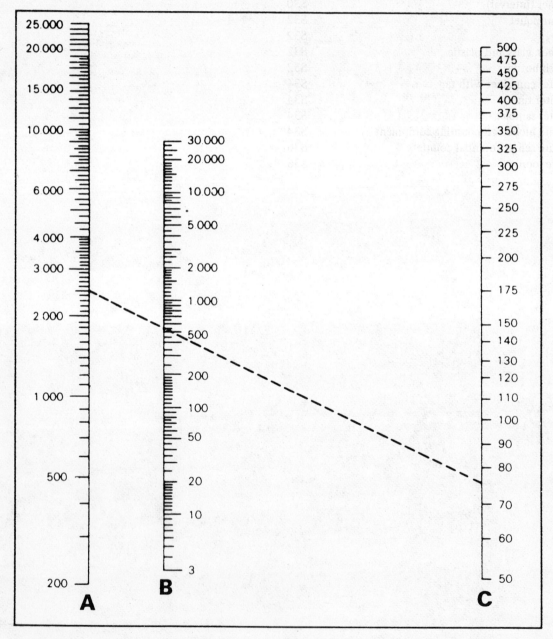

A   Speed of centrifuge spindle in rpm.
B   Relative centrifugal force (× g).
C   Radius in mm from centre of centrifuge spindle to point along tube or flask.

INDEX